HEALTH PSYCHOLOGY

Sara Miller McCune founded SAGE Publishing in 1965 to support the dissemination of usable knowledge and educate a global community. SAGE publishes more than 1000 journals and over 800 new books each year, spanning a wide range of subject areas. Our growing selection of library products includes archives, data, case studies and video. SAGE remains majority owned by our founder and after her lifetime will become owned by a charitable trust that secures the company's continued independence.

Los Angeles | London | New Delhi | Singapore | Washington DC | Melbourne

HEALTH PSYCHOLOGY

THEORY, RESEARCH AND PRACTICE

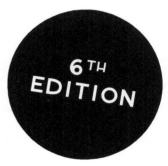

6TH EDITION

DAVID F. MARKS
MICHAEL MURRAY
EMEE VIDA ESTACIO

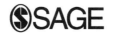

Los Angeles | London | New Delhi
Singapore | Washington DC | Melbourne

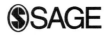

Los Angeles | London | New Delhi
Singapore | Washington DC | Melbourne

SAGE Publications Ltd
1 Oliver's Yard
55 City Road
London EC1Y 1SP

SAGE Publications Inc.
2455 Teller Road
Thousand Oaks, California 91320

SAGE Publications India Pvt Ltd
B 1/I 1 Mohan Cooperative Industrial Area
Mathura Road
New Delhi 110 044

SAGE Publications Asia-Pacific Pte Ltd
3 Church Street
#10-04 Samsung Hub
Singapore 049483

© David F Marks, Michael Murray and Emee Vida
Estacio 2021

First edition published 1999; reprinted 2002, 2003.
Second edition published 2005; reprinted 2008, 2009, 2010.
Third edition published 2010; reprinted 2011, 2013, 2014.
Fourth edition published 2015; reprinted 2016, 2017.
Fifth edition, published 2018; reprinted 2018 (twice), 2019
(three times). This, sixth edition, published 2021.

Editor: Donna Goddard
Editorial assistant: Marc Barnard
Assistant editor, digital: Sunita Patel
Production editor: Imogen Roome
Marketing manager: Camille Richmond
Proofreader: Leigh C. Smithson
Cover design: Wendy Scott
Typeset by: C&M Digitals (P) Ltd, Chennai, India
Printed in the UK

Library of Congress Control Number: 2020935695

British Library Cataloguing in Publication data

A catalogue record for this book is available
from the British Library

ISBN 978-1-5297-2308-3
ISBN 978-1-5297-2307-6 (pbk)

At SAGE we take sustainability seriously. Most of our products are printed in the UK using responsibly sourced
papers and boards. When we print overseas we ensure sustainable papers are used as measured by the PREPS
grading system. We undertake an annual audit to monitor our sustainability.

CONTENTS

AUTHOR BIOGRAPHIES

DAVID F. MARKS was born in Petersfield, England and lives in Provence, France. David graduated from the University of Reading and completed his PhD in mathematical psychology at the University of Sheffield. He held positions at the University of Otago, New Zealand and at University College London. He served as Head of the School of Psychology at Middlesex Polytechnic, and as Head of the Department of Psychology at City, University of London, UK. As a Visiting Professor, he carried out research in the Department of Neurosurgery at Hamamatsu School of Medicine and at the Department of Psychology, Kyushu University, Japan, at the Universities of Oregon and Washington, USA, and taught at the Universities of Cambridge, UK, and Tromsø, Norway. In addition to five previous editions of this book, David has published 25 books including: *The Psychology of the Psychic* (1980, with R. Kammann), *Theories of Image Formation* (1986), *Imagery: Current Developments* (1990, with J.T.E. Richardson and P. Hampson), *The Quit For Life Programme: An Easier Way to Stop Smoking and Not Start Again* (1993), *Improving the Health of the Nation* (1996, with C. Francome), *Dealing with Dementia: Recent European Research* (2000, with C.M. Sykes), *The Psychology of the Psychic* (revised edition, 2000), *The Health Psychology Reader* (2002), *Research Methods for Clinical and Health Psychology* (2004, with L. Yardley), *Overcoming Your Smoking Habit* (2005), *Obesity: Comfort vs. Discontent* (2016), *Stop Smoking Now* (2017), *A General Theory of Behaviour* (2018) and *Psychology and the Paranormal: Exploring Anomalous Experience* (2020).

David served as Chair of the British Psychological Society's Health Psychology Section and Special Group in Health Psychology and as Convenor of the European Task Force on Health Psychology when he was instrumental in establishing the first postgraduate health psychology training programmes at Master's and Doctoral levels in the UK. With Michael Murray, David is a founding member of the International Society of Critical Health Psychology. He is the founder and Editor of the *Journal of Health Psychology* and founder of *Health Psychology Open*. David is a specialist in theories, methods and psychometrics.

MICHAEL MURRAY is Emeritus Professor of Psychology at Keele University, UK, where he was Head of the School of Psychology. Previously, he was Professor of Social and Health Psychology at Memorial University, Canada, and held positions at St Thomas' Hospital Medical School, London, UK and at the University of Ulster, Northern Ireland. He has published many books, chapters, journal articles and reports on various issues in social and health psychology. His previous books include *Smoking Among Young Adults* (1988, with

L. Jarrett, A.V. Swan and R. Rumen), *Qualitative Health Psychology: Theories and Methods* (1999, with K. Chamberlain) and *Critical Health Psychology* (2004, 2015). He also edited with Kerry Chamberlain the collection *New Directions in Health Psychology (Vols 1–5)* (2015) and with Liz Peel and Carol Holland *Psychologies of Ageing: Theory, Research and Practice* (2018). Michael has been Associate Editor of the *Journal of Health Psychology* and of *Psychology and Health* and an editorial board member of *Health Psychology Open*, *Health Psychology Review*, *Psychology, Health and Medicine* and *Arts and Health*. He was Chair of the Health Psychology Section of the Canadian Psychological Association for which he edited *Canadian Health Psychologist/Psychologue Canadien de la Santé* and a founding member of the International Society of Critical Health Psychology. He is a Fellow of the British Psychological Society, the Canadian Psychological Association and the Academy of Social Sciences. In 2017 he was elected an Honorary Fellow of the British Psychological Society. His current research interests include the use of participatory and arts-based methods to promote social engagement among older people.

EMEE VIDA ESTACIO is a chartered psychologist, author, speaker, and life transformation and health promotion specialist. Originally from the Philippines, she completed her Bachelor's degree in Psychology (magna cum laude) from the University of the Philippines, Diliman and her MSc and PhD in Health Psychology at City University London. She previously held positions at the University of East London and Keele University. Emee specialises in health promotion and community development and has facilitated action research projects in some of the most deprived areas in the UK and in the Philippines. As a scholar activist, she became actively involved in supporting activities for Oxfam, the Association for International Cancer Research, CRIBS Philippines and Save the Children UK. In addition to previous editions of this book, Emee is also the author of the 'Psychology in Your Life' Book Series (2019), including titles such as *The Imposter Syndrome Remedy*, *Change Your Life for Good* and *Fear is Not My Enemy*. She also sits on the editorial board of the *Journal of Health Psychology*, *Health Psychology Open* and *Community, Work and Family*.

COPYRIGHT ACKNOWLEDGEMENTS

The authors and publishers wish to thank the following for permission to use copyright material:

CHAPTER 1

The Institute of Futures Studies for Figure 1.5, 'A framework for the determinants of health' Dahlgren, G., Whitehead, M. (1991). *Policies and Strategies to Promote Social Equity in Health*. Stockholm, Sweden: Institute for Futures Studies.

CHAPTER 2

Terese Winslow for Figure 2.5, The brain, brainstem, medulla, pons and other important brain structures.

Springer Nature for Figure 2.10, Gamble, K.L., Berry, R., Frank, S.J. and Young, M.E. (2014). Circadian clock control of endocrine factors. *Nature Reviews Endocrinology*, 10 (8): 466–75.

Oxford University Press, for Figure 2.11, Neuman, H., Debelius, J.W., Knight, R. and Koren, O. (2015). Microbial endocrinology: the interplay between the microbiota and the endocrine system. *FEMS Microbiology Review*, 39 (4): 509–21. doi:10.1093/femsre/fuu010.

CHAPTER 3

Springer Nature, for Figure 3.5, Polderman, T.J., Benyamin, B., De Leeuw, C.A., Sullivan, P.F., Van Bochoven, A., Visscher, P.M. et al. (2015). Meta-analysis of the heritability of human traits based on fifty years of twin studies. *Nature Genetics*, 47 (7): 702–9.

John Wiley and Sons, for Figure 3.6, Hadas, Y., Katz, M.G., Bridges, C.R. and Zangi, L. (2017). Modified mRNA as a therapeutic tool to induce cardiac regeneration in ischemic heart disease. *Wiley Interdisciplinary Reviews: Systems Biology and Medicine*, 9 (1). doi:10.1002/wsbm.1367.

Springer Nature, for Figure 3.7, Bowers, M.E. and Yehuda, R. (2016). Intergenerational transmission of stress in humans. *Neuropsychopharmacology*, 41 (1): 232–44.

Elsevier, for Figure 3.8, Klengel, T. and Binder, E.B. (2015). Epigenetics of stress-related psychiatric disorders and gene × environment interactions. *Neuron*, 86 (6): 1343–57.

CHAPTER 5

Publication for Figure 5.1, Reproduced with permission from Elsevier, Journal *Public Health* 'Why the Scots die younger: synthesizing the evidence', June, 2012, Vol/Iss: 126 (6) pp.459–70.

CHAPTER 14

Figure 14.3, 'Examples of loss-framed and gain-framed messages for smoking cessation' (source: www.yalescientific.org).

Figure 14.4, 'Health literacy levels in eight European nations' (HLS-EU Consortium, 2012, *Comparative Report of Health Literacy in Eight EU Member States: The European Health Literacy Survey*, http://ec.europa.eu/eahc/documents/news/Comparative_report_on_health_literacy_in_eight_EU_member_states.pdf).

Elsevier, for Figure 14.5, Schulz, P.J. and Nakamoto, K. (2013). Health literacy and patient empowerment in health communication: the importance of separating conjoined twins. *Patient Education and Counseling*, 90 (1): 4–11.

CHAPTER 15

Oxford University Press, for Figure 15.1, von Wagner, C., Good, A., Whitaker, K.L., Wardle, J. (2011). Psychosocial determinants of socioeconomic inequalities in cancer screening participation: a conceptual framework. *Epidemiol Rev*, 33: 135–47. doi:10.1093/epirev/mxq018

The World Health Organisation for Figure 15.2.

CHAPTER 16

Figure 16.1, Protesters outside of St Paul's Cathedral in London (source: http://en.wikipedia.org/wiki/Occupy_London).

CHAPTER 17

John Wiley and Sons, for Figure 17.1, Joseph, J.J., and Golden, S.H. (2017). Cortisol dysregulation: the bidirectional link between stress, depression, and type 2 diabetes mellitus. *Annals of the New York Academy of Sciences*, 1391 (1), 20–34.

Taylor & Francis, for Figure 17.2, Cox, T. (1978). *Stress*. London: Macmillan Press.

Every effort has been made to trace the copyright holders but if any have been inadvertently overlooked the publishers will be pleased to make the necessary arrangement at the first opportunity.

PREFACE

Welcome to *Health Psychology: Theory, Research and Practice (Sixth Edition)*. This textbook provides an in-depth introduction to the field of health psychology. It is designed for all readers wishing to update their knowledge about psychology and health, especially undergraduates and postgraduates taking courses in health psychology, medicine, nursing, public health, and other subjects allied to medicine and health care. The authors strive to present a balanced view of the field and its theories, research and applications. We aim to present the mainstream ideas, theories and studies within health psychology and to examine the underlying theoretical assumptions and critically analyse methods, evidence and conclusions. This edition updates all content from previous editions and adds significant, core topics from the biological and clinical domains.

All mainstream domains and topics relevant to health psychology are included. A key feature of this textbook is the equal priority given to the three aspects of the biopsychosocial (BPS) approach: biological, social and psychological determinants of health, illness and health care. The authors argue that both social embeddedness and psychological influences are as important to health and illness as genes and 'germs'. In this book we attempt to locate health psychology within its global, social and political contexts. We attempt to provide a snapshot of the 'bigger picture' using a wide-angle lens, as well as giving detailed, critical analyses of the 'nitty-gritty' of theory, research and practice.

This textbook introduces readers to the field of health psychology, the major foundations and theoretical approaches, contemporary research on core topics, and how this theory and evidence is being applied in practice. This more streamlined sixth edition includes a new chapter on stress as well as brand new online case studies. The outbreak of the coronavirus pandemic (**COVID-19**) occurred as this book was being prepared for production in the first months of 2020. As we were checking the proofs, in May 2020, almost 6 million people had been infected with COVID-19, 2.5 million people had recovered, but, sadly, 350,000 people had died. Around 4 billion people are estimated to have been living under some form of restriction of movement. Unfortunately these numbers will continue to rise (for an interactive dashboard, see Johns Hopkins University, 2020). Unless a vaccine is developed, or we discover medicines to treat the virus, our means of controlling the spread of infection depend entirely upon behavioural changes. Unfortunately,it was impossible here to include an in-depth discussion of the COVID-19 pandemic. However, the COVID-19 pandemic will be a major new topic within the next (7th) edition.

Health psychology is still relatively young, having developed as a sub-discipline in the 1970s and 1980s. The primary mainstream focus has been theories and models about social-cognitive processes concerned with health beliefs and behaviours. This approach has yielded thousands of research publications of a mainly empirical nature to study issues, test theories and models about the causes of health behaviour change, and investigate interventions. The growth of interest in this subject has been truly amazing. Similar to psychology more generally, the primary focus of health psychology has been the behaviour, beliefs and experiences of individuals.

The book introduces alternative, critical approaches to health psychology which are not yet part of the mainstream. We advance the case that psychological issues are embedded in human social structures in which economics and social justice play crucial roles. The mainstream socio-cognitive framework appears to us to be of limited relevance in a world where issues of poverty, social injustice and conflict exist for millions of people, and psychological processes are conditioned by basic limitations of capability, freedom and power (Marks, 1996, 2002a, 2004; Murray and Campbell, 2003; Murray, 2014a, 2014b). We evaluate and critique contemporary psychological theories and models in that context.

In our view, to make a contribution to society, theory, research and practice in health psychology must engage with the real economy, develop approaches for industrial-scale behaviour change, and work with communities and the struggles of the dispossessed. An agenda for health psychology needs to include 'actionable understandings of the complex individual–society dialectic underlying social inequalities' (Murray and Campbell, 2003: 236). Preliminary thoughts on 'actionable understandings' and of the 'individual–society dialectic' are presented in this book. By having access to mainstream and alternative perspectives in a single volume, lecturers and students can reach an assessment of the field and how it could make more progress in the future.

We explain the significance of the biological and social contexts, and review theory and methods (Part 1), analyse the complexity and diversity of health behaviour (Part 2), discuss health promotion and disease prevention (Part 3), and explicate the significance of clinical health psychology for some of the major afflictions of the age (Part 4).

Table P1   A multi-level framework or 'Onion Model' for health psychology

Level	Description	Where covered
Core	Age, sex and hereditary factors	Part 1
Level 1	Individual lifestyle	Part 2
Level 2	Social and community influences	Whole book
Level 3	Living and working conditions; health care system	Parts 3 and 4
Level 4	General socio-economic, cultural and environmental conditions	Part 1

Source: Adapted from Dahlgren and Whitehead (1991: 23)

The book uses a multi-level framework that takes into account both the biological determinants and the social context of health-related experience and behaviour. This multi-level framework, the 'Onion Model', assumes different levels of influence and mechanisms for bringing about change (see Table P1 and Chapter 1 for details).

Health psychology is a potentially rich field, but, if it is to become more than a 'tinker', it is necessary to master an appreciation of the cultural, socio-political and economic roots of human behaviour. In this book, we aim to apply an international, cultural and interdisciplinary perspective. We wish to demonstrate the great significance of social, economic and political changes. As the gaps between the 'haves' and the 'have-nots' widen, and the world population grows larger, the impacts of learned helplessness, poverty and social isolation are increasingly salient features of contemporary living.

Those concerned with health promotion and disease prevention require in-depth understanding of the lived experience of health, illness and health care. By integrating research using quantitative, qualitative and action-oriented approaches, we take a step in that direction.

THE BIOPSYCHOSOCIAL MODEL

The dominance of the biomedical system has been challenged by figures in the scientific establishment and by certain patient groups. These challenges are reflected in a call for more attention to the psychological and social aspects of health and, in particular, in the so-called 'biopsychosocial model' (BPSM) proposed by Engel (1977, 1980). According to Engel (1980) all natural phenomena can be organized into a hierarchy of systems ranging from the biosphere at one end of the hierarchy, to society and the individual level of experience and behaviour towards the middle, and then to the cellular and subatomic levels at the other end of the hierarchy. These different levels need to be considered if we are to fully understand health and illness. The BPSM has become the conceptual status quo of contemporary psychiatry (Ghaemi, 2009) and a banner for health psychology. Yet it is far from being established as a paradigm in medicine and health care where the biomedical model remains resiliently in force.

Long before Engel, William Osler (1849–1919) had stated: 'The good physician treats the disease; the great physician treats the patient who has the disease.' He also stated: 'Listen to your patient, he is telling you the diagnosis.' The traditional biomedical model remains the core of medical education, although there may have been a slight shift in the thinking of doctors in primary care and in liaison psychiatry towards a more holistic, BPS view of the patient (see Chapter 1). The BPSM remains a fertile idea for a transformed biomedical model by including the psychological and social aspects of illness along with the biological aspects. The BPSM has been influential, for example, in providing an account of the influence of racism on health outcomes (Clark et al., 1999) and in understanding adolescent conduct problems (Dodge and Pettit, 2003).

However, the BPSM has not been free of controversy – for example, when it has been extended as a cognitive behavioural theory of illness such as myalgic encephalomyelitis (ME) or chronic fatigue syndrome (CFS) by asserting that cognitions and behaviours perpetuate the fatigue and impairment in individuals suffering from the condition(s) (Wessely et al., 1991; Chapter 23). In psychiatry Engel's BPSM became associated with a particular socio-cognitive model for illness experience. We argue that the socio-cognitive formulation has tended to constrain theorizing within health psychology (Chapter 8) and narrowed thinking about clinical conditions and stigma to the presumption of incorrect beliefs and attitudes (Chapter 22). It is important to distance Engel's generic BPSM as a schematic approach to health care from specific formulations of the socio-cognitive model. In truth, there is a multitude of biopsychosocial theories and models that should not be lumped together under a single umbrella, because the devil is in the detail. The adoption of the BPSM by general practitioners can meet with resistance or even hostility by patients, either because they feel more comfortable with the traditional 'doctor knows best' model of biomedicine or because they deem the BPSM is not a good fit for their illness (e.g., myalgic encephalomyelitis/chronic fatigue syndrome (ME/CFS)).

Seventy years ago the World Health Organization (WHO) proposed a definition of health as: 'a state of complete physical, mental and social well-being, not the mere absence of disease or infirmity'. This definition widened the scope of health care to consider well-being more holistically. The WHO definition has not been revised since its original publication in 1948. In Chapter 1 we suggest a wider definition, encompassing the economic, political and spiritual domains of daily living for these are also contributing conditions of well-being. Currently, some areas of health care are shifting from a concern with purely bodily processes to an awareness of broader concepts of quality of life and subjective well-being.

Another recent trend has been an ideological emphasis on patient choice and individual responsibility for health. Crawford (1980: 365) argued that 'in an increasingly "healthist" culture, healthy behaviour has become a moral duty and illness an individual moral failing'.

HUMAN RIGHTS AND THE RESPONSIBILITY TO 'DO NO HARM'

The universal human rights of freedom of speech, thought and action within the law are an essential principle in health care. Health care is at the interface between policy and practice and as such must have a strong foundation in the rights of patients and populations as human beings. In recent years there has been a political shift wherein hate speech and divisive rhetoric by key political leaders have served to 'unleash the dark side of human nature'. This political shift has been the subject of a report by Amnesty International (2017), which has brought to stark attention the 'dark forces' which are changing the geo-political environment … wherein more and more politicians call themselves anti-establishment and wield a politics of demonization that hounds, scapegoats and dehumanizes entire groups of people to win the support of voters.

> This rhetoric will have an increasingly dangerous impact on actual policy. In 2016, governments turned a blind eye to war crimes, pushed through deals that undermine the right to claim asylum, passed laws that violate free expression, incited murder of people simply because they use drugs, legitimized mass surveillance, and extended draconian police powers. (Amnesty International, 2017: https://www.amnesty.org/en/latest/research/2017/02/amnesty-international-annual-report-201617/)

The report also refers to the fact that some countries have implemented intrusive security measures, such as prolonged emergency powers in France and unprecedented surveillance laws in the UK. Another feature of 'strongman' politics has been the rise of anti-feminist and anti-LGBTI rhetoric, such as efforts to roll back women's rights in Poland (Amnesty International, 2017).

Changes to the geo-political framework towards an openly political agenda that supports division, inequality, discrimination, scapegoating and stigma are likely to ripple across into health and social care. All who work in health care face everyday difficult decisions that profoundly impact upon people's lives. The embedding of such decisions in a human rights-based ethical foundation of 'do no harm' becomes ever more relevant if the current climate continues.

MAKING THE BEST USE OF THIS BOOK

This sixth edition has been streamlined in order to focus on the core issues pertinent to students. A new chapter on stress has also been added. Lecturers may recommend the chapters in any order, according to the requirements of any particular course and their personal interests and preferences. Chapters are written as free-standing documents. No prior reading of other chapters is assumed.

Each chapter begins with an **Outline** and ends with a detailed **Summary** of key ideas and suggestions for **Future Research**. Each chapter contains tables, figures and boxes, and recent examples of key studies to guide student understanding. International studies present works by key people living in different parts of the world, showing how context, culture and the environment affect health and behaviour.

Key terms are identified by **bold** and defined in the **Glossary** at the end of the book.

A useful companion reader to this textbook is *The Health Psychology Reader* (Marks, 2002a), which reprints and discusses 25 key articles, accompanied by introductions to the main themes. Readers can also refer to the 85 key articles in *New Directions in Health Psychology* (Murray and Chamberlain, 2015).

ONLINE RESOURCES

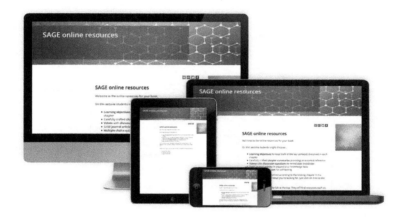

The following online resources in support of *Health Psychology* can be found at **https://study.sagepub.com/Marks6e**

STUDENT RESOURCES

- **Learning objectives** for each chapter to help structure your learning and summarise key points.
- Useful **multiple choice questions** to test your understanding of important information.
- Extra **case studies** to see how health psychology is applied in real world contexts.
- **Video links** that offer a fresh perspective on the concepts covered in the book.
- **eFlashcards** to aid your revision of key terms and ideas.

LECTURER RESOURCES

- A **testbank** of questions which can be used to help student progress and understanding.
- Downloadable and customisable **PowerPoint** slides for use in class.

ACKNOWLEDGEMENTS

DFM: Over 20 years, many talented people have created this textbook and I wish to acknowledge their contributions. To Michael and Emee, my co-authors, for friendship and collaboration; specifically, to MM for his unstinting support and lively humour; to EVE for cake, songs and smiles. To Brian Evans, co-author of four previous editions, for walks and talks over heath and by river. To Ziyad Marar for his enthusiastic skills of persuasion that drew me into the SAGE fold more than two decades ago. To colleagues at SAGE: Michael Carmichael, the original commissioning editor, Luke Block, Amy Jarrold, Donna Goddard and Katie Rabot and the complete editorial team for editing this sixth edition. To Alice Vallat, for a happy home in Arles, Provence. Thank you all warmly – this book couldn't and wouldn't have happened without you.

MM: Thanks to David for initiating and sustaining this project over the years and to the various other co-authors (Brian, Carla, Catherine, Cailine and Emée) who have added so much to it. Thanks, as well, to my wonderful and loving wife (Anne) and sons (Matthew and Daniel) for their continuing support, kindness and inspiration.

EVE: To my parents for life, to my Andy for love, to my mentor, DFM, for guidance, and to my son, Vas, for purpose – thanks!

HEALTH PSYCHOLOGY IN THE CONTEXT OF BIOLOGY, SOCIETY AND METHODOLOGY

This book provides an in-depth, critical overview of the field of health psychology. In Part 1 we are concerned with the biological and psychosocial context of the health and illness experience. This part covers the most relevant aspects of the biological and social sciences that contribute to an in-depth knowledge of health psychology.

In Chapter 1 we review the meaning of the concept of 'health' and the development of health psychology as a field of inquiry. Health and health psychology are defined and issues of measurement and the scaling of subjective well-being are presented. Frameworks, theories and models are discussed and a framework we call the 'Health Onion' is introduced.

In Chapter 2 we introduce the role of the nervous, endocrine and immune systems and the important principle of homeostasis in human health and well-being. These are the key biological systems for the preservation of equilibrium in mind, body and spirit.

In Chapter 3 we focus on the influence of genetics, epigenetics and development across the lifespan. Development is life-long and multi-dimensional with biological, cognitive, psychosocial, economic and spiritual aspects.

In Chapter 4 we discuss the contextual factors of the macro-social environment: the demographic, economic and societal factors which operate globally to structure the health experience of populations, communities and individuals. The chapter uses a wide-angle lens to explore the bigger picture of the global context for human health and suffering.

In Chapter 5 we examine the associations of social inequalities and social injustice with health outcomes. Measures to tackle social injustice are required at political and policy levels and health psychologists can play a role as agents and facilitators of change.

In Chapter 6 we examine the ways in which health and illness have been construed across time and place. Western biomedicine often tends to be accepted as 'scientific' and 'evidence based', while the medical systems of other cultures and indigenous populations, including 'complementary' therapies, are often written off as 'unscientific mumbo-jumbo', 'supernatural' or 'magical'. These alternative systems at least deserve to be fairly evaluated in the light of studies conducted with participants from different cultures and ethnic groups.

In Chapter 7 we present an A–Z of relevant research issues and methods for carrying out research in health psychology. Three categories of methods are quantitative, qualitative and action research methods. These types of method all have potential in assessing, understanding and improving health, illness and health care outcomes.

HEALTH PSYCHOLOGY: AN INTRODUCTION

1

'Cell, organ, person, family each indicate a level of complex integrated organization about the existence of which a high degree of consensus holds. ... In no way can the methods and rules appropriate for the study and understanding of the cell as cell be applied to the study of the person as person or the family as family.'

George Engel (1980)

OUTLINE

In this chapter, we introduce health psychology as a field of inquiry. At the beginning, we introduce the concept of 'health' from a historical perspective. We define health psychology and review theories of need-satisfaction and subjective well-being. We present a new Theory of Well-Being that includes the constructs of attachment, life satisfaction, subjective well-being, affect and consumption. Problems with measurement are examined. Finally, a framework we call the 'Health Onion' is described.

WHAT DO WE MEAN BY 'HEALTH'?

It seems logical – although few textbooks do it – to discuss what is meant by the term '**health**' in a book about health psychology. Otherwise, how do we understand the subject? It seems slightly bizarre that few textbooks ever consider it. We must never take the meaning of 'health' for granted.

Ancient links exist between the concepts of 'health', 'wholeness', 'holiness', 'hygiene', 'cleanliness', 'goodness', 'godliness', 'sanitary', 'sanity' and 'saintliness', as in: 'Wash you, make you clean; put away the evil of your doings from before mine eyes; cease to do evil' (Isaiah, 1:16, King James Bible) and: 'O you who believe! when you rise up to prayer, wash your faces and your hands' (Quran). The concept of health as wholeness existed in ancient China and classical Greece where health was seen as a state of 'harmony', 'balance', 'order' or 'equilibrium' with nature. Related ideas are found in many healing systems today. On the other hand, there are traditional associations between concepts of 'disease', 'disorder', 'disintegration', 'illness', 'crankiness' (or 'krankheit' in German), 'uncleanness', 'insanity', 'chaos' and 'evil'.

Galen (CE 129–200), the early Roman physician, followed the Hippocratic tradition with *hygieia* (health) or *euexia* (soundness) as a balance between the four bodily humours of black bile, yellow bile, phlegm and blood. Galen believed that the body's 'constitution', 'temperament' or 'state' could be put out of equilibrium by excessive heat, cold, dryness or wetness. Such imbalances might be caused by fatigue, insomnia, distress, anxiety, or by food residues resulting from eating the wrong quantity or quality of food. Human moods were viewed as a consequence of imbalances in one of the four bodily fluids. Imbalances of humour corresponded to particular temperaments (blood–sanguine, black bile–melancholic, yellow bile–choleric, and phlegm–phlegmatic). The theory was also related to the four elements: earth, fire, water and air (Table 1.1).

In the winter, when it is chilly and wet, people might worry about catching a cold, caused by a build-up of phlegm. In summer, when a person is hot and sweaty, they may worry about not drinking enough water or they could otherwise become 'tetchy' or 'hot and bothered' (bad tempered). It is remarkable that some common beliefs today are descendants of early Greek and Roman theories of medicine from 2,000-plus years ago. It is significant that the concept of balance/equilibrium and the idea that a basic bodily process exists to restore balance (homeostasis) are as much core issues in Science today as in Classical times.

Table 1.1 Galen's theory of humours

Humour	Season	Element	Organ	Qualities	Personality type	Characteristics
Blood	spring	air	liver	warm and moist	sanguine	amorous, courageous, hopeful
Yellow bile	summer	fire	gall bladder	warm and dry	choleric	easily angered, bad tempered
Black bile	autumn	earth	spleen	cold and dry	melancholic	despondent, sleepless, irritable
Phlegm	winter	water	brain/lungs	cold and moist	phlegmatic	calm, unemotional

Universal interest in health is fuelled by a continuous torrent of content in the media about health and medicine, especially concerning the 'dread' diseases. In 1946 the **World Health Organization (WHO)** defined health as: 'the state of complete physical, social and spiritual well-being, not simply the absence of illness'. It is highly doubtful whether 'complete physical, social and spiritual well-being' can ever be reached by anyone. Apart from this idealism, the WHO definition overlooks the *psychological*, *cultural* and *economic* aspects of health. Psychological processes, the main subject of this book, are a key factor in health and are embedded in a social context. For this reason, the term 'psychosocial' is often used to describe human behaviour and experience as an influence on well-being. Social inequalities and poverty are also strongly associated with health outcomes and warrant explicit inclusion in any definition of health. With these thoughts in mind, we define health in the light of five key elements (Box 1.1).

BOX 1.1

Definition of health

Health is a state of well-being with satisfaction of physical, cultural, psychosocial, economic and spiritual needs, not simply the absence of illness.

NEED SATISFACTION, HAPPINESS AND SUBJECTIVE WELL-BEING

To be useful, the above definition of health needs to be unpacked. Philosophers, psychologists, poets, songsters and others have had much to say about what makes a person feel well. A key concept is that of **need satisfaction**. In Maslow's (1943) more academic **hierarchy of needs** (Figure 1.1), a person is healthy if all of their needs are satisfied, starting with the most basic needs for air, food, water, sex, sleep, homeostasis and excretion. Then as need satisfaction moves towards the top of the pyramid, the epitome of need satisfaction, a person becomes more and more 'satisfied', and thus physically and mentally healthy to the point of 'self-actualization'.

Maslow's hierarchy framework has been influential. It puts the concept of **'self-actualization'** at the top of the pyramid, a state in which the person feels they have achieved a so-called 'peak experience' of meaningful and purposeful existence. Maslow's needs hierarchy emphasizes the great importance of safety, love and belonging, and self-esteem. For every good principle in psychology, there are always exceptions, and human needs do not always fall into any fixed hierarchy. For example, an extreme sports enthusiast who is into mountain climbing may put 'esteem' and 'self-actualization' ahead of 'safety'. We read about it in the news the next morning. Few would disagree about the existence of the five levels of need within the pyramid. However, there are also key elements of human fulfilment that are not explicitly mentioned in Maslow's hierarchy, for example, **agency** and **autonomy** – the freedom to choose – and the often-neglected **spirituality** – the subjective intuition that lacks any hard empirical proof that not all that is significant is of the physical world.

Homeostasis is a core concept within Physiology, a regulating property of the organism wherein the stability of the internal environment is actively maintained. The function of cells, tissues and organs are organized into negative feedback systems. Homeostasis operates at cellular, organismic and ecosystems levels. At organismic level, homeostasis regulates core body temperature and the levels of pH, sodium, potassium and calcium, glucose, water, carbon dioxide and oxygen in the body.

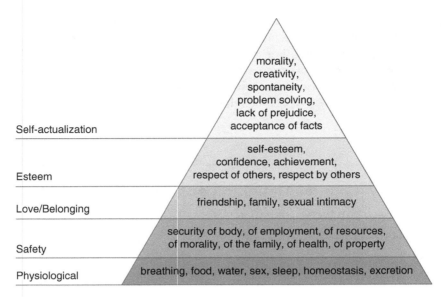

Figure 1.1   Maslow's hierarchy of human needs

In Chapter 2 we present a Homeostasis Theory of Behaviour which can be applied across all areas of health psychology. If homeostasis breaks down, a person can suffer a variety of life-threatening conditions, including diabetes, obesity, starvation, chronic thirst and insomnia (Marks, 2015, 2016a, 2016b). Homeostasis is not actually a 'need' as suggested by Maslow's pyramid; it is the process that works towards the restoration of equilibrium, as we shall see in Chapter 2. A broad spectrum of evidence from many scientific fields suggests that homeostasis is an organizing principle of considerable generality, not simply at the level of physiological need, but throughout the psychological universe of regulation of thought, feeling and action (Marks, 2018).

Throughout history, philosophers have discussed the nature of a *good and happy life* or what, in health care, is termed '**quality of life' (QoL)**. For Aristotle, happiness was viewed as 'the meaning and the purpose of life, the whole aim and end of human existence'. For utilitarians such as Jeremy Bentham, happiness was pleasure without pain. To individuals suffering from cancer or other conditions with pain, unpleasant physical symptoms and treatment options, and an uncertain prognosis, QoL has special relevance.

QoL has been defined by WHO as (take a deep breath):

> An individual's perception of their position in life, in the context of the culture and value systems in which they live, and in relation to their goals, expectations, standards, and concerns. It is a broad ranging concept, affected in a complex way by the person's physical health, psychological state, level of independence, social relationships, and their relationship to salient features of their environment. (WHOQoL Group, 1995: 1404)

A sixth domain, concerning spirituality, religiousness and personal beliefs, was later added by the WHOQoL Group (1995). The Collins dictionary defines QoL more simply as: 'The general well-being of a person or society, defined in terms of health and happiness, rather than wealth.' The QoL concept overlaps with that of **subjective well-being (SWB)**, which has been defined by a leader in the field, Ed Diener ('Dr Happiness'), as: 'An umbrella term for different valuations that people make regarding their lives, the events happening to them, their bodies and minds, and the circumstances in which they live' (Diener, 2006: 400). The evidence linking SWB with health and longevity is strong and plentiful.

With a global population of more than seven billion unique individuals of diverse cultures, religions and social circumstances, one wonders whether QoL can ever be assessed using a single yardstick. A few courageous individuals and organizations have given it a try and, since the 1970s, many scales and measures have been constructed. A few examples are listed in Table 1.2.

By far, the most utilized scale to date has been the SF-36, which accounts for around 50% of all clinical studies (Marks, 2013). These 'happiness scales' are diverse and consist of items about what makes a 'good life'. For example, Diener et al.'s (1985) brief *Satisfaction with Life Scale* (SWLS) uses a seven-point Likert scale with five items:

In most ways my life is close to my ideal.

The conditions of my life are excellent.

I am satisfied with my life.

So far I have gotten the important things I want in life.

If I could live my life over, I would change almost nothing.

Table 1.2   Examples of QoL, subjective well-being and happiness scales

Authors	Year	Title	Domains	Samples
Andrews and Withey	1976	Social indicators of well-being	Job satisfaction	Adults
Flanagan	1978	The QoL scale (QoLS)	Material and physical well-being Relationships Social, community and civic activities Personal development and fulfilment Recreation	Healthy adults and patients with chronic illnesses
Kammann	1979	Affectometer 1	Happiness/subjective well-being	Adults
Kammann and Flett	1983	Affectometer 2		
Diener et al.	1985	Satisfaction with Life Scale (SWLS)	Satisfaction with life	Adults
European Organization for Research and Treatment of Cancer (EORTC)	1986	QLQ-C30	Physical Role Cognitive Emotional Social Global QoL	Patient samples

(Continued)

7

Table 1.2   (Continued)

Authors	Year	Title	Domains	Samples
Ware and Sherbourne	1992	Short-Form Health Survey (SF-36)	Vitality Physical functioning Bodily pain General health perceptions Physical role functioning Emotional role functioning Social role functioning Mental health	Healthy adults and patients with chronic illnesses
WHOQoL group	1995	WHOQoL	Physical Psychological Level of independence Social relationships Environment Spirituality	Healthy adults and patient groups
International Wellbeing Group	2013	Personal Wellbeing Index Percentage Scale Maximum	Allows results from different scales to be compared,	Healthy adults and patient groups

Using the 1–7 scale below, testees indicate their agreement with each item by placing the appropriate number on the line preceding that item. They are asked to 'be open and honest' in their responding.

7   Strongly agree

6   Agree

5   Slightly agree

4   Neither agree nor disagree

3   Slightly disagree

2   Disagree

1   Strongly disagree

For the vast majority of people, SWB is relatively stable over the long term. Using longitudinal data, Headey and Wearing (1989) reported that when the level of SWB changed following a major event, it tended to return to its previous level over time. To account for this, the authors proposed that each person has an 'equilibrium level' of SWB, and that 'personality' restores equilibrium after change by making certain kinds of events more likely. Restoration of equilibrium is nothing to do with personality; it's a fundamental stabilizing process across all living systems, called 'homeostasis'.

Diener and Chan (2011) review evidence that *having high SWB adds four to ten years to life*. The evidence for an association between SWB and all-cause mortality is mounting. As always, there could be a mysterious third variable influencing both SWB and mortality (e.g., foetal nutrition, social support, lifestyle) and, if the relationship between SWB and mortality did prove to be causal, the possible mediating processes would be a matter for speculation and further research. For the time being, it seems safe to assume that happy people live longer.

SUBJECTIVE WELL-BEING HOMEOSTASIS

The most basic property of SWB is that it is normally positive. On a rating scale from 'feeling very bad' to 'feeling very good', only a few people lie below the scale mid-point. General population data from over 60,000 people gathered over 13 years by the Australian Unity Wellbeing Index surveys (Cummins, 2013) found that only 4% of scores lie below 50 percentage points. Feeling good about yourself is the norm.

While it has been generally agreed that SWB consists of both affect and cognition, it is thought that SWB mainly comprises mood (Cummins, 2016). Russell (2003) coined the term 'Core Affect' to describe a neurophysiological state experienced as a feeling, a deep form of affect or mood. Russell considered it analogous to felt body temperature in that it is always present, can be accessed when attended to, existing without words to describe it.

Robert A. Cummins introduced the idea that homeostasis is operating on SWB, as it does in biological systems of the body: 'It is proposed that life satisfaction is a variable under homeostatic control and with a homeostatic set-point ensuring that populations have, on average, a positive view of their lives' (Cummins, 1998: 330). Cummins suggested the concept of 'Homeostatically Protected Mood' (HPMood) as the most basic feeling state of SWB (Cummins, 2010). The concept of 'HPMood' places the regulation of mood in the same framework as physiological homoeostasis, which controls body temperature, blood pressure, and a thousand and one other bodily systems (Cannon, 1932). Cummins' describes HPMood as follows:

1. It is neurophysiologically generated consisting of the simplest, constant, non-reflective feeling, the tonic state of affect that provides the underlying activation energy, or motivation, for routine behavior.

2. It is not modifiable by conscious experience, yet it is a ubiquitous, background component of conscious experience. It is experienced as a general feeling of contentment, but also comprises aspects of related affects, including happy and alert.

3. When SWB is measured using either the Satisfaction with Life Scale (Diener et al., 1985) or the Personal Wellbeing Index (International Wellbeing Group, 2013), HPMood accounts for over 60% of the variance.

4. Under normal conditions of rest, the average level of HPMood for each person represents their 'set-point', a genetically determined, individual value. Within the general population, these set-points are normally distributed between 70% and 90% along the 0–100-point scale.

5. For each person's set-point there is a 'set-point-range', the limits within which homeostatic processes normally maintain HPMood for each individual.

6. HPMood 'perfuses all cognitive processes to some degree, but most strongly the rather abstract notions of self (e.g., I am a lucky person). Because of this, these self-referent

perceptions are normally held at a level that approximates each set-point range' (Cummins, 2016: 63).

7. Under resting conditions, SWB is a proxy for HPMood. However, SWB can vary outside the set-point-range for HPMood when a strong emotion is generated by momentary experience. 'When this occurs, homeostatic forces are activated, which attempt to return experienced affect to set-point-range. Thus, daily affective experience normally oscillates around its set-point' (Cummins, 2016: 64).

One of the principal goals of health psychology is to understand the links between subjective well-being and health. The application of the concept of homeostasis from Physiology in the discipline of Psychology holds significant potential. A general homeostasis theory of well-being, physical health and life satisfaction is summarized in Box 1.2.

BOX 1.2

Homeostasis Theory of Well-Being

The Homeostasis Theory of Well-Being (HTWB) shows causal links between some significant determinants of physical and mental well-being (see Figure 1.2). In addition to emotion, and the role of income, restraint and consumption, the HTWB places emphasis on the developmentally important construct of attachment (Bowlby, 1969, 1973, 1980). The manner in which a baby attaches to its mother, father and/or other caregiver is assumed to create a template for life based on the infant's need to maintain proximity to an anchor person who provides a 'secure base' for exploring the environment. The availability and responsivity of the anchor person to attachment are internalized as mental models that are generalized to relationships throughout life until the individual's death (Ainsworth et al., 1978). The different ways of attaching to anchor figures is termed 'attachment style'.

Of relevance to the GTWB is the basic construct SWB. The hedonic conception of SWB of Diener and Chan (2011) can be contrasted with the **eudaimonic** approach, which focuses on meaning and self-realization and defines well-being in terms of the degree to which a person is fully functioning (Ryan and Deci, 2001). Waterman (1993) has argued that eudaimonic well-being occurs when people are living in accordance with their 'daimon', or authentic self. Eudaimonia is thought to occur when people's life activities mesh with deeply held values and are fully engaged in authentic personal expression.

An important aspect of life satisfaction is the search for eudaimonic meaning. Empirical studies suggest that there exists a strong and stable relationship between meaning in life and subjective well-being (Zika and Chamberlain, 1992). People who believe that they have meaningful lives tend to be more optimistic and self-actualized (Compton et al., 1996), and experience more self-esteem (Steger et al., 2006) and positive affect (e.g., King et al., 2006), as well as less depression and anxiety (Steger et al., 2006) and less suicidal ideation (Harlow, 1986). The 'Salutogenic Theory' of Antonovsky (1979) also emphasized the relationship between meaning and purpose in life, assessed by the Sense of Coherence scale, and positive health outcomes (Eriksson and Lindström, 2006).

THE NATURE OF HEALTH PSYCHOLOGY

The importance of psychosocial processes in health and illness is an established part of health care. The evidence on the role of behaviour and emotion in morbidity and mortality has been steadily accumulating over the last century. By the end of the First World War, the British Army had dealt with 80,000 cases of shell shock, including those of poets Siegfried Sassoon and Wilfred Owen. Millions of men and women suffered psychological trauma as a result of their war experiences. Since that time, and the experiences of many other wars, much research has been conducted to investigate the possible role of trauma, stress and psychological characteristics on the onset, course and management of physical illnesses. Health psychology has grown rapidly, and psychologists are increasingly in demand in health care and medical settings. Psychologists have become essential members of multidisciplinary teams in rehabilitation, cardiology, paediatrics, oncology, anaesthesiology, family practice, dentistry, and other fields, including defence, intelligence, policing and justice.

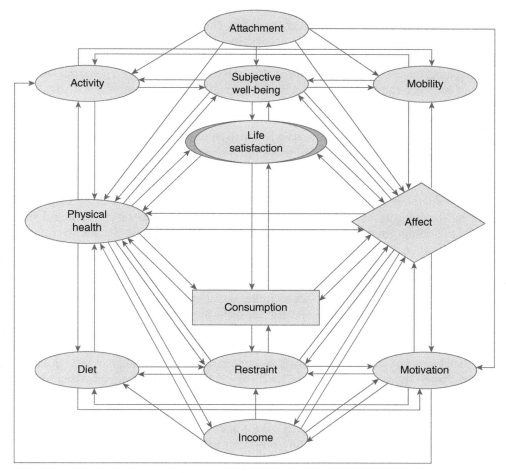

Figure 1.2   General Theory of Well-Being (GTWB)

Source: Marks (2015)

11

Increasing interest is being directed towards disease prevention, especially with reference to sexual health, nutrition, smoking, alcohol, inactivity and stress. A current ideology is '**individualism**', in which individual 'agents' are deemed responsible for their own health. From this neoliberalist viewpoint, a person who smokes 40 a day and develops lung cancer is responsible for causing their own costly, disabling and terminal illness. Traditional health education has consisted of campaigns providing a mixture of exhortation, information and advice to persuade people to change their unhealthy habits. By telling people to 'Just say no', policy makers expect people to make the 'right' choices and change 'unhealthy' choices into 'healthy' ones. There has been notable success in tobacco control, which provides a benchmark for what may be achieved through health education, and policy in other clinical areas, such as coronary artery disease, obesity, diabetes and metabolic syndrome.

Against the 'healthist' view that keeping ourselves healthy means making responsible choices, there is little convincing evidence, beyond the example of smoking, that people who change their lifestyle actually *do* live longer or have a greater quality of life than people who 'live and let live' and make no real attempt to live healthily. Consider an example: a prospective study suggests that vegetarians live longer than meat eaters. But vegetarians may differ from the meat-eaters in many ways other than their choice of diet (e.g., religious beliefs, use of alcohol, social support). A statistical association between two variables, such as a vegetarian diet and longevity, does not prove causality or allow a prediction about any particular individual case. A vegetarian can still die of stomach cancer and becoming vegetarian does not necessarily lengthen the life of any specific individual. Epidemiology is a statistical science. It provides a statistical statement to which there will always be inconvenient exceptions, such as 90-year-old smokers.

The healthist assumption that a person must 'live well to be well' is prevalent today in industrialised countries and it can lead to victim blaming. If people become ill, it is seen as possibly being 'their own fault' because they smoke, drink, eat poorly, fail to exercise or use screening services, do not jog or join a gym, and so on. Health policy is run through with blaming and shaming individuals for their own poor health. The 'smoking evil' has been replaced by the 'obesity evil'. More recently we have seen cases of blaming and shaming of people, including government advisors, for not following social distancing rules in the COVID-19 emergency.

Health campaigns are often based on the idea that by informing people they can make responsible choices. People are presumed to be free agents with self-determination. Yet human behaviour is influenced by so many factors in the social and economic environment, and especially by role models among family and friends or in the mass media. The herd instinct is as strong in humans as it is in bees, birds or sheep. Christakis and Fowler (2007) reported evidence that behaviour changes such as quitting smoking or putting on weight are associated with similar changes in networks of friends. Imitation is an important influence in human behaviour and one significant change approach, social cognitive theory, is based on this principle (Bandura, 1995).

The built environment, the sum total of objects placed in the natural world by human beings, is another influence on behaviour. Included within this are the images and messages from advertisers in mass media, and the digital environment. A 'toxic environment' has been engineered to draw people towards unhealthy products, habits and behaviours (Brownell, 1994). The **obesogenic** environment contains affordable but nasty, fatty, salty and sugary foods that readily cause weight gain and obesity on an industrial scale. Items for sale include foods such as 'hot dogs' containing 'mechanically recovered meat' and 0% real meat, and 'chicken nuggets' with 0% chicken. The proliferation of such low-priced items in supermarkets and 24/7 stores offer low-income consumers an unhealthy selection of options. A reliance on meat-eating and careless practices in markets has contributed to the spreading of dangerous viruses such as Ebola and COVID-19, with devastating impact.

In this book, arguments are presented on different sides of the 'freedom and choice' debate. It is accepted that our present understanding of health behaviour is far from definitive. However, we also need to adopt a critical position towards the discipline. Health psychology is still relatively young as a sub-discipline and there are many issues to be addressed. For the most part, health psychology has been formulated within an individualistic ideological formulation which is part of neoliberalist mass culture. The evidence presented in this book suggests that socio-cognitive approaches to behaviour change that target internalized processes in the form of hypothetical 'social cognitions' are ineffectual, inefficient and too small in scale (Marks, 1996, 2002a, 2002b). Apart from their theoretical shortcomings, mass dissemination of individualized therapeutic approaches through the health care system is unsustainable and unaffordable. Like it or not, in spite of the many critiques, the biomedical model remains the foundation stone of clinical health care.

Health psychologists work at different levels of the health care system: carrying out research; systematically reviewing research; designing, implementing and evaluating health interventions; training and teaching; doing consultancy; providing and improving health services; carrying out health promotion; designing policy to improve services; giving scientific advice to government; and advocating social justice for people and communities to act on their own terms. In this book we give examples of all these activities, and suggest opportunities to make further progress.

A community perspective on health work offers an alternative prospect for intervention. Community approaches are less popular within mainstream health psychology and have been the mainstay of community psychology. There could be valuable synergies between health and community psychology working outside the health care system. In working towards social justice and reducing inequalities, people's rights to health and freedom from illness are, quite literally, a life and death matter; it is the responsibility of planners, policy makers and leaders of people wherever they may be to fight for a fairer, more equitable system of health care (Marks, 2004; Murray, 2014a).

Our definition of health psychology is given in Box 1.3. In discussing this definition, we can say that the objective of health psychology is the promotion and maintenance of well-being in individuals, communities and populations.

BOX 1.3

Definition of health psychology

Health psychology is an interdisciplinary field concerned with the application of psychological knowledge and techniques to health, illness and health care.

Although there are diverse points of view, health psychologists generally hold a holistic perspective on individual well-being, that all aspects of human nature are interconnected. While the primary focus of health psychology is *physical* rather than *mental* health, the latter being the province of clinical psychology, it is acknowledged that mental and physical health are actually 'two sides of one coin'. When a person has a physical illness for a period of time, then it is not surprising if they also experience worry (= anxiety) and/or sadness (= depression). If serious enough, 'negative affect' (sadness and/or worry) may become classified as 'mental illness' (severe depression and/or anxiety), and be detrimental to subjective well-being and to aspects of physical health. Each side of the 'well-being coin' is bound to the other. The distinction between 'health psychology' and 'clinical psychology' is an unfortunate historical accident that is difficult to explain to non-psychologists (or even to psychologists themselves). There is also significant overlap between health and clinical psychology and 'positive psychology' as an integrative new field (Seligman and Csikszentmihalyi, 2000; Seligman et al., 2005), although not without critiques of exaggerated claims and poor methodology (e.g., Coyne and Tennen, 2010).

RATIONALE AND ROLE FOR HEALTH PSYCHOLOGY

There is a strong rationale and role for the discipline of health psychology. First, the behavioural basis for illness and mortality requires effective methods of behaviour change. Second, a holistic system of health care requires expert knowledge of the psychosocial needs of people.

In relation to point 1, *all* the leading causes of illness and death are *behavioural*. This means that many deaths are preventable if effective methods of changing behaviour and/or the environment can be found.

BOX 1.4

KEY STUDY: The Global Burden of Disease study

An important epidemiological perspective comes from measures of 'disability' or 'disablement'. The Global Burden of Disease (GBD) study projected mortality and disablement over 25 years. The trends from the GBD study suggest that disablement is determined mainly by ageing, the spread of HIV, the increase in tobacco-related mortality and disablement, psychiatric and neurological conditions, and the decline in mortality from communicable, maternal, perinatal and nutritional disorders (Murray and Lopez, 1997).

The GBD study was repeated in 2010 and figures were prepared by age, sex and region for changes that had occurred between 1990 and 2010. Global figures for life expectancy show increases for all age groups (Figure 1.3).

The GBD uses the disability-adjusted life year (DALY) as a quantitative indicator of the burden of disease. It reflects the total amount of healthy life lost that is attributed to all causes, whether from premature mortality or from some degree of disablement during a period of time. The DALY is the sum of years of life lost from premature mortality plus years of life with disablement, adjusted for the severity of disablement from all causes, both physical and mental (Murray and Lopez, 1997).

The data in Table 1.3 indicate that nearly 30% of the total global burden of disease is attributable to five risk factors. The largest risk factor (underweight) is associated with poverty (see Chapters 4 and 5). The remaining four risk factors are discussed in Part 2 of this book (see Chapters 8–13).

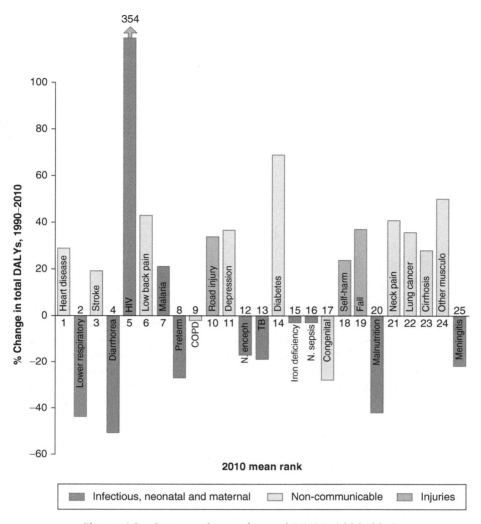

Figure 1.3   Percent change in total DALYs, 1990–2010

Source: Institute for Health Metrics and Evaluation (2014), www.healthdata.org/infographic/percent-change-total-dalys-1990-2010

There were changes in the total DALYs attributable to different causes between 1990 and 2010, as shown in Figure 1.3. Good progress is evident in DALYs for the lower respiratory tract and diarrhoea, but a huge increase of 354% occurred in DALYs for HIV patients. Moderate but significant increases in DALYs occurred for heart disease, stroke, low back pain, depression and diabetes.

The statistics on death and disablement indicate the significant involvement of behaviour and therefore provide a strong rationale for the discipline of health psychology in all three of its key elements: theory, research and practice. If the major risk factors are to be addressed, there is a pressing need for effective programmes of environmental and behavioural change. This requires a sea change in policy. The dominant ideology that makes individuals responsible for their own health may not be the most helpful approach. The environment is a hugely important factor. In our opinion, a psychological approach in the absence of environmental change is like whistling in the wind.

Table 1.3   The five leading risk factors for global disease burden computed in DALYs

Risk factor	Number of DALYs (millions)	Percentage of DALYs
Childhood and maternal underweight	138	9.5
Unprotected sex	92	6.3
High blood pressure	64	4.4
Tobacco	59	4.1
Alcohol	58	4.0
Totals	411	28.3

Health psychologists are at the 'sharp end' of the quest to produce health behaviour change on an industrial scale. The fact that people are highly constrained by their environment and socio-economic circumstances militates against such change. In a sense, without adaptations of the environment, this effort is disabled. There are strong constraints on the ability of health care systems to influence health outcomes at a population level because of the significant social and economic determinants that structure the health of individuals and communities. The environment must change, and by that route there can be behaviour change on a societal scale. Attempting to change behaviour without first attending to the environment is akin to 'the tail wagging the dog', mission impossible.

A second rationale for health psychology is growing recognition that a purely medical approach to health care is failing to meet the psychosocial needs of many patients. This has led to a search for an alternative perspective that values holistic care of patients and attempts to improve services through higher quality psychosocial care. In spite of their very high costs, health care systems are often perceived to be inefficient, ineffective and unfit for purpose. This is especially the case in the USA, where the largest per capita expenditure is producing some unimpressive outcomes.

The **biomedical model** has been criticized since the 1970s (Illich, 1976). While medical experts want to give modern medicine the credit for the decline of disease in the twentieth century, critics have suggested that health improvements are due mainly to better hygiene, education and reduced poverty (McKeown, 1979). In addition, there has been a growing awareness of psychological and social influences in health and illness which has been formulated as the **biopsychosocial model** (BPSM) (Engel, 1977). Following in the footsteps of Weiss and von Bertalanffy, Engel observed that nature is a 'hierarchically arranged continuum with its more complex, larger units superordinate on the less complex smaller units' (Engel, 1980: 536). He represented the hierarchy either as a vertical stack or as a nest of squares, with the simplest at the centre and the most complex on the outside (Figure 1.4). At the very beginning of this chapter, we print a quotation from Engel (1980), part of which states: 'In no way can the methods and rules appropriate for the study and understanding of the cell as cell be applied to the study of the person as person or the family as family.'

Our review of the core construct of homeostasis in the next chapter will prove this part of Engel's statement to be 100% false. Homeostasis is a unifying principle across the continuum of natural systems from the molecule at one end to the biosphere at the other.

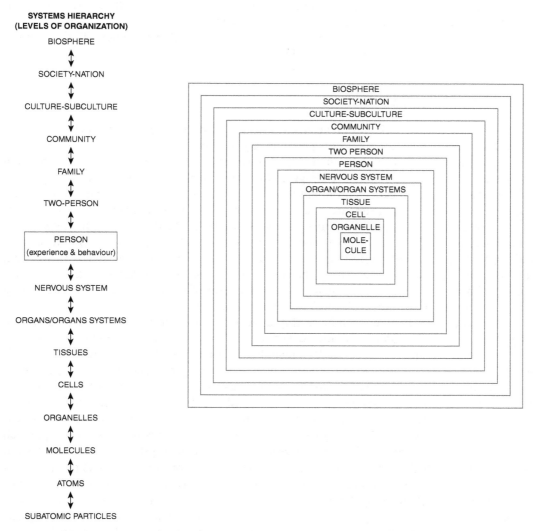

Figure 1.4   Continuum of nature from the simplest unit to the most complex
Adapted from Engel (1980)

The vertical stack was sub-divided into two stacks, the first starting with subatomic particles and ending with the individual person, the second starting with the person and finishing with the biosphere. The first is an organismic hierarchy, the second a social hierarchy. The constructs of a biological/organismic and a social universe are both integral to the study of health psychology. There has been a lot of discussion in health psychology about the adoption of the BPSM. However, the evidence of this adoption in medical education is meagre.

A majority of US physicians reported not receiving effective training regarding the role of the BPSM, and thus have feelings of low self-efficacy in addressing and managing biopsycho-social issues (Moser and Stagnaro-Green, 2009). Some reference to the BPSM occurs in the nursing research literature on patient-centred care, but the specific influence of the BPSM on nursing is not significant (e.g., Mead and Bower, 2002; Kitson et al., 2013). The paradigm shift that Engel proposed for health care is yet to happen.

One crucial tool in the development of the BPSM and of health psychology as a discipline is the need for measurement of psychological variables.

MEASUREMENT

In the natural sciences, attributes of the physical world, such as space, time, temperature, veloc-ity and acceleration, are all measured quantitatively. Psychologists, concerned with behaviour and experience, are unable to measure many of the most interesting psychological attributes in the same objective manner and have struggled to justify the discipline as a science.

Psychology's early years as an infant science were spent developing psychophysics and ability testing. Despite some apparent successes in these two areas, the measurement problem in psychology had not been satisfactorily resolved. In the 1950s the influential *Handbook of Experimental Psychology* was published by a professor at Harvard, Stanley Smith Stevens (1951). Stevens proposed a solution, or so he hoped, to the measurement problem by invoking the principle of **operationism**. Since that time, psychologists have assumed that measure-ment is simply what Stevens said it was: the assignment of numbers to attributes according to rules. Unfortunately, Stevens' solution is purely illusory.

It is apparent that numbers can be readily allocated to attributes using a non-random rule (the operational definition of measurement) that would generate 'measurements' that are not quantitatively meaningful. For example, numerals can be allocated to colours: red = 1, blue = 2, green = 3, etc. The rule used to allocate the numbers is clearly not random, and the allocation therefore counts as measurement, according to Stevens. However, it would be patent nonsense to assert that 'green is 3 × red' or that 'blue is 2 × red', or that 'green − blue = red'. Intervals and ratios cannot be inferred from a simple ordering of scores along a scale. Yet this is how psychological measurement is usually carried out. Despite its obvious flaws, Stevens' approach circumvented the requirement for quantitative measurement that only quantitative attributes can be measured (Michell, 1999). This is because psychological constructs, such as the quality of life, are nothing at all like physical variables that are quantitative in nature. However, psycholo-gists have routinely treated psychological constructs *as if they are quantitative in nature and as amenable to measurement as physical characteristics*. For more than 60 years, psychology has been living in a make-believe world where making rules for applying numbers to attributes has been treated as if it were proper measurement. This fundamental issue cuts off at its very roots the claim that psychology is a quantitative science on a par with the natural sciences.

However, this would be a very short textbook if we were to give up at this point! We must soldier on as if we have solid ground to walk upon rather than boggy sand.

Measurement can be defined as the estimation of the magnitude of a quantitative attribute relative to a unit (Michell, 2003). Before quantification can happen, it is first necessary to obtain evidence that the relevant attribute is quantitative in structure. This has rarely, if ever, been car-ried out in psychology. Unfortunately, it is arguably the case that the definition of measurement within psychology since Stevens' (1951) operationism is incorrect and psychologists' claims about being able to measure psychological attributes can be questioned (Michell, 1999, 2002). Contrary to common beliefs within the discipline, psychological attributes may not actually be quantitative at all, and hence not amenable to coherent numerical measurement and statistical analyses that make unwarranted assumptions about the numbers collected as data.

The situation is akin to the 'Emperor has no clothes' story. Psychometricians are forced to pretend/make the inference that the ordering of scores is a reflection of an underlying quantity and therefore that psychological attributes are measurable on interval scales. Otherwise there would be no basis for quantitative measurement in psychology. Michell (2012: 255) argued that: 'the most plausible hypothesis is that the kinds of attributes psychometricians aspire to measure are merely ordinal attributes with impure differences of degree, a feature logically incompatible with quantitative structure. If so, psychometrics is built upon a myth.' This view is supported by Sijtsma (2012), who argued that the real measurement problem in psychology is the absence of well-developed theories about psychological attributes and a lack of any evidence to support the assumption that psychological attributes are continuous and quantitative in nature. This fundamental measurement problem exists as much within health psychology as it does within psychology as a whole.

BOX 1.5

Measuring a psychological attribute – what the majority of textbooks don't tell you and about which you are not supposed to ask

A typical study requires participants to complete a set of ratings on questionnaire scales that are designed to measure a psychological attribute. The essential issue is whether the total score obtained from the numbers (ratings) provided by an individual is in any way a measure of an attribute along a quantitative scale, like the readings from a tape measure, which reflect the quantity of distance. Distance has an absolute zero and different objects can be placed at equal distances from each other or in fixed ratios. Now let's consider the example of Diener's *Satisfaction with Life Scale* (SWLS) (Table 1.2). The total scores on the SWLS are obtained by summing the seven-point ratings of each of five items. Thus, a maximum score is 35 and the minimum score is 5. The scoring scheme is given here:

31–35   Extremely satisfied

26–30   Satisfied

21–25   Slightly satisfied

20   Neutral

15–19   Slightly dissatisfied

10–14   Dissatisfied

5–9   Extremely dissatisfied

(Continued)

Is there any basis for assuming the total scores on the SWLS are measures of a quantitative attribute 'Life Satisfaction' such that there is an absolute zero (as there would be in any ratio scale) and a person with a score of 20 has exactly double the life satisfaction of a person who has a score of 10 and/or that two people with scores of 30 and 25 have a life satisfaction that is the same 'distance' apart (5 points) as in the case of two people with scores of 20 and 15? If the 5-point differences were shown to be the same, then the SWLS would be an interval scale. However, *neither of the hypotheses is plausible.* We can only infer a person's life satisfaction from their answers to items on the SWLS. *This is because we have no independent definition of life satisfaction, and no evidence that life satisfaction is a quantitative attribute, apart from the SWLS scores themselves.*

The total scores on the SWLS really only allow respondents to be placed along an ordinal scale, yet it is common practice to treat the scores as if they were interval scale data that can be added together, subtracted, averaged and compared between groups using standard deviations and variance scores in statistical analyses.

This measurement problem cuts through the entire discipline of psychology. We infer or, in truth, are forced to act on the unproven assumption (i.e., prejudice) that a person's score on a questionnaire is a measure on a continuous quantitative interval scale. That assumption has never been tested and psychometrics, therefore, has been challenged as a form of 'pathological science' (Michell, 2008).

[Nobody promised you a rose garden! We said at the outset that we would adopt a critical stance, and the measurement problem we have described here, which, for obvious reasons, is not normally talked about, is a good start. The situation is not completely hopeless, however, so please do read on.]

Fortunately, for a practical domain like health psychology, it is possible to 'get by' without any proper solution to the measurement problem. Yes, it's a fudge, but a necessary fudge, because otherwise psychological science would be no more advanced today than it was in 1900. One of the main goals of health psychologists is to design interventions that are effective solutions to health problems. Normally we can find ways to objectively compare different interventions to see what works and what doesn't work. The associations between interventions and outcomes can be observed and measured in quantitative terms. Additionally, a patient seeking treatment for an unpleasant condition can express their thoughts, feelings and motives using plain words by answering questions or items on a questionnaire. In the vast majority of cases, either psychological measures are assumed, for the sake of convenience, to lie along an interval scale or the data are purely categorical.

Health psychologists are concerned with patient–practitioner interactions, public health promotion, or working in communities where actions are carried out, all with observable inputs and outputs. Outcomes in these various scenarios are all objectively observable and measurable, even if the measurements themselves are not shown to have an underlying quantitative attribute. In addition, it is the experiences of the actors that are important, and these are amenable to qualitative methods where the presumption of quantitative attributes and the associated measurement problem do not apply.

A FRAMEWORK FOR HEALTH PSYCHOLOGY

Theoretical thinking in any scientific discipline consists of four broad types that vary according to their level of generality: paradigms, **frameworks**, **theories** and **models**. Paradigms explicitly state assumptions, laws and methods in a complete system of thinking about a field of inquiry (Kuhn, 1970). Frameworks have some of the characteristics of paradigms, but are smaller-scale and much looser, although they are a way of organizing information about a field. Figure 1.5 shows a framework about the main influences on the health of individual human beings that we find quite helpful. It has been adapted from the work of Dahlgren and Whitehead (1991) and we call this the 'Health Onion'.

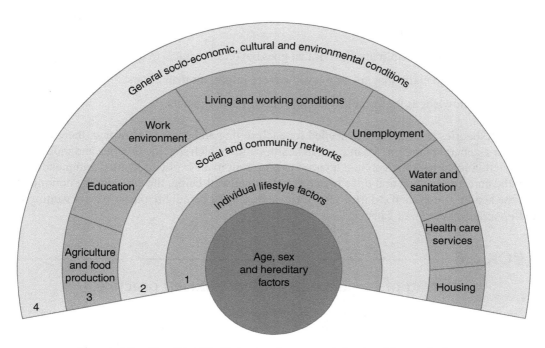

Figure 1.5   The 'Health Onion': a framework for health psychology

Source: Dahlgren and Whitehead (1991)

The 'Health Onion' has a multi-layered structure of 'rings', with the individual person at its core, surrounded by four layers of influence, 'systems' or 'rings'

Core: age, sex and hereditary factors (Part 1 of this book).

Level 1: individual lifestyle (Part 2 of this book).

Level 2: social and community influences (Part 1 of this book).

Level 3: living and working conditions, and health care services (Parts 3 and 4 of this book).

Level 4: general socio-economic, cultural and environmental conditions (Part 1 of this book).

The Health Onion is a systems framework with seven characteristics:

1. It is holistic – all aspects of human nature are interconnected.

2. It is concerned with all health determinants, not simply with events during the treatment of illness.

3. The individual is at the core with health determinants acting through the community, living and working conditions, and the socio-economic, cultural and physical environment.

4. It places each layer in the context of its neighbours, including possible structural constraints upon change.

5. It has an interdisciplinary flavour that goes beyond a medical or quasi-medical approach.

6. It makes no claim that any one level is more important than others.

7. It acknowledges the complex nature of health determinants.

Different theories and models are needed for each setting and context. However, there is also a need for a general paradigm for individual health within which specific theories and models can be nested. Such a paradigm should attempt to represent in an explicit, detailed and meaningful way the constraints upon and links between individual well-being, the surrounding community and the health care system (Marks, 1996). No such general paradigm exists. We are waiting for a Hippocrates, Darwin or Einstein.

BOX 1.6

Filtering of evidence in evidence-based practice

Some methodological purists believe we have a paradigm for all of health care in the form of evidence-based medicine or **evidence-based practice (EBP)**. In EBP, randomized controlled trials are used to produce conclusions about the effectiveness of different methods and treatments. In theory, the approach sounds wonderful. In practice, it is far from perfect. Evidence on effectiveness in EBP is assumed to have an objective, inviolable status that reflects 'reality'. It is given an iconic status. In some undefined ways, this evidence about 'reality' not only aids decision-making, but also determines it. In truth, evidence is never absolutely certain. It rests on subjective elements consisting of negotiable, value-laden and contextually dependent beliefs that are given the status of 'facts' when all they really are items of information. Until the Magellan–Elcano circumnavigation of 1519–22 the Earth was assumed by everybody to be completely flat. The flat-Earth was a belief masquerading as fact. Flat-earthers still exist, but their numbers are dwindling.

The nature of evidence, and the methods by which evidence is gained, are contentious issues in the history of science. In health care, evidence (= new knowledge) for a technique or treatment is not an accident, but the product of a series of 'gates' or 'filters' that must be passed before the technique is deemed to be useful.

Consider the sequence of processes through which evidence must pass if it is to be considered admissible in EBP. The filtering is so selective that, typically, systematic reviewers will be able to find only a dozen or fewer primary studies that fulfil the inclusion criteria from a field of several thousand. It's not unlike making a pot of filter coffee – the stronger the filtering, the less fresh and flavourful the coffee or using a tea-bag to make a cup of tea. There are no guarantees the end product will be fit for purpose. The final product is almost certainly inferior to the genuine article. The filtering process in EBP consists of seven levels: current knowledge, theory and paradigms taught in universities and schools; funding priorities of government, industry and charities; hypotheses considered important by the funders; methodology approved by funders; journal publication; systematic reviews; translated into EBP.

To be judged 'sound', evidence must pass through these seven filters, which are biased towards the preservation of existing practices, knowledge and myths. In confirming the 'sound' status of the techniques that have passed through the filters, the 'unsoundness' of the unfiltered techniques occurs by default. Undeniably, evidence filtering is systematic and biased towards the status quo. Evidence is considered 'sound' or 'unsound' according to established criteria.

However, EBP is contentious on a number of grounds. First, it is wasteful that so much evidence is 'thrown away'. Many unfiltered techniques are quite possibly as effective as techniques that have been filtered. Second, the filtering process gives a high weighting to techniques that conform to beliefs and values of the knowledge establishment. For example, pharmacotherapy will be established ahead of psychological therapies (pharmaceutical industry sponsorship at filters 1–4), quantitative techniques will be preferred to qualitative techniques (filters 5–6), and patient treatment care will be about outputs and outcomes, rather than feeling they have been cared for as human beings (filters 7). Third, innovation may have difficulty breaking through.

In this book, we review the results of many studies using the approach of EBP, but many studies that have *not* been based on EBP are also reviewed. Many such studies have been in settings where EBP would be unethical, impractical or impossible. We also include qualitative studies because the findings illuminate the lived experience of health and illness.

Source: Marks (2005, 2009)

FUTURE RESEARCH

1. Psychology requires a solution to the measurement problem (if there is one): there is no evidence that psychological attributes are continuous quantitative variables of the kind studied in the natural and physical sciences.

2. Trans-cultural studies of health, illness and health care are needed to facilitate communication and understanding of systems of healing among different cultural, ethnic and religious groups.

3. Evidence needs to be gathered to confirm that lifestyle changes cause positive changes to life expectancy and quality of life.

4. The limits of evidence-based practice require innovative evaluation methods of interventions.

SUMMARY

1. Health is a state of well-being with physical, cultural, psychosocial, economic and spiritual attributes, not simply the absence of illness.

2. The fundamental sociality of individual behaviour demands a social orientation to health psychology, which must be studied in the context of society and culture.

3. To be healthy in body and mind a person's needs to interconnect and to act autonomously as an agent must both be satisfied as well as his/her biological needs.

4. Subjective well-being is normally positive for the majority of individuals. It fluctuates around a set-point inside a range and is regulated by homeostasis.

5. Behavioural and environmental changes need to be given equal priority in interventions.

6. Health psychology has grown rapidly, with increasing evidence that much illness and mortality is caused by behaviour, and there is a growing awareness of the psychosocial aspects of health and illness.

7. The 'Health Onion' is a useful framework for the investigation of health and illness. The core of the onion is an individual's current health status, including age, sex, genetic and epigenetic factors. Four layers of analysis surrounding this core are: (1) individual lifestyle, (2) social and community influences, (3) living and working conditions, and (4) general socio-economic, cultural and environmental conditions.

8. Concepts about health and disease are embedded in culturally diverse ways, with significant differences in experience and behaviour between cultures and places.

9. The organization of knowledge in health psychology is structured within frameworks, theories and models. It is helpful to notice the difference between these three types of structure and to treat them differently.

10. The nature of evidence and the methods by which evidence is gained are contentious issues in science. In health care, new knowledge about a theory, technique or intervention is the product of a series of evidence 'gates' or 'filters' that must be passed before it is deemed to be useful.

THE NERVOUS, ENDOCRINE AND IMMUNE SYSTEMS AND THE PRINCIPLE OF HOMEOSTASIS

'... almost all aspects of behaviour can be fully understood in terms of the concept of homeostasis.'

Curt Richter (1967)

OUTLINE

In this chapter, we outline three interacting biological systems with a primary role in the regulation of health and illness: the nervous system, endocrine system and immune system. These three systems together control and coordinate the body's responses to changes in the internal and external environment. We outline each system in turn and examine interactions between the nervous system, endocrine system and immune system with examples of recent research on psychoneuroimmunology. We conclude with a description of two kinds of homeostasis, both physiological and psychological.

BIOLOGICAL SYSTEMS

Three biological systems of relevance to health psychology are the nervous system (NS), the endocrine system (ES) and the immune system (IS). These three systems communicate within the body using electrical and chemical signals. They activate and de-activate tissues, organs and muscles to control and regulate the body, the emotions and the mind. The principal objective of the three systems is to preserve homeostasis. The three systems and their relationships to the brain and behaviour are illustrated in Figure 2.1.

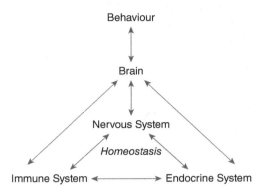

Figure 2.1   The nervous system (NS), endocrine system (ES) and immune system (IS) and their relationships to brain and behaviour

Constant reciprocated interaction between the three systems – the brain, organs and gut – is required to enable the control and coordination of behaviour. Endocrine substances directly affect the nervous and immune systems. The NS innervates every organ and tissue of the IS with reciprocal connections. The continuous interactions among the nervous, endocrine and immune systems was named 'neuroimmunomodulation' by Spector and Korneva (1981). Other related terms for these interactions include 'psychoimmunology', '**psychoneuro-immunology**' (Kiecolt-Glaser and Glaser, 1992), 'immunoendocrinology', 'behavioural immunology' and 'mind and immunology'. We review research on psychoneuroimmunology later in the chapter.

The three biological systems provide an essential foundation for the understanding of health and illness. Interest in the NS, however, is more than an academic one; it is also economic. The burden on health care and the economy from neurological disease is massive and rapidly increasing. For example, in the USA nearly 100 million people are ill with neurological disease. The combined annual costs of Alzheimer's and other dementias, low back pain, stroke, traumatic brain injury, migraine, epilepsy, multiple sclerosis, spinal cord injury and Parkinson's disease totals nearly $800 billion, and this figure is rapidly rising due to the ageing population (Gooch et al., 2017). This huge sum suggests a pressing need to expand knowledge and training in neuroscience. One necessary step is to begin with a basic grounding in the nature and function of the NS, a foundation stone for everything that follows.

THE NERVOUS SYSTEM

Neurones and microglial cells

It has been estimated that the human body consists of 37.2 trillion cells plus or minus around 0.81 trillion (Bianconi et al., 2013) and there are hundreds of different cell types (Mescher, 2016). The cells in one body have identical DNA but carry out a coordinated myriad functions to enable the maintenance of a near-stable internal environment. Only by communicating with one another can the necessary high level of coordination be possible. The two primary organizations for cell–cell communication are the NS, using **neurotransmitters** such as acetyl-choline, and the ES, which transports **neuromodulators** and **hormones** (e.g., cortisol) around the entire body. Most cell–cell communication occurs using intracellular enzymes, molecules that speed up chemical reactions (Michael et al., 2017). We outline here the basic structure and functions of the NS.

There are two main cell types in the NS, **neurones** and **glial cells**. Both cell types are absolutely necessary for neurological health. Glial cells provide support and nutrition, maintain local homeostasis, produce myelin and participate in signal transmission. The total number of glial cells roughly equals the number of neurons. Of particular importance are **microglial cells**, a type of glial cell accounting for 10–15% of all cells found within the brain. Microglial cells are highly plastic and act as **macrophage** ('big eater') cells, the main form of active immune defence in the central nervous system (CNS).

As both unique immune cells and unique brain cells that constantly change shape and have numerous different functions, microglial cells could stake a claim to being the 'smart' cells of the body. Microglia travel independently, unattached to any structure, circling a territory with extended arms seeking suboptimal functioning. This constant system of microglial surveillance protects the brain against any microbe invaders, demyelination, trauma and cancerous or defective cells (Lieff, 2013). When glial cells go wrong, all sorts of chaos can break loose, including brain inflammation and neurodegeneration, which can cause chronic pain (McMahon et al., 2005), Alzheimer's disease (Paresce et al., 1996), Parkinson's disease (Kim and Joh, 2006) and, according to some research, myalgic encephalomyelitis/chronic fatigue syndrome (**ME/CFS**) (Morris and Maes, 2014). It can be seen already that intimate connections exist between the immune and nervous systems, and so far we have only mentioned the 'foot soldiers' of the NS and not the command structures.

Neurones provide the main 'wiring' of the NS; they are communication devices that connect with other neurones, tissues, organs and muscles. How the neuronal communication works can best be explained by looking at the structure of the neurone (Figure 2.2).

The brain contains around 86 billion neurones, 20% in the cerebral cortex and 80% in the **cerebellum** (Lent et al., 2012). Each neurone can connect with up to 1–10,000 other neurons so there may be as many as *860 trillion* **synaptic connections** in total. Each neurone consists of a cell body or 'soma', dendrites and an axon. Dendrites are thin structures that arise from the cell body. They may be hundreds of micrometres in length and branch multiple times to produce a complex 'dendritic tree'. An axon, or 'nerve fibre' when myelinated, arises from the soma at the axon hillock and travels for a distance which can be as far as one metre in humans (connecting the toe to the spinal column).

Most excitatory synapses are formed between the axon of one neuron and a dendritic spine on another. When two neurons on either side of a synapse are active simultaneously, that synapse becomes stronger, a form of memory. The dendritic spine also becomes larger to accommodate the extra molecular machinery needed to support a stronger synapse.

Myelin is a fatty white substance that surrounds the axon of some neurones, providing electrical insulation. Multiple sclerosis (MS) occurs when an abnormal IS response produces chronic inflammation, which damages or destroys myelin.

Synapses and neurotransmission

One major form of communication in the NS uses neurotransmitters which are 'squirted' across an inter-cell channel called a 'synapse' or 'synaptic cleft'. This feature is illustrated in Figure 2.3.

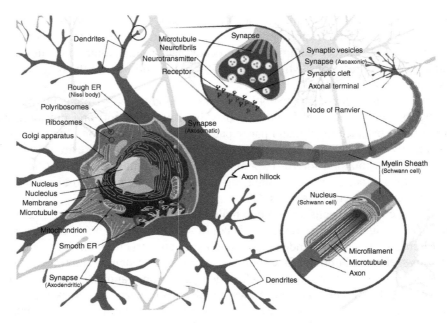

Figure 2.2   A schematic neurone and synapse

Source: Yurana's portfolio, IMG ID:214981837, acquired via Shutterstock

A wave of electrochemical excitation called an action potential travels along the membrane of the presynaptic cell, until it reaches the synapse. Channels that are permeable to calcium ions then open and calcium ions flow through the presynaptic membrane, increasing the calcium concentration in the interior. The increased calcium concentration activates a set of calcium-sensitive proteins attached to vesicles which contain a neurotransmitter. These proteins change shape, causing the membranes of some 'docked' vesicles to fuse with the membrane of the presynaptic cell, thereby opening the vesicles and dumping their neurotransmitter molecules into the synaptic cleft, the narrow space between the membranes of the pre- and postsynaptic cells.

To use an analogy, think of a couple of crazy kids having some fun in the school cafeteria when the teacher is nowhere to be seen. In a mêlée of hundreds of children all waiting for lunch, one kid picks up a bottle of ketchup and squirts it at the other kid's face. If the ketchup squirt hits the target, and lands squarely in the other kid's mouth, we have a successful 'transmission'. If he misses, he'll have to have another go, or another kid from the crowd will need to have a squirt to achieve a successful transmission. This is the kind of thing that goes on in neurotransmission across the synapse. The first kid with the ketchup bottle is the neurone, the bottle is the synaptic vesicle, the ketchup is the neurotransmitter, the first kid's squeezy hand is the neurotransmitter transporter, and the second kid with ketchup all over his face is the receptor. The more ketchup on the face, the better the communication. Once the ketchup has done its job, it magically returns to the bottle. Job done! Unless, of course, that tomato ketchup is the 'wrong' kind of neurotransmitter and the receptor kid demands a certain flavour of ice-cream instead! These 'ketchup kid fights' are going on trillions of times every day in each and everyone of us.

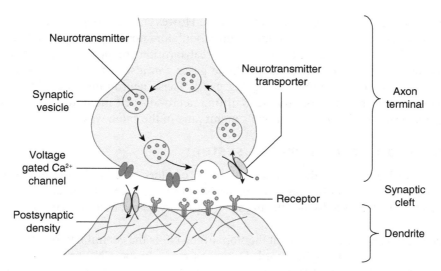

Figure 2.3   The synapse, axon terminal, dendrites and associated processes

Source: Thomas Splettstoesser, Wikimedia Commons, CC 4.0 International license

There are at least 60 different kinds of ketchup – sorry, I mean neurotransmitter – to choose from. To be a neurotransmitter, a molecule must: (1) be red, sticky and taste like ketchup [*no cancel that, just checking whether you're concentrating*], be produced inside a neurone, be found in the neurone's terminal button, and be released into the synaptic gap upon the arrival of an action potential; (2) produce an effect on the postsynaptic neurone; (3) be deactivated rapidly, after it has transmitted its signal to this neurone; (4) have the same effect on the postsynaptic neurone when applied experimentally as it does when secreted by a presynaptic neurone. The best-known neurotransmitters are:

- acetylcholine

- serotonin

- catecholamines, including epinephrine, norepinephrine and dopamine

- excitatory amino acids, such as aspartate and glutamate (half of the synapses in the CNS are glutamatergic)

- inhibitory amino acids, such as glycine and gamma-aminobutyric acid (GABA; one-quarter to one-third of the synapses in the CNS are GABAergic)

- histamine

- adenosine

- adenosine triphosphate (ATP).

Peptides form another large family of neurotransmitters, with over 50 known members, including: substance P, beta endorphin, enkephalin, somatostatin, vasopressin, prolactin, angiotensin II, oxytocin, gastrin, cholecystokinin, thyrotropin, neuropeptide Y, **insulin**, glucagon, calcitonin, neurotensin and bradykinin. However, many peptides act more as neuromodulators than as neurotransmitters. Neuromodulators do not propagate nerve impulses, but instead affect the synthesis, breakdown or reabsorption (reuptake) of neurotransmitters (more on this later). Curiously, certain soluble gases can also act as neurotransmitters, for example nitrogen monoxide (NO, 'laughing gas'). These neurotransmitters have their own distinctive mechanism: they exit the transmitting neurone's cell membrane by simple diffusion and penetrate the receiving neurone's membrane in the same way.

Organization of the nervous system

Having outlined aspects of the 'wiring' of small clusters of cells in the NS, we need to consider how the 86 or so billion cells of the NS are organized into functional subsystems (Figure 2.4). This diagram divides the highly complex system into a framework of functional domains.

The command and control centre at the 'top' of the NS is the central nervous system (CNS), consisting of the brain and spinal cord. Decisions made in the CNS are communicated via the peripheral NS, the cranial and spinal nerves, to the motor (effector) division of the NS. Communication back to the CNS is conducted by the sensory (afferent) division. There are two branches of the efferent division, the autonomic nervous system (ANS), which deals with cardiac muscles, smooth muscles and glands, and the somatic nervous system, which deals with skeletal muscular actions (speech and behaviour).

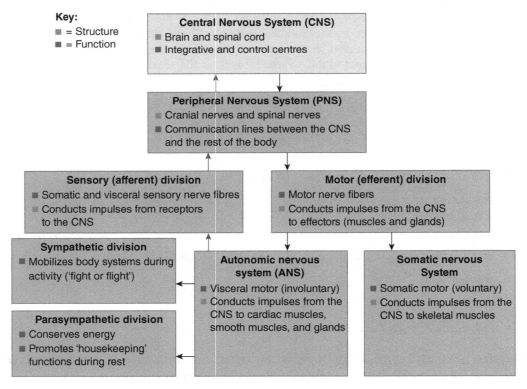

Figure 2.4   Organizational framework of the nervous system

The brain[1]

The brain and associated structures are shown in Figure 2.5. The cortex controls information input, synthesis and comparison, and output and action. Information input comes through receptors that are sensitive either to variations in the outside world or to variations within the body, such as changes in body position. Before the nerve fibres emerging from a sensory organ reach the primary cortex, where inputs are processed, almost all make at least one connection in subcortical centres such as the thalamic nuclei.

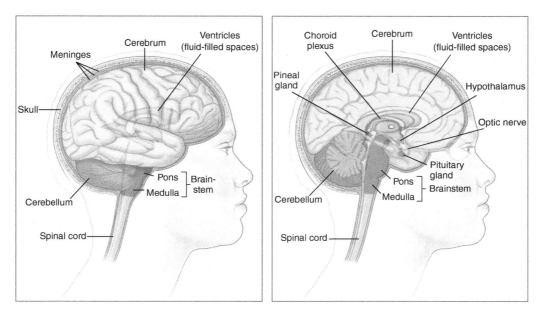

Figure 2.5 The brain, brainstem, medulla, pons and other important brain structures

Source: © 2010 Terese Winslow, U.S. Govt.

Another cortical input consists of fibres from the cortex itself, from either the same hemisphere or the opposite one. Once sensory signals arrive in their primary cortical area, they diverge into various local circuits responsible for information processing. These cortical microcircuits comprise the same types of cell distributed in the same six layers of the cortex. The results of 'computations' performed by these microcircuits ultimately converge at pyramidal neurons whose axons are the only output pathways from the cortex. A high proportion of axons that leave the cortex return to it, on the same or the opposite side. Other axons emerging from the cortex terminate in subcortical centres such as the thalamic nuclei, where they come into contact with the sensory fibres that send their axons to the cortex.

'Feedback looping' is a fundamental characteristic of information processing by the brain. At every stage, some of the fibres and connections loop back to the preceding stage to provide feedback that helps to control it. For instance, feedback loops enable the brain's motor control centres to correct and adjust their signals to the muscles, right up to the moment these signals are sent. Feedback

---

[1]Some illustrations and content are from 'The Brain from Top to Bottom', available at: http://thebrain.mcgill.ca/

loops like these let us keep our balance while walking against sudden gusts of wind. Feedback loops are also found in bodily reflexes, such as the leg withdrawal reflex. A complex task, such as playing a piano, involves highly complex connections because it requires the pianist to contract and relax many different muscles simultaneously, which is controlled by the cerebellum.

Neuromodulation

Neuromodulation occurs when a neurone uses a chemical to regulate diverse populations of neurones. Neuromodulators are secreted by a small group of neurons and diffused through large areas of the NS, instead of into a synaptic gap, affecting multiple neurones at the same time. Just one of these neurones can influence over 100,000 others through the neuromodulators that it secretes into the brain's extracellular space.

Neuromodulators spend significant amounts of time in the cerebrospinal fluid (CSF), 'modulating' the activity of several other neurones. Some of the same chemicals that act as neurotransmitters are also neuromodulators, specifically serotonin, acetylcholine, dopamine and norepiniphrene. The neurons of the 'hormonal brain' differ from those of the 'wired brain' in several ways. The hormonal neurones are concentrated mainly in the brainstem and the central region of the brain. They form small masses of thousands of cells, but these cells project their axons into large areas of the forebrain and the midbrain. Many drugs and medications, including those prescribed for affective disorders and schizophrenia, act on the neuromodulators of the diffuse projection neurons in the brainstem. For this reason, the function and distribution of the projections of these neurons have been the subject of much research using tracing techniques, because the axons of these neurons are not myelinated and do not form readily identifiable bundles. The results have confirmed how widely diffused these projections are. For example, a single axon from one of these neurons may subdivide and innervate both the cortex and the cerebellum.

The four main neuromodulators are norepinephrine (diffused by the locus coereleus), serotinin (diffused by the Raphe nuclei), acetylcholine (diffused by the basal nucleus of Meynert, pedunculopontine and pontine nuclei) and dopamine (diffused by the substantia nigra and ventral tegmental area). Each of these groups of neurones projects axons into large areas of the CNS and thus modulates numerous behaviours. The diffusion of the four main neuromodulators is illustrated in Figure 2.6.

THE SOMATIC AND AUTONOMIC NERVOUS SYSTEMS

The **somatic nervous system** is the organism's apparatus for responding to the external environment. It sends information to the brain from the body's various sensory detectors. The somatic nerves enable us to respond to these stimuli by moving through our environment, taking voluntary action, reacting and speaking. One of the principal roles of the somatic NS is maintaining homeostasis in the external environment, as discussed later in this chapter.

The **autonomic nervous system** (ANS) maintains homeostasis in the internal environment by regulating vital organs, such as those involved in digestion, respiration, blood circulation, excretion, and the secretion of hormones. The ANS is divided into two subsystems, the sympathetic and parasympathetic systems. The two branches of the ANS generally work in opposite directions, enabling a continuous upward or downward control of the internal organs to maintain homeostasis in the internal environment.

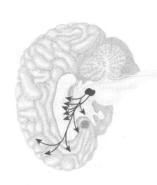

A. The **locus coeruleous** contains most of the neurons that produce **norepinephrine** in the brain. They send projections to just about every part of the central nervous system. Located in the dorsal portion of the pons, these cells are strongly activated by new sensory stimuli. They play a role in regulating vigilance and attentiveness and are inactive during sleep. Overactivity of this system can cause anxiety, while underactivity can lead to depression.

B. The neurons of the **Raphe nuclei** release **serotonin** as a neurotransmitter. These neurons are grouped into about nine pairs, distributed along the entire length of the brainstem. They project very widely throughout the central nervous system. The more rostal nuclei innervate thee cortex and the thalamus, while the more caudal nuclei innervate the cerebellum and the spinal cord. These latter nuclei appear to work in conjunction with the norepinergic neurons: they are active during waking periods and quiet during waking periods and quiet during sleep. In addition to being involved in the sleep/wake cycle, they also appear to affect mood.

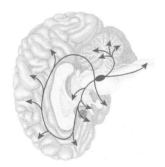

C. Diffuse projection neurons that use **acetylcholine** as a neurotransmitter are found in the ventral region of the telencephalon and the rostral portion of the pons. Nearly three-quarters of all acetylcholine in the cortex comes from the **basal nucleus of Meynert**, while the **pedunculopontine nucleus** and the **lateral tegmental pontine nucleus** project to the thalamus. The limbic system also receives acetylcholine from the medial septal nucleus (not shown here). This nucleus is believed to contribute to vigilance and neuronal plasticity, and would therefore play an important role in learning and memory. The memory loss associated with Alzheimer's disease is probably linked to the deterioration of this cholinergic system.

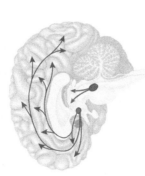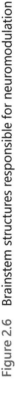

D. The two groups of neurons that diffuse **dopamine** are located in the lower portion of the midbrain. The **substantia nigra** (black substance) projects to the striatal structures (caudate nuclei and putamen). The degeneration of this nigrostriatal pathway that accompanies Parkinson's disease produces the trembling and the difficulty in initiating movement that characterize this illness. Other dopamine-producing cells project from the **ventral tegmental area** to the frontal cortex and to most of the structures in the limbic system. This system appears to be involved in reinforcing certain behaviours by associating them with pleasurable sensations. It also seems to be associated with the mechanisms involved in substance dependencies and in schizophrenia.

Figure 2.6   Brainstem structures responsible for neuromodulation

The **sympathetic nervous system** (SNS) goes into action to prepare the organism for physical or mental activity of 'fight or flight'. When the organism faces a major stressor, it is the SNS that orchestrates the fight-or-flight response. It dilates the bronchi and the pupils, accelerates heart rate and respiration, and increases perspiration and arterial blood pressure, but reduces digestive activity. Two neurotransmitters are primarily associated with this system: epinephrine and norepinephrine. The **parasympathetic nervous system** (PNS), on the other hand, causes a general slowdown in the body's functions in order to conserve energy. Whatever was dilated, accelerated or increased by the SNS is contracted, decelerated or decreased by the PNS. The only things that the PNS augments are digestive functions and sexual appetite. One neurotransmitter is primarily associated with this system: acetylcholine. The two divisions of the ANS and their functions are illustrated in Figure 2.7.

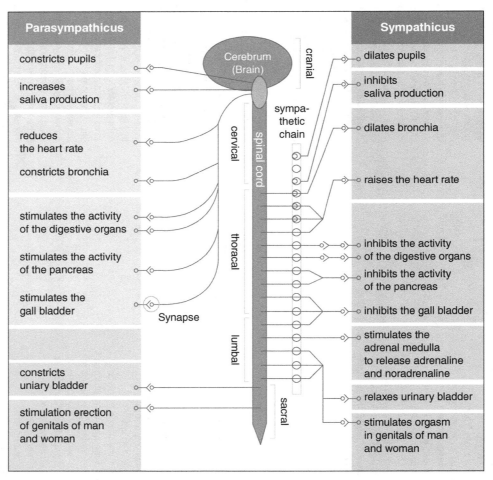

Figure 2.7   Schematic diagram of the autonomic nervous system

Source: Adapted from Geo-Science-International

EMOTION, REWARD, PUNISHMENT AND INHIBITION

The earliest scientific studies of human emotion were by Cannon (1915). Both in language and behavioural terms, we differentiate distinctive emotional responses. For example, in fear, humans go through basically the same steps: we stop what we are doing, turn towards the source of the threat, and initially show behavioural inhibition while trying to assess the threat. If this assessment confirms a threat, typically we try to flee or hide rather than engage in confrontation. If confrontation is unavoidable, fighting the threat becomes the last remaining option.

Attempts have been made to identify NS activity components associated with different emotions. The amygdala triggers bodily responses to emotional events, including the release of adrenalin by the adrenal glands. Adrenalin helps memories to be encoded more effectively in the hippocampus and the temporal lobe. We are better at remembering things that trigger our emotions. A review by Kreibig (2010) concerning emotion in healthy individuals suggested some level of response specificity in the ANS to different emotions, with some overlaps. See Box 2.1 for a few examples.

BOX 2.1

Differentiation of human emotions in the autonomic nervous system

Anger: reciprocal sympathetic activation and increased respiratory activity, particularly faster breathing.

Anxiety: sympathetic activation and vagal deactivation, a pattern of reciprocal inhibition, together with faster and shallower breathing (overlaps with anger).

Disgust (A) in relation to contamination and pollution: sympathetic–parasympathetic co-activation and faster breathing, particularly decreased inspiration.

Disgust (B) in relation to mutilation, injury and blood: sympathetic cardiac deactivation, increased electrodermal activity, unchanged vagal activation and faster breathing.

Embarrassment: largely overlaps with anger and anxiety but includes facial blushing.

Fear: broad sympathetic activation, including cardiac acceleration, increased myocardial contractility, vasoconstriction and increased electrodermal activity.

Sadness: a heterogeneous pattern of sympathetic–parasympathetic coactivation.

Affection, love, tenderness or sympathy: decreased heart rate (similar to sadness), unspecific increase in skin conductance.

Amusement: increased cardiac vagal control, vascular-adrenergic, respiratory and electrodermal activity, together with sympathetic cardiac-adrenergic deactivation.

(Continued)

Contentment: a strong sympathetically deactivating component.

Happiness: increased cardiac activity due to vagal withdrawal, vasodilation, increased electrodermal activity and increased respiratory activity.

Joy: increased cardiac vagal control, decreased-adrenergic, increased-adrenergic and increased cholinergically mediated sympathetic influence as well as increased respiratory activity.

Source: Kreibig (2010)

Another approach has been to identify the brain areas and circuits responsible for reward and punishment (Figure 2.8).

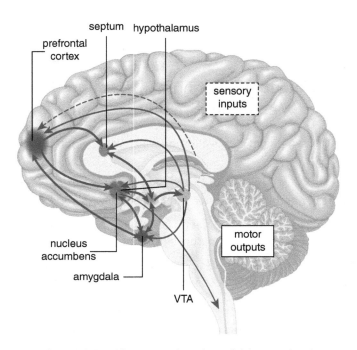

Figure 2.8   The reward and punishment circuits

The main centres of the brain's **reward circuit** are located along the medial forebrain bundle (MFB). The ventral tegmental area (VTA) and the nucleus accumbens are the two major centres in this circuit, but it also includes several others, such as the septum, the amygdala, the prefrontal cortex and parts of the thalamus. All of these centres are interconnected and innervate the hypothalamus, informing it of the presence of rewards. The lateral and ventromedial nuclei of the hypothalamus are especially involved in this reward circuit. The hypothalamus then acts in return not only on the ventral tegmental area, but also on the autonomic and endocrine functions of the entire body, through the pituitary gland.

Turning from rewarding to aversive stimuli, fight-or-flight responses activate the brain's **punishment circuit** (the periventricular system, or PVS), which enables us to cope with unpleasant situations. The PVS was identified by De Molina and Hunsperger (1962). It includes the hypothalamus, the thalamus and the central grey substance surrounding the aqueduct of Sylvius. Some secondary centres of this circuit are found in the amygdala and the hippocampus. The punishment circuit functions by means of acetylcholine, which stimulates the secretion of adrenal cortico-trophic hormone (ACTH). ACTH in turn stimulates the adrenal glands to release adrenalin to prepare the body's organs for fight-or-flight actions.

The MFB and the PVS provide two motivational systems that enable people to suppress their instinctive impulses and avoid painful experiences. A third circuit is known as the 'behavioural inhibition system' (BIS). The BIS is associated with the septo-hippocampal system, the amygdala and the basal nuclei. It receives inputs from the prefrontal cortex and transmits its outputs via the noradrenergic fibres of the locus coeruleus and the serotininergic fibres of the medial Raphe nuclei. The BIS is activated when both fight and flight seem impossible and the only remaining option is to passively submit by doing nothing. Long-term behavioural inhibition can be stressful, with an increased probability of long-term illness (Pennebaker, 1985). Large individual differences are observed in behavioural inhibition which, in adolescents, can be associated with anxiety and depression (Muris et al., 2001).

Neuroplasticity, learning and memory

The hippocampus has been a focus for research on synaptic plasticity, the ability to potentiate transmission at the synapse by repeated stimulation, providing a neural foundation for learning and memory in terms of 'long-term potentiation' (LTP) (Bliss and Lømo, 1973). When we learn something, the efficiency of hippocampal synapses increases, facilitating the passage of nerve impulses along a particular circuit. For example, when exposed to a new word, we have to make new connections among certain neurones to deal with it: some neurones in the visual cortex to recognize the spelling, others in the auditory cortex to hear the pronunciation, and still others in the associative regions of the cortex to relate the word to our existing knowledge. All memories of events, words and images correspond to particular activities of neuronal networks that have strengthened interconnections with one another.

As noted, at least half of the synapses in the CNS are glutamatergic. Glutamate is the major excitatory neurotransmitter in the NS. Glutamatergic pathways are linked to many other neurotransmitter pathways, and receptors are found throughout the brain and spinal cord in neurons and glia. As an amino acid and neurotransmitter, glutamate has multiple normal physiological functions and any dysfunction can have profound effects both in disease and injury. At least 30 proteins at, or near, the glutamate synapse control or modulate neuronal excitability. The N-methyl-D-aspartate receptor (NMDA receptor) is a glutamate receptor found in nerve cells. It is activated when glutamate and glycine (or D-serine) bind to it, and when activated it allows positively charged ions to flow through the cell membrane. These are especially important in synaptic plasticity and the encoding and intermediate storage of memory traces, while AMPA (α-amino-3-hydroxy-5-methyl-4-isoxazolepropionic acid) receptors mediate fast synaptic transmission necessary for memory retrieval (Tsien et al., 1996).

Collingridge and Singer (1990) discovered that excitatory amino acid receptors mediate synaptic transmission at many synapses that display LTP-type synaptic efficiency. These amino acids are one mechanism of synaptic plasticity in health and disease, and alterations in these processes may lead to brain disorders, such as Alzheimer's disease.

THE ENDOCRINE SYSTEM

The endocrine system consists of the ductless glands of the body and the hormones produced by those glands. Endocrine glands release their secretions directly into the intercellular fluid or into the bloodstream. Hormones act as 'messengers' carried by the bloodstream to different cells in the body, which interpret these messages and act on them. In regulating the functions of organs in the body, the ES maintains physiological homeostasis. Cellular metabolism, reproduction, sexual development, sugar and mineral homeostasis, heart rate and digestion are processes regulated by the actions of hormones.

Without hormones we could not grow, maintain a constant temperature, produce offspring, or perform the essential actions and functions of our everyday lives. The ES provides an electrochemical connection from the hypothalamus to the organs that control the metabolism, growth, development and reproduction. The ES operates 24/7 for the entire lifespan. It operates throughout sleep and waking – without tea breaks, weekends or holidays.

The main endocrine glands are the pituitary (anterior and posterior lobes), thyroid, parathyroid, adrenal (cortex and medulla), pancreas and gonads. The pituitary gland is attached to the hypothalamus of the lower forebrain. The thyroid gland consists of two lateral masses, connected by a cross bridge, that are attached to the trachea. They are slightly inferior to the larynx. The parathyroid glands are four masses of tissue, two embedded posterior in each lateral mass of the thyroid gland. One adrenal gland is located on top of each kidney. The cortex is the outer layer of the adrenal gland. The medulla is the inner core. The pancreas is along the lower curvature of the stomach, close to where it meets the first region of the small intestine, the duodenum. The gonads are in the pelvic cavity.

Many studies indicate that hormonal changes influence cognition. For example, research by Sherwin (1997) suggested that estrogen helps to maintain verbal memory and enhances the capacity for new learning in women, whereas other cognitive functions, such as verbal memory, are seemingly unaffected by this steroid hormone. Even the human imagination is related to hormones. Drake et al. (2000) found evidence that both estrogen and testosterone have associations with cognitive performance and that estrogen may enhance, and depress, specific cognitive skills. Wassell et al. (2015) found that the strength and vividness of imagery is greater for females in the mid-luteal phase (second half of menstrual cycle) than for both females in the late follicular phase (first half of cycle) and males. The changes in hormone concentrations over time provide a possible basis for individual differences in visual mental imagery, cognitive functions and mental disorders.

Endocrine glands release hormones as a response to three kinds of stimuli: (1) hormones from other endocrine glands; (2) chemical characteristics of the blood (other than hormones); and (3) neural stimulation. Most hormone production is managed by a negative feedback system. The NS and certain endocrine tissues monitor the internal condition of the body. If action is required to maintain homeostasis, hormones are released, either directly by an endocrine gland or indirectly through the action of the hypothalamus of the brain, which stimulates other endocrine glands to release hormones. When homeostasis is restored, the corrective action is ceased. Thus, in negative feedback, when the subnormal condition has been rebalanced, the corrective action is stopped. One of the many vital functions that is taken care of by the ES is the circadian rhythm and clock.

The circadian clock

The ES regulates the circadian rhythm and sleep/waking cycle with a variety of hormone releases. Melatonin is produced in the pineal gland, under the control of the **central circadian pacemaker**

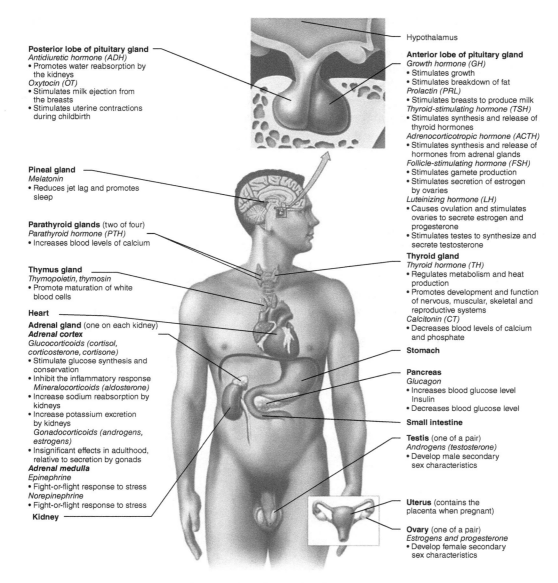

Posterior lobe of pituitary gland
Antidiuretic hormone (ADH)
• Promotes water reabsorption by
  the kidneys
Oxytocin (OT)
• Stimulates milk ejection from
  the breasts
• Stimulates uterine contractions
  during childbirth

Pineal gland
Melatonin
• Reduces jet lag and promotes
  sleep

Parathyroid glands (two of four)
Parathyroid hormone (PTH)
• Increases blood levels of calcium

Thymus gland
Thymopoietin, thymosin
• Promote maturation of white
  blood cells

Heart

Adrenal gland (one on each kidney)
Adrenal cortex
*Glucocorticoids (cortisol,
corticosterone, cortisone)*
• Stimulate glucose synthesis and
  conservation
• Inhibit the inflammatory response
  Mineralocorticoids (aldosterone)
• Increase sodium reabsorption by
  kidneys
• Increase potassium excretion
  by kidneys
  *Gonadocorticoids (androgens,
  estrogens)*
• Insignificant effects in adulthood,
  relative to secretion by gonads
Adrenal medulla
Epinephrine
• Fight-or-flight response to stress
Norepinephrine
• Fight-or-flight response to stress

 Kidney

Hypothalamus

Anterior lobe of pituitary gland
Growth hormone (GH)
• Stimulates growth
• Stimulates breakdown of fat
Prolactin (PRL)
• Stimulates breasts to produce milk
Thyroid-stimulating hormone (TSH)
• Stimulates synthesis and release of
  thyroid hormones
Adrenocorticotropic hormone (ACTH)
• Stimulates synthesis and release of
  hormones from adrenal glands
Follicle-stimulating hormone (FSH)
• Stimulates gamete production
• Stimulates secretion of estrogen
  by ovaries
Luteinizing hormone (LH)
• Causes ovulation and stimulates
  ovaries to secrete estrogen and
  progesterone
• Stimulates testes to synthesize and
  secrete testosterone

Thyroid gland
Thyroid hormone (TH)
• Regulates metabolism and heat
  production
• Promotes development and function
  of nervous, muscular, skeletal and
  reproductive systems
Calcitonin (CT)
• Decreases blood levels of calcium
  and phosphate

Stomach

Pancreas
Glucagon
• Increases blood glucose level
  Insulin
• Decreases blood glucose level

Small intestine

Testis (one of a pair)
Androgens (testosterone)
• Develop male secondary
  sex characteristics

Uterus (contains the
placenta when pregnant)

Ovary (one of a pair)
Estrogens and progesterone
• Develop female secondary
  sex characteristics

Figure 2.9   The endocrine system

in the suprachiasmatic nucleus (SCN) region of the hypothalamus (Gamble et al., 2014). Melatonin relays information about the light–dark cycle in response to day-length changes, triggering endocrine changes. Melatonin production is low in the presence of light and increases during the night when it induces and supports sleep. Melatonin supplementation is used for the treatment of winter depression and sleep disorders, and as an adjuvant therapy for epilepsy.

The **hypothalamo-pituitary-adrenal (HPA) axis** produces corticotropin releasing hormone (CRH) from the hypothalamus and conveys it to the anterior pituitary gland. There, CRH triggers release of adrenocorticotropic hormone (ACTH) into the general circulation whereupon ACTH binds to receptors in the adrenal gland and stimulates **cortisol** release. Cortisol levels exhibit a robust ultraradian rhythm normally peaking during the morning (0700–0800), preparing the body for the energetic demands of waking.

Growth hormone (GH) is produced in the anterior pituitary in response to the integrated stimulatory and inhibitory effects of GH releasing hormone (GHRH) and somatostatin (SMS), respectively, from the hypothalamus. GH has powerful metabolic effects in opposition to insulin (e.g., decreasing glucose utilization). Circulating GH levels exhibit both circadian and ultradian variation, as well as sexual dimorphism. GH is secreted throughout the day with an increased secretion during sleep.

Adiponectin exhibits a time-of-day-dependent rhythm, peaking between 1200 and 1400 and is best known as an insulin sensitizer, whose circulating levels vary inversely with body mass index (BMI). Hypoadiponectinemia is associated with metabolic syndrome, but conversely, elevated levels are seen in chronic heart failure and chronic renal failure. Insulin is secreted by beta cells of pancreatic islets in response to increased levels of circulating nutrients, particularly glucose. Insulin stimulates glucose utilization and protein synthesis by the liver, skeletal muscle and fat. It displays a diurnal rhythm which peaks at around 1700 hours, suggestive of nutrient storage during the awake/fed state and mobilization during the fast period of sleep.

The EC responds in a complex manner during sleep (Van Cauter and Tasali, 2011). The secretion of some hormones increases during sleep (e.g., growth hormone, prolactin and luteinizing hormone), while the secretion of other hormones is inhibited (e.g., thyroid stimulating hormone and cortisol). Some hormones are directly linked to a particular sleep stage. Growth hormone is typically secreted in the first few hours after the onset of sleep and generally occurs during slow-wave sleep. Cortisol is tied to the circadian rhythm and peaks in late afternoon, regardless of the person's sleep status or the darkness/light cycle. Melatonin is released in the dark and is suppressed by light (Buxon et al., 2002). Thyroid hormone secretion occurs in the late evening

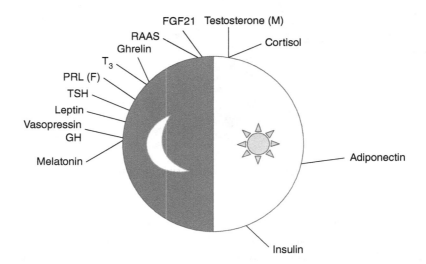

Figure 2.10   Circadian clock control of endocrine factors

Time of day at which circulating levels of key endocrine factors peak in humans. Abbreviations utilized include: GH, growth hormone; TSH, thyroid stimulating hormone; PRL, prolactin; T_3, triiodothyronine; RAAS, renin-angiotensin-aldosterone system; FGF21, fibroblast growth factor 21; (F), females only; (M), males only

Source: Reproduced by permission from Gamble et al. (2014)

(Institute of Medicine, 2006). Endocrine dysfunction has been linked to sleep disturbances such as insomnia (Institute of Medicine, 2006). It has been suggested that over-activity of the HPA axis in response to stress affects sleep and subsequently increases the secretion of cortisol and norepinephrine (Buckley and Schatzberg, 2005).

Diabetes is associated with the ES's ability to produce the insulin which is affected by sleep. Adults who report having 5 or fewer hours of sleep a night are 2.5 times more likely to have diabetes, compared to people who sleep 7–8 hours per night. People who sleep 6 hours a night are 1.7 times more likely to have diabetes than their peers who sleep longer. People who sleep for 9 or more hours also have higher rates of diabetes (Institute of Medicine, 2006). A European epidemiological study followed sleep patterns and illness among 23,630 people for up to 8 years (von Ruesten et al., 2012). Short sleep, defined as less than 6 hours in a 24-hour period, was associated with a 31% increased risk of overall chronic disease, including stroke, myocardial infarction and cancer. In non-hypertensive people, the overall risk of chronic disease, primarily cancer, was reduced by a daytime nap. Sleep duration of less than 6 hours is a 'risky behaviour' for the development of chronic disease.

The regular daily oscillations in hormone releases do not appear to be solely a response to the sleep/wake and feeding/fasting cycles, but are 'orchestrated in part by a timekeeping mechanism called the circadian clock' (Gamble et al., 2014: 466). Recent studies suggest that the circadian clock has been a feature of evolution for at least 2.5 billion years. Disruption of the clock through genetic or environmental means can precipitate disorders, including cardio-metabolic diseases and cancer. Realigning circadian rhythms can be beneficial in the treatment of endocrine-related disorders.

Gender, sexual dimorphism and identity

The biological basis for gender identity, if there is one, is unknown. The basis of biological sex is better understood. A single factor – the steroid hormone testosterone – accounts for most, and perhaps all, of the known sex differences in neural structure (Morris et al., 2004). Testosterone is said to 'sculpt' the developing NS by inhibiting or exacerbating cell death and/or by modulating the formation and elimination of synapses. Testosterone masculinizes both the brain and the body, yet experience can interact with testosterone to enhance or diminish its effects on the CNS.

The steps leading to masculinization of the body appear to be consistent across mammals. The Y chromosome contains the sex-determining region of the Y (*Sry*) gene and induces the undifferentiated gonads to form as testes (rather than as ovaries). The testes secrete hormones to masculinize the rest of the body. Two masculinizing testicular hormones are antimullerian hormone, a protein that suppresses female reproductive tract development, and testosterone, a steroid that promotes the development of the male reproductive tract and masculine external genitalia (Morris et al., 2004). In masculinizing the body, testosterone binds to the androgen receptor protein and then this steroid-receptor complex binds to DNA, promoting differentiation as a male. If the *Sry* gene is absent (as in females, who receive an X chromosome from the father), the gonad develops as an ovary, and the body, unexposed to testicular hormones, forms a feminine configuration. The genitalia will only respond to testicular hormones during a particular time in development, which constitutes a sensitive period for hormone action: hormonal treatment of females in adulthood is claimed to have negligible effects on genital morphology (Morris et al., 2004).

Contrary to the mainstream hormonal accounts of gender identity, the concept of sexual neutrality at birth, after which infants differentiate as masculine or feminine as a result of social experiences, was proposed by John Money and colleagues (Money and Erhardt, 1972). In the human brain, structural differences have been described that seem to be related to gender identity and sexual orientation (Swaab, 2004). However, the evidence is highly equivocal. Solid evidence for the importance of postnatal social factors in gender identity is lacking. The truth is we simply do not know.

Vitamin D and its deficiency

The importance of the molecule **vitamin D** has been recognized since its discovery by Edward Mellanby in 1920. The chemical structure of vitamin D was determined in 1932, and it was only then found to be a **steroid** hormone, more specifically, a secosteroid. Vitamin D normally arises in the skin from sunlight or it can come from food, such as oily fish, or from supplements. It is metabolized in the liver and kidney. Vitamin D metabolites appear to be involved in a host of cellular processes, including calcium homeostasis, immunology, cell differentiation and regulation of gene transcription (Bouillon et al., 1995). Vitamin D is the main hormone regulating calcium phosphate homeostasis and mineral bone metabolism. A variety of tissues can express vitamin D receptor (VDR) and vitamin D is implicated in the regulation of the IS, the cardiovascular system, oncogenesis and cognitive functions (Halfon et al., 2015).

Hormones can act as **immunomodulators**, altering the sensitivity of the IS. **T cells** have a symbiotic relationship with vitamin D, by binding to the steroid hormone version of vitamin D, calcitriol, but T cells express the gene CYP27B1, the gene responsible for converting the pre-hormone version of vitamin D, calcidiol, into the steroid hormone version, calcitriol. The decline in hormone levels with age is partially responsible for the weakened immune responses in older people. Conversely, some hormones are regulated by the IS, notably thyroid hormone activity. The age-related decline in immune function is also related to decreasing vitamin D levels in the elderly. As people age, two things happen that negatively affect their vitamin D levels. First, they stay indoors more due to decreased activity levels. This means that they get less sun and therefore produce less vitamin D via solar radiation. Second, as a person ages the skin produces less vitamin D.

Hypovitaminosis D is associated with decreased muscle function and performance and an increase in disability. On the other hand, vitamin D supplementation improves muscle strength and gait, especially in elderly patients. A reduced risk of falls has been attributed to vitamin D supplementation due to direct effects on muscle cells. Finally, a low vitamin D status is associated with a frail phenotype. Many authorities recommend vitamin D supplementation for frail patients.

Vitamin D deficiency is a factor in a variety of illnesses. Pereira-Santos et al. (2015) found that the prevalence of vitamin D deficiency was 35% higher in obese people and 24% higher in overweight people. Vitamin D deficiency was associated with obesity irrespective of age, latitude, cut-offs to define vitamin D deficiency and the Human Development Index of the study location. Altered vitamin D and calcium homeostasis are also associated with the development of Type 2 diabetes mellitus. Pittas et al. (2007) reviewed observational studies and clinical trials in adults with outcomes related to glucose homeostasis. Observational studies showed an association between low vitamin D status, calcium or dairy intake and prevalent Type 2 diabetes mellitus or metabolic syndrome. There are inverse associations with the incidence of Type 2 diabetes mellitus or metabolic syndrome. Trials with vitamin D and/or calcium supplementation suggest that combined vitamin D and calcium supplementation may have a preventive role for Type 2 diabetes mellitus only in populations at high risk (i.e., those with glucose intolerance).

Microbiome research

The new field of microbiome research studies the microbes within the gut and the effects of these microbes on the host's well-being. Microbes influence metabolism, immunity and behaviour. One mechanism appears to involve hormones because specific changes in hormone levels correlate with the presence of the gut **microbiota**. The microbiota produce and secrete hormones, respond to host hormones and regulate expression levels of host hormones (Neuman et al., 2015). Increasing evidence links both hormones and the microbiome to immune responses under both healthy conditions and autoimmune disease. There are many interconnections and the microbiome and hormones may work through shared pathways to affect the immune response (Neuman et al., 2015).

Organisms within the gut play a role in the early programming and later responsivity of the stress system. The gut is inhabited by 10^{13}–10^{14} micro-organisms, which is ten times the number of cells in the human body, and contains 150 times as many genes as our genome (Dinan and Cryan, 2012) or, according to Verdino (2017), 360 times. When pathogens such as Escherichia coli enter the gut, the HPA can be activated. Stress can induce an increased permeability of the gut, allowing bacteria and bacterial antigens to cross the epithelial barrier and activate a mucosal immune response, which in turn alters the composition of the microbiome and leads to an enhanced HPA drive. Research indicates that patients with irritable bowel syndrome and major depression show alterations of the HPA which are induced by increased gut permeability. In the case of irritable bowel syndrome, the increased permeability can respond to probiotic therapy. The gut microbiota play a role in regulating the HPA. In a double-blind, placebo-controlled trial, participants were given a fruit bar that contained either the probiotic formula or a similarly tasting placebo bar for 30 days (Messaoudi et al., 2011). The experimental fruit bar group reported significantly lower levels of anxiety, anger, depression and somatization, on a number of self-report measures. Lower levels of cortisol were also evident in the fruit bar condition compared to the control group. Verdino (2017) cautiously concludes his review of the growing connection between gut health and emotional well-being as follows: "… it is crucial not to oversimplify the idea that nutritional intervention and a healthy gut will be the panacea for profound psychological difficulties. Severe mood and paralyzing anxiety disorders are not going to be cured with probiotic yogurt and prebiotic fiber, alone" (Verdino, 2017: 4).

The immune and neuroendocrine systems share a common set of hormones and receptors. **Glucocorticoids**, such as corticosterone and cortisol, regulate inflammation levels and have effects both on the innate and adaptive immune responses. Additionally, vitamin D affects immune cell responses by enhancing antigen presentation. Moreover, sex hormones affect the immune response in numerous ways. The effects of hormones on microbiota are summarized in Figure 2.11.

THE IMMUNE SYSTEM

The immune system (IS) is a network of cells, tissues and organs that protects the body against disease or other potentially damaging foreign bodies. When properly functioning, the IS identifies and attacks a variety of threats using billions of diverse **antibodies**, including viruses, bacteria and parasites, while distinguishing them from the body's own healthy tissue. For each type of invader the body needs a distinct antibody. Antibodies are made by **B cells** using a combination of 20,000 genes and an enzyme called 'RAG', which is a DNA shuffler. This enables

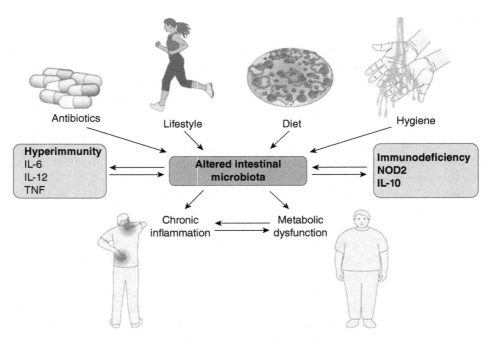

Figure 2.11   Host effects on gut microbiota

A variety of host factors (such as diet, exercise, mood, general health state, stress and gender) lead to alterations in hormonal levels, which in turn lead to a variety of effects on the microbiota (including growth, virulence and resistance)

Source: Reproduced with permission from Neuman et al. (2015)

the immune system to create a vast diversity of antibodies and respond to diseases it has never encountered before.

The IS is composed of two parts: the innate IS and the adaptive IS. Both change as people get older. The main features of the IS are illustrated in Figure 2.12.

Our innate IS is made up of barriers and cells that keep harmful germs from entering the body. These include our skin, the cough reflex, mucous membranes and stomach acid. If germs are able to pass through these physical barriers, they encounter a second line of innate defence, composed of specialized cells that alert the body to the impending danger.

The IS changes over the lifespan. Newborn babies have an immature IS. Immunological competence is gained after birth partly as a result of maturation factors present in breast milk and partly as a result of exposure to **antigens** from food and environmental micro-organisms. Early encounters with antigens help the development of tolerance, and a breakdown in 'immune education' can lead to disease (Calder, 2013). At the end of the life-cycle, older people experience progressive dysregulation of the IS, leading to decreased acquired immunity and a greater susceptibility to infection. Innate immunity appears to be less affected by ageing than acquired immunity.

A healthy, young person's body produces numerous T cells and is able to fight off infections and build a storehouse of memory T cells. With age, people produce fewer naïve T cells, which makes them less able to combat new health threats. This also makes older people less

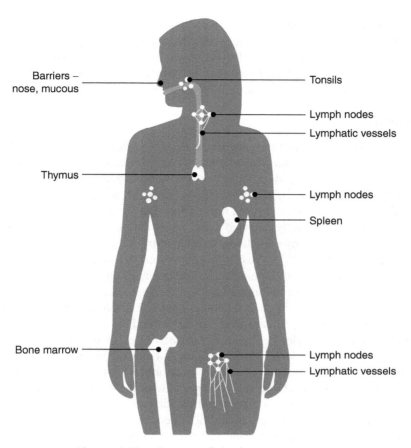

Figure 2.12   Organs of the immune system

responsive to vaccines because vaccines generally require naïve T cells to produce a protective immune response (except in the case of the shingles vaccine). Negative, age-related changes in our innate and adaptive immune systems are known as **immunosenescence**. A lifetime of stress on our bodies is thought to contribute to immunosenescence. Radiation, chemical exposure and exposure to certain diseases can also speed up the deterioration of the IS.

The adaptive IS is more complex than the innate IS and includes the thymus, spleen, tonsils, bone marrow, circulatory system and lymphatic system. These different parts of the body work together to produce, store and transport specific types of cells and substances to combat health threats. **T cells**, a type of white blood cell (called **lymphocytes**), attack infected or damaged cells directly or produce powerful chemicals that mobilize an army of other IS substances and cells. Before a T cell is programmed to recognize a specific harmful germ, it is in a 'naïve' state. After a T cell is assigned to fight off a particular infection, it becomes a 'memory' cell. Because these cells remember how to resist a specific germ, they help to fight a second round of infection faster and more effectively. Memory T cells remain in our systems for many decades.

An important part of our adaptive IS is the **lymphatic system**, consisting of bone marrow, spleen, thymus and lymph nodes. Bone marrow produces white blood cells, or **leukocytes**. The spleen is the largest lymphatic organ in the body and contains white blood cells that fight infection or disease. The thymus is where T cells mature. T cells help destroy infected or cancerous cells. Lymph nodes produce and store cells that fight infection and disease. Lymphocytes and leukocytes are small white blood cells that play a large role in defending the body against disease. The two types of lymphocyte are B cells, which make antibodies that attack bacteria and toxins, and T cells, which help destroy infected or cancerous cells.

Inflammation

Inflammation is a critical defence response in our innate IS wherein white blood cells protect us from infection by foreign organisms, bacteria and viruses. Inflammation occurs following infection or tissue damage when a rapid and complex series of reactions takes place to prevent tissue damage, isolate and destroy the infective organism, conserve and protect some micronutrients and activate the repair processes to restore normal function (Thurnham, 2014). Inflammation is a homoeostatic process that is only intended to last a few days but, if it is continued indefinitely, there is a poor prognosis in many conditions. Inflammatory responses take precedence over normal body metabolism with the objective of restoring normality as quickly as possible.

In a young person, bouts of inflammation are vital for fighting off disease. As people age, they tend to have mild, chronic inflammation, which is associated with an increased risk for heart disease, arthritis, frailty, Type 2 diabetes, physical disability and dementia. Whether inflammation leads to disease, disease leads to inflammation, or whether both scenarios are true currently remains uncertain. Centenarians and other people who have grown old in relatively good health generally have less inflammation and more efficient recovery from infection and inflammation when compared to people who are unhealthy or have average health. Acute inflammation on a timescale of seconds to days allows the host to heal and protect damaged tissue from disease. Chronic inflammation lasting weeks or months is linked to many pathologies and age-related diseases, including sleep apnea, insomnia, neurodegeneration, Alzheimer's disease, atherosclerosis, cancer, kidney and lung diseases, metabolic syndrome and Type 2 diabetes mellitus.

Disorders of the IS can result in autoimmune diseases, inflammatory diseases and cancer. When the IS is less active than normal, which is called **immunodeficiency**, recurring and life-threatening infections can occur. Immunodeficiency can result from a genetic disease, acquired conditions such as HIV infection (see Chapter 22), or the use of an immunosuppressive medication.

The opposite situation of **autoimmunity** results from a hyperactive IS attacking normal tissues as if they were foreign organisms. Common autoimmune diseases include Hashimoto's thyroiditis, rheumatoid arthritis, Type 1 diabetes mellitus (see Chapter 23) and systemic lupus erythematosus. Autoimmune diseases are chronic conditions with no cure. Treatment requires controlling the disease process to decrease the symptoms, especially during flare-ups. The following actions can alleviate symptoms of autoimmune disease: a balanced and healthy diet, regular exercise, plenty of rest, vitamin supplements (especially A and D), a decrease of stress, and the avoidance of any known triggers of flare-ups. Sound familiar? Hippocrates knew about them and your doctor's waiting room has a poster.

Circadian rhythm of the immune system

Circadian variation occurs in immunocompetent cells and **cytokines** as an anticipatory process for the preservation of body homeostasis and defence (Cermakian et al., 2013). Cytokines are small protein cells responsible for cell signalling. The IS shows reliable daily variations, for example immunocompetent cell counts and cytokine levels vary according to the time of day and the sleep–wake cycle. Different immune cell types, such as **macrophages**, **natural killer (or NK) cells**, and **lymphocytes**, all contain circadian molecular clockwork.

The biological clocks of immune cells and lymphoid organs, together with the central pacemaker of the suprachiasmatic nuclei via humoural and neural pathways, regulate the IS, including its response to signals and their effector functions. There is a diurnal variation in the response to immune challenges (e.g., a bacterial injection) and circadian control of allergic reactions. The circadian–immune connection is bidirectional, and immune challenges and immune mediators (e.g., cytokines) affect circadian rhythms at the molecular, cellular and behavioural levels. Cross-talk between the circadian and immune systems has implications for disease, as shown by the higher incidence of cancer and the exacerbation of autoimmune symptoms upon circadian disruption (Cermakian et al., 2013).

Sleep and rest

Sleep and rest are necessary for a properly functioning IS. Feedback loops involving cytokines in response to infection participate in the regulation of non-rapid eye movement sleep. In sleep deprivation, active immunizations may have a diminished effect, resulting in lower antibody production and a lower immune response than for well-rested individuals. Proteins such as NFIL3, which are closely intertwined with both T-cell differentiation and our circadian rhythms, are affected by disturbances of natural light and dark cycles through instances of sleep deprivation, travelling across time zones or shift work. Such disruptions on a regular and frequent basis can lead to an increase in chronic conditions such as heart disease, chronic pain and asthma.

Sleep, sleep loss and disrupted sleep are strongly linked to acute and chronic inflammation (Opp and Krueger, 2015). People suffering from sleep deprivation demonstrate changes in circulating pro-inflammatory and anti-inflammatory cytokines, soluble receptors, inflammatory signalling pathways and innate immunity. Circadian misalignment also induces inflammation, which has ramifications for shift workers. Shift work is a risk factor for inflammatory diseases, including cancer and diabetes. In addition to the negative consequences of sleep deprivation, sleep and the circadian system have regulatory effects on immunological functions in both innate and adaptive immunity.

Chronic diseases that are associated with suboptimal sleep are inflammatory diseases. Chronic insufficient sleep is a risk factor in part because of the inflammatory state that results from sleep disruption. Inflammation, defined by elevated local and systemic cytokines and other pro-inflammatory mediators, occurs in response to many stimuli, including pathogen exposure, cellular damage, irritants, cellular dysregulation and waking activity.

Nutrition and diet

Consumption of high-fat (e.g., ice cream – 11g fats per 100g serving) and high-sugar (e.g., tomato ketchup – 23.6g sugar per 100g serving) foods is associated with conditions such as diabetes and obesity, which can affect immune function. Moderate malnutrition, as well as certain specific trace mineral and nutrient deficiencies, also can compromise the immune response. Undernutrition-associated impairment of immune function can be due to insufficient intake of energy and macronutrients and/or due to deficiencies in specific micronutrients. Foods rich in certain fatty acids may foster a healthy IS. Foetal undernourishment is especially risky as it can cause a lifelong impairment of the IS. A variety of micronutrients have been implicated in improving the immune response, especially Vitamin A, Vitamin D, Vitamin E, zinc, iron and selenium.

PSYCHONEUROIMMUNOLOGY

The study of the interactions between psychological, neurological and immunological processes constitutes the field of 'psychoneuroimmunology', but 'PNI' will do just fine. As we have already seen, the immune system and CNS maintain extensive communications. The brain modulates the IS by hardwiring sympathetic and parasympathetic nerves to lymphoid organs. The IS modulates brain activity, including sleep and body temperature. Based on close functional and anatomical links, the immune and nervous systems act in a highly reciprocal manner. From fever to stress, the influence of one system on the other has evolved in an intricate manner to help sense danger and to mount an appropriate adaptive response. Research over recent decades suggests that these brain-to-immune interactions are highly modulated by psychological factors that influence immunity and IS-mediated disease.

The brain and the IS are involved in functionally relevant cross-talk, with homeostasis being the main function. The CNS is without lymphatic drainage and so lacks the immune surveillance available for the rest of the body. However, there are mechanisms to exclude the potentially destructive lymphoid cells from the brain, spinal cord and peripheral nerves, ranging from small molecules, such as nitric oxide, to large proteins, including cytokines and growth factors, which tie the two systems together.

Recent studies in PNI are indicating many empirical links between the psychological, endocrinological and immunological systems. PNI research remains at a relatively early stage of development, with many publications having an empirical rather than a theoretical focus.

In a randomized controlled experiment, people who performed kind acts for others showed favourable changes in immune cell gene expression profiles (Nelson-Coffey et al., 2017). High sensitivity C-reactive protein (hs-CRP) has emerged as a marker of inflammation in atherosclerotic vascular disease.

Tayefi et al. (2017) measured symptoms of depression and anxiety and serum hs-CRP levels in 9,759 participants (40% males and 60% females) aged 35–65 years in north-eastern Iran. They found that depression and anxiety are associated with serum levels of hs-CRP, higher BMI in women, and smoking in men.

Blair et al. (2017) analysed a prospective longitudinal sample of 1,292 infants in predominantly low-income and rural communities from infancy through to age 60 months. For children with relatively low cortisol levels between the ages of 7, 15, 24 and 48 months, those illustrating *moderate* fluctuations in their cortisol levels over this span tended to show subsequently better executive function (EF) performance at 60 months than did children with either highly stable or highly variable temporal profiles. This curvilinear function did not extend to children whose cortisol levels were high on average, who tended to show lower EF performance, irrespective of the stability of their cortisol levels over time.

PNI research suffers from the same ailments as most other areas of health psychology: it is underpowered with small sample sizes, cross-sectional designs and lack of replication. It is a field that has been hyped but is yet to reach its full potential.

HOMEOSTASIS

Homeostasis refers to the principle by which the internal environment of the body is kept in a state of equilibrium by a multitude of fine adjustments at a hierarchy of levels ranging from the molecular level to the level of the organism as a whole. Claude Bernard (1865) first described what he called the 'internal milieu' and showed that this internal environment was ordinarily maintained within fixed limits. Walter Cannon (1932), in *The Wisdom of the Body*, coined the term 'homeostasis' for the coordinated physiological processes by which an organism maintains an internal steady state. Both Bernard and Cannon focused almost entirely on physiological homeostasis. Curt Richter (1942) expanded the idea of the protection of the internal milieu to include behavioural or 'total organism regulators'. From this viewpoint, behaviour lies on a continuum with physiological events. Richter combined the perspective of Bernard with that of Cannon and he added behavioural regulation.

Behaviour, for Richter, was broadly conceived to include all aspects of identification, acquisition and ingestion of the substances needed to maintain the internal environment. The current theory extends the homeostasis concept one step further in suggesting that not only feeding, but all human behaviour, follows the principle of homeostasis. **Psychological homeostasis** is best explained in two stages, starting with the classic version in Physiology, followed by the new version extended to Psychology. Physiological homeostasis is illustrated in Figure 2.13.

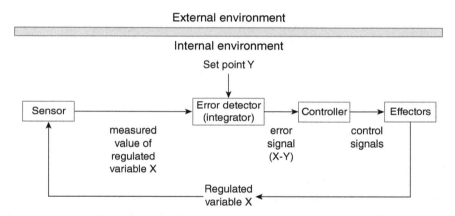

Figure 2.13   A complete representation of physiological homeostatic mechanisms (adapted from Modell et al., 2015)

There are five critical components that a regulatory system must contain in order to be counted as homeostasis:

1. It must contain a sensor that measures the value of the regulated variable.

2. It must contain a mechanism for establishing the 'normal range' of values for the regulated variable. In the model shown in Figure 2.13, this mechanism is represented by the 'Set point Y'. Arguably, the term 'set range' would be more appropriate than 'set point'.

3. It must contain an 'error detector' that compares the signal being transmitted by the sensor (representing the actual value of the regulated variable) with the set point or range. The result of this comparison is an error signal that is interpreted by the controller.

4. The controller interprets the error signal and determines the value of the outputs of the effectors. In the vast majority of cases, the controller is an automatic, nonconscious process.

5. The effectors are those elements that determine the value of the regulated variable.

We turn next to consider psychological homeostasis. Identical principles to those described above for physiological homeostasis apply to the regulation of behaviour and experience (Figure 2.14). For psychological homeostasis, however, the internal effectors remain active but *the boundary between the internal and external environments lies between the controller and the outward effectors of the somatic nervous system, i.e., the muscles that control speech and action.*

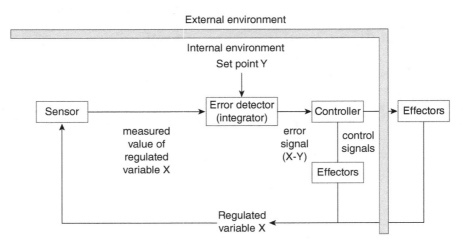

Figure 2.14   A complete representation of psychological homeostatic mechanisms (adapted from Modell et al., 2015)

Let us consider how psychological homeostasis works in practice. All people are oriented towards seeking and/or preserving physical and subjective well-being at a set point that is kept at the highest possible level. Hence, we tend to approach new resources in the hope of finding a reward for this behaviour and equally to avoid punishing or confrontational situations. If we do encounter threat, our behavioural options include either 'fight or flight' or inhibiting our behaviour so as to go unnoticed and to avoid confrontation. One can easily imagine the adaptive value of behavioural inhibition. A mouse scurrying through the grass suddenly notices a buzzard flying overhead. Out of fear, the mouse freezes, thus avoiding attracting the buzzard's attention. Playing dead until a predator has passed can be beneficial, as long as the tension of waiting does not have to go on for too long. Figure 2.15 shows a homeostatic strategy for choosing optimal behaviours and the brain structures that may be involved in the process. The diagram shows the feedback loops whereby our memories associate positive or negative connotations with situations that we experience, and then guide behaviour the next time they arise.

Life isn't always this simple, however. The whole process could fall apart if you're not a mouse hiding from a buzzard but, for example, you're a worker dealing with an exploitative boss. The worker cannot fight or flee, or they would be out of a job. So they can either join a labour union and talk to the union representative or they can let months and years go by while they inhibit their behaviour. This 'do-nothing' strategy ultimately can have disastrous effects on their health. For one thing, such inhibition causes hormonal changes that produce high blood levels of glucocorticoids, whose depressive effect on IS function is well known. This weakening of the IS is why remaining in a prolonged state of behavioural inhibition can cause all kinds of health problems.

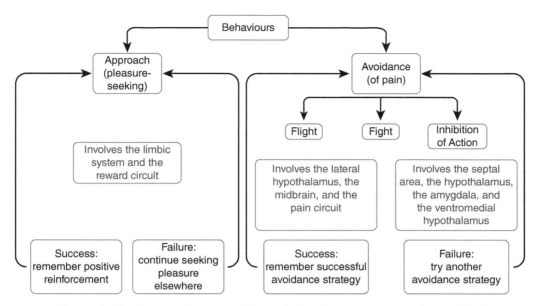

Figure 2.15   Approach and avoidance behaviours that maximize well-being

Source: Copyleft, http://thebrain.mcgill.ca

One source of inhibition is our imagination – our fear of failure. This can lead us to foresee so many potentially negative scenarios that we end up doing nothing. To do nothing, and to maintain a dream, may be a better option than to act and to fall flat on one's face. Whichever way one looks at the issue of inhibition, it has an obvious connection with homeostasis, a striving towards equilibrium.

Initiated by the brain, homeostasis also can act in an anticipatory mode. The preprandial (prior to having a meal) secretion of insulin, ghrelin and other hormones enables the consumption of a larger nutrient load with only minimal postprandial homeostatic consequences. When a meal containing carbohydrates is to be consumed, a variety of hormones is secreted by the gut that elicit the secretion of insulin from the pancreas *before* the blood sugar level has actually started to rise. This starts lowering the blood sugar level in anticipation of the influx of large quantities of glucose from the gut into the blood. This has the effect of blunting the blood glucose concentration spike that would otherwise occur. The relevance of psychological homeostasis has been underestimated in the study of behaviour, health and illness. In this book, psychological homeostasis is given its rightful position at the 'hightable' of psychological constructs.

Quack's corner and the placebo effect

The **placebo effect** can be viewed as *a form of anticipatory homeostasis*. When a patient feels unwell, for example with depression, and seeks help from a trusted medical practitioner, (s)he is given a prescription. Upon receiving the medicine, (s)he anticipates feeling better and, after swallowing the allegedly curative pill, sits back and looks for the signs of increased well-being and improvement. Lo and behold, in many such cases (s)he actually does feel better, and her/his well-being is restored. If it is an active placebo with somatic side effects, then even better (Thomson, 1982). To the degree that any treatment is perceived to be effective, then expectancy must play a role. Homeopathic medicine, which has no active content by definition, provides a cogent example of anticipatory homeostasis with no harmful side effects. Homeopathic medicine is a 100% placebo masquerading as active medicine. Yet this form of medicine is used worldwide by hundreds of millions of people who swear by its efficacy.

Homeopathy has two principal 'laws', the first being '*similia similibus curentur*' or '*let likes be cured by likes*'. This 'law' means that treatments that cause specific symptoms (e.g., onions cause runny eyes and nose) can cure conditions that cause the same symptoms (e.g., a bad cold). As if that isn't kooky enough, there is the '*law of infinitesimal doses*' that when treatments are diluted in water or alcohol, they actually *increase* in therapeutic potency. This means that a 1-in-1,000 solution should be *more* effective than a 1-in-100 dilution. It's an inverted dose response curve.

The anticipatory phenomena of placebos are certainly not confined to complementary and alternative medicines. The placebo effect has wide application in all areas of medicine. There is no harm in it whatsoever, as long as one doesn't swallow the quack claims that come along as part of the package with the pills.

Consider antidepressants. These are supposed to work by fixing a chemical imbalance, specifically, a lack of serotonin in the brain. Irving Kirsch (2015) reviews analyses of published and unpublished data that were hidden by drug companies, revealing that:

> most (if not all) of the benefits are due to the placebo effect. Some antidepressants increase serotonin levels, some decrease it, and some have no effect at all on serotonin. *Nevertheless, they all show the same therapeutic benefit. Even the small statistical difference between antidepressants and placebos may be an enhanced placebo effect, due to the fact that most patients and doctors in clinical trials successfully break blind.* The serotonin theory is as close as any theory in the history of science to having been proved wrong. Instead of curing depression, popular antidepressants may induce a biological vulnerability making people more likely to become depressed in the future. (Kirsch, 2015: 128, italics added)

Whatever people may believe will help them to feel better may indeed help them to feel better, at least for a short while. Long-term, however, placebo effects almost always fade. This isn't being snootily cynical. It's a brutal fact about human nature. All the more reason, then, to apply 'hard-nosed', sceptical analysis to outlandish treatment claims. Carl Sagan and other wise people have suggested that 'Extraordinary claims require extraordinary evidence'. There can be nothing more extraordinary or outlandish than the claims of homeopathic medicine. To turn our discussion full circle, *there is not a single replicated piece of scientific evidence of a homeopathic remedy influencing the NS, ES or IS.* The biological systems of the body carry the traces of every physical and mental stimulus we encounter. Homeopathic medicine leaves no trace. QED.

FUTURE RESEARCH

1. Advanced imaging techniques such as 'serial section electron microscopy' could be applied to study the mechanisms of inflammation.

2. We need to know more about misalignments of the circadian clock, emotion, and susceptibility to inflammation and acute and chronic conditions.

3. PNI research is needed to investigate the relationships between individual differences in cognitive ability, such as IQ test scores and changes in the immune system.

4. We need more studies of the impact of psychological homeostasis on the development of physical illnesses.

SUMMARY

1. Three important biological systems in health and illness are the nervous system (NS), the endocrine system (ES) and the immune system (IS). They activate and deactivate tissues, organs and muscles to control and regulate action, emotion and mental activity.

2. The NS uses neurotransmitters and the ES uses neuromodulators and hormones. The brain modulates the IS by hardwiring sympathetic and parasympathetic nerves to lymphoid organs. The IS modulates brain activity, including sleep and body temperature.

3. Two important classes of cell in the NS are neurones and microglial cells. Microglial cells are highly plastic and act as macrophage ('big eater') cells, the main form of active immune defence in the CNS.

4. Decisions made by the CNS are communicated via the peripheral NS to the effector division and inputs to the CNS are conducted by the afferent division. The autonomic nervous system deals with the non-conscious control of cardiac muscles, smooth muscles and glands, while the somatic nervous system deals with skeletal muscular responses in speech and behaviour.

5. The hypothalamo-pituitary-adrenal (HPA) axis produces corticotropin releasing hormone from the hypothalamus and conveys this to the anterior pituitary gland. The HPA axis has a primary role in emotion and stress. The amygdala triggers bodily responses to emotional events, including the release of adrenalin by the adrenal glands.

6. The endocrine system consists of the ductless glands and the hormones produced by those glands. Endocrine glands release their secretions directly into the intercellular fluid or into the bloodstream. Cellular metabolism, reproduction, sexual development, sugar and mineral homeostasis, heart rate and digestion are all regulated by hormones.

7. The ES regulates the circadian rhythm and sleep/waking cycle with a variety of hormone releases. Melatonin is produced in the pineal gland, under the control of the central circadian pacemaker in the suprachiasmatic nucleus (SCN) region of the hypothalamus.

8. The IS protects the body against disease or other potentially damaging foreign bodies. When functioning properly, the IS identifies and attacks a variety of threats, including viruses, bacteria and parasites, while distinguishing them from the body's own healthy tissue.

9. Psychoneuroimmunology is the study of the interactions and relationships between psychological, neurological and immunological processes. Research over recent decades suggests that brain-to-immune interactions are highly modulated by psychological factors which influence immunity and IS-mediated disease.

10. The principle of physiological homeostasis is extended to psychological homeostasis. Identical mechanisms exist in both forms of homeostasis. In seeking to maximize physical and subjective well-being to a high set point, we approach new sources of potential reward and try to avoid aversive or confrontational situations.

GENETICS, EPIGENETICS AND EARLY LIFE DEVELOPMENT

3

'Health will be defined as a function of gene–environmental homeostasis.'

Dover (2009)

'The brain is an extraordinary organ showing high levels of epigenetic features.'

Delgado-Morales and Esteller (2017)

'While undernutrition kills in early life, it also leads to a high risk of disease and death later in life. This double burden of mal-nutrition has common causes, inadequate foetal and infant and young child nutrition followed by exposure (including through marketing practices) to unhealthy energy dense nutrient poor foods and lack of physical activity. The window of opportunity lies from pre-pregnancy to around 24 months of a child's age.'

United Nations System Standing Committee on Nutrition (2006)

OUTLINE

The passage from the gametes to a fully functioning adult human involves a matrix of intricate, interacting genetic and environmental processes. All living organisms store genetic information using DNA and RNA, with different genes having their expression switched on or off by DNA methylation. Genetic processes lay down scripts that are edited by epigenetic processes that produce lifelong alterations in individual development, health and disease. Early life development is a formative and critical stage that requires nurturing care for optimal outcomes and maximum protection from sources of adversity.

The 1971 novel *The Dice Man* by Luke Rhinehart tells of a psychiatrist who decides to make life decisions based on the rolling of dice. *The Dice Man* is based on a reckless and scary conceit which, due to its subversive content, with issues such as rape, murder and sexual experimentation, led to the banning of the novel in several countries, no doubt increasing sales. It is alleged that the author wrote the book based on his experiences of using dice to make decisions while studying psychology. The cover bore the confident sub-heading: 'Few novels can change your life. This one will.' However, another, more profound truth does not feature in *The Dice Man* story. That is the fact that the most crucial 'dice of life' are cast long before we can say 'ABC' – the dice of biological determination and early life development (Figure 3.1), the topics of this chapter.

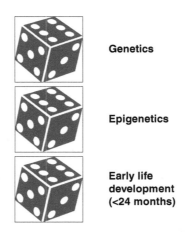

Genetics

Epigenetics

Early life development (<24 months)

Figure 3.1   The 'dice of life' – genetics, epigenetics, and early life development

GENETICS AND HERITABILITY

The science of genetics began with Hippocrates. His theory of 'pangenesis' suggested that heredity material in the form of 'pangenes', collected from around the body, enters the sperm and ovaries. Information from specific parts of the parents' bodies were communicated to the offspring to create the corresponding body part. For example, information from the parents' hearts, lungs and limbs was believed to transmit directly from these body parts to create the offspring's heart, lungs and limbs. The theory that inheritance was based on the 'blending' of parental traits was also popular and could not be dismissed until the research by Gregor Mendel (1822–1884), an Austrian monk. Mendel cultivated and tested the physical characteristics of 28,000 pea plants, which made excellent study items as they have easily recognizable and constant features, such as seed texture, colour and height. Mendel observed seven traits that existed in one out of two possible forms, for example the flower colour is white or purple, the seed shape is either round or wrinkled, and the seed colour and pod colour are both green or yellow. With only one of two possible results from cross-pollination, Mendel could determine which traits were passed down to the offspring with what frequency. The modern-day science of genetics was born.

A world-wide survey of human mitochondrial DNA (mtDNA)[1] led to the claim that 'all mitochondrial DNAs stem from one woman' and that she probably lived around 200,000 years

---

[1]Mitochondria are structures within cells that convert the energy from food into a usable form.

ago in Africa (Cairn et al., 1987). This prolific woman has been called 'Mitochondrial Eve' or 'African Eve'. Allowing 25 years per generation, that is just 8,000 generations to create the entire human population of more than 7.5 billion people alive today. How does the science of genetics explain the huge diversity of descendants from Mitochondrial Eve?

First, the blending theory of the ancients was found to be inadequate. In his study of peas, Mendel proposed that there can be no blending because the gene alternate for yellow is 'dominant' over the gene alternate for green. The dominant trait is observed whenever a single copy of its gene is inherited. When Mendel crossed the hybrid offspring, green seeds would reappear in one-quarter of plants in the next generation. Mendel concluded that the 'recessive' green trait appears only when a copy of the recessive gene form is inherited from each parent. Although Mendel published his discoveries in 1866, his ideas were not appreciated until the early twentieth century (Figure 3.2).

In 1905, the study of meiosis revealed that gender is based on **chromosomes**, threadlike structures inside the nucleus of animal and plant cells. Each chromosome is made of protein and a single molecule of DNA. Chromosome keeps DNA tightly wrapped around spool-like proteins called **histones**. Without this tight packaging, DNA molecules would be too long to fit inside cells. For example, if all of the DNA molecules in a single human cell were unwound from their histones and placed end-to-end, they would stretch six feet. Bearing in mind that the body contains 37.2 trillion cells, one can appreciate the need for histones.

In humans, each cell normally contains 23 pairs of chromosomes, a total of 46. Of these pairs, called autosomes, 22 look the same in both males and females. The twenty-third pair, the sex chromosomes, differ between males and females. One sex chromosome (X) is much bigger than the other (Y). A mismatched pair of one X and one Y chromosome occurs in male cells, while a matched pair of X chromosomes occurs in female cells. Females produce eggs with only X chromosomes, while males produce sperm with an X or a Y chromosome.

Thomas Morgan studied inheritance in the common fruit fly by crossing white-eyed male flies with red-eyed female flies which produced only red-eyed offspring. However, white-eyed mutants reappeared in the following generation, indicating a recessive trait, but only in males of the second generation. Morgan correctly concluded that being white-eyed must be a sex-linked recessive trait, with the gene for eye colour being physically located on the X chromosome.

Recessive inheritance has explained genetic disorders such as alkaptonuria and albinism, while other disorders are based on dominant genes such brachydactyly (short fingers), congenital cataracts and Huntington's chorea. Duchenne muscular dystrophy, red-green colour blindness and haemophilia are also sex-linked disorders.

Mendel's ideas were exploited and taken into a scientific cul-de-sac by the **eugenics** movement, which proposed that the human species could be improved by breeding from 'superior' white stock, while reproduction of the 'genetically unfit' was to be stopped. Eugenicists misused ideas of dominant and recessive genes to explain in simplistic terms complex human behaviours and mental illnesses, and failed to take account of environmental effects in human development. Eugenics reached its lowest point in the 'Final Solution' of Nazism and the Holocaust of Jewish and Romani people in the Second World War.

As early as 1881 Albrecht Kossel had isolated five nucleotide bases – adenine, cytosine, guanine, thymine and uracil – which were all later shown to be basic building blocks of DNA and RNA in all living things. **Deoxyribonucleic acid (DNA)** carries the instructions used in the growth, development, functioning and reproduction of all known living organisms and many

57

viruses. DNA is composed of nucleotide deoxyribose sugar, a phosphate group and one of four nitrogen bases — adenine (A), thymine (T), guanine (G) and cytosine (C). Phosphates and sugars of adjacent nucleotides link to form a long polymer. The ratios of A to T and G to C are found to be constant in all living things. Uracil is only present in RNA, replacing thymine.

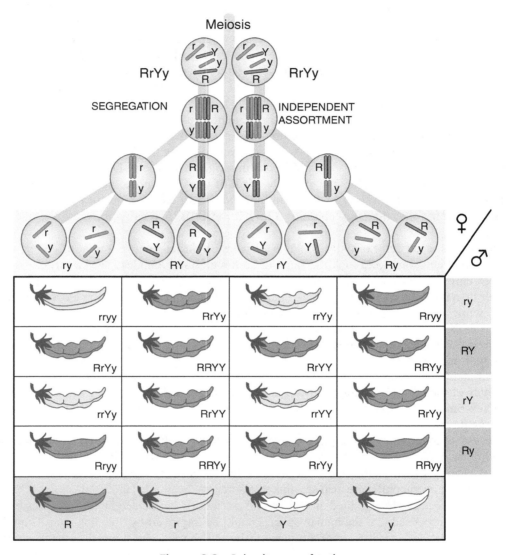

Figure 3.2   Inheritance of traits

In Mendel's research with round and wrinkled peas, he observed that a quarter of the peas were wrinkled in the second generation, suggesting that the characteristic is produced by two 'factors' (genes)

Source: Public domain, Mariana Ruiz Villarreal, 12 September 2008

In 1953, an American, James Watson, and an Englishman, Francis Crick, described the structure of DNA as a double helix, shaped like a twisted ladder. This discovery was in part based on an image produced by Raymond Gosling and Rosalind Franklin using X-ray crystallography, 'Photo 51'. On 28 February 1953 in a pub in Cambridge, Crick allegedly announced that he and Watson had 'discovered the secret of life'. Two months later the discovery was reported in *Nature* (Watson and Crick, 1953). Crick and Watson demonstrated that alternating deoxyribose and phosphate molecules formed the twisted uprights of the DNA ladder, while the rungs of the ladder are formed by complementary pairs of nitrogen base, with A always paired with T and G always paired with C, an elegant and beautiful structure (Figure 3.3).

An important molecule related to DNA is ribonucleic acid (RNA), which carries out coding, decoding, regulation and expression of genes. As noted above, RNA and DNA are both nucleic acids, and, along with proteins and carbohydrates, constitute the four macromolecules that are necessary for all known forms of life. The type of RNA that transcribes information from DNA as a sequence of bases and transfers it to a ribosome is called messenger RNA. Messenger RNA translates instructions from DNA to make proteins, without which we would not have evolved from the slime that we apparently evolved from.

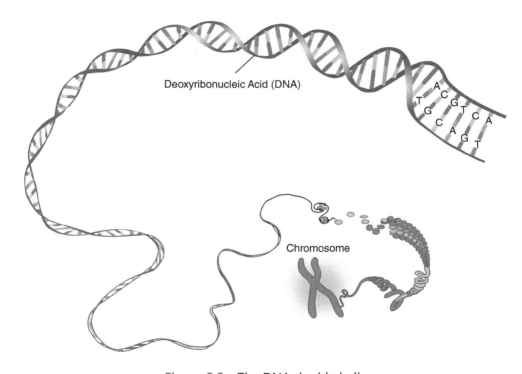

Deoxyribonucleic Acid (DNA)

Chromosome

Figure 3.3   The DNA double helix

Source: Reproduced from National Institutes of Health/National Human Genome Research Institute (2017). Public domain

THE HUMAN GENOME

A **genome** is any organism's complete set of DNA, including all of its genes. An organism's genome contains all of the information needed to build and maintain the organism. Accompanied by much fanfare and hype as a 'landmark in science', the first draft of the human genome appeared on 12 February 2001. In humans, a copy of the genome with all of its 3,234.83 mega-basepairs is contained in each and every one of the body's cells.

Knowing the complete sequence of the human genome is similar to having a manual on how to construct the human body. However, this manual has more than 3 billion pages and is not easy to read. Great expectations were raised by the scientists involved with the human genome project. However, understanding how the 3.4 billion complex parts work to create human life, health and disease is a challenge. It is currently estimated that there are 19,000–20,000 human protein-coding genes, although this estimate may be reduced over time. Figure 3.4 gives a graphical representation of the idealized human **karotype** showing the organization of the genome into chromosomes. The drawing shows both the female (XX) and male (XY) versions of the twenty-third chromosome pair.

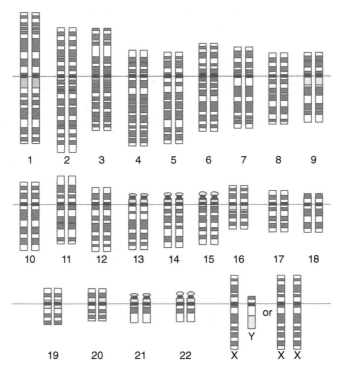

Figure 3.4   The idealized human karotype divided into 23 chromosome pairs

Source: Public domain

With the human genome project came the formation of new organizations to capitalize on the project. The National Institutes of Health/National Human Genome Research Institute is steering many research programmes on the human genome. One objective is to identify any gene suspected of causing an inherited disease. More than 2,000 genetic tests enable patients and families to be informed about their genetic risks for disease and to help professionals diagnose disease. The cost of sequencing an individual's genome is being reduced to below US$1,000. When this cost eventually falls, people will be able to carry copies of their karotype on their smart phones. Comparative genomic studies are identifying the causes of rare diseases. These scientific advances do not come without consequences for human liberty, privacy and rights.

Ethical, legal and social implications may affect individuals, families and the whole of society in four areas:

- Privacy and fairness in the use of genetic information, including the potential for genetic discrimination in education, employment, immigration and insurance. There is potential for a new, indelible type of stigmatization.

- The integration of new genetic technologies, such as genetic testing, into the practice of clinical medicine.

- Ethical issues surrounding the design and conduct of genetic research with people, including the process of informed consent. People will need the right to refuse the holding of their genome in databases.

- The education of health care professionals, policy makers, students and the public about genetics and the complex issues that result from genomic research.

We inherit from our parents all of the information necessary to create the proteins that make up our bodies. This inherited information, together with the influence of the environment, creates the complete human being. Much research has focused on the obvious question: How important is heredity and how important is the environment in human behaviour, health and well-being?

Heritability of human traits

Finding answers to the nature/nurture question has kept many scientific minds busy for over a century. Yet despite all of this research, the specific nature of the influences of genes and environment on human traits remains controversial. In part, this may rest on the fact that the question implies a dichotomy that in reality is a continuum of genetic-plus-environmental influence. The study of the influence of genetics on behaviour is called 'behaviour genetics'. One of the main techniques for unravelling nature and nurture has been the study of identical (monozygotic) and non-identical (dizygotic) twins, either reared together or reared apart. Such studies require meticulous attention to detail and the recruitment of large samples of twin participants, which tends to be time-consuming. Data from twin studies are open to interpretation and have often led to controversy.

In discussing heritability, we need to distinguish between a person's genotype and phenotype. The genotype is the part of the genetic makeup of an individual which determines their potential characteristics, for example eye colour, height, weight, general intelligence and personality traits. The phenotype is the set of observable characteristics of an individual resulting from the interaction of the genotype with the environment. A particular person's phenotype is the sum of genetic and environmental effects:

Phenotype (P) = Genotype (G) + Environment (E)

Likewise, the phenotypical variance in the trait – Var (P) – is the sum of effects, as follows:

Var(P) = Var(G) + Var(E) + 2 Cov(G,E)

In a planned experiment $\text{Cov}(G,E)$ can be controlled and held at 0. In this case, heritability, H2, is defined as:

$$H^2 = Var(G)/Var(P)$$

An H2 estimate is the proportion of trait variation among individuals that is a consequence of genetic factors; it is not the degree of genetic influence on that trait in any particular individual. For example, if the heritability of personality traits is .60, we can *not* say that 60% of an individual's personality is inherited from her/his parents and 40% from the environment. In most usual circumstances, the proportions of genetic and environmental influence for any individual and trait are unknown. In rare cases, when there is an autosomal dominant condition such as Huntington's disease (1 in 15,000 births) or familial hypercholesterolemia (1 in 500 births), then there is a 50% chance of inheritance in each new birth, providing there is only one affected parent.

There has been a large amount of research using the monozygotic versus dizygotic twin design. Polderman et al. (2015) reported a mammoth meta-analysis of twin correlations with variance estimates for 17,804 traits from 2,748 publications based on 14,558,903 partly dependent twin pairs, i.e., virtually all published twin studies of complex traits. Estimates of heritability were found to cluster strongly within different functional domains. Across all traits the reported, heritability was 49%, indicating an almost exactly equal contribution of genes and environment. For 69% of traits, the observed twin correlations were consistent with a simple, parsimonious model in which twin resemblance is solely due to additive genetic variation (Figure 3.5). The authors concluded that the dataset was 'inconsistent with substantial influences from shared

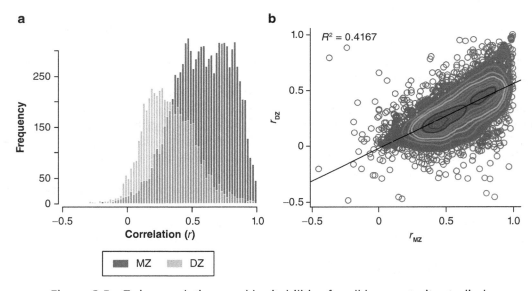

Figure 3.5 Twin correlations and heritabilities for all human traits studied

(a) Distribution of rMZ and rDZ estimates across the traits investigated in 2,748 twin studies published between 1958 and 2012. rMZ estimates are based on 9,568 traits and 2,563,628 partly dependent twin pairs; rDZ estimates are based on 5,220 traits and 2,606,252 partly dependent twin pairs. (b) Relationship between rMZ and rDZ, using all 5,185 traits for which both were reported

Source: Reproduced by permission from Polderman et al. (2015)

environment or non-additive genetic variation' (Polderman et al., 2015). In other words, nurture and nature were independent and equal contributors to individual differences in traits.

On the basis of the Polderman et al. (2015) study, it can be concluded that nature and nurture are of equal importance in determining human abilities and character. However, the relative proportions of influence differ from 50:50 for specific functions and characteristics. The largest heritability estimates were for traits in the ophthalmological domain (H2 = 0.71, s.e.m. = 0.04), followed by the ear, nose and throat (H2 = 0.64, s.e.m. = 0.06), dermatological (H2 = 0.60, s.e.m. = 0.04) and skeletal (H2 = 0.60, s.e.m. = 0.02) domains. The lowest heritability estimates were found for traits in the environmental, reproductive and social value domains (Polderman et al., 2015). Nature is more important for structural and anatomical differences, while nurture has greater influence on psychological and social differences.

One example of a psychological variable is emotional overeating (EOE), the tendency to eat more in response to negative emotions. Herle et al. (2017) examined the relative genetic and environmental influences on EOE in toddlerhood and early childhood in 2,402 British twins born in 2007. Genetic influences on EOE were found to be minimal, while shared environmental influences explained most of the variance. Herle et al. (2017) stated that EOE is 'moderately stable from 16 months to 5 years and continuing environmental factors shared by twin pairs at both ages explained the longitudinal association'.

A new approach to the study of nature and nurture has been the **genome-wide association studies (GWAS)**. GWAS examine a genome-wide set of genetic variants in a large sample of individuals to see whether any variant is associated with a trait. GWAS typically focus on associations between **single nucleotide polymorphisms** (SNPs, pronounced 'snips') and traits or major human diseases. A SNP is a DNA sequence variation occurring when a single nucleotide adenine (A), thymine (T), cytosine (C) or guanine (G) in the genome (or other shared sequence) differs between individuals or between paired chromosomes in an individual. SNPs occur throughout a person's DNA once in every 300 nucleotides on average, which means there are roughly 10 million SNPs in one human genome. Most commonly, SNP variations are found in the DNA lying between genes.

One approach in GWAS is the case-control design, which compares two large groups of individuals, one healthy control group and one case group affected by a disease. Initially, all individuals are genotyped for commonly known SNPs. The exact number of SNPs varies but is typically 1 million or more. For each SNP, the investigators examine whether the allele frequency is significantly altered between the case and the control group. The statistic for reporting effect sizes is the odds ratio, the ratio of disease for individuals having a specific allele and the odds of disease for individuals who do not have that allele. A p-value is calculated using a chi-squared test. An odds ratio that departs significantly from 1.0 indicates that a SNP is associated with disease.

In spite of the precision of the method, GWAS findings have been disappointing. There is a lack of consistency in findings across studies and the amount of variance explained in traits or diseases is very low. For example, known SNPs explain less than 2% of the variation in body mass index (BMI) despite the evidence of greater than 50% heritability from twin and family studies, a phenomenon termed 'missing heritability'. Llewellyn et al. (2013) used a novel method (Genome-wide Complex Trait Analysis, GCTA) to estimate the total additive genetic influence due to common SNPs on whole-genome arrays. This study provided the first GCTA estimate of genetic influence on adiposity in children. Participants were from the Twins Early Development Study (TEDS), a British twin birth cohort. Selecting one child per family (n = 2,269), GCTA results from 1.7 million DNA markers were used to quantify the additive genetic influence of common SNPs. For direct comparison, a standard twin analysis in the same families estimated the additive genetic influence as 82%. GCTA explained 30% of the variance in BMI-SDS. These results indicate that 37% of the twin-estimated heritability (30/82%) were explained by additive effects of multiple common SNPs, which is indicative of a strong genetic influence on adiposity in childhood. To fully explain this 'missing heritability', larger sample sizes are required to improve statistical power. Also, most variants that are associated with obesity from current GWAS are correlational, not causative (Xia and Grant, 2013).

In discussing obesity, Marti and Ordovas (2011: 190) reflected on the lack of progress on the tenth anniversary of the publications that reported the initial human genome sequence: 'It was stated that the complete genome sequence would "revolutionize the diagnosis, prevention, and treatment of most, if not all, human diseases." Whereas this is probably true, the question remains about "when" and "how"'. Ten years later the situation remains the same, and it is apparent that the human genome project has yet to reach its full potential. New approaches are required to identify the causative genes for the late onset and progressive nature of most common diseases, complex traits, and the mechanism by which the environment can modulate genetic predisposition to commonly occurring diseases.

Genetic counselling

Genetic counselling provides patients or relatives at risk of an inherited disorder (such as certain types of cancer) with advice and support concerning the consequences and nature of the disorder, the probability of developing or transmitting it, and the options open to them in management and family planning. The main elements of genetic counselling have been described by Harper (2010) as follows:

- Diagnostic and clinical aspects
- Documentation of family and pedigree information
- Recognition of inheritance patterns and risk estimation
- Communication and empathy
- Information of available options and further measures
- Support in decision-making and for decisions already taken.

During a first appointment, the counsellor will draw a family tree using information about grandparents, aunt/uncles, and cousins on both sides of the family.

When an inherited condition is diagnosed in an individual there are potential consequences for other family members. However, privacy legislation and ethical considerations restrict health professionals' ability to communicate the diagnosis with other family members, and it is normally the person who first receives the diagnosis who is responsible for sharing the news with their relations. There are many possible barriers to sharing this information, including stigma, fear, guilt and shame (James et al., 2006).

Owing to the complexity of genetic counselling as an intervention, there have been few randomized controlled trials (RCTs) to evaluate it. A trial of telephone genetic counselling conducted in Australia obtained a non-significant treatment effect. Hodgson et al. (2016) conducted an RCT in six public hospitals to assess whether a telephone counselling intervention improved family communication about a new genetic diagnosis. Only 26% (142/554) of the intervention group relatives made contact with genetic services, compared with 21% (112/536) of the control group relatives ($P = 0.40$).

A systematic review by Mendes et al. (2016) examined the dissemination of information within families, finding it to be actively encouraged and supported by genetic counselling professionals, following guidelines and recommendations from professional bodies. People requiring support or showing difficulties can receive psycho-educational guidance and written information aids as 'cues for action'. A more direct approach is for genetics services to send letters to at-risk relatives informing them of their risks and the availability of counselling services. According to Mendes et al. (2016), this direct approach is acceptable to relatives and effective in promoting clarification of relatives' genetic status.

We now turn to consider the second of the three 'dice of life', epigenetics.

EPIGENETICS AND INTERGENERATIONAL TRANSMISSION

Epigenetics is the study of heritable changes in a chromosome other than changes in the underlying DNA sequence. The epigenetic inheritance system has been described as 'soft inheritance' in comparison to genetics, which is 'hard inheritance' (Mayr and Provine, 1980). The inheritance of traits in genetics occurs as a result of rare genetic mutations that involve DNA mutation, but selection is slow in making adaptations to the constantly changing environment. The soft inheritance system of epigenetics, on the other hand, is able to adapt to fluctuations in the environment, such as changes in nutrition, stress and toxins (Wei et al., 2015).

Epigenetics at the cellular level produces cell differentiation by determining the functional types of cell, such as hepatocytes in the liver, neurones in the brain, or skin cells, as well as influencing whether or not they become cancerous. Within the CNS, epigenetics are involved in various neurodegenerative disorders and physiological responses, such as Alzheimer's disease, depression, schizophrenia, glioma, addiction, Rett syndrome, alcohol dependence, autism, epilepsy, multiple sclerosis and stress. As neurones are incapable of dividing and cannot be replaced after degeneration, epigenetic alterations that cause neuronal dysfunction have to be targeted and modified to prevent chronic kinds of neurodegeneration, which can prove fatal (Adwan and Zawia, 2013).

Epigenetic changes include DNA methylation and histone modification, both of which regulate gene expression without altering the linear sequence of DNA. DNA methylation adds methyl groups to the DNA molecule, which can change the activity of a DNA segment without changing the sequence. DNA methylation typically acts to repress or switch off gene transcription. DNA methylation is implicated in a wide range of processes, including chromosome instability, X-chromosome inactivation, cell differentiation, cancer progression and gene regulation. The flexibility in gene expression is seen early in childhood and can be demonstrated in identical twins, who, even when raised in the 'same' environment, can have a different expression of genes. Essentially, DNA methylation is a switch that switches genes in the genotype on or off to produce the phenotype, the human being we actually become, rather than the one determined by a random mix from the gene bank of 'Mum and Dad' (Figure 3.6).

Epigenetics can be viewed as a set of bridging processes between the genotype and the creation of the all-important phenotype – a phenomenon that changes the final outcome of a locus or chromosome without changing the underlying DNA sequence (Goldberg et al., 2007). We turn to consider the role of epigenetics in developmental plasticity and the 'Foetal Origins Hypothesis', which is concerned with the role of nutrition and malnutrition in healthy foetal development.

Developmental plasticity and the Foetal Origins Hypothesis

Malnutrition during foetal life and infancy have been linked to the development of coronary heart disease, stroke, Type 2 diabetes, hypertension, osteoporosis and certain cancers, including breast cancer. All of these conditions can originate through the developmental plasticity process of foetal life. Geographical studies led David Barker (2007) to propose the 'Foetal Origins Hypothesis', that undernutrition *in utero* and during infancy permanently changes the body's structure, physiology and metabolism, causing coronary heart disease and stroke in adult life:

> Like other living creatures in their early life human beings are 'plastic' and able to adapt to their environment. The development of the sweat glands provides a simple example of this. All humans have similar numbers of sweat glands at birth but none of them function. In the first three years after birth a proportion of the glands become functional, depending on the temperature to which the child is exposed. The hotter the conditions, the greater the number of sweat glands that are programmed to function. After three years the process is complete and the number of sweat glands is fixed. Thereafter, the child who has experienced hot conditions will be better equipped to adapt to similar conditions in later life, because people with more functioning sweat glands cool down faster. This brief description encapsulates the essence of developmental plasticity: a critical period when a system is plastic and sensitive to the environment, followed by loss of plasticity and a fixed functional capacity. For most organs and systems, the critical period occurs *in utero.* (Barker, 2013: 5)

Developmental plasticity has been described as the phenomenon by which one genotype can give rise to a range of different physiological or morphological states in response to different environmental conditions during development (West-Eberhard, 1989). One area in which to explore the developmental origins of chronic disease is cardiovascular disease. Barker's team had earlier identified groups of men and women in middle or late life whose birth size had been recorded. Their birthweight could be related to the later occurrence of coronary heart disease (CHD). In Hertfordshire, UK, from 1911 onwards, women with babies were attended by a midwife, who recorded the birthweight. After the birth, a health visitor went to the baby's home at intervals throughout infancy, and the weight at 1 year was recorded. In 10,636 men born between 1911 and 1930, hazard ratios for CHD fell with increasing birthweight. There were stronger trends with weight at 1 year. A later study found a similar trend of decreased hazard ratios for CHD with increasing birthweight among women born during this time but no trend with weight at 1 year. The association between low birthweight and CHD has since been replicated in Europe, North America and India. Because the associations are independent of the duration of gestation, they can be assumed to be the result of slow foetal growth (Barker, 2007). The findings from ecological studies have been confirmed in studies with individuals. Barker (2007: 416) concluded that the 'orthodox view that cardiovascular disease results from adult lifestyles and genetic inheritance has not provided a secure basis for prevention of these disorders. The developmental model of the origins of chronic disease now offers a new way forward'. If true, Barker's hypothesis means that the majority of work in public health and in much of health psychology, which is designed to help adults change 'lifestyles', is redundant. [*Hmmm. No need for this textbook then! However, Barker's hypothesis is only true to a certain extent. Adults' behaviours, such as smoking, drinking and unhealthy eating, are all examples of known risk factors for cancers and cardiovascular disease.*]

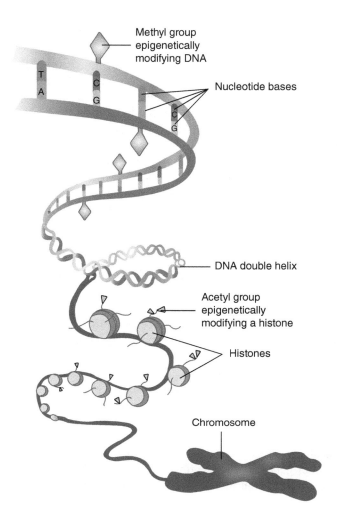

Methyl group
epigenetically
modifying DNA

Nucleotide bases

DNA double helix

Acetyl group
epigenetically
modifying a histone

Histones

Chromosome

Figure 3.6 A schematic diagram of DNA pulled from a chromosome, showing the double helix wrapped around histones, and some epigenetic modifications to both the DNA and the histones

Source: Reproduced by permission from Hadas et al. (2017)

The *intrauterine* period of development certainly is important in development because it includes stimuli such as nutrients, stress, drugs, trauma and smoking. A healthy intrauterine environment enables the mother to impart a rich 'maternal forecast' for her developing foetus, predicting a healthy post-birth environment where resources will be plentiful and negative exposures are expected to be minimal. However, a relatively adverse intrauterine environment may result in a poor maternal forecast for her developing foetus, a so-called 'thrifty phenotype' (Hales and Barker, 1992) that becomes a small, low-weight baby, preparing the child to survive in a poor post-birth environment. Maternal forecasts that inaccurately predict the post-birth environment are hypothesized to lead to ill health over the child's later life, for example an increased risk for metabolic diseases and decreased cognitive functioning in offspring that had received a poor maternal forecast but were born into a rich environment (Knopik et al., 2012).

There can be few times in the lifespan that are more significant than the period of prenatal development. At this time there appear to be 'critical windows' where disturbances may alter foetal growth and development, leading to health and behavioural consequences across the life course. Early life programming can have long-term effects on metabolism (Tarry-Adkins and Ozanne, 2011) via mechanisms that include: (1) permanent structural changes resulting from suboptimal concentrations of an important factor during a critical period of development (e.g., the permanent reduction in B cell mass in the endocrine pancreas); (2) persistent alterations in epigenetic modifications that lead to changes in gene expression (e.g., several transcription factors are susceptible to reprogrammed gene expression); and (3) permanent effects on the regulation of cellular ageing (e.g., increases in oxidative stress that lead to macromolecular damage, including that to DNA and specifically to telomeres[2]). Prevention and intervention to combat the burden of common diseases such as Type 2 diabetes and cardiovascular disease may be developed as a consequence of improved understanding of early life programming.

INTERGENERATIONAL TRANSMISSION, SOCIAL EPIGENETICS AND MATERNAL STRESS

'Intergenerational transmission' occurs when enduring epigenetic changes in parental biological systems in response to maternal exposure are transmitted to the offspring and to the offspring of the offspring. Nutritional status, exposure to toxins and drugs, and the experiences of interacting with varied environments can all modify an individual's epigenome. Epigenetic programming changes how and when certain genes are turned on or off and triggers temporary or enduring health problems. Research suggests that epigenetic changes occurring in the foetus can be passed on to later generations, affecting children, grandchildren and their descendants. For example, turning on genes that increase cell growth, while at the same time switching off genes that suppress cell growth, can cause cancer. Repetitive, stressful experiences can cause epigenetic changes that alter the biological systems that manage one's response to adversity later in life. We illustrate these ideas with recent examples of epigenetic research on maternal stress.

Stress exposures of parents may occur before conception, at the time of conception, at the time of pregnancy, or in the early postnatal period, where the environment of mothers influences the epigenetic patterning of their offspring, which can have a life-long influence on their behaviour, emotions and well-being, both mental and physical. Children of mothers who are exposed to poverty, hunger, poor diet, smoking, stress, war or violence prenatally are prone to epigenetic influences on their offspring's later well-being.

Research from Moshe Szyf and colleagues has provided significant findings on the epigenetic influences of prenatal maternal stress. This work has been labelled 'social epigenetics' (Szyf, 2013). One study looked at the offspring of mothers exposed to severe ice storms in southern Quebec, Canada, in 1998. For several days freezing rain storms covered everything

---

[2]A telomere is a region of repetitive nucleotide sequences at each end of a chromosome, which protects the end of the chromosome from deterioration or from fusion with neighbouring chromosomes.

in layers of ice, resulting in power outages which ranged from a few hours to as long as six weeks for 3 million Québécois. Security forces went door to door to rescue isolated individuals in danger from cold and hypothermia, asphyxiation from unconventional heating devices, and fire due to blocked chimneys.

The investigators of a research project called 'Project Ice Storm' have reported that maternal hardship and subjective distress predicted a variety of developmental outcomes. One focus for the project was the potential influence of prenatal maternal stress (PNMS) on the offspring (Box 3.1).

Intergenerational transmission to offspring from parental exposures and characteristics can be more specific than the general links that occur between parental problems and offspring outcomes (Bowers and Yehuda, 2016). Parents can model behaviours, and children can learn to react to their environments in a manner similar to their parents. Phenotypic changes can also occur as a consequence of child rearing and offspring can also experience parental trauma vicariously or by imagining traumas that they know their parents experienced from parents' stories. The observation of biological changes in offspring associated with parental trauma may indicate similar genetic risks in both generations, rather than intergenerational transmission of biological sensitivity. The idea that an observed biological change in offspring may be transmitted from the parent first arose following studies of pregnant women exposed to starvation during the Dutch famines (Barker, 1990, 1998). Adult offspring of Holocaust survivors were found to be at greater risk for the development of post-traumatic stress disorder (PTSD), depression and anxiety disorders (Yehuda et al., 2008). Women who develop PTSD as a result of trauma during pregnancy, for example having to evacuate the World Trade Center on 9/11, also give birth to affected offspring with evidence of a trimester effect (Yehuda et al., 2005). The evidence suggests that the third trimester is a more sensitive period for *in utero* effects in intergenerational transmission of risk than the second trimester.

BOX 3.1

Prenatal maternal stress predicts a wide variety of behavioural and physical outcomes in the offspring

Although epigenetic processes may be responsible for prenatal maternal stress (PNMS) effects, human research is hampered by the lack of experimental methods that parallel controlled animal studies. Disasters, however, provide natural experiments that can present models of prenatal stress. This study took advantage of a natural disaster to carry out fundamental research on prenatal maternal stress.

Five months after the 1998 Quebec ice storm Cao-Lei and colleagues recruited women who had been pregnant during the disaster and assessed their degrees of objective hardship and subjective distress. Thirteen years later, they investigated DNA methylation profiling in T cells obtained from 36 of the children, and compared selected results with those from saliva samples obtained from the same children at age 8.

Prenatal maternal objective hardship was correlated with DNA methylation levels in 1,675 CpGs (or 'CGs' – CGs are regions of DNA where a cytosinenucleotide is followed by a guanine nucleotide) affiliated with 957 genes predominantly related to immune function; maternal

(Continued)

69

subjective distress was uncorrelated. DNA methylation changes in SCG5[3] and LTA,[4] both of which highly correlated with maternal objective stress, were comparable in T cells, peripheral blood mononuclear cells and saliva cells.

These data provide the first evidence in humans supporting the idea that PNMS results in a lasting, broad and functionally organized DNA methylation in several tissues in offspring. By using a natural disaster model, the investigators could infer that the epigenetic effects found in Project Ice Storm were due to objective levels of hardship experienced by the pregnant woman rather than to her level of sustained distress.

Source: Cao-Lei et al. (2014)

Figure 3.7 indicates three levels at which biological stress effects in parents can potentially have a direct impact on offspring (Bowers and Yehuda, 2016). Other relevant mechanisms are

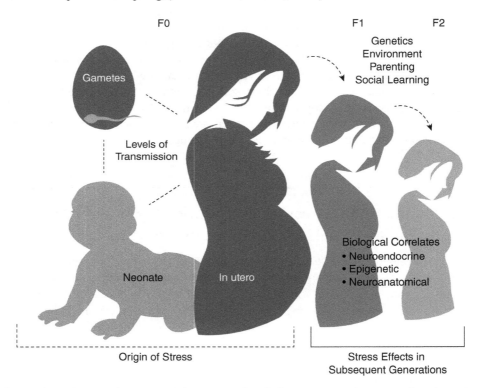

Figure 3.7   Parental stress can be transmitted via gametes, the gestational uterine environment, and early postnatal care

Source: Reproduced by permission from Bowers and Yehuda (2016)

---

[3]The SCG5 gene encodes the neuroendocrine protein 7B2 in humans; 7B2 is widely distributed in neuroendocrine tissues.

[4]The LTA gene encodes lymphotoxin-alpha (LT-α) or tumour necrosis factor-beta; LT-α has a significant role in the maintenance of the immune system.

genetics, social learning, parenting and shared environmental contexts. 'Intergenerational transmission' of stress effects that are inherited is reflected in biological changes in the offspring, consisting of neuroendocrine, epigenetic and neuroanatomical changes.

Theoretical models are needed to explain how early life adversities are epigenetically programmed towards life-long alteration in hormonal responses to stressors. Acute stress normally produces a biobehavioural response which, following its removal, is corrected by homeostasis, which restores the system to baseline functioning. Reactivity to acute stress is a trait that is both genetically and epigenetically determined. The effects of acute stressors can persist over time due to long-term changes in thresholds to stress triggers.

Figure 3.8 illustrates a theory of epigenetic processes suggested by Klengel and Binder (2015: 1344), as follows:

> Stress and, in particular, early life adversities activate the stress hormone system and may epigenetically program the system toward a lifelong alteration of the hormonal response to even minor stressors. The neuropeptides corticotrophin-releasing hormone (CRH) and vasopressin (AVP), released from the hypothalamus in response to stress, activate the release of adrenocorticotropic hormone (ACTH) from the anterior pituitary gland, finally leading to an increased systemic cortisol secretion from the adrenal gland. Cortisol binds to steroid receptors, the mineralocorticoid receptor (MR) and the glucocorticoid receptor (GR), that act as transcriptional activators or repressors in the nucleus through binding to glucocorticoid response elements. This influences the expression of numerous genes involved in the stress response, immune function, and metabolism. Binding of the GR and transcriptional activation of, for example, FKBP5 provide an ultrashort feedback to the GR, terminating the stress response and secretion of cortisol.

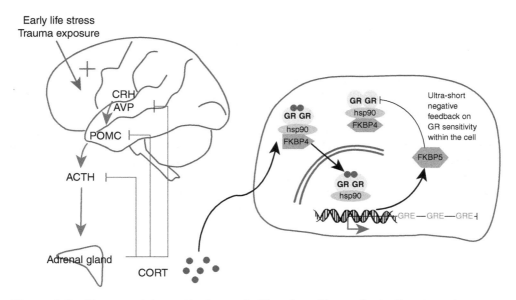

Figure 3.8 Stress and, in particular, early life adversities activate the stress hormone system and may epigenetically programme the system towards a life-long alteration of the hormonal response to even minor stressors

Source: Reproduced by permission from Klengel and Binder (2015)

Figure 3.8 is based on evidence suggesting that the effects of parental stress can be directly transmitted to offspring via gametes (*oocytes* and sperm), the uterine environment during pregnancy, or during early postnatal care of newborns. In Holocaust and Dutch Famine survivors' offspring, the parental trauma occurred years before conception, suggesting that effects in offspring might be due in part to some biological change in gametes. Stress effects that are inherited via an 'intergenerational transmission' mode are reflected in offspring biological changes, including neuroendocrine, epigenetic and neuroanatomical changes.

Although there have already been a number of significant findings, our knowledge of the role of the epigenome in shaping human behaviour across generations is at the beginning stages and very little is yet certain. Epigenetics has the potential to provide a foundation for the hypothesis that interventions to promote nurturing care, and to improve the cognitive and socio-emotional well-being of children, have positive transgenerational consequences. We await new developments with great interest.

EARLY LIFE DEVELOPMENT

Two profound changes over recent decades have produced a dramatically altered landscape for early childhood in many countries (Phillips and Shonkoff, 2000). First, research reviewed in this chapter has advanced our understanding of early development. Second, there have been changes in the social and economic circumstances in which families with young children are living: (1) work patterns of parents with young children; (2) high levels of economic hardship among families; (3) increasing cultural diversity and the persistence of significant racial and ethnic disparities in health and developmental outcomes; (4) growing numbers of young children spending considerable time in childcare settings; and (5) greater awareness of the negative effects of stress on young children. Britto et al. (2017) collated the findings of many thousands of studies on the characteristics of nurturing care in a systematic review (see Box 3.2).

Early environmental experiences can have a lasting impact on a child's later success in school and life more generally. It has been claimed that differences in the size of children's vocabulary first appear at 18 months of age, based on whether they were born into a family with high education and income or low education and income (Hart and Risley, 1995). By age 3, children with college-educated parents or primary caregivers have vocabularies two to three times larger than those whose parents had not completed high school. Unless they are engaged in a language-rich environment in early life by school age, children are already behind their peers.

Adverse living circumstances impair a child's development in the first 24–36 months of life, and the greater the degree of adversity, the greater the odds of developmental delay. Risk factors include poverty, caregiver mental illness, child maltreatment, single parenthood and low maternal education, which can collectively have a cumulative impact. Maltreated children who are exposed to up to six additional risks face a 90–100% likelihood of having one or more delays in their cognitive, language or emotional development (Barth et al., 2008).

BOX 3.2

Nurturing care: promoting early childhood development

Advances in basic and intervention science indicate that early childhood is a period of special sensitivity to experiences that promote development, and that critical time windows exist when the benefits of early childhood development interventions are amplified.

The most fundamental promotive experiences in the early years of life come from nurturing care and protection received from parents, family and community, which have lifelong benefits including improved health and wellbeing, and increased ability to learn and earn.

Nurturing care and protection are supported by a range of interventions delivered pre-pregnancy and throughout birth, the newborn period, infancy and early childhood. Many of these interventions (centred around the areas of parenting support, attachment and bonding, breastfeeding, micronutrients and child feeding, prevention of child maltreatment and out-of-home interventions) have shown benefits for child development, nutrition and growth, and reductions in morbidity, mortality, disability and injury.

Interventions that integrate nurturing care and protection can target multiple risks to developmental potential at appropriate times, and can be integrated within existing preventive and promotive packages.

Preventive and promotive packages can build on existing platforms, such as community-based strategies and social safety nets, for delivering parental and child services at scale to vulnerable and difficult-to-reach populations, enhancing their effectiveness and sustainability.

Source: Britto et al. (2017: 91). Reproduced by permission

Early experiences can actually get 'under the skin' and have life-long effects on cognitive and emotional well-being, and on long-term physical health as well. Significant childhood adversity is a predictor of adult health problems, including diabetes, hypertension, stroke, obesity and some forms of cancer. Adults who recall having seven or eight serious adverse experiences in childhood are three times more likely to have cardiovascular disease as an adult (Dong et al., 2004).

FUTURE RESEARCH

1. The developmental model of the origins of chronic disease suggested by Barker and others offers an important alternative approach to disease prevention based on the provision of nurturing care and the protection of the foetus and neonate. Economic studies of the benefits of early life prevention versus the traditional approach, which targets adult lifestyle change, are needed to inform policy and prevention.

2. Improved understanding of the epigenetic mechanisms of early life development, especially those associated with the initial critical phases, will make it possible to design effective interventions.

3. The ethical and legal implications of epigenetic embryonic forecasting need to be studied so that guidelines can be devised prior to implementation.

4. There is a need for more research to validate the GWAS approach and to examine the reasons for the high amounts of missing heritability.

SUMMARY

1. Humans have 23 pairs of chromosomes, and thus a total of 46 chromosomes. One copy of each chromosome is inherited from the female parent and the other from the male parent. Chromosomes are made of protein and a single molecule of deoxyribonucleic acid (DNA), which contains the instructions making each human being unique.

2. It is necessary to distinguish between a person's genotype and phenotype. The genotype is the part of the individual's genetic makeup that determines their potential characteristics. The phenotype is the observable characteristics of an individual resulting from the interaction of the genotype with the environment.

3. Nature and nurture are of equal importance in determining human abilities and character. However, the relative proportions of influence can differ from a 50:50 split for specific functions and characteristics. Nature is more important for structural and anatomical differences, while nurture has greater influence on psychological and social differences.

4. Epigenetics is the study of heritable changes caused by mechanisms other than changes in the underlying DNA sequence. The epigenetic inheritance system has been described as 'soft inheritance' because it is amenable to adaptation to fluctuations in environments, such as changes in nutrition, stress and toxins.

5. The 'Foetal Origins Hypothesis' of David Barker proposed that undernutrition in utero and during infancy permanently changes the body's structure, physiology and metabolism, causing coronary heart disease and stroke in adult life.

6. Orthodox thinking about chronic disease suggests that it results from adult lifestyles and genetic inheritance. The developmental model of the origins of chronic disease suggested by Barker and others offers an important alternative approach to disease prevention based on the provision of nurturing care and the protection of the foetus and neonate.

7. Breastfeeding has clear short-term benefits for child health, reducing mortality and morbidity from infectious diseases, encouraging healthy food preferences and promoting the establishment of a healthy gut microbiome.

8. Stress exposures of parents may occur before conception, at the time of conception, at the time of pregnancy, or in the early postnatal period. Children of mothers who are exposed to poverty, hunger, poor diet, smoking, stress, war or violence prenatally are prone to epigenetic influences on their offspring's later well-being.

9. Maltreatment during childhood is associated with reduced volume of both the midsaggital area and the hippocampus, the two brain regions involved in learning and memory. Epigenetic changes in the CNS may be responsible for observed delays in cognitive development.

10. Children who receive inadequate care, especially in the first 24 months of life, are more sensitive to the effects of stress and display more behavioural problems than children who receive nurturing care.

MACRO-SOCIAL INFLUENCES

'As in earlier times, advances in the 21st century will be won by human struggle against divisive values – and against the opposition of entrenched economic and political interests.'

Human Development Report (2000: 6)

OUTLINE

We employ a wide-angle lens to explore the macro-social context for human health. We discuss the fact that what individuals can do to change their lives is not simply a matter of personal choice; choices are constrained biologically, culturally, economically and environmentally. In spite of medical and technological advances, population growth, the globalized promotion of unhealthy commodities, increasing poverty and the shrinking availability of natural resources, especially safe drinking water, are acting to worsen health globally. Universal gradients both within and between nations are persistent over time and space. The 'doom and gloom' prospects for human beings described in this chapter are not an inevitability, however. The prospects can be improved if elected governments take appropriate action to intervene independently from corporate interests.

FACTS OF LIFE AND DEATH

Where a baby is born and the mother's access to water, food and education determine whether the baby lives or dies. A baby in Sierra Leone has a 72% chance, while a Japanese baby has a 96% chance of reaching the age of 5. Health inequalities have always existed; in this chapter, we examine why.

Each individual human is a creation of genetics, environmental experience and the interaction between the two (see Chapter 3). The environment can be broken down into macro and micro levels. The macro-social environment affects health and well-being in a huge variety of ways. The term **macro-social** refers to large-scale social, economic, political and cultural forces that influence the life course of masses of people simultaneously. Macro-social influences include actions and policies of governmental organizations, non-governmental organizations (NGOs), cultures, historical legacies, organized religions, multinational corporations and banks, and unpredictable, large-scale environmental events, all of which have the potential to influence huge sectors of the entire human race.

First, devastating 'acts of God' can have severe consequences for individuals and communities. The short- and long-term health impacts of these events are moderated by international readiness to respond, and Interdisciplinary Emergency Response Teams can ameliorate the impact of natural disaster and extreme weather events. Microblogging on Twitter and other social media is helpful in expediting rapid disaster response (Tapia et al., 2013).

Second, a variety of pandemics that spread across continents include typhoid, cholera, avian flu (Shinya et al., 2006), influenza (Karademas et al., 2013; Mo and Lau, 2014; Flowers et al., 2016), COVID-19 (Matias, Dominski, & Marks, 2020) and HIV infection (Pellowski et al., 2013; Rohleder, 2016).

Third, the scourges of war, genocide, sectarian violence and terrorism take a significant toll, with multiple deaths, injuries and trauma (De Jong and Kleber, 2007; Medeiros, 2007; Ciccone et al., 2008; Maguen et al., 2010; Zerach et al., 2013).

Fourth, the legacies of colonial genocide take centuries to heal. Indigenous 'First Nation' communities have consistently disproportionate rates of psychiatric distress that are associated with historical experiences of European colonization (Gone, 2013). Aboriginal children experience a greater burden of ill health compared with other children, and these health inequities have persisted for hundreds of years (Greenwood and de Leeuw, 2012).

Fifth, human recklessness with fossil fuels is causing global warming, climate change, rising sea temperatures, acid rain, coral bleaching, global dimming, ozone depletion, biodiversity loss and rising water levels, all transforming life on this planet as we know it (Pearce, 2009).

Sixth, the use of fossil fuels is peaking and, as oil and gas reserves run out, have become more costly; the world economy could go into decline, with significantly decreased agriculture and food production (Murphy and Hall, 2011; Pfeiffer, 2013).

Seventh, increasing poverty makes life a struggle for survival for a billion people. In spite of progress, almost 870 million people were chronically undernourished in 2010–12, the majority living in developing countries, where 850 million people, or 15% of the population, were estimated to be undernourished (Food and Agriculture Orgwanization, 2012).

Eighth, lack of clean drinking water is a major cause of suffering, disease and early deaths: 3.4 million people die each year from a water-related disease, with 780 million people lacking access to clean drinking water; 2.5 billion people have no access to a toilet (water.org, 2014: http://bit.ly/1aa4eri).

The message of this chapter is summarized thus: what individuals can do to change their lives is not simply a matter of personal choice – such changes are constrained politically, economically and culturally. In the globalized economy, everything is interconnected. Macro-social economic, political and cultural factors create the context for everything else, including health, illness and health care.

POLICY, IDEOLOGY AND DISCOURSE

The dominant discourse within neoliberal health policy has been that of the autonomous individual, in which each individual is an agent, responsible for his/her own health. The ideology of *individualism* dictates that each person is motivated by self-interest to elevate his/her well-being with the least effort and resources possible. Deep within the ideological substratum of modern culture lurks the credo of individualism – 'each man for himself' – making his/her choices, and taking the consequences, as in: 'You made your bed, now lie in it.' Theories in health psychology are imbued with this cultural presumption. The existential truth of 'do or die' is embellished in polite language as 'making informed choices'.

The cult of the individual has spawned the notion of the **responsible consumer** (RC). The RC is an active processor of information and knowledge concerning health and illness. He/she makes rational decisions and responsible choices to optimize well-being. The epitome of the RC is the hypothecated 'anything in moderation' person who eats five-a-day, never smokes, drinks alcohol in moderation, exercises vigorously for at least 30 minutes three times a week, always uses a condom when having sex, and sleeps eight hours a day. The stereotype of the more common 'irresponsible consumer' (IC) is the so-called 'couch potato' who enjoys beer and cola, smokes, eats junk food, watches TV for many hours each day, and rarely takes exercise. Accordingly, responsibility for illness relating to personal lifestyle is seen as the fault of the individual, not an inevitable facet of a social, corporate, economic environment designed to maximize shareholder profits.

Using a mixture of well-intentioned pleading, information and advice, the traditional approach to health education aimed to persuade people to change their habits and lifestyles. Information campaigns designed to sway consumers into healthier living were the order of the day. Combined with policy and taxation, health education justifiably can claim some limited success over the last 50 years, e.g., the fall in lung cancer rates. Tobacco control has become a benchmark for what may be achieved through consistent public policy, educational campaigns and behaviour change. A major public health call today is for a vigorous campaign to halt the obesity epidemic. If similar methods are deployed to those used for tobacco (i.e., voluntary controls, advertising restrictions, product labelling, health education), then the evidence suggests that it could take at least 50–70 years before obesity rates can be expected to go into any noticeable decline (Marks, 2016b).

In recent decades, appealing to the right-minded 'anything in moderation' consumer has been prevalent throughout health care. The prescription to live well has always had a distinctively moral tone. Health promotion policy has been portrayed as a quasi-religious quest, a war against the deadly old sins of gluttony, laziness and lust. Discourse analysis of public health policy statements makes this fact all too clear (Sykes et al., 2004).

The demise of the construct of the RC is imminent within health policy. Common observation and decades of research show that people are really pushed and pulled in different directions while exercising their 'freedom of choice'. Emotions and feelings are as important in making choices as cognition. The beneficial satisfaction of needs and wants must be balanced against perceived risks and costs. Health policy is beginning to acknowledge both the complexity of health and the power of the market. Human activity is a reflection of the physical, psychosocial and economic environment. The built environment, the sum total of objects placed in the natural world, dramatically influences health. The 'toxic environment' propels people towards unhealthy behaviours, directly causing mortality and illness (Brownell and Fairburn, 1995).

Government policy documents in the UK indicate that the reliance on consumers as responsible decision-makers has been waning, but it remains a primary strategy. The environment and corporations are being given a larger role. In *Healthy Lives, Healthy People: Our Strategy for Public Health in England* (Department of Health, 2010: 29), the government stated:

> 2.29 Few of us consciously choose 'good' or 'bad' health. We all make personal choices about how we live and behave: what to eat, what to drink and how active to be. We all make trade-offs between feeling good now and the potential impact of this on our longer-term health. In many cases, moderation is often the key.
>
> 2.30 All capable adults are responsible for these very personal choices. At the same time, we do not have total control over our lives or the circumstances in which we live. A wide range of factors constrain and influence what we do, both positively and negatively.
>
> 2.31 The government's approach to improving health and wellbeing – relevant to both national and potential local actions – is therefore based on the following actions, which reflect the Coalition's core values of freedom, fairness and responsibility. These are:
>
> * strengthening self-esteem, confidence and personal responsibility;
>
> * positively promoting 'healthier' behaviours and lifestyles; and
>
> * adapting the environment to make healthy choices easier.

In the above policy document, *personal responsibility* remains at the top of the agenda. The statement that 'we do not have total control over our lives or the circumstances in which we live' is a small step forward but, unfortunately, taking two steps back negates this. Only holistic public policies can lower the toxicity of the environment, and to declare otherwise is a cop-out. Yet large corporations are engaged as the new allies of health promotion in the twenty-first century. The UK government enlisted the food industry, including McDonald's and Kentucky Fried Chicken, among other corporations, to help to write policy on obesity, alcohol and diet-related disease (MailOnline, 2010). Processed food and drinks manufacturers, including PepsiCo, Kellogg's, Unilever, Mars and Diageo, were contributors to five 'responsibility deal' networks set up by then Health Secretary Andrew Lansley. In a similar sponsorship arrangement to previous Olympic Games, McDonald's and Coca-Cola sponsored the 2012 London Olympics. This is putting foxes in charge of the hen house!

In the USA there has been a similar shift in thinking: the 'anything in moderation' philosophy of responsible consumption is no longer the principal foundation for public health interventions. *The Surgeon General's Vision for a Healthy and Fit Nation* states:

> Interventions to prevent obesity should focus not only on personal behaviors and biological traits, but also on characteristics of the social and physical environments that offer or limit opportunities for positive health outcomes. Critical opportunities for interventions can occur in multiple settings: home, child care, school, work place, health care, and community. (US Surgeon General, 2010: 5)

In twenty-first-century health care, the opportunities for health psychological interventions to assist within the major settings has never been greater. But one must ask whether the discipline is fit to meet these challenges. Alternative methods must be tried and tested if we are to make in-roads into the massive scale of issues on the public health agenda.

Economic analyses use **gross domestic product (GDP)** as a measure of *output* and, to a degree, an indicator of welfare also (Oulton, 2012). GDP measures the value of goods and services produced for final consumption, private and public, present and future. Across countries, GDP per capita is highly correlated with important social indicators. GDP is positively correlated with life expectancy and negatively correlated with infant mortality and inequality. One of the most traumatic events in anybody's life is the loss of a child, and infant mortality rates might be thought of as a proxy indicator of happiness. Figure 4.1 plots infant mortality against per capita GDP for a large sample of countries. The graph shows that richer countries tend to have greater life expectancy, lower infant mortality and lower inequality. As always, it is important to state that correlation is not necessarily causation, although there is strong evidence that higher GDP per capita leads to improved health (Fogel, 2004).

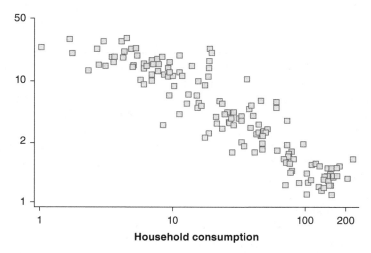

Figure 4.1   Infant mortality versus household consumption per head across 146 countries

Source: Oulton (2012)

A key component of subjective well-being and quality of life is employment. A strong relationship exists between these factors. Unemployment brings stigma, lowered self-esteem and mental health problems, especially depression and feelings of low self-worth (Warr et al., 1988). In some cultures, for example in Japan, a particularly strong correlation exists between the suicide rate and unemployment rate among men (Chen et al., 2012). Under a blanket of statistics lies a multitude of individual calamities.

Population growth and the scourges of unhealthy commodities, unemployment, poverty and inequality place their fingerprints over human existence. In charting the macro-social environment for health, we consider the transitions that have accompanied the globalization of unhealthy commodities, population growth and widespread poverty; we briefly discuss inequalities both within and between societies, and the inequities that exist between genders and ethnic groups. In the following chapters, we take up social justice issues in more detail (Chapter 5) and explore the significance of culture (Chapter 6).

EPIDEMIOLOGICAL TRANSITION AND GLOBALIZATION

Epidemiology is concerned with the distribution of disease and death and their determinants and consequences. Diseases can be divided into two broad categories: communicable and non-communicable. Communicable diseases spread from one person to another or from an animal to a person. This spread may happen via airborne viruses or bacteria, but also through blood or other bodily fluid. The terms 'infectious' and 'contagious' are used to describe communicable disease. Major examples are influenza, HIV infection, hepatitis, polio, malaria and tuberculosis. Non-communicable, or chronic, diseases are generally diseases of long duration and have a slow progression. Major examples are cardiovascular diseases (e.g., heart attacks and stroke), cancer, chronic respiratory diseases (e.g., chronic obstructed pulmonary disease and asthma) and diabetes. Non-communicable diseases (NCDs) are currently the leading cause of death in the world, representing 63% of all annual deaths (World Health Organization, 2014b). NCDs kill at least 36 million people each year, some 80% of which occur in low- and middle-income countries.

Omran (1971) described what he termed the **'epidemiological transition'**. This refers to a reduction in prevalence of communicable diseases and an increase in the prevalence of NCDs that occur as a country becomes economically stronger. NCDs are lifestyle-related chronic diseases that accompany increased usage of unhealthy commodities such as alcohol, tobacco and processed foods. During this transition, countries that have low or middle incomes face a heavy burden from both communicable and non-communicable diseases. In industrial countries such as the USA, Germany, the UK and Japan, the prevalence of communicable diseases is much lower compared to chronic NCDs. In India, and other low- and middle-income countries, while communicable diseases are still present, the rise of NCDs has been rapid (Anjana et al., 2011). Low- and middle-income countries like India, therefore, are currently facing an epidemiological transition with a 'double burden' of disease.

The major driver of the transition towards widespread prevalence of NCDs is corporate globalization. From the point of view of human health, **globalization** flies a banner of progress and freedom yet brings illness and an early death to millions of people. Transnational corporations are indeed the major drivers of NCD 'pandemics' as they scale up their promotion of, and huge profits from, tobacco, alcoholic and other beverages, ultra-processed food and other unhealthy commodities throughout low- and middle-income countries.

Stuckler et al. (2012) observed that the sales of unhealthy commodities across 80 low- and middle-income countries are strongly interrelated. They argue (see Figure 4.2) that:

> in countries where there are high rates of tobacco and alcohol consumption, there is also a high intake of snacks, soft drinks, processed foods, and other unhealthy food commodities. The correlations of these products with unhealthy foods suggest they share underlying risks associated with the market and regulatory environment. (Stuckler et al., 2012: 3)

Referring to these data, Moodie et al. (2013: 670) argued in *The Lancet* that:

> Alcohol and ultra-processed food and drink industries are using similar strategies to the tobacco industry to undermine effective public health policies and programmes.

Unhealthy commodity industries should have no role in the formation of national or international policy for non-communicable-disease policy.

Despite the common reliance on industry self-regulation and public–private partnerships to improve public health, there is no evidence to support their effectiveness or safety.

In view of the present and predicted scale of NCD epidemics, the only evidence-based mechanisms that can prevent harm caused by unhealthy commodity industries are public regulation and market intervention.

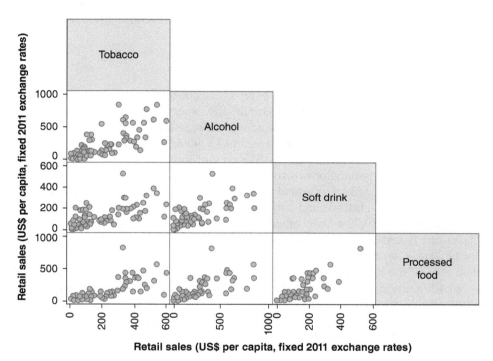

Figure 4.2   Associations of sales of tobacco, alcohol, soft drink and processed food markets, 80 countries, 2010

Source: Stuckler et al. (2012)

POPULATION GROWTH

The US Census Bureau (2017) publishes online a continuous, second-by-second update of the world's population on its website (https://www.census.gov/popclock/). According to the Bureau, the total world population, at 05:07 GMT on 28 October 2017, was 7,430, 555, 770. That figure was increasing at *a rate of 2.4 extra people every second*. By 2025 there will be 8 billion people on Earth.

Dividing the globe into regions, the most populous region is China. With 1.379 billion people in 2017, China contains 19% of all people on Earth. The second most populous country is India, with 1.282 billion in 2017. It is expected that India's population will surpass China's, with around 1.5 billion by 2040. Fertility is falling in most of the developing world but there is a huge variation between countries.

One intervention for population growth, birth control, is practised in many countries. However, religious edicts influence sexual and reproductive practices, leading to population growth. This issue is difficult to ignore. Consider the position of the Roman Catholic Church as one example. The human failure to practise abstinence as the *only* acceptable method for birth control in South America and Africa is adding to population growth, poverty and the spread of HIV infection. Fertility is highest in sub-Saharan Africa, the poorest region in the world where the prevalence of AIDS is maximal. Birth control is also cheaper than other methods of reducing carbon emissions (Wire, 2009). Failing to prevent unwanted births increases the population and causes poverty and malnutrition, and the physical climate becomes more unstable.

INCREASING LIFE EXPECTANCY

Life expectancy has been increasing almost everywhere due to dramatic decreases in infant and adult mortality from infectious diseases. In Britain, life expectancy is currently around 75 years for men and 80 years for women. Life expectancy is increasing by three months every year in developed countries. If life expectancy increases to 85, 90 or even 100, social, health and pension systems will be difficult to maintain in their present form.

The age profile of any population is displayed as a '**population pyramid**', in which numbers in each age group are plotted on a vertical axis. In the UK, the number of people older than 85 is increasing dramatically. Inflows and outflows suggest that by 2050 the UK will be the largest country in Europe. In 2050, like many other places, the country will be both crowded and warm.

China has the fastest-changing demographic profile in the world, with the largest population of senior citizens. Currently, China has more than 130 million senior citizens aged above 60, more than 10% of the total population. By the middle of this century senior citizens in China will exceed 400 million, one-quarter of the total population. There will be a significant shift in the demographic profile of the Chinese population between 2010 and a projection for 2050. The population pyramids show the ageing process is changing China's pyramid, with much larger segments in the higher age brackets.

POVERTY

Of 7.2 billion people alive in 2014, approximately 5 billion (70%) live in so-called 'developing' countries, i.e., low- and middle-income countries, the word 'developing' being a polite euphemism for 'poor'. **Poverty**, by whatever name, exists on a massive scale: 1 billion to 1.5 billion people live on less than US$1.25 per day – i.e., more than one person in every five. For them, clean drinking water, flushing toilets, health services and modern medicines are completely out of reach. Initiatives that have attempted to improve the health of people in extreme poverty mostly have failed.

The UN Development Programme defined poverty as 'a level of income below that people cannot afford a minimum, nutritionally adequate diet and essential non-food requirements' (United Nations Development Programme, 1995). Half of the world's population lacks regular access to medical care and most essential drugs. International organizations such as the UN state with some justification that poverty is the greatest cause of ill health and early mortality.

The health effects of poverty are tangible and the biological and economic mechanisms are the same everywhere. The major impacts of poverty on health are caused by the absence of:

- safe water;

- environmental sanitation;

- adequate diet;

- secure housing;

- basic education;

- income-generating opportunities;

- access to medication and health care.

These are familiar themes. The most common health outcomes of poverty are infectious diseases, malnutrition and reproductive hazards (Anand and Sen, 2000). Poverty implies a lack of access to necessary medicines. HIV infection and AIDS provide a good example. A major killer disease is **AIDS (acquired immune deficiency syndrome)**. In 2004, 6 million people living with HIV infection and AIDS in developing countries urgently needed access to highly active antiretroviral therapy (HAART). The World Health Organization (WHO) began the '3 by 5 Initiative' in 2004 when less than 10% of sufferers had access to HAART. The WHO set a target of providing HAART to 3 million people living with HIV infection or AIDS by the end of 2005. The data show that this figure was half met. However, the number of people accessing antiretroviral therapy in low- and middle-income countries has risen, and reached an estimated 6.6 million at the end of 2010. The major barrier to increasing access to HAART is cost. The pharmaceutical industry holds the patents and loses profits if patent rights are relinquished to enable the generic production of HAART medication. Further discussion of HAART can be found in Chapters 8 and 22.

Economic growth refers to the rate of increase in the total production of goods and services within an economy. Such growth increases the capacity of an economy to produce new goods and services, allowing more needs and wants to be satisfied. A growing economy increases employment, and stimulates business enterprise and innovation. Sustained growth is fundamental to the raising of living standards and to providing greater quality of life (QoL). A key concept is **gross national income (GNI)**, which is the monetary value of all goods and services produced in a country over a year. GNI is therefore a useful indicator for measuring growth.

BOX 4.1

INTERNATIONAL EXAMPLE: Reducing poverty in Brazil

The Brazilian economy came under the media spotlight in June 2014 when it hosted the FIFA World Cup. In spite of its anti-hunger programme, protests and strikes in Brazil's cities were a prominent feature of the 2014 World Cup. Life in the favelas was shown in TV documentaries as exotic, entrepreneurial and exciting, in spite of the child prostitution, drug trafficking and

(Continued)

extremely impoverished communities. Graffiti art was used to draw attention to the contradiction between the lavish expenditure on 12 new stadia and the chronic levels of extreme poverty among a large proportion of the Brazilian population.

At the United Nations in 2000, 189 countries adopted the 'Millennium Development Goals', including halving poverty rates by 2015, reducing child mortality, decelerating the growth of AIDS and educating all children. In the early 2000s Brazil was working towards, and expected to reach, these targets using the *Bolsa Família* (family stipend) and *Fome Zero* (zero hunger) programmes (Galindo, 2004). Doctors at a local health clinic in Brazil observed that their patients, who regularly came in with health problems related to poverty, were visiting less often. This can be reasonably attributed to the national, anti-hunger *Fome Zero* (zero hunger) programme that aimed to give every Brazilian at least three meals a day. With one-quarter of Brazil's 170 million people below the poverty line, this goal was a challenge. To date, the government has provided emergency help to 13 million families.

The scheme involved giving 'something for something' by making cash transfers conditional upon regular school attendance, health checks, and participation in vaccination and nutrition programmes. Almost three-quarters of benefits reached the poorest 20% of the population and absolute poverty halved from 21% in 2001 to 11% in 2008 (Hall, 2012). Opinions vary about the success of the programme. Commentators suggested that the Workers' Party gained many extra votes as one consequence of *Bolsa Família*, and also that there was shift in policy towards short-term solutions to poverty rather than long-term investments in health and education (Hall, 2008, 2012).

The production of good population health requires much more than simply providing doctors, nurses and hospital services. Basic economic, educational and environmental foundations need to be put into place. This means that some fairly dramatic economic changes are needed if we are to see health improvements during the twenty-first century. Among these changes, the cancellation of unpaid debts of the poorest countries and trade justice have the potential to bring health improvements to match those of the last 50 years.

A case can be made that health improvements are a necessary precondition of economic growth. This was suggested by the WHO Commission on Macroeconomics and Health. The Commission Report stated: 'in countries where people have poor health and the level of education is low it is more difficult to achieve sustainable economic growth' (World Health Organization, 2002). If current trends continue, health in sub-Saharan Africa will worsen over the next decades. If the Millennium Development Goals are going to have any chance of success in Africa, health must be given a higher priority in development policies. Sub-Saharan Africa contains 34 of the 41 most indebted countries, and the proportion of people living in absolute poverty (on under US$1 per day) is growing. The health of sub-Saharan Africans is among the worst in the world. Consider the following indicators:

Two-thirds of Africans live in absolute poverty.

More than half lack safe water.

A total of 70% are without proper sanitation.

Forty million children are not in primary school.

Infant mortality is 55% higher than in other low-income countries.

Average life expectancy is 51 years.

The incidence of malaria and tuberculosis is increasing.

These figures indicate the very large gaps that exist between the 'haves' and 'have-nots' on the international stage. International debt is a significant factor in poverty. Rich nations will need to honour pledges they have given to cancel debts and establish fair trade to produce reductions in poverty and hunger in Africa.

INEQUALITIES WITHIN A COUNTRY

The existence of health gradients within health care is a universal constant. Many of the determinants of ill health were identified by Edwin Chadwick in his studies of public health in Victorian England: poverty, housing, water, sewerage, the environment, safety and food. In addition, we recognize today that illiteracy, tobacco, AIDS/HIV, immunization, medication and health services are also important (Ferriman, 2007).

Recent studies of the social determinants of health have pinpointed various kinds of inequity. The first of these is based on **socio-economic status (SES)**: people who are higher up the 'pecking order' of wealth, education and status have better health and live longer than those at the lower end of the scale. To illustrate this, Figure 4.3 shows a map of the Jubilee Line, which travels along an east–west axis across London. If you travel eastwards along this tube line from Westminster to Canning Town, the life expectancy of the local population is reduced by one year for every stop.

Health gradients are found in all societies. Wealthier groups always have the best health; poorer groups have the worst health. These differentials occur in both illness and death rates, and health gradients are equally dramatic in both rich and poor countries. The majority of studies have been carried out in rich countries.

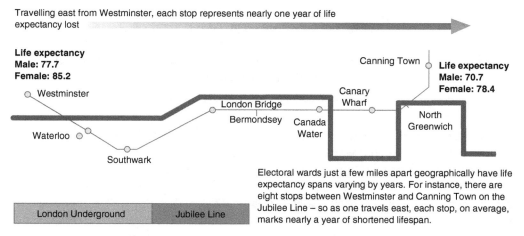

Figure 4.3 Differences in life expectancy within a small area of London

Source: Department of Health (2008)

BOX 4.2

KEY STUDY: The Whitehall studies

The Whitehall studies investigated social class, psychosocial factors and lifestyle as determinants of disease. The first Whitehall study of 18,000 men in the Civil Service was set up in the 1960s. The Whitehall I study showed a clear gradient in which men employed in the lowest grades were much more likely to die prematurely than men in the highest grades.

The Whitehall II study started in 1985 with the aim of determining the causes of the social gradient and also included women, including potential psychological mediators. A total of 10,308 employees participated, two-thirds men and one-third women. The cohort was followed up over time with medical examinations and surveys. Most participants are now retired or approaching retirement.

There have been many phases of data collection, alternating postal self-completion questionnaires with medical screenings and questionnaires. In addition to cardiovascular measures, blood pressure, blood cholesterol, height, weight and ECGs were taken, along with tests of walking, lung function and mental functioning, questions about diet, and diabetes screening.

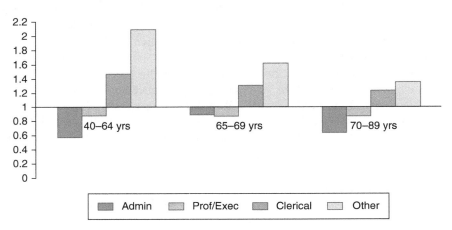

Figure 4.4   Death rates (%) vs. employment grades over a 25-year period in the Whitehall studies

Source: Ferrie (2004). Reproduced with permission

The Whitehall studies found that an imbalance between demands and control lead to illness. Control is less when a worker is lower in the hierarchy and so a worker in a lower position is unable to respond effectively if demands are increased, supporting Karasek and Theorell's (1990) demand–control model. Other mechanisms can buffer the effect of work stress on mental and physical health: **social support** (Stansfeld et al., 2000), **effort–reward balance** (Kuper and Marmot, 2003), **job security** and organizational stability (Ferrie et al., 2002). Figure 4.4 shows the gradient of death rates versus employment grades over a 25-year period in men from the Whitehall studies. The death rate is shown relative to the whole Civil Service population (reproduced from Ferrie, 2004).

Virtanen et al. (2015) examined whether midlife adversity predicts post-retirement depressive symptoms in 3,939 Whitehall II participants (mean age 67.6 years at follow-up). Strong associations occurred between midlife adversities and post-retirement depressive symptoms, including low occupational position, poor standard of living, high job strain and few close relationships. Associations between socio-economic, psychosocial, work-related or non-work-related exposures and depressive symptoms were of similar strength. The data suggest that socio-economic and psychosocial risk factors for symptoms of depression post-retirement can be detected in midlife.

Source: Ferrie (2004)

There are relatively few studies of health gradients in poor countries. The data are cross-sectional rather than longitudinal, but show a similar pattern to those observed with Whitehall civil servants. One of the authors analysed data from the Demographic and Health Surveys (DHS) programme of the World Bank (2002) (Marks, 2004). These are large-scale household sample surveys carried out periodically in 44 countries across Asia, Africa, the Middle East, Latin America and the former Soviet Union. Socio-economic status was evaluated using answers about assets given by the head of each household. The asset score reflected the household's ownership of consumer items ranging from a fan to a television and car, dwelling characteristics such as flooring material, type of drinking water source and toilet facilities used, and other characteristics related to wealth. Each household was assigned a score for each asset and scores were summed for each household; individuals were ranked according to the total score of the household in which they resided. The sample was divided into population wealth quintiles – five groups with the same number of individuals in each.

The gradient of under-5 mortality rates (U5MRs) for 22 countries in sub-Saharan Africa are shown collectively in Figure 4.5. The U5MR indicator is the number of deaths of children under 5 years of age per 1,000 live births. This figure shows gradients in all countries. A wide gap in health outcomes exists between the rich and the poor even within these very poor countries. Similar gradients exist for countries in Latin America and the Caribbean and throughout the 44 countries included in the DHS. Infant mortality is halved between quintiles 1 and 5, representing the poorest of the poor and the wealthiest of the poor.

An interesting set of relationships was observed between the U5MRs, literacy and resources (Marks, 2004). The U5MRs in 44 countries were positively correlated with female illiteracy rates and the proportion of households using bush, field or traditional pit latrines, and negatively correlated with the proportion of households having piped domestic water, national health service expenditure, the number of doctors per 100,000 people, the number of nurses per 100,000 people and immunization rates.

The most important predictors of infant survival are educational and environmental. The most effective long-term structural interventions to combat inequality are to improve the educational opportunities for women and to improve the supply of drinking water. High literacy among mothers and access to water supplies and toilets are highly associated with low infant mortality.

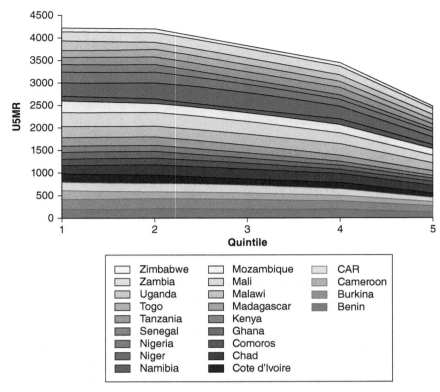

Figure 4.5 Under-5 mortality gradients for sub-Saharan Africa plotted against asset quintile. The area under each line represents the individual country rates. Quintile 1 has the least assets, quintile 5 the most

Source: Marks (2004)

High numbers of doctors and nurses, immunization rates and health service expenditure are associated with lower mortality rates, but these health service variables are less influential, statistically speaking, than literacy, domestic water and sanitation. The latter provide the foundations of good health, while health services are the bricks and mortar.

GENDER

Significant differences exist in health outcomes between men and women. Attitudes have changed a little over the last 100 years. A medical textbook from the nineteenth century stated: 'child-bearing is essentially necessary to the physical health and long life, the mental happiness, the development of the affections and whole character of women. Woman exists for the sake of the womb' (Holbrook, 1880: 13–14; cited in Gallant et al., 1997).

In industrialized societies men die earlier than women, but women generally have poorer health (Macintyre and Hunt, 1997). Men in the USA suffer more severe chronic conditions, have higher death rates for all 15 leading causes of death, and die nearly seven years younger than women (Courtenay, 2000). Similar figures exist in the UK. In 1996, UK males had a life expectancy of 74.4 years compared with 79.7 years for females. This excess mortality of 5.3 years in males in 1996 increased over the course of the twentieth century from only 3.9 years in 1900–1910.

Evidence suggests that from the Paleolithic period to the industrial revolution men lived longer than women, 40 years as compared to 35. Also, in less developed countries (e.g., India, Bangladesh, Nepal and Afghanistan) men still live longer than women (World Health Organization, 1989). To complicate the picture further, the health gradient is steeper for men than for women, while illness rates, treatment rates, absenteeism and prescription drug use are generally higher for women (Macintyre and Hunt, 1997). Women suffer more non-fatal chronic illnesses and more acute illnesses. They also make more visits to their family physicians and spend more time in hospital. Women suffer more from hypertension, kidney disease and auto-immune diseases such as rheumatoid arthritis and lupus (Litt, 1993). They also suffer twice the rate of depression. Men, on the other hand, have a shorter life expectancy, and suffer more injuries, suicides, homicides and heart disease.

Psychosocial and lifestyle differences play a role in gender-linked health differences. In industrialized societies women suffer more from poverty, stress from relationships, childbirth, rape, domestic violence, sexual discrimination, lower status work, concern about weight and the strain of dividing attention between competing roles of parent and worker. Financial barriers may prevent women from engaging in healthier lifestyles and desirable behaviour change (O'Leary and Helgeson, 1997).

Gender is a social construction, and social constructions of masculinity and femininity have relevance in particular to young men's and young women's health-seeking behaviour. The concept of 'hegemonic masculinity' as a locally dominant ideology of masculinity has been a focus of research (Connell, 2005). Hegemonic masculinity includes the demonstration of 'machismo' through the possession of physical and emotional strength, predatory heterosexuality, being a breadwinner and being unafraid of risk. Studies have focused on the health of men, why they suffer more from alcoholism and drug dependency, and why they are so reluctant to seek health from professionals. Gender-specific beliefs and behaviours are likely contributors to these differences (Courtenay, 2000). Men are more likely than women to adopt risky beliefs and behaviours, and less likely to engage in health-protective behaviours that are linked with longevity. Practices that undermine men's health are used to signify masculinity and to negotiate power and status. Social and institutional structures often reinforce the social construction of men as the 'stronger sex'.

One of the cornerstones of masculinity is violence, especially violence against women. This violence cuts across culture and, with only a few exceptions, is a near-universal constant. Kaufman (1987) argues that violence by men against women is one corner of a triad of men's violence. The other two corners are violence against other men and violence against self.

Alternative constructions that subvert normative ideas of masculinity include non-drinking. A study of non-drinkers' discourse examined the manner in which not drinking alcohol is construed in relation to the masculine identity. Three prominent discourses about non-drinking were revealed: (1) as something strange requiring explanation; (2) as simultaneously unsociable yet reflective of greater sociability; and (3) as something with greater negative social consequences for men than for women (Conroy and de Visser, 2013).

Constructions of masculinity extend to young men's help-seeking and health service use online. In one study, 28 young men took part in two online focus groups investigating understandings of health, help-seeking and health service use. Discourse analysis was used to explore the young men's framing of health-related practices. Young men are interested in their health and construct their health practices as justified, while simultaneously maintaining masculine identities surrounding independence, autonomy and control over their bodies (Tyler and Williams, 2014).

ETHNICITY

The health of minority ethnic groups is generally poorer than that of the majority of the population. This pattern has been consistently observed in the USA between African-Americans ('blacks') and Caucasian-Americans ('whites') for at least 150 years (Krieger, 1987). There has been an increase in income inequality in the USA that has been associated with a levelling-off or even a decline in the economic status of African-Americans. The gap in life expectancy between blacks and whites widened between 1980 and 1991 from 6.9 years to 8.3 years for males and from 5.6 years to 5.8 years for females (National Center for Health Statistics, 1994). Under the age of 70, cardiovascular disease, cancer and problems resulting in infant mortality account for 50% of the excess deaths for black males and 63% of the excess deaths for black females (Williams and Collins, 1995). Similar findings exist in other countries. Analyses of three censuses from 1971 to 1991 have shown that people born in South Asia are more likely to die from ischaemic heart disease than the majority of the UK population (Balarajan and Soni Raleigh, 1993).

There are many possible explanations for these persistent health differences between people of different races who live in the same country and are served by the same educational, social, welfare and health care systems (Williams and Collins, 1995; Williams et al., 1997). First, the practice of **racism** means that minority ethnic groups are the subject of discrimination at a number of different levels. Such discrimination could lead directly or indirectly to health problems additional to any effects related to SES, poverty, unemployment and education. Discrimination in the health care system exacerbates the impacts of social discrimination through reduced access to the system and poorer levels of communication resulting from language differences.

Second, **ethnocentrism** in health services and health promotion unofficially favours the needs of majority over minority groups. The health needs of members of minority ethnic groups are less likely to be appropriately addressed in health promotion, which in turn leads to lower adherence and response rates in comparison to the majority population. These problems are compounded by cultural, lifestyle and language differences. For example, if interpreters are unavailable, the treatment process is likely to be improperly understood or even impaired and patient anxiety levels will be raised. The lack of permanent addresses for minority ethnic group families, created by their high mobility, makes communication difficult so that screening invitations and appointment letters are unlikely to be received.

Third, health status differences related to race and **culture** are to a large extent mediated by differences in SES. Studies of race and health generally control for SES, and race-related differences frequently disappear after adjustment for SES. Race is strongly correlated with SES and is even sometimes used as an indicator of SES (Williams and Collins, 1995; Modood et al., 1997).

Fourth, differences in health-protective behaviour may occur because of different cultural or social norms and expectations. Fifth, differences in readiness to recognize symptoms may also occur as a result of different cultural norms and expectations. Sixth, differences can occur in access to services. There is evidence that differential access to optimal treatment may cause poorer survival outcomes in African-Americans who have cancer, in comparison with other ethnic groups (Meyerowitz et al., 1998). Seventh, members of minority ethnic groups are more likely to inhabit and work in unhealthy environments because of their lower SES. Eighth, there are genetic differences between groups that lead to differing incidences of disease, and some diseases are inherited. There are several well-recognized examples, including sickle cell disorder affecting people of African-Caribbean descent; thalassaemia, another blood disorder that affects people of the Mediterranean, Middle Eastern and Asian descent; and Tay–Sachs disease, which affects Jewish people.

Other possible mechanisms underlying **ethnicity** differences in health are differences in personality, early life conditions, power and control, and stress (Williams and Collins, 1995; Taylor et al., 1997). Research is needed with large community samples so that the influence of the above variables and the possible interactions between them can be determined. Further research is needed to explore the barriers to access to health care that exist for people from different groups. We will return to this topic in other chapters.

FUTURE RESEARCH

1. The causes of poverty and interventions to ameliorate poverty should be *the* priority for economic and social policy and research.

2. Studies in psychology and sociology are necessary to understand humanitarian values, altruism, oppression, fear, aggression and cross-cultural issues.

3. Possible mechanisms underlying ethnicity differences in health, such as differences in early life conditions, racism, power, control and stress, must be explored.

4. Research is needed with large community samples so that the influence of the above variables and their possible interactions can be determined.

SUMMARY

1. The world population is increasing dramatically. From 1 billion in 1800, it is expected to climb to 9 billion by 2050, while the amount of drinkable water available per person over the same period will fall by 33%. The increasing shortage will affect mainly the poor in countries where water shortage is already chronic. Conflict about water will become as prominent as the conflict about oil today.
2. The consumption of tobacco, alcohol, ultra-processed food, drink and other unhealthy commodities is increasing throughout the low- and middle-income countries and is driving a huge increase in the prevalence of non-communicable diseases.
3. The greatest influence on health for the majority of people is poverty. Half of the world's population lacks regular access to treatment of common diseases and most essential drugs. Globally, the burden of death and disease is much heavier for the poor than for the wealthy.

(Continued)

4. In developed countries, life expectancy is increasing by three months every year. If this trend continues, life expectancy will approach 100 years by 2060, placing social, health and pension systems in a perilous position.
5. Economic growth does not reduce disparities in wealth across a society. 'Trickle-down' is a myth. Health gradients remain a universal feature of the health of populations in both rich and poor countries.
6. Gender differences in health, illness and mortality are significant and show striking interactions with culture, history and socio-economic status.
7. The health of minority ethnic groups is generally poorer than that of the majority of the population. Possible explanations include racial discrimination, ethnocentrism, SES differences, behavioural and personality differences, cultural differences and other factors.
8. 'Doom and gloom' is not inevitable. Prospects can significantly improve if policy makers intervene. The future health of populations depends upon actions taken by governments, corporations and opinion leaders supported by improved education about the social, political and economic determinants of health and illness.

SOCIAL JUSTICE

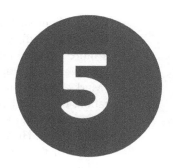

'To love life is to risk it,

to live it fully

means being ready always

to lose it

giving it over entirely to solidarity.'

Miguel D'Escoto Brockmann (1933–2017)

OUTLINE

There is substantial evidence linking poor social conditions with ill health. The explanations for this include material, behavioural and psychosocial factors. In this chapter we consider health inequalities in the context of social justice, the competing explanations and the role of health psychologists in creating a healthier society. The explanation of health inequalities creates many important challenges for theory and research in health psychology.

SOCIAL INEQUALITIES AND HEALTH

As shown in Chapter 4, substantial evidence from dozens of countries has linked social inequalities with health. Consistently, these studies show that people of lower **socio-economic status (SES)** have more illness and lower longevity than those in higher socio-economic groups. There is a gradient such that those one step down the ladder are unhealthier than those above. This persistent gradient is often referred to as a '**health gradient**'. When mortality is the measure, a more apposite term would be 'mortality' or '**death gradient**'. 'Death gradients' have been observed in all human societies in both rich/developed countries and poor/developing countries (Marks, 2004). Such gradients are normally continuous throughout the range of economic variation. If the gradient were stepped or flat at one end of the range and steep at the other, it could be inferred that the causative mechanism(s) had a threshold value before any of the 'ill-effects' could appear. However, there is no evidence of such thresholds; the gradient is a continuous one.

One of the earliest reports on the health gradient was by the French physician Louis-René Villermé (1782–1863) who, in the 1820s, examined the health of residents in different neighbourhoods of Paris. From a careful review of the data, Villermé concluded that there was a relationship between the wealth of the neighbourhood and the health of its residents. Those living in the poorer neighbourhoods had a higher death rate, and military conscripts from those neighbourhoods were smaller and had more illnesses and disabilities (Krieger and Davey Smith, 2004). Shortly afterwards, Friedrich Engels published his classic work on *The Condition of the Working Class in England in 1844* (Engels, 1845/1958). This book provided a detailed description of the appalling conditions and the limited health care of working-class residents of Manchester.

When Engels compared death rates within the city he found that they were much higher in the poorer districts. Further, he realized the importance of early development and noted: 'common observation shows how the sufferings of childhood are indelibly stamped on the adults' (1845/1958: 115). Although these early researchers realized the importance of the impact of adverse social conditions, interest in the social aspects of health was marginalized with the rise of germ theory and the growth of **Social Darwinism** and eugenics (e.g. Krieger and Davey-Smith, 2004). The former theory focused on controlling specific pathogens rather than social reform, whereas the second argued that innate inferiority, not social injustice, was the cause of ill health (see also Chapter 3). However, the growth of social movements in the 1960s rekindled interest in social justice.

The foundation of the National Health Service (NHS) in the UK in 1947 was an attempt to remove inequalities that existed in health care provision. Health services were provided for all – free at the point of delivery. Titmuss (1968: 196) observed, after 15 years' experience of the NHS, that the higher income groups:

> know how to make better use of the service; they tend to receive more specialist attention; occupy more of the beds in better equipped and staffed hospitals; receive more elective surgery, have better maternal care, and are more likely to get psychiatric help and psychotherapy than low-income groups – particularly the unskilled.

These continued disparities led Tudor Hart (1971) to describe the 'inverse care law': the availability of good medical care tends to vary inversely with the need for the population served.

In 1977 the UK government established a working group to further investigate social inequalities in health. The subsequent **Black Report** (Townsend and Davidson, 1982), named after Sir Douglas Black, the working group's chair, summarized the evidence on the relationship between occupation and health. It showed that those classified as unskilled manual workers (Social class V) consistently had poorer health status compared with those classified as professionals (Social class I). Further, the report graphically portrayed an inverse relationship between mortality and occupational rank for both sexes and at all ages. A class 'gradient' was also observed for most causes of death, particularly respiratory, infective and parasitic diseases. Inequalities in terms of utilization of health care, especially among preventive services, were also apparent.

In a follow-up study, similar trends persisted in the 1980s as social inequalities in health continued to widen (Townsend et al., 1992). As discussed in Chapter 4, the Whitehall studies provided supporting evidence on the relationship between SES and health. As Marmot and Allen (2014: S517) explained:

> To reduce health inequalities requires action to reduce socioeconomic and other inequalities. There are other factors that influence health, but these are outweighed by the overwhelming impact of social and economic factors—the material, social, political, and cultural conditions that shape our lives and our behaviours [...] In fact, so close is the link between social conditions and health, that the magnitude of health inequalities is an indicator of the impact of social and economic inequalities on people's lives. Health then becomes an important further cause for concern about the rapid increase in inequalities of wealth and income in our societies. Increasingly, we are using the language of health inequity to describe those health inequalities that, though avoidable, are not avoided and hence are unfair.

Tackling health inequalities is not just about combatting the growing social inequalities, but also about understanding and addressing the material, behavioural and psychosocial pathways by which these inequalities impact health.

In understanding and dealing with health inequalities, it is important to recognize all determinants of health – from micro to macro levels – and to consider how many of these are within the control of individuals in society. The idea of capabilities is related to the actual freedom and rights enjoyed by people (Sen, 1999). In this respect, freedom does not only entail one's freedom to choose; rather, it also involves freedom from the barriers that restrain people from reaching their fullest human potential. Only when individuals have the 'capability' to exert control over the factors that influence their health can they truly exercise their 'right to health'. The vast levels of social inequalities pose serious questions regarding the capacity of individuals to exercise their human rights. The emergence of new centres of power extends the issue to the international scale where the capacity of nation states to protect and promote their citizens' right to health is also being threatened.

The Acheson Report (1998) outlined recommendations to address health and social inequalities in the UK. In 2008, the WHO Global Commission on the Social Determinants of Health published a report to address health equity by taking action regarding the social determinants of health. In the same year, the Scottish government (2008) published the *Equally Well* report, which provided substantial evidence on the relationship between health and socio-economic deprivation in Scotland. The UK government commissioned Sir Michael Marmot to review current trends and to propose the most effective evidence-based strategies to reduce health inequalities in England. In 2010, Marmot's report entitled *Fair Society, Healthy Lives* recognized the reduction of health inequalities as a matter of fairness and social justice (Marmot, 2013). The report underlined that solely focusing action on the most disadvantaged would be inadequate. Fair distribution of health, well-being and sustainability are more important measures of success than economic growth. As expressed in the final report of the Commission on Social Determinants of Health, inequities in power, money and resources were to blame for many of the inequities in health within and between countries.

In order to address inequities in health effectively, cross-government commitment to action is needed across all of the social determinants of health (for more details see http://www.institu-teofhealthequity.org and https://www.podsocs.com/podcast/health-inequalities).

EXPLANATIONS FOR SOCIAL INEQUALITIES IN HEALTH

Health inequalities can be considered from an **ecological approach** or **systems theory approach**. Bronfenbrenner's (1979) ecological approach conceptualized developmental influences in terms of four nested systems:

microsystems: families, schools, neighbourhoods;

mesosystems: peer groups;

exosystems: parental support systems, parental workplaces;

macrosystems: political philosophy, social policy.

These systems form a nested set, like a set of Russian dolls: microsystems within mesosystems, mesosystems within exosystems and exosystems within macrosystems.

Ecological theory assumes that human development can only be understood in reference to the structural ecosystems. The 'Health Onion', a general systems framework for understanding the determinants of health and illness, was presented in Chapter 1 (Figure 1.5). Of key importance is the *perceived environment*, not the so-called 'objective' environment. In Box 5.1 we list some of the characteristics of low SES using Bronfenbrenner's (1979) systems approach. The box shows the many different disadvantages across all four systems of the social, physical and economic environment. In addition, we can add the high levels of perceived injustice that many people with low SES may feel.

SCIENTIFIC EXPLANATIONS

Any explanation of the SES–health gradient needs to consider psychosocial systems that structure inequalities across a broad range of life opportunities and outcomes – health, social and educational. As illustrated in Box 5.1, in comparison to someone at the high end of the SES scale, the profile of a low SES person is one of multiple disadvantages. The disadvantages of low SES accumulate across all four ecosystems. It is this kind of *accumulation* and *clustering* of adverse physical, material, social and psychological effects that could explain the health gradient. While each factor alone can be expected to produce a relatively modest impact on mortality, the combination and interaction of many kinds of ecosystem disadvantage are likely to be sufficiently large to generate the observed gradient. The socio-economic conditions that contribute to the health gradient can also be experienced by individuals across the life course (Pavalko and Caputo, 2013).

While the Black Report (Townsend and Davidson, 1982) clearly documented the link between social position and health, it also detailed four possible explanations for health inequalities:

An artefact: the relationships between social position are an artefact of the method of measurement.

Natural and social selection: the social gradient in health is due to those who are already unhealthy falling downwards while those who are healthy rise upwards.

Materialist and structuralist explanations: emphasize the role of economic and socio-structural factors.

Cultural and/or behavioural differences: 'often focus on the individual as the unit of analysis emphasizing unthinking, reckless or irresponsible behaviour or incautious lifestyle as the moving determinant' (Townsend and Davidson, 1982: 23).

BOX 5.1

Behaviours and experiences associated with low SES

Microsystems: families, schools, neighbourhoods

Low birthweight

Family instability

Poor diet/nutrition

Parental smoking and drinking

Overcrowding

Poor schools and educational outcomes

Poor neighbourhoods

Mesosystems: peer groups

Bullying, gangs and violence

Smoking

Drinking

Drugs

Unprotected sex

Exosystems: parental support systems, parental workplaces

Low personal control

Less social support

Unemployment or unstable employment

(Continued)

High stress levels

Low self-esteem

Poorer physical and mental health

Macrosystems: political philosophy, social policy

Poverty

Poor housing

Environmental pollution

Unemployment or unstable employment

Occupational hazards

Poorer access to health services

Inadequate social services

While accepting that each explanation may contribute something, the report emphasized the importance of the materialist explanations and developed a range of policy options that could address the inequalities. Contemporary research into explanations for social inequalities in health has been reviewed by Macinko et al. (2003). Their classification extends the four-fold explanation developed in the Black Report.

Psychosocial explanations are considered at the individual (micro) and social (macro) levels. At the micro level, it is argued that 'cognitive processes of comparison', in particular perceived relative deprivation, contribute to heightened levels of stress and subsequent ill health. Additionally, the Whitehall studies suggested that it was the lack of perceived control over working conditions that increases stress at the lower end of the social scale. At the macro level, psychosocial explanations focus on the impairment of social bonds and limited civic participation, so-called social capital (see below), that flows from income inequality.

The **neo-material explanations** have drawn increased support in critiques of the psychosocial approaches (see Macleod and Davey Smith, 2003; Marks, 2004; Stephens, 2014). They focus on the importance of income and living conditions. At the micro level, it is argued that in more unequal societies those worse off have fewer economic resources, leading to increased vulnerability to various health threats. At the macro level, high income inequality contributes to less investment in the social and physical environment. In addition, it has been argued that sustained exposure to stress from various sources, including financial hardships and poor living conditions, can have adverse biological effects and subsequently lead to various health problems (Taylor et al., 1997). Those who favour the neo-material explanations argue that the psychosocial explanations ignore the broad political context within which social and health inequalities are nested.

There are also the artefact and selection explanations of the social inequalities in health. Although these initially attracted attention, there is less support for these arguments today.

Contemporary research has focused on the relationship between the extent of social inequality in a particular society and the extent of ill health. Wilkinson (1996) argued that health was poorer in more unequal societies. In their book *The Spirit Level*, Wilkinson and Pickett (2010) provided a comprehensive analysis of the empirical association that exists between health/social problems and inequality among rich countries. For example, higher infant mortality rates were shown in countries where income inequality is high. The same index of health/social problems was found to be only very weakly related to national income but strongly related to inequality. Wilkinson and Pickett (2010) hypothesized that the structural inequality in society causes people to become more anxious, stressed, ashamed, untrusting and unhappy. In the same year that *The Spirit Level* was published, the Equality Trust (https://www.equalitytrust.org.uk/) was founded by the authors and Bill Kerry. This charity aims to develop and promote policies to reduce social inequalities.

Torre and Myrskylä (2014) examined the relationship between income inequality and health using data from 21 developed countries over a 30-year period. Findings suggested that income inequality was positively related to the mortality of males and females at ages 1–14 and 15–49 years. The positive correlation between income inequality and mortality of females was also found at ages 65–89 years, although this relationship was weaker than for the younger age groups. These findings suggest that narrowing the income inequality gap may be an effective way to promote health, especially among children and young to middle-aged groups. However, we need to remember, once again, that correlation does not mean causation. As previously argued, the relationship between income inequality and health is not as straightforward as was initially conjectured (Lynch et al., 2004). However, as Lynch and Davey Smith (2002) also warned, we should be careful not to throw the 'social inequality baby' out with the 'income inequality bathwater'. There is much more to social inequality than inequality of income.

SOCIAL JUSTICE

Critics of research into social inequalities in health often charge that social inequalities are an inevitable part of life and are also necessary for social progress. An alternative perspective is to consider not simply inequalities *per se* but inequities in health. According to Dahlgren and Whitehead (1991), health inequalities can be considered as inequities when they are avoidable, unnecessary and unfair. The issue of fairness leads us to consider the issue of **social justice**.

A useful starting point is the theory of 'justice as fairness' developed by the moral philosopher John Rawls (1999). He identified certain underlying principles of a just society, as follows:

> Assure people equal basic liberties, including guaranteeing the right of political participation.
>
> Provide a robust form of equal opportunity.
>
> Limit inequalities to those that benefit the least advantaged.

Daniels et al. (2000) argued that adhering to these principles would address the basic social inequalities in health. They detailed a series of implications for social organization that flow from the acceptance of these principles. First, assuring people equal basic liberties implies that everyone has an equal right to fully participate in politics. In turn, this will contribute to improvements in health since, according to social capital theory, political participation is an important determinant of health.

Second, providing measures actively to promote equal opportunities implies the introduction of measures to reduce socio-economic inequalities and other social obstacles to equal opportunities. Such measures would include comprehensive childcare and childhood interventions to combat any disadvantages of family background (Daniels et al., 2000). They would also include comprehensive health care for all, including support services for those with disabilities.

Finally, a just society would allow only those inequalities in income and wealth that would benefit the least advantaged. This requires direct challenge to the contemporary neoliberal philosophy that promotes the maximization of profit and increasing the extent of social inequality. A Framework Convention on Global Health (FCGH) grounded in the human right to health could help to reconstruct global governance for health and offer a new vision post-Millennium Development Goals (Gostin and Friedman, 2013).

To an increasing extent, psychological organizations have been recognizing the links between poor social conditions and physical and mental health. Somewhat belatedly, they are catching up with Villermé's and Engels' findings from the 1840s. But why is awareness of social justice issues among the psychology profession so slow in the making? The American Psychological Association was founded in 1892, but it took more than 100 years for the Association to pass a resolution on 'Poverty and Socio-economic Status' in the year 2000. The resolution called for a programme of research on the causes and impact of poverty, negative attitudes towards people living in poverty, strategies to reduce poverty, and the evaluation of anti-poverty programmes. The resolution has been followed by a few new initiatives, including interventions facilitated by critical and community health psychologists (see Chapter 16). A special issue on poverty reduction was published in the *Journal of Health Psychology* in October 2010.

Much more could be achieved if psychologists were more willing to engage with social justice issues 'in their own backyards'. Shamefully, in our opinion, societies like the British Psychological Society (BPS) have maintained a stance of neutrality on the grounds that the society is a charity and that it is prohibited from engaging in political issues. But times are changing. At the 2017 Annual Conference, the outgoing President Peter Kinderman delivered an address entitled 'Psychology is action, not thinking about oneself' (Kinderman, 2017). In this he called on psychologists 'to speak out about those social, economic and political circumstances that impact on our clients and the general public, and to bring such evidence to politicians and policy makers'. More recently the BPS agreed that a priority for research and practice should be poverty and ways of addressing it (https://www.bps.org.uk/blogs/chief-executive/focus-poverty). Social justice isn't simply a political issue; it is a life and death issue, affecting the mental and physical well-being of billions of people. It is a problem that is too important to leave to politicians. It affects everybody; everybody can do something towards creating a more just society.

A focus on individual change to the neglect of the broader social determinants of health and illness accepts the status quo instead of challenging it and only leads to victim blaming. There is a need for what Horrocks and Johnson (2014) have described as a 'socially-situated' approach to promoting health and preventing illness. The continued focus on individual behaviour-change strategies reflects powerful ideological interests (Braun and Fisher, 2013). Health psychologists can challenge the current dominant neoliberal ideology through, for example, aligning with popular health movements for change (e.g., People's Health Movement, 2000).

THE UNIVERSAL RIGHT TO HEALTH

Justice is about rights and freedoms. People talk about rights and freedoms of different kinds, e.g., the freedom of expression, the right to vote, having equal rights, and so on. 'Human rights' refers to the fundamental moral and legal social norms necessary for people to live a minimally good life. Every individual is entitled to human rights simply because that person is human. International declarations and legal conventions have been issued by governments and international organizations to ensure that such rights are respected and protected. The Universal Declaration of Human Rights (UDHR) is an example of an international standard that outlines our most basic human rights (United Nations General Assembly, 1948). It affirms that all human beings are 'born free and equal in dignity and rights' (Article 1). These rights are universal and indiscriminate of 'race, color, sex, language, religion, political or other opinion, national or social origin, property, birth or other status' (Article 2).

Can we talk about rights to health in a similar way? In 1946, the World Health Organization first expressed the right to health as a fundamental human right. Although not legally binding, the UDHR two years later provided the foundation for succeeding laws and policies adopted by governing bodies and states around the world. It is formed of 30 articles consisting of the most comprehensive statements concerning human rights and includes security, liberty, political, equality, economic and social rights. In particular, Article 25 affirmed the human right to a standard of living for adequate health and well-being through the provision of food, clothing, housing, and medical and social services. The promotion and protection of these rights are prerequisites to a dignified, free and secure way of living.

The right to health is intricately linked with other civil liberties and freedoms. To illustrate this link, it is worth considering the effects of human rights violations on the health and well-being of its victims. Just think of the consequences of ethnic cleansing, slavery, war, genocide and other forms of social aggression and cruelty. The histories of countries such as the USA and the UK and other European powers show many well-known examples of these kinds of abuses. These crimes against humanity reflect how violations of human rights can lead to debilitating consequences for the physical, psychological and social well-being of others. As shown in Box 5.2, the development of effective interventions in the context of violence and conflict need to take into account historical and psychosocial factors that influence health and well-being.

BOX 5.2

INTERNATIONAL CASE STUDY: Using a psychosocial and participatory approach to health in the context of violence and conflict

Background

While several studies have been conducted to explore the relationship between health and physical activity, most of these have been conducted in Western contexts. In communities where violence and conflict are prevalent, it is important to also consider the impact of

(Continued)

historical and socio-cultural factors and the prevailing incidence of racism, violence, sexual abuse and discrimination experienced by community members.

The programme

The project described by Ley and Rato Barrio (2013) was called *Acción Psicosocial a través del Movimiento, Juego y Deporte* (Psychosocial Action through Movement, Play and Sport). This project was based in a rural area of Guatemala with two groups of women who had suffered from violence. It used a psychosocial and participatory approach to develop the use of sports and games as educational and therapeutic tools. The methods of movement, games and sports used in the project included *physical* (e.g., progressively increased physical activity of middle–low intensity, stretching and relaxation exercises) and *psychosocial and educative activities* (e.g., cooperative games, modified sports, role-play, verbalization of experiences and perceptions). A mixed method approach was used combining questionnaires, participatory observation and interviews to examine the effectiveness of the programme in promoting health.

Findings

Quantitative findings reflected improvements in a sense of coherence and self-esteem among participants. Results suggest that the programme provided opportunities for women who suffered from violence to socialize and offer mutual support. Modified sport, games and participatory group activities that were conducted in an active and enjoyable way also facilitated group interaction. By enabling participants to share their experiences of violence and domestic conflicts in a safe and protective space, they were able to express their feelings and to explore potential solutions with others. This process contributed to mutual learning and enabled participants to reconstruct their perceptions of the world and to reflect on how their circumstances could be improved.

Conclusion

Using a psychosocial and culturally grounded use of games and sports as participatory tools may be useful in promoting health in the context of violence and conflict.

Source: Ley and Rato Barrio (2013)

People with poor health may also suffer from an increased vulnerability to human rights violations due to their fragile state. The stigma associated with their condition may increase their vulnerability to discrimination and maltreatment, as discussed below.

STIGMA

Stigma refers to unfavourable reactions towards people when they are perceived to possess attributes that are denigrated. Stigmatization is universal; it is found in all cultures throughout history. The majority of people will experience it at some time, as both the young and the elderly are stigmatized groups. In addition, people can be multiply stigmatized, as in the case of HIV infection and AIDS, which is associated with certain highly stigmatized groups (e.g., homosexuals, sex workers, intravenous drug users) and adds a further source of stigma as well as intensifying existing stigma(s) (see Chapter 22). Stigma involves a pattern of discrediting, discounting, degradation and discrimination, directed at stigmatized people and extending to their significant others, close associates and social groups. Link and Phelan (2014) used the term 'stigma power' to refer to instances whereby exploitation, control and exclusion of others enable people to obtain what they want. They argued that stigmatization is most effective in achieving its prejudiced aims when it is hidden or 'misrecognized'.

Stigmatization devalues the whole person, ascribing them a negative identity that persists (Miles, 1981) even when the basis of the stigma disappears (e.g., when someone recovers from mental illness they remain characterized forever as a person who had mental health problems). It is a form of social oppression and operates to disqualify and marginalize stigmatized individuals from full social acceptance and participation. Health care professionals are as likely to stigmatize as any other group, influencing their behaviour and decision-making in the provision of health care. The consequences of stigma include physical and psychological abuse, denial of economic and employment opportunities, non-seeking or restricted access to services, and social ostracism. It is not surprising, then, that individuals frequently expend considerable effort to combat stigmatization and manage their identities, including passing (acting as if they do not have the stigmatized attribute), covering (de-emphasizing difference), resistance (e.g., speaking out against discrimination) and withdrawal. They may also internalize the stigmatization, feeling considerable guilt and shame and devaluing themselves. Kadianaki (2014) argued that coping with stigma could be seen as a meaning-making effort to enable those who are being stigmatized to transform the way they see themselves and to orient themselves in society.

The pervasive Western idealization of physical perfection, independence and beauty may play an important role in the constant devaluation of disabled people and people who are ill. Particular characteristics of illness or disablement increase stigmatization, including perceptions that the condition is the person's own fault (e.g., obesity), is incurable and/or degenerative (e.g., Alzheimer's disease), is intrusive, compromises mobility, is contagious (e.g., HIV infection and AIDS) and is highly visible.

The lower value placed on the lives of disabled people can be seen in the way disabled people are segregated from the general population, including in education, housing, employment and transportation. It is also apparent in the way crimes against disabled people are minimized (e.g., discourses of abuse rather than theft/fraud/rape; acquittals and light sentences in cases of 'acceptable' euthanasia). For both disabled people and those with severe or terminal illness, stigma may be central to debates around suicide/euthanasia and abortion (see below). Stigma is a powerful determinant of social control and exclusion. By devaluing certain individuals and groups, society can excuse itself for making decisions about the rationing of resources (e.g., HIV antiretroviral drugs), services (e.g., health insurance exclusions), research funding/efforts and care (e.g., denying operations to individuals who are obese) to these groups. In terms of the social model of disablement, stigmatization may be the main issue concerning disablement.

Multidisciplinary research is needed to further explore how stigma is related to health, disablement and social justice. Why is recognition of the similarities between stigmatized and non-stigmatized individuals overridden and obscured by perceived differences that are devalued? How do different stigmas, particularly health-related stigmas, interact? How is stigma manifested by health care professionals and what interventions might mitigate the negative effects of stigma?

LIVES WORTH LIVING VERSUS THE RIGHT TO DIE

The pervasive devaluation of people with disabilities, and the negative assumptions about their lower quality of life, are central to the current debates about the abortion of impaired foetuses and the legalization of assisted suicide/euthanasia or the right to die. Disablement rights organizations champion the argument that abortion decisions should not be made on the basis of foetal impairment indicators, whereas they challenge the 'right-to-die' rhetoric on the basis of disablement.

The disablement movement argues against abortion on the grounds of potential impairment due to the eugenic implications of such a practice (Sharpe and Earle, 2002). The reason for their concern is encapsulated in Singer's quote: 'the killing of a defective infant is not morally equivalent to the killing of a person; very often it is not morally wrong at all' (Singer, 1993: 184). The new genetic testing and selection technologies allow the identification of suspected foetal impairment during pregnancy and subsequent foetal termination. Shakespeare (1998: 669) argues that such technologies operate as a weak form of eugenics 'via non-coercive individual choices' based on the assumed unacceptable quality of life of disabled people. The rationales for screening and termination include assumptions that people with disabilities are more costly to society, that the lives of children with disabilities are harmful to their families, and that some impairments involve a level of suffering and misery that makes life not worth living.

The way professionals describe test results and the influence of the advice they give is also a concern. There is substantial evidence that the advice given, while often subtle, most frequently encourages termination in response to potential impairment results, and most testing takes place within a plan-to-abort context. There is a tension between this argument and the feminist position that women have a categorical right to make decisions about their own bodies, including the decision to terminate an unwanted pregnancy. However, the disablement movement position is not against abortion itself; rather, it revolves around the basis upon which the decision is made. Aborting a specific foetus on the basis of a devalued attribute is different from aborting any foetus on the basis of not wanting to have a child at that time (Fine and Asch, 1982). It is unlikely that a woman would be encouraged to terminate a pregnancy because a test indicated the child is likely to have ginger hair; however, the same is not true when a test suggests a possibility of impairment. It is this difference that makes it an issue of discrimination. The disablement movement also asserts the rights of disabled women to have children. This fundamental human right is denied to many women, particularly those with cognitive and emotional impairments, as the additional support and resources that they need to allow them to raise a child are often not available. In some countries forced sterilization still occurs, including Australia, Spain and Japan.

The right-to-die debate revolves around the argument that people with severe or terminal illness and people with disabilities have the right to end their lives when they feel life has become unbearable, and that assisting them to do so should not be illegal. We discuss this issue in more detail in Chapter 24.

The argument against the right-to-die lobby, although implicitly anti-suicide, is not necessarily about whether suicide is right or wrong *per se*. It should be viewed as being about the differential treatment of the issue for people with disabilities and severe illnesses as opposed to 'healthy' people. Morally sanctioning assisting people with incurable terminal or non-terminal conditions to end their lives or withholding life-sustaining treatment/support, while morally opposing the right of suicidal 'healthy' individuals to end their lives (and offering them suicide prevention interventions), equates to a severe form of discrimination based on the stigmatization of these individuals.

REDUCING INEQUALITIES

If inequalities can be reduced at all, the evidence suggests that this will only happen by adopting a thoroughly multi-layered approach. Dahlgren and Whitehead (1991) identified four different levels for tackling health inequalities:

Strengthening individuals.

Strengthening communities.

Improving access to essential facilities and services.

Encouraging macroeconomic and cultural change.

These four levels correspond to the four layers of influence in Whitehead's 'Onion Model' of the determinants of health outlined in Chapter 1 (see Figure 1.5). Extra microsystem and mesosystem levels, as in Bronfenbrenner's model, could perhaps be added to Whitehead's list. Psychologists do not usually talk quite so simplistically about 'strengthening' individuals; they analyse the personal characteristics and skills associated with positive health (e.g., self-efficacy, hardiness, sense of coherence, social skills). Developing interventions aimed at individual health beliefs and behaviours is a core feature of psychological theory, research and practice.

Interventions aimed at tackling inequalities at an individual level have shown mixed results. There are four possible reasons. First, people living and working in disadvantaged circumstances have fewer resources (time, space, money) with which to manage the process of change. Second, health-threatening behaviours, such as smoking, tend to increase in difficult or stressful circumstances as they provide a means of coping. Third, there may have been a lack of sensitivity to the difficult circumstances in which people work and live that constrain the competence to change. Fourth, there has been a tendency to blame the victim. For example, cancer sufferers may be blamed for the disease if they are smokers on the grounds that they are responsible for the habit that caused it.

Overall, efforts directed at the individual level have been inconclusive and small-scale. Because most health determinants are beyond the control of the individual, psychological interventions aimed at individuals have limited impact on public health problems when considered on a wider scale. There is a need for psychologists to work beyond the individual level, with families, communities, work sites and community groups. We are not alone in thinking that structural changes at a societal level are ultimately required if the prevalent inequities are ever going to be reduced. Anything else is simply tinkering, a case of 'fiddling while Rome burns'.

SOCIAL CAPITAL

There is increasing interest in **social capital** as an aid to explaining social variations in health. The concept was especially promoted by Robert Putnam, who used it to characterize civic life in Italy (Putnam et al., 1993). He argued that certain communities had higher degrees of civic engagement, levels of interpersonal trust and norms of reciprocity. Together, these characteristics contributed to a region's degree of social capital. Putnam (2000) subsequently explored the extent of social capital in the USA, and argued that over the past generation there has been a steady decline in participation in social organizations and thus a steady decline in social capital. An important distinction that Putnam (2000) makes is that between 'bridging' and 'bonding' social capital. 'Bridging' social capital refers to links with diverse groups and provides an opportunity for community members to access power and resources outside their community, whereas 'bonding' social capital refers to inward-looking social ties that bond the community together. Campbell (2004) stresses that both forms of social capital are essential in building healthy communities.

There has been a series of studies investigating variations in social capital and its connection with health. For example, in a national cohort of Open University adults in Thailand ($n = 82,482$), self-assessed health was shown to be significantly associated with social trust and social support (Yiengprugsawan et al., 2011). Gilbert et al. (2013) conducted a meta-analysis of social capital, self-reported health and mortality. A total of 39 studies were included in the analysis. Findings suggested that high social capital can increase the odds of good health by 27%. Furthermore, social capital variables, such as reciprocity and trust, increased the odds of good health by 39% and 32%, respectively.

Studies have explored the pathways linking social capital with health. In a study with church-going Latinas in California, Martinez et al. (2013) explored the relationship between leisure/physical activity and social cohesion. Leisure/physical activity and neighbourhood cohesion were assessed at baseline, three months and six months after the implementation of a *promotora*-delivered pilot intervention. *Promotoras* are community health leaders who help with the dissemination of health information to community members. They are locally based and have very similar characteristics to the target population. They were given training on how to lead walking groups, general information on the health benefits of physical activity, and information on the barriers to and facilitators of physical activity, especially among the Latino community. Evaluation of this intervention showed that social cohesion was an important predictor of physical activity (i.e., social cohesion at three months can predict levels of physical activity at six months). The authors suggested that it is possible that the *promotoras* enhanced social cohesion by providing participants with a sense of belonging and friendship while facilitating these activities. Considering the effectiveness of this approach in promoting leisure-time physical activity, it was argued that intervention coordinators can learn to maximize the benefits of working with community-based facilitators to promote health and well-being.

Participatory and community-based approaches can help to address issues related to poverty and health by empowering individuals and communities more widely (Ng, 2010). For example, Lawson et al. (2014) explored the benefits of participating in a community arts project among people living with mental health problems. The community members selected artwork and curated a public exhibition. Interviews suggested that participants had improved self-worth and lost some of the stigma associated with mental health issues. The project also offered a sense of belonging and helped participants to develop new knowledge and skills.

Scheib and Lykes (2013) facilitated a participatory action and photo elicitation research project in post-Katrina New Orleans from 2007 to 2010. Eleven African-American and Latina women took part in the project. Findings suggested that in developing ties and new ways to respond to the consequences of an 'unnatural disaster', the participants developed intra- and inter-group empathy and the capacity to critically examine the social and structural determinants of health inequities.

Social capital, or its lack, has been linked with health inequalities. Uphoff et al. (2013) systematically reviewed evidence on the associations and interactions between social capital and socio-economic inequalities in health. Of the 60 studies that met the inclusion criteria, 56 showed significant correlations between social capital and socio-economic inequalities in health. Twelve studies showed how social capital can act as a buffer against the negative effects of low SES on health, while five concluded that social capital has a stronger positive effect for people with a lower SES.

There has been a wide range of criticisms of social capital as an explanatory concept (e.g., Lynch et al., 2000). These include confusion over what exactly the term implies, debates over ways of measuring it, and ignorance of the broader political context. Bjørnskov and Sønderskov (2013) argued that social capital is not a good concept since contemporary research either conceptualizes it as several distinct phenomena or constructs it using other terms. Baum (2000: 410) also emphasizes caution in the use of the concept in that 'there are dangers that the promotion of social capital may be seen as a substitute for economic investment in poor communities particularly by those governments who wish to reduce government spending'.

COMMUNITY MOBILIZATION AND POWER

Considering that current global economic processes restrain the capacity of grassroots organizations to respond to structural challenges in health, it is important for future interventions to develop new methods to leverage power for such organizations (Campbell, 2014; Campbell and Cornish, 2014; Speer et al., 2014). It is important to recognize the need to transform power relationships, not just at individual and community levels, but also at macro levels (Ansell, 2014). As shown in the case presented in Box 5.3, developing strategic alliances can help grassroots organizations to strengthen their political power to affect policy change. Developing partnerships for health and community development 'must be understood not as a tool for intervention, but as part of the interventions and definition of success' (Aveling and Jovchelovitch, 2014: 34). The process of building partnerships involves critical reflection and is influenced by institutional and socio-cultural contexts.

BOX 5.3

INTERNATIONAL CASE STUDY: Creating social alliances to influence positive policy change

Speer et al. (2014) presented the case of ISAIAH, a faith-based community organizing group based in the Minneapolis–St Paul metropolitan area. It was formed in 2000 when three faith-based groups merged after recognizing that small groups do not have sufficient political power to influence change. It is now composed of 90 different organizations and uses a social action approach to affect positive policy change to address social inequity. The group had been instrumental in preventing the elimination of three stops for a light rail line being built in Minneapolis–St Paul. The communities that would potentially benefit from these transit stops were predominantly ethnic minority groups. The group influenced planning

(Continued)

---

decisions and funding legislations by collaborating with neighbourhood groups and high-lighting the link between transportation and health. As the authors noted:

> Pursuing a deeper appreciation of the connection between health and trans-portation led ISAIAH leaders to policy professionals who emphasized the role of transportation for community vitality – through access to grocery stores, employ-ment, schools, and affordable neighborhoods. Simultaneous to this discernment, ISAIAH responded to the Governor's vetoes by revisiting state legislators and pushing back against the Governor's neoliberal articulation of scarcity and limited resources. (Speer et al., 2014: 165)

To maintain the momentum of the group's efforts, ISAIAH and its allies are currently working on a health-impact assessment to explore land-use policies to prevent the negative consequences of the rail line on marginalized neighbourhoods.

Source: Speer et al. (2014)

Campbell et al. (2010) showed that it is possible for people from disadvantaged communities to mobilize themselves to demand better social and economic conditions to improve health. They presented three successful pro-poor social movements in Brazil, India and South Africa wherein social groups demanded access to land, health services and life-saving medical treatment. A similar case is presented in Box 5.4, wherein *pobladores* successfully mobilized themselves to demand better living and working conditions in Chile (Hadjez-Berrios, 2014). In these case studies, although enabling disadvantaged groups to make their concerns heard was an important aspect of the movement, the willingness of those in power to take these demands seriously proved crucial to the success of these campaigns. As Stephens (2010) argued, health promotion research and practice need to recognize how those in more advantaged social positions maintain and perpetuate unequal power relations in society. She noted:

> Using social theories will enable us to develop research questions with a focus on making visible the practices of those with privilege that work to simultaneously preserve and increase power and access to resources while denying access to other groups. (Stephens, 2010: 997)

BOX 5.4

INTERNATIONAL CASE STUDY: Community participation in health during the Unidad Popular Government – Santiago de Chile (1970–1973)

Context

The organization and mobilization of popular classes had a significant impact on the improvement of living and working conditions in overcrowded cities in Chile. In addition to the creation of the National Health System in 1952 and its later institutional development until 1973, the active participation of disadvantaged and marginalized communities, also known as *pobladores*, had mobilized social action to address local health problems in poor urban settlements. Community participation in health in Chile saw its peak with the arrival of the Unidad Popular Government in 1970. This ended abruptly in September 1973 due to a military coup that lasted for 17 years.

Method

This qualitative study aimed to explore the experiences of community participation in health during the Unidad Popular Government in Santiago de Chile from 1970 to 1973. Participants included three former health government officials, three primary health care workers and six *pobladores*, who were directly involved with the movement.

Findings

Participants constructed community participation in health programmes from 1970 to 1973 as a multiple and dynamic response to the health and political challenges faced by communities. Three different moments in community participation in health were highlighted in the analysis. The first moment aimed to expand health care coverage, prevent diseases, educate pregnant women and prevent alcoholism through the development of 'Health Brigades' inside settlements. 'Health Brigades' were relatively autonomous organizations (mostly composed of young women) that were trained by health workers. The second moment was characterized by improvements in autonomy and widening of the scope of participation through grassroots participation in health decisions. In this context, health issues were no longer conceptualized in biomedical terms. Finally, the third moment in community participation in health was characterized by a growing understanding of the wider determinants of health and the development of comprehensive definitions of health related to the democratization of health services.

Conclusion

Community participation in health in Chile during the Unidad Popular Government contributes to a critical understanding of community participation, conceived as a dialectic and transformative action. In this context, the *pobladores* constituted themselves as social subjects who actively transformed Chilean health institutions by challenging the dominant and oppressive hierarchies in society.

Source: Hadjez-Berrios (2014)

In a review of what it would take to eradicate health inequalities, a report for NHS Scotland (Scott et al., 2013: 6) concluded that this can only be achieved 'if the underlying differences in income, wealth and power across society are reduced'. In a similar report, McCartney et al. (2012) reviewed the evidence for the higher rate of mortality in Scotland.

They concluded that the continued high rates of mortality, despite improvements in health care, can be accounted for by a 'synthesis that begins from the changed political context of the 1980s, and the consequent hopelessness and community disruption experienced' (2012: 459). Their summary of this synthesis of the evidence is presented in Figure 5.1.

It is a challenge for health psychologists to position themselves within this movement for change, but it is something that we need to reflect on as scholars and activists (Murray, 2012b). The life of Miguel D'Escoto Brockmann (1933–2017), whose frequently quoted exhortation opened this chapter, reminds us of this challenge. D'Escoto was a priest, a member of Nicaragua's Sandinista government in the 1980s and ex-president of the UN General Assembly, whose commitment to social justice leaves a legacy and an inspiration. There is a need for a more social and political health psychology that is informed by contemporary debates about social change, but is also committed to the ideals of social justice (Murray, 2012; Tileaga, 2013).

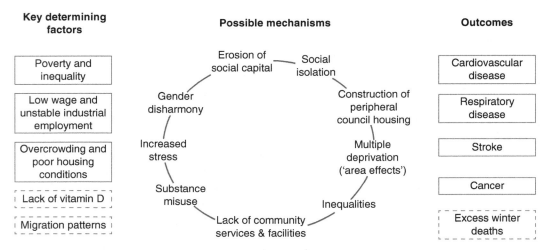

Figure 5.1   Representation of the synthesis of evidence of the cause of the higher rate of mortality in Scotland

Source: Reproduced with permission from McCartney et al., 2012

FUTURE RESEARCH

1. There is a need to clarify the character of the psychosocial explanations for the social inequalities in health.

2. Research on social inequalities needs to be combined with further research on ethnic and gender inequalities in health. Qualitative studies of the health experiences of people from different socio-economic backgrounds are of particular importance to our understanding of the psychological mechanisms underlying health variations. Further qualitative studies are also needed to explore the relationship between social positioning and health experience.

3. Forms of research on social inequalities in health need to explicitly consider how they can contribute to reducing them.

4. An essential aspect of future research is to consider the social and psychological obstacles to movements to alleviate social inequalities in health.

SUMMARY

1. Health and illness are determined by social conditions.
2. There is a clear relationship between income and health, leading to the development of a social gradient.
3. Psychosocial explanations of these social variations include perceived inequality, stress, lack of control and less social connection.
4. Material explanations of the social gradient in health include reduced income and reduced access to services.
5. Political factors connect both psychosocial and material explanations in a broader causal chain.
6. Social environment includes the character of people's social relationships and their connection with the community.
7. Social justice is concerned with providing equal opportunities for all citizens. Socio-economic status (SES) and wealth are strongly related to health, illness and mortality. These gradients may be a consequence of differences in social cohesion, stress and personal control.
8. A health psychology committed to social justice needs to orient itself towards addressing the needs of the most disadvantaged in society.

CULTURE AND HEALTH

'There is no such thing as human nature independent of culture.'

Clifford Geertz (1973)

OUTLINE

The way people think about health, become ill and react to illness is rooted in broader health belief systems that are immersed in culture. In this chapter, we provide examples of different health belief systems that have existed historically and popular belief systems of today. We consider several indigenous health systems and those of complementary and alternative medicine. Finally, we discuss some issues related to rapid cultural change in contemporary society, including racism and how culturally competent health care systems help to bridge cultural, social and linguistic barriers.

WHAT IS CULTURE?

We are cultural beings, and an understanding of health beliefs and practices requires an understanding of the historical and socio-cultural context that gives human lives meaning.

Culture has been viewed principally in two different ways: (1) as a fixed system of beliefs, meanings and symbols that belong to a group of people who speak a common language and may also adhere to a common religion and system of medicine; (2) as a developmental and dynamic system of signs that exists in continuously changing narratives or stories. People's reactions to illness are driven by a constant struggle for meaning in light of beliefs that are evolving across space and time. These two approaches yield very different kinds of psychological investigation.

Within psychology, the study of culture that uses the first approach is that of **cross-cultural psychology**. Samples of populations said to be from different cultures are compared in terms of attitudes, beliefs, values and behaviours that are viewed as stable and essential characteristics of particular cultures. This approach is illustrated by research on individualism versus collectivism by Triandis (1995) and Hofstede and Bond (1988). The study of culture that uses the second approach is that of **cultural psychology** and is illustrated by the work of Valsiner (2013), who views cultural psychology as:

> a science of human conduct mediated through signs from beginning to end, and from one time moment to the next in irreversible time. … All phenomena of manifest kind – usually subsumed under the blanket term behavior – are subordinate to that cultural process of irresistible meaning-making (and re-making). Behavior is not objective, but subjective – through the meanings linked with it. … Human psychology is the science of human conduct and not of behavior, or of cognition. (2013: 25)

The concept of belief is a core concept in health psychology but rarely is it defined. Beliefs are viewed as:

> durable and implicit; as associated with practices, choices and activities; and as bearing personal significance and import. … Belief tends to reproduce cultural norms, the precepts, expectations and values of particular times and places. … Simultaneously, within such broad cultural patternings, the belief of any given individual is produced through the mediation of that person's particular history of social relations – with parents, carers, teachers, significant others – with which these acquired norms get inflected. (Cromby, 2012: 944–6)

Belief is viewed in social cognition models such as the theory of planned behaviour (TPB; Ajzen, 1985) as a fundamental theoretical construct, with each of the TPB's three core constructs – attitude, subjective norm and perceived behaviour control – being underpinned by belief, an enduring, cognitive entity employed in rational thought and detached from feelings. It is often constructed and expressed as a part of discourse and narrative when asked for an account of one's views about a topic in conversation. Beliefs are therefore constructed 'on the hoof' as much as they are a fixed piece of dogma that underlies decisions and actions.

Yet, as we argue elsewhere in this book, beliefs are almost always associated with affect. This is the view of Cromby (2012: 954), who states:

> Belief arises when social practice works up structures of feeling in contingent association with discourse and narrative. … Believing is not merely information-processing activity, and belief is not an individual cognitive entity. Belief is the somewhat contingent, socially co-constituted outcome of repeated articulations between activities, discourses, narratives and socialized structures of feeling.

Beliefs are at the core of what we mean when we talk of culture.

HEALTH BELIEF SYSTEMS

As societies evolve, **health belief systems** develop as bodies of knowledge are constructed and exchanged among those who undergo specialized training. This gives rise to the separation of *expert* or *technical* beliefs systems from *traditional, folk* or *indigenous* systems. These two types of system are not discrete but interact, and are in a process of constant evolution. Although the majority of people in any society organize meaning-making through the use of loosely organized indigenous belief systems, the character of these is connected in some form with expert belief systems.

Kleinman (1980) described three overlapping sectors of any health care system:

- The *popular sector* refers to the lay cultural arena where illness is first defined and health care activities initiated.

- The *professional sector* refers to the organized healing professions, their representations and actions.

- The *folk sector* refers to the non-professional, non-bureaucratic, specialist sector that shades into the other two sectors.

Although this three-fold division is widely cited, other researchers (e.g., Blumhagen, 1980) have preferred a simpler two-fold division into professional and popular realms. The former are said to consist of systematicity, coherence and interdependence (Blumhagen, 1980: 200). Conversely, a lay health belief system can appear disconnected, inconsistent and at times plainly contradictory. This broad classification avoids an accusation that certain specialized health belief systems are classified as 'folk' when they have limited status in society, although they may offer an extensive classification of health complaints and treatments. These two broad kinds of belief systems interact such that the lay person can draw upon more specialized knowledge but also the specialist will make use of more popular knowledge. Further, both ways of thinking about health draw upon a more general worldview located within particular local socio-political contexts. Blumhagen (1980) argues that these two kinds of health belief systems should be considered distinct from an individual belief system that a person employs to understand their personal experience of illness. Dominant expert health belief systems have the tendency to become doctrinal in nature, with principles and guidelines that inform practitioners and specialists in systems of treatment for different illnesses.

WESTERN HEALTH BELIEF SYSTEMS

Classical views of health

The classical view of health and illness in the West is derived from the Graeco-Arabic medical system known as **Galenic medicine**. This provided an expert system developed from the Greeks, in particular the work of Hippocrates and his colleagues. We discussed the central concepts in Galen's formulation in Chapter 1.

Besides focusing on understanding natural processes, the Galenic tradition placed responsibility on individuals to look after themselves. Ill health was viewed as one consequence of natural processes, not a result of divine intervention. In many ways Galen's ideas not only prefigured but also continue to influence much of contemporary health beliefs in industrialised societies.

Christian ideas

Galenic ideas dominated medicine in Europe for almost two millennia. However, during the Middle Ages in Europe, Galen's work became confined more to the learned few and other ideas based upon religion became more commonplace. Illness was often seen as punishment for humankind's sinfulness. The Church's *seven deadly sins* came to be associated with pathological conditions of the body. For example, pride was symbolized by tumours and inflammations, while sloth led to dead flesh and palsy (Thomas, 1979).

Christianity drew upon different traditions. The *ascetic tradition* scorned concern for the body and instead promoted acts such as fasting and physical suffering, which supposedly led to spirituality. With the *Protestant Reformation* this belief was replaced with the idea that the body had been given to humans by God. It was the individual's religious duty to look after and care for the body. Illness was seen as a sign of weakness and neglect. To honour God required living a healthy life and abstaining from excess, especially in terms of sex and diet.

Despite the authority of the Church, these religious interpretations began to decline with the growth of medical science. While in terms of the expert belief system there has been increasing acceptance of a naturalistic view of disease, the moral basis of health continues to underlie much of contemporary health belief. Externalizing religious health beliefs has also been shown to influence health and well-being outcomes. For example, in a US survey of religion and health (n = 2948), belief in divine control over health has been shown to impact negatively upon health outcomes, while also contributing to a better sense of life satisfaction (Hayward et al., 2016)

Biomedicine

Two streams of thought in knowing the world dominated during the Enlightenment. The first was the acceptance of the distinction between superstition and reason. The second was the emergence of **positivism**, which emphasized that science based upon direct observation, measurement and experimentation gave direct access to the real world. This approach concentrated attention on material reality and a conception of the body as distinct from the mind. A central figure was Descartes (1596–1650), who conceived the human being as composed of mind and body. The former was not open to scientific investigation, whereas the latter could be conceived as a machine.

The eighteenth century saw the rise of **individualism** in Western society. In previous eras the group or collective organized ways of thinking and acting, which in turn was interconnected with the physical and spiritual world. Professional understanding of health and illness became more closely entwined with knowledge of the individual physical body. Foucault (1976) described how between the mid-eighteenth and mid-nineteenth centuries the 'medical gaze' came to focus on the interior of the human body. The symptoms of illness now became signs of underlying pathophysiology. Foucault noted that the change in perspective of the physician was illustrated in the change in the patient query from 'How do you feel?' to 'Where does it hurt?'. For this new physician the stethoscope became the symbol of having insight into the bodily interior. Treatment centred on changing the character of this physiology by either medical or surgical means.

This approach to the study of health and illness has become known as **biomedicine**, or 'cosmopolitan' or 'allopathic' medicine (Leslie, 1976). It came to dominance for several reasons, including the fact that it was in accord with a broader view of humans, its alliance with physical science and the steady improvement in the health of the population that was attributed to medical intervention. The focus on the body is in accord with the Western emphasis on the individual. Further, the separation of mind and body 'offers a subtle articulation of the person's alienation from the body in Western society, but this alienation is found, as well, in every sphere of economic and political life' (Benoist and Cathebras, 1993: 858). Biomedicine separates the person from the body.

NON-WESTERN VIEWS OF HEALTH

Chinese views of health

Traditional Chinese Medicine (TCM) is greatly influenced by the religion and philosophy of **Taoism**. According to this view, the universe is a vast and indivisible entity and each being has a definite function within it. The balance of the two basic powers of yin and yang governs the whole universe, including human beings. *Yang* is considered to represent the male, positive energy that produces light and fullness, whereas the *yin* is considered the female, negative force that leads to darkness and emptiness. A disharmony in yin and yang leads to illness. A variety of methods including *acupuncture* and *herbal medicines* can be used to restore this harmony. There are at least 13,000 medicinal substances with 50 fundamental herbs, including the roots, twigs and leaves of cannabis, ginseng, ginger, licorice, peony and rhubarb.

Confucianism is influential in the traditional Chinese views on health. Within this culture, human suffering is traditionally explained as the result of destiny or *ming*. Cheng (1997: 740) quotes the Confucian teacher Master Meng: 'A man worries about neither untimely death nor long life but cultivates his personal character and waits for its natural development; this is to stand in accord with Fate. All things are determined by Fate, and one should accept what is conferred.' An important part of your destiny depends upon your horoscope or *pa-tzu*. During an individual's life, his or her pa-tzu is paired with the timing of nature. Over time these pairings change and create the individual's luck or *yun*.

Buddhist beliefs are also reflected in Chinese medical belief systems. Good deeds and charitable donations, for example, are promoted. Heavenly retribution is expected for those who commit wrongs. This retribution may not be immediate, but it will be inevitable. An important concept in this respect is *pao*, which has two types: (1) reciprocity and (2) retribution (Cheng, 1997). In mutual relationships reciprocity is expected. When this does not occur some form of retribution will take place.

These influences are not only codified within Chinese medicine, but also influence everyday lay beliefs about health and illness in Chinese communities around the world. For example, Rochelle and Marks (2010) explored the extent of medical pluralism among Chinese people in London. The thematic analysis suggests that Chinese medicine and Western medicine were perceived as two systems of health provision and that these two systems could be used concurrently. Generally, the National Health Service was perceived to be difficult to use and concerns were expressed around communication and trust with health care providers due to language barriers. Similarly, qualitative research by Jin and Acharya (2016) suggests that yin–yang balance and 'qi' still influence practices related to medication adherence among people of Chinese descent in the USA. Narratives also suggest that Western and Chinese medicine have strengths and limitations that can counteract each other. Participants also discussed the importance of social support and how they coped with acculturation stress, especially when health care providers failed to understand their cultural practices and beliefs.

Like orthodox medicine, TCM raises ecological and ethical concerns. TCM is a private industry worth billions of dollars and the efficacy of the treatments is largely unknown. Many rare and endangered species currently face extinction owing to the harvesting of animal parts such as tiger bone, rhinoceros horn, turtle shell and seahorses, and the cruel conditions in which the animals used as a source of medicines are kept causes suffering, e.g., the harvesting of bile from thousands of captive Asiatic black bears, which are held in small cages. The bile is the main source of ursodeoxycholic acid, which is used to treat kidney problems and stomach and digestive disorders (Lindor et al., 1994). Cruelty to animals to generate medicines within TCM is paralleled by the use of animals in the testing of new medicines in orthodox medicine.

Islamic views on medicine

Islam is derived from the Arabic words *istaslama*, which means surrender, and *salam*, which means peace. As such, Islam, in its religious sense, means submission and obedience to the will of God. During sickness, Muslims are expected to seek Allah's mercy and help through prayer. They also believe that death is an inevitable part of life and that the whole creation belongs to Allah and to him is the final return.

There are specific health-related practices which Muslims follow. Health care providers need to have an understanding of general Islamic beliefs and practices to enable them to provide quality care for Muslim patients. For example, health care professionals need to be aware of the need for modesty, privacy, the appropriate use of touch and clothing, dietary requirements (e.g., Halal and fasting during Ramadan), the availability of prayer rooms, interactions with opposite-sex patients, the use of medications, shared decision-making and its impact on the family (Rassool, 2000; Mataoui and Sheldon, 2016).

Awareness and respect for spiritual and cultural values are important in clinical practice since these have implications on patients' choices and engagement in health care. For example, it is Islamic practice to visit the sick. Culturally sensitive health care establishments find ways that enable such visits from families, friends and other well-wishers. Health care professionals need to be aware that there is Islamic guidance on end-of-life care and funeral arrangements. When treating migrant Muslims from non-English speaking countries, health care providers need to consider health literacy and linguistic barriers, which may interfere with the patient's comprehension and ability to implement health advice when given in their non-native language (see Chapter 14).

Ayurvedic medicine

The Ayurvedic system of medicine is based upon the Sanskrit words *ayus* (life) and *veda* (science). This system is practised extensively in India. It is estimated that 70% of the population of India and hundreds of millions of people throughout the world use Ayurvedic medicine, which is based on Hindu philosophy (Schober, 1997). Both the cosmos and each human being consist of a female component, *Prakrti*, which forms the body, and a male component, *Purusa*, which forms the soul. While the Purusa is constant, the Prakrti is subject to change. The body is defined in terms of the flow of substances through channels. Each substance has its own channel. Sickness occurs when a channel is blocked and the flow is diverted into another channel. When all channels are blocked, the flow of substances is not possible and death occurs. At this stage, the soul is liberated from its bodily prison. The task of Ayurvedic medicine is to identify the blockages and to get the various essences moving again. The different forms of imbalance can be corrected through both preventive and therapeutic interventions based on diet, yoga, breathwork, bodywork, meditation and/or herbs (Schober, 1997). The use of herbs plays a major role in the treatment and prevention of illnesses (see Table 6.1 below).

As in TCM, the Ayurvedic system informs beliefs about health and illness through the Indian sub-continent and among Indian communities everywhere. However, Ayurvedic medicine has not dominated Western biomedicine, even within India. There is a variety of other competing health belief systems in a pluralistic health culture. In an interview study of a community in northern India, Morinis and Brilliant (1981) found evidence not only of Ayurvedic beliefs, but also beliefs on 'unami' (another indigenous health system), allopathic, homeopathic, massage, herbalist, folk, astrologic and religious systems. They note that while these systems may formally seem to conflict, participants can draw on some or all of them to help explain different health problems. Further, the strength of these beliefs is related to the immediate social situation and the roles and expectations of the community. For example, for women in some parts of Pakistan, the health belief system is a mixture of biomedicine and unami medicine, which is a version of Galenic medicine.

African health beliefs

A wide range of traditional medical systems continues to flourish in Africa. These include a mixture of herbal and physical remedies intertwined with various religious belief systems.

Two dimensions are paramount in understanding African health beliefs: *spiritual influences* and a *communal orientation*. It is common to attribute illness to the work of ancestors or to supernatural forces. Inadequate respect for ancestors can supposedly lead to illness. In addition, magical influences can be both negative and positive, contemporary and historical. Thus, illness can be attributed to the work of some malign living person. The role of the spiritual healer is to identify the source of the malign influence. African culture has a communal orientation. Thus, the malign influence of certain supernatural forces can be felt not just by an individual, but also by other members of his/her family or community. Thus intervention may be aimed not only at the sense of balance of the individual, but also at the family and community.

Nemutandani et al. (2015) explored HIV- and tuberculosis-related beliefs among traditional practitioners in South Africa. Findings suggest that the belief that HIV/AIDS and tuberculosis patients were bewitched was still prevalent. In particular, it is believed that HIV is caused by sexual promiscuity and that transmission of this disease is a punishment from God. Similarly, in a study exploring beliefs on family planning in Kenya, Nigeria and Senegal, it was suggested that the most prevalent beliefs were that modern contraceptives are dangerous and can harm women's wombs (Gueye et al., 2015).

Using the 2010 Malawi Demographic and Health Survey, Sano et al. (2016) found that knowledge about prevention was associated with a lower likelihood of endorsing misconceptions around HIV transmission. Socio-demographic factors such as marital status, ethnicity, income, religion and urban or rural residence also showed significant associations with misconceptions around HIV transmission. Thus, it is important that cultural and ethnic considerations are taken into account when developing and implementing HIV education programmes in the region. (Further discussion on community-based health promotion and education on HIV can be found in Chapter 22.)

Although cultural beliefs play a crucial role in shaping health behaviour, it is important to recognize the social and structural barriers that impact upon people's ability to utilize health education and services. For example, Lim and Ojo (2017) explored the barriers preventing women from utilizing cervical screening services in sub-Saharan Africa. Findings from this systematic review suggest that despite cultural and linguistic diversity in the region, participants reported similar barriers, such as fear of the procedure and the possibility of a negative outcome, lack of awareness, embarrassment and stigma, lack of spousal support, and other factors such as cost of accessing the service, travel costs, waiting times and negative staff attitudes. Similarly, Skinner and Claassens (2016) explored the factors that influenced initiation and adherence to tuberculosis treatment in South Africa. Poor knowledge, lack of awareness and stigma around tuberculosis and its connection to HIV were raised as key issues. Structural factors such as poverty, lack of access to transport, the need to continue working, and problems related to the poor functioning of health systems were also raised as major constraints to long-term adherence.

POPULAR VIEWS OF HEALTH

Evidence from a series of studies of popular beliefs about health and illness in Western society illustrates the interaction of what can be described as the 'classic', the 'religious', the 'biomedical' and the 'lifestyle' approaches to health and illness. Probably the most influential study of Western lay health beliefs was carried out by Herzlich (1973, 2017). She conducted interviews with a sample of French adults and concluded that health was conceived as an attribute of the individual – a state of harmony or balance. Illness was attributed to outside forces in our society or way of life. Lay people also referred to illness in terms of both organic and psychosocial factors. On their own, organic changes did not constitute illness. Rather, for the layperson, 'physical facts, symptoms and dysfunctions have, of course, an existence of their own, but they only combine to form an illness in so far as they transform a patient's life'. The ability to participate in everyday life constitutes health, whereas inactivity is considered the true criterion of illness. Herzlich's study was seminal because it provoked further research into popular health beliefs.

Blaxter (1990) analysed the definitions of health provided by over 9,000 British adults in a health and lifestyle survey. She classified the responses into nine categories:

1. Health as not-ill (the absence of physical symptoms).
2. Health despite disease.
3. Health as reserve (the presence of personal resources).
4. Health as behaviour (the extent of healthy behaviour).
5. Health as physical fitness.
6. Health as vitality.
7. Health as psychosocial well-being.
8. Health as social relationships.
9. Health as function.

In analysing the responses across social classes, Blaxter (1990) noted considerable agreement in the emphasis on behavioural factors as a cause of illness. She commented on the limited reference to structural or environmental factors, especially among those from working-class backgrounds.

However, health beliefs go beyond descriptive dimensions to consider underlying aetiology. In a discussion of **social representation theory**, Moscovici (1984) suggested that people rarely confine their definition of concepts to the descriptive level. Rather, lay descriptions often include reference to explanations. Lay perceptions of health and illness can be rooted in the social experience of people, in particular sub-cultures. A study of East and West German workers found similar findings to those of Herzlich, but with an added emphasis on health as lifestyle (Flick, 1998). Similarly, in a study of Canadian baby-boomers, Murray et al. (2003) found a very activity-oriented conception of health. In another study, Campbell (2015) explored the meaning of health among older adults in the United Arab Emirates. The narratives suggest that health was embedded in culture and represented as something that is valuable and coming from God. Health was also attributed to the food they eat and was generally perceived to be better in the past.

COMPLEMENTARY AND ALTERNATIVE MEDICINE

The biomedical perspective has come to a position of dominance throughout the world, reflecting 'globalization' more generally. Alternative health care systems tend to be disparaged and marginalized by advocates of biomedicine. Based on a positivist, reductionist perspective, practitioners of biomedicine believe that the material existence of medical science is independent of any patient's psychological search for meaning, understanding and control. As such, alternative perspectives are seen as basically flawed. In spite of this resistance from orthodoxy, alternative professional systems of health care continue to exist in large parts of the world, especially in Asia. As migrants have moved to other countries they have taken their health beliefs with them. In the major Western metropolitan centres, the availability of health care systems other than biomedicine is extensive. This has fed back into Western ways of thinking about health and illness, especially among those who are disenchanted with biomedicine. Increasingly, **complementary and alternative medicine (CAM)** is gaining popularity and respectability in Western health care. CAM encompasses all health systems and practices other than those of the established health system of a society.

In the USA, the National Center for Complementary and Alternative Medicine (NCCAM, 2013) categorizes CAM into two sub-groups: (1) natural products and (2) mind and body practices. *Natural products* often include the use of herbs, vitamins, minerals and probiotics. These products are marketed widely and are commonly sold as dietary supplements. *Mind and body practices* cover a diverse range of procedures that are often administered by a trained practitioner. Examples include acupuncture, massage therapy, meditation techniques, movement therapies (e.g., Feldenkrais method, Alexander technique, Pilates), relaxation techniques, spinal manipulation, tai chi, qi gong, reiki and hypnotherapy.

Harris et al. (2012) reviewed the 12-month prevalence of CAM use by the general public. They reviewed 51 published reports from 49 surveys in 15 countries. Estimates of CAM use ranged from 9.8% to 76%, and from 1.8% to 48.7% for visits to CAM practitioners. In surveys using consistent measurement methods, CAM rates have been stable, particularly in Australia (49% in 1993, 52% in 2000 and 52% in 2004) and in the USA (36% in 2002 and 38% in 2007). The three highest rates of CAM use in this systematic review were reported in Japan (76%), South Korea (75%) and Malaysia (56%). Posadzki et al. (2013a) conducted a systematic review to examine the prevalence of CAM use among patients in the UK. The review included 89 surveys, with a total of 97,222 participants between January 2000 and October 2011. Findings showed that the average one-year prevalence of CAM use was 41.1%, while the average lifetime prevalence was 51.8%. Herbal medicine was the most popular CAM, followed by homeopathy and aromatherapy.

Herbal medicine

Herbal medicine involves the use of plants and plant extracts to treat illnesses or to promote well-being. This practice has been used for thousands of years, with the first recorded use in China in 2800 BC (Brown, 2007). It is believed that this practice was derived from the Ayurvedic tradition and then later adopted by the Chinese, Greeks and Romans. With the growth of the pharmaceutical industry, herbal medicine can now be produced and marketed on a massive scale. In the UK, about one in three adults takes herbal medicine (Posadzki et al., 2013b), while in the USA it is about 20% (Bent, 2008). Some of the most commonly used herbal products, and their purpose, efficacy and risks, are summarized in Table 6.1.

Table 6.1 Commonly used herbal medicines

Herb	Purpose[†]	Evidence for efficacy[†]	Risks	References
Echinacea	Upper respiratory tract infection	Inconclusive	Side effects similar to placebo	Lindeet et al. (2006)
Ginseng	Physical and cognitive performance	Inconclusive	Limited data; hyperactivity and restlessness in case reports	Vogler et al. (1999)
Ginkgo biloba	Dementia	Likely effective	Side effects similar to placebo; case reports of bleeding	Oken et al. (1998); Pittler and Ernst (2000); Bentet al. (2005); Birks and Grimley Evans (2009)
	Claudication	Likely effective		
Garlic	Hyper-cholesterolaemia	Likely effective	Mild gastro-intestinal side effects and garlic odour; case reports of bleeding	Rose et al. (1990); Burnham (1995); Stevinson et al. (2000)
St. John's wort	Depression	Likely effective for mild–moderate depression	Drug interactions	Hammerness et al. (2003); Linde et al. (2008)
Peppermint	Upset stomach/ irritable bowel syndrome	Inconclusive	Limited data, but side effects appear to be mild	Pittler and Ernst (1998)
Ginger	Nausea	Inconclusive	No known side effects	Ernst and Pittler (2000); Rotblatt and Ziment (2002)

Herb	Purpose[†]	Evidence for efficacy[‡]	Risks	References
Soy	Menopausal symptoms	Not effective	Concerns regarding long-term estrogenic effects	Lethaby et al. (2007); Taku et al. (2007)
	Hyper-cholesterolaemia	Effective		
Chamomile	Insomnia/ gastrointestinal problems	No high-quality data	Rare allergic reactions	Ulbricht and Basch (2005)
Kava kava	Anxiety	Likely effective	Case reports of severe hepatotoxicity	CDC (2002); Pittler and Ernst (2003)

Source: Adapted from Bent (2008: 856)

Data sources: [†] Rotblatt and Ziment (2002), Fugh-Berman (2003) and Ulbricht and Basch (2005); [‡] systematic review by Bent and Ko (2004)

Systematic reviews show inconsistent evidence on the efficacy of herbal medicine in treating various conditions. While some reviews did not have substantial evidence to support the use of herbal supplements during pregnancy (Dante et al., 2013) or to treat depression (Butler and Pilkington, 2013), others showed support for treatment of tic disorders (Kim et al., 2014), gout (Li et al., 2013) and irritable bowel disease (Ng et al., 2013). A systematic review by Li et al. (2014) showed how the use of herbal medicine can help to improve the quality of life among chronic heart failure patients. However, reviews that showed substantial findings also raised concerns regarding small sample sizes, high clinical heterogeneity, and poor methodological quality in some trials. We return here to a refrain from other chapters concerned with the evidence base for treatments: more large-scale randomized controlled trials (RCTs) are required to provide robust evidence on the efficacy of herbal medicine. At present, there is limited support for a few specific treatments but the evidence is inconclusive for many of the most popular herbal remedies.

Homeopathy

Homeopathy is a form of CAM which involves the use of highly diluted substances to trigger the body's natural healing system. It is based on the Latin principle *similia similibus curentur*, which means 'let like be cured by like'. This means that a substance that can cause symptoms when taken in large doses can also be used to treat the same symptoms when taken in smaller doses. Its origins can be traced back to the work of the German physician Samuel Hahnemann (1755–1843). During his time, medical treatments often relied on harsh procedures such as blood-letting, purging and the use of poisons. Hahnemann refused to use these techniques and experimented on himself and other healthy volunteers. He recorded the physiological effects of toxic materials such as mercury, arsenic and belladonna and then collated reports of 'cured symptoms' based on homeopathic prescriptions of these substances. See also the discussion of placebos in Chapter 2.

Homeopathic medicine is particularly popular in Europe and in India. In the UK there are currently four homeopathic hospitals, in London, Bristol, Liverpool and Glasgow. It is much more widely used on the European continent, especially in France and Germany. Homeopathy has been used for a variety of health conditions, including asthma, ear infections, hay fever, allergies, dermatitis, arthritis and high blood pressure, and for mental health conditions such as depression, stress and anxiety. However, systematic reviews on the effectiveness of homeopathy showed inconclusive results and trials are of poor quality (Ernst, 2012; Peckham et al., 2013; Saha et al., 2013). Posadzki et al. (2012) have also commented on the potential harm of homeopathy to patients in direct and indirect ways.

Aromatherapy

Aromatherapy involves the use of essential oils from plant extracts for therapeutic purposes. This practice dates back to ancient Egyptian, Chinese and Indian traditions. French chemist and scholar René-Maurice Gattefossé (1881–1950) is considered to be the father of modern aromatherapy. He discovered the healing properties of lavender when he accidentally burned his hand while working in his laboratory. He continued to experiment on essential oils, including thyme, lemon and clove, and used these with First World War soldiers as antiseptics. In recent years, aromatherapy is being used for stress and pain relief, headaches, and digestive and menstrual problems. The essential oils can be massaged into the skin, added to warm bath water, blended into lotions or creams, or inhaled through a diffuser, vaporizer or candles. Consumers can buy oils at pharmacies or health shops or attend an aromatherapy session with a trained therapist. However, as with other CAMs, systematic reviews on the efficacy of aromatherapy have produced inconclusive results (Hur et al., 2012; Lee et al., 2012).

Perspectives on CAM

Debates around the efficacy of CAM have polarized researchers. The most basic explanation for the popular appeal of CAM is the **placebo effect**. The generous time, warm glow of personal attention and friendly conversation received by each individual patient with many CAM practitioners compares favourably to the brief and business-like encounters of mainstream medicine. This aspect seems particularly true in the case of cancer. For example, one Australian study found that 'CAM use appeared to be associated with high patient acceptance and satisfaction which was not related to either cancer diagnosis or prognosis' (Wilkinson and Stevens, 2014: 139). Another positive factor in favour of CAM is that patients 'find these health care alternatives to be more congruent with their own values, beliefs, and philosophical orientations toward health and life' (Astin, 1998: 1548). Arguably, the specific treatment effects *per se* are of marginal relevance. In light of the inconclusive evidence base, Segar (2012) outlined two main discussions around this topic. First, there were concerns regarding evidence-based medicine and whether CAM can be assessed appropriately using the currently available methods, which are based on positivist, biomedical approaches that may be incongruent with the underlying principles of CAM. Second, there were questions about whether CAM should be advocated considering that its effect may be no different from a placebo. While some commentators are concerned that CAM is pseudo-scientific, MacArtney and Wahlberg (2014: 114) argued that 'this form of problematization can be described as a flight from social science' and could negatively represent CAM users as 'duped, ignorant, irrational or immoral'. While there is insufficient evidence from RCTs to support the efficacy of CAM, findings from qualitative research suggest that the use of CAM can promote feelings of control, empowerment and agency (Sointu, 2013).

In the UK, the Department of Health provides clinical guidelines for health care professionals on CAM. A systematic review by Lorenc et al. (2014) showed that a total of 60 guidelines have been produced in relation to CAM therapies. About 44% were inconclusive, mostly due to insufficient empirical evidence, while there was almost an equal proportion of guidelines either recommending or advising against CAM (19%). The World Health Organization launched a Strategy on Traditional Medicine (2014–2023) to support the development of policies and action plans to strengthen the role of CAM to improve health, well-being and people-centred health care, and to promote quality and safety of CAM through regulation and better training and skills development of practitioners. The strategy aims to build a knowledge base around CAM, regulate products, therapies and practitioners, and integrate CAM into national health care systems.

CHANGING CULTURES AND HEALTH

In a world of rapid change and interpenetration of cultural groups and belief systems and an increasingly globalized society, health psychologists need to recognize the complexity and diversity of dynamic and interlocking systems rather than assume that our health belief systems are fixed (MacLachlan, 2000).

BOX 6.1

The false stereotype of the 'Drunken Aboriginal'

Traditionally, Aboriginal people consumed weak alcohol made from various plants. Their problems with alcohol began with the colonial invasions of the eighteenth century. Contrary to all popular stereotypes, surveys find that roughly similar proportions of Aboriginal people drink alcohol to the European colonial population. The media distort the facts and reinforce stereotyping.

Evidence shows that the lifetime risk of alcohol consumption for Australian Aboriginal and Torres Strait Islanders is similar to that of the non-indigenous population for both males and females. Similar proportions of Aboriginal and Torres Strait Islander people and non-indigenous people of the same age and sex exceed lifetime risk guidelines, apart from women aged 55-plus where Aboriginal and Torres Strait Islanders are significantly *less* likely than non-indigenous women to exceed lifetime risk guidelines (7% compared to 10%) (Australian Bureau of Statistics, 2014).

So where did the false stereotyping come from? One answer lies in early colonial art. A lithograph was created by Augustus Earle (1793–1838) and printed by C. Hullmandel, London, in 1830. A group of bedraggled indigenous Australians are sitting in a Sydney street. They wear ragged remnants of European clothing or simply material wraps. Empty 'grog' bottles are scattered on the ground. Behind them there is a two-storey hotel with a kangaroo sign and another sign on the side of the building says 'George Street'. Fashionably dressed British settlers promenade down the street or stand near the hotel. Beyond is a glimpse of Sydney Harbour, with masts and rigging of sailing ships. The picture references the 'grog culture' of the early colonial years – 'grog' being a mid-eighteenth-century term meaning cheap alcohol. Two men gather round a bucket of 'bull', a cheap source of alcohol made by soaking and fermenting old sugar bags.

Indigenous health

There are about 370 million indigenous people from thousands of different cultures in all continents of the planet (United Nations, 2017). While indigenous communities cannot be encapsulated within a single definition, the United Nations (2009) used Martinez Cobo's (1987) conceptualization of indigenous groups as:

> peoples and nations which, having a historical continuity with pre-invasion and pre-colonial societies that developed on their territories, consider themselves distinct from other sectors of the societies now prevailing on those territories, or parts of them. They form at present non-dominant sectors of society and are determined to preserve, develop and transmit to future generations their ancestral territories, and their ethnic identity, as the basis of their continued existence as peoples, in accordance with their own cultural patterns, social institutions and legal system.
> (United Nations, 2009: 4)

Globally, indigenous peoples experience poorer health outcomes, reduced quality of life and higher mortality rates from specific diseases, such as heart disease, tuberculosis, cancer, respiratory disease, stroke and diabetes, than their non-indigenous counterparts. Indigenous populations are six times more likely to die from injuries and are disproportionately more affected by forced displacement caused by natural disasters, armed conflict and loss of their ancestral domains. They also have worse access to education, health care and social services. This trend can be observed among indigenous groups around the world, including those in North America (Ramraj et al., 2016), Australia (Marmot, 2016), New Zealand and the Pacific (Anderson et al., 2006), Latin America and the Caribbean (Montenegro and Stephens, 2006) and Africa (Ohenjo et al., 2006).

The alleged health profile of indigenous groups has been distorted by racism and racial stereotypes. This is illustrated by the alleged alcoholism rates of Australian Aboriginals (Box 6.1). Similar stereotyping occurs regarding the alcohol use of Native Americans. Direct comparisons to published alcohol consumption data from other US populations indicated that American Indians in two reservation samples may be *less likely to use alcohol* than are others in the USA. However, among American Indian drinkers, more alcohol was consumed per drinking occasion (Beals et al., 2003).

Governmental efforts aim to address inequalities that disadvantage indigenous communities, but in some instances these efforts are tokenistic or symbolic in nature. Living with a legacy of conquest and culture, they may even continue to subjugate indigenous people to unjust and unfair economic and educational systems (Fredericks et al., 2014). It is important to recognize indigenous ways of knowing and to value indigenous stories and narratives within their socio-cultural context to bring to the surface knowledge that is relevant, insightful and meaningful for community members. **Participatory action research** can be used to facilitate this process (see Chapters 7 and 16). Genuine participation, instead of tokenistic participation, can foster a sense of ownership for community members and can strengthen personal and community capabilities.

For example, Thompson et al. (2013) facilitated an arts-based participatory action research project to explore the experiences and meaning of physical activity in two remote Northern Territory communities in Australia. Semi-structured interviews were conducted with community members ($n = 23$) and supplemented by five commissioned paintings by community-based artists and ethnographic observations. Physical activities were often linked with work, diet, social relationships and being active 'on country'. They also were associated with educating younger generations about indigenous traditions.

Culturally appropriate physical activities such as bush walking, dancing and art making contribute to health promotion of the community. It is important that indigenous beliefs, knowledge and traditions are considered in the process. Furthermore, social and political issues, including those that are related to racism and discrimination, need to be taken into account since these may compound experiences and access to health care and promotion (Denison et al., 2014).

Racism and health

Racism contributes to poor mental and physical health among migrants, ethnic minority groups and indigenous peoples. Research evidence suggests that everyday experiences of discrimination are related to stress that can potentially lead to chronic illnesses. Even after controlling for factors such as perceived neighbourhood unsafety, food insecurity and financial stress, these associations were consistent across various ethnic groups (Clark et al., 1999; Earnshaw et al., 2016b). Strong associations were also shown between racial discrimination and psychological distress (Halim et al., 2017). Anderson (2013) used data from the 2004 Behavioral Risk Factor Surveillance System (BRFSS) to examine the relationship between stress symptoms from perceived racism and overall health ($n = 32,585$). The analyses suggest that stress from perceived racism can have substantial negative consequences that contribute to poor mental and physical health in adults. Among young people, Grollman (2012) used data from the African-American Youth Culture Survey ($n = 1,052$) to examine the prevalence, distribution, and mental and physical health consequences of multiple forms of perceived discrimination. Findings suggest that young people from disadvantaged backgrounds are more susceptible as a result of experiencing multiple forms of discrimination than their more privileged counterparts. As with the findings from the adult population, a systematic review showed that the relationship between perceived racial discrimination and mental health can be observed among children and young people from minority ethnic groups (Priest et al., 2013).

Health-limiting behaviours, such as poor diet, smoking and increased alcohol intake, can also manifest as a response to the chronic stress of racism. For example, low socio-economic status, racial discrimination and low acculturation (i.e., being immersed in African-American culture and communities) are known to be the major socio-cultural correlates of smoking among African-American adults (Landrine and Corral, 2014). Bermudez-Millan et al. (2016) also found that while lower income predicted lower physical activity as well as poorer sleep quality and medical adherence, racial discrimination was associated with increases in food intake and alcohol consumption.

Landrine et al. (2016) tested whether racial discrimination can negatively influence a person's self-reported health and whether they will rate it in terms of social instead of health indicators. They surveyed 2,118 African-Americans and found that the majority of their respondents (81.8%) rated their health as good/excellent, while only a relatively small proportion (18.2%) rated it as poor/fair. They also found that racial discrimination did not contribute to poor self-reported health, even after controlling for demographic factors. Findings also indicate that self-reported health was associated with objective health and was more strongly linked in the low- than the high-discrimination group.

Imposing culturally insensitive health promotion activities may exacerbate the social exclusion that is already being experienced by minority ethnic groups. Ochieng (2013) conducted a qualitative study exploring the beliefs and perceptions of healthy lifestyle practices among African-Caribbean men and women. In-depth interviews were conducted with 18 participants from the north of England. Findings suggest that participants felt that messages around healthy lifestyle practices were not applicable to their everyday lived experiences since these often ignored issues related to their experiences of social exclusion, racism and ethnic identity. Health promotion programmes that use individualistic approaches are inappropriate for, and isolate, those from ethnic minority communities who practise more collectivist traditions to express their beliefs, values and identity. Thus campaigns that try to promote healthy lifestyles need to consider socio-economic and cultural contexts, including issues related to disadvantage, racism and marginalization, to enable African-American and other minority ethnic groups to incorporate these messages and practices into their everyday lives (see Chapter 16).

Refugees and asylum seekers

According to the United Nations Report (2017), over 65.3 million people were forcibly displaced worldwide in 2015. Nearly 21.3 million were refugees, the majority of whom were under the age of 18. More than half of the refugees came from war-stricken countries such as Syria (4.9 million), Afghanistan (2.7 million) and Somalia (1.1 million), with nearly 34,000 people fleeing their homes as a result of violence and conflict every day. This is the highest level of displacement on record.

The living conditions of refugees are bleak. Based on a study of 150,000 Syrian refugees living in camps in Jordan in 2014, nearly two-thirds were living below the national poverty line. Access to heating, reliable electricity and adequate sanitation were also problematic (United Nations High Commissioner for Refugees (UNHCR), 2014). It is no wonder that the physical and psychological well-being of refugees are impeded by these circumstances.

Communicable diseases are major causes of morbidity among refugees. Children under the age of 5 are most vulnerable, with cases of measles, respiratory tract infections, diarrhoea and severe acute malnutrition soaring at high levels. The risk of anaemia is also a challenge for refugee women and children. The psychological and social well-being of refugees is also a cause for concern. A systematic review exploring the psychosocial challenges of Syrian refugees in Jordan showed that psychological distress was generally experienced by refugees and was often exacerbated by environmental (e.g., financial, housing, employment) issues and psychosocial outcomes (e.g., loss of role and social support, inactivity) (Wells et al., 2016). Furthermore, in a recent study investigating the prevalence of insomnia among refugees in Jordan, it was found that the majority of refugees had moderate to severe insomnia. Incidence of insomnia was predicted by factors such as older age, living in the city of Mafraq, poor education, unemployment, and lack of access to medication (Al-Smadi et al., 2017).

Understanding the experiences of refugees and asylum seekers is important in informing plans to alleviate these issues. Participatory engagement and ethical reporting are necessary to ensure that recommendations are based on evidence that is meaningful and useful on the ground. For example, McCarthy and Marks (2010) facilitated participatory action research to explore the health and well-being of refugee and asylum-seeking children. The research process suggests that although young refugees often face many challenges in their new life, they are able to find enough strength and resilience to cope with these issues. Similarly, Haaken and O'Neill (2014) used participatory visual methods to explore the experiences of women migrants and asylum seekers in the UK. Through photography and videography, participants were able to share their stories of seeking refuge in the UK. As an outcome of the project, a 10-minute video was developed which conveyed the complexities of the asylum process and also reflected historical and social dynamics of their experiences.

CULTURALLY COMPETENT HEALTH CARE SYSTEMS

In the ever-changing demographic and cultural trends of 'globalized' society, health care systems need to be able to adapt flexibly to such changes and develop **cultural competence**. Culturally competent health care involves developing (1) *culturally sensitive staff* who are able to reflect on their own beliefs and practices and acknowledge diversity in the community, and (2) *culturally appropriate materials, activities and systems* that address linguistic, cultural and social barriers. Cultural competence in health care asserts the importance of health service users and providers being able to communicate clearly with each other. Training health care professionals to develop skills that enable them to deal with communication issues associated with cultural, linguistic and health literacy differences may be a good way to reduce inequities in health (Lie et al., 2012). Culturally competent health care systems can do this by helping health care professionals to develop cultural sensitivity, knowledge and skills and by instilling processes that will enable them to engage meaningfully with culturally diverse patients. Systematic reviews suggest that interventions that aim to improve cultural competence among health care professionals can help to increase their knowledge of cultural issues in health care (Renzaho et al., 2013) and improve patient and clinical health outcomes (Truong et al., 2014).

In addition to culturally competent health care, diversity and inclusivity can be promoted in other social contexts. For example, Andreouli et al. (2014) explored the role of schools in promoting inclusive communities. The authors argued that intercultural exchange can be promoted by examining how communities resist stigma and discrimination on a local level. While starting on a micro level, such approaches can be endorsed to build the foundations of health-promoting communities.

FUTURE RESEARCH

1. Through access to historical documents, research psychologists can assist our understanding of the evolution of health beliefs.

2. Understanding popular health beliefs requires an appreciation of their social and cultural context.

3. The increasing development of alternative health care in Western society requires ongoing research.

4. The comprehensive and accurate measurement of perceived discrimination and its mechanisms, which contribute to poor health, require examination.

SUMMARY

1. Human thought and practices are culturally immersed.
2. The Western view of health has moved through various stages from the classic to the religious and then the scientific.
3. The scientific view of health, or biomedicine, is the dominant view in contemporary society but other health belief systems remain popular.
4. Traditional Chinese Medicine remains popular in China and among Chinese migrants in other societies.
5. Ayurvedic medicine remains popular in parts of Southern Asia.
6. In Africa a wide variety of health belief systems emphasize spiritual aspects and a communal orientation.
7. In contemporary society there is increasing interest in various complementary and alternative (CAM) therapies, such as herbal medicine, homeopathy, aromatherapy and reflexology.
8. While debates are ongoing about the efficacy of CAM, guidelines and policies are being developed to ensure quality and safety.
9. Interventions aiming to promote indigenous health need to reflect the holistic notion of health among these communities and the voice of the community itself.
10. Racism continues to contribute to poor health among migrants, ethnic minority groups and indigenous peoples.
11. Culturally competent health care must aim to adapt to changing demographic and cultural trends.

AN A–Z OF RESEARCH METHODS AND ISSUES RELEVANT TO HEALTH PSYCHOLOGY

'Be curious.'

Anon

OUTLINE

In this chapter, we present an A–Z of methods and issues within health psychology research in four categories: quantitative, qualitative, action research, or mixed. Quantitative researchers place an emphasis on reliable and valid measurement in controlled experiments, trials and surveys. Qualitative researchers use interviews, focus groups, narratives, diaries, texts or blogs to explore health and illness concepts and experiences. Action researchers facilitate change processes, improvement, empowerment and emancipation. Mixed methods researchers combine methods from different traditions. This chapter also introduces issues that are crucial to the progression of the field, such as replication, power and repeatability.

INTRODUCTION

Curiosity is the overarching motive for any piece of research. We always want to know more, to better understand how things work. Researchers are generating an increasingly diverse array of questions that require equally diverse methods to answer them. Inevitably publications end with more questions than answers and conclude with the statement that more research is needed. Theories play a crucial role in guiding our curiosity along worthwhile avenues. We need to go where the field is most fertile, and avoid sterile ground, error and false conclusions. We would not know where to start without theories, models and hypotheses to guide us. Using sound methodology and analysis is of equal importance in testing theories and models, putting theory into practice, and evaluating the consequences of doing so. In interventions and actions to produce change, we need to know what works and doesn't work, and why. The process is as important as the outcome. In an ideal situation we understand both, and can repeat the process and achieve the same outcome on multiple occasions.

Many traditional methods and research designs are quantitative, placing an emphasis on reliable and valid measurement in controlled investigations with experiments, trials and surveys. Multiple sources of such evidence are integrated or synthesized using systematic reviews and meta-analysis. Case studies are more suited to unique, one-off situations that merit investigation. Qualitative methods use interviews, focus groups, narratives or texts to explore health and illness concepts and experiences. Action research enables change processes to feed back into plans for improvement, empowerment and emancipation. Interest in qualitative methods and action research has been increasing. These different kinds of method complement each other, and are necessary if we want a complete picture of psychology and health. Which method is appropriate in any given situation depends entirely upon the question being asked and the context.

The sections below present an A–Z of the most commonly used research methods and issues that arise in health psychology.

ACTION RESEARCH

Action research is about the process of change and what stimulates it. The investigator acts as a facilitator, collaborator or change-agent who works with the stakeholders in a community or organization to help develop a situation or make a change of direction happen. Action research is particularly suited to organizational and consultancy work when a system or service requires improvements. In a community it aims to be emancipatory, helping to empower members to take more control over the way things work in their local community.

Action research can be traced back to the Gestalt psychology of Kurt Lewin (1936: 12): 'Every psychological event depends upon the state of the person and at the same time the state of the environment. … One can hope to understand the forces that govern behaviour only if one includes in the representation the whole psychological situation.' Lewin later wrote about what he called 'Feedback problems of social diagnosis and action' (1947) and presented a diagram of his method (see Figure 7.1). A series of action steps with feedback loops allows each action step to be 'reconnoitred' before further action steps.

Participant action research (PAR) is a prominent method in community health psychology (Campbell and Cornish, 2014). In PAR, researchers share power and control with participants and need to tolerate the uncertainty that rolls out of power-sharing. PAR is a suitable research approach in direct social actions that are organized to create change in entrenched scenarios where power imbalances are disadvantaging many of the actors. For example, Yeich (1996) described how housing campaigns with groups for homeless people involved assisting in the organization of demonstrations and working with the media to raise awareness of people's housing needs.

Action research takes time, resources, creativity and courage. It requires collaboration with different agencies. It is an approach that does not follow a straight line but proceeds in a halting, zig-zag format. Often there are personal challenges and disappointments for the researcher, who must devote substantial emotional and intellectual energy to the project (Brydon-Miller, 2004). Cornish et al. (2014) proposed the Occupy movement as a paradigm example of community action that they labelled 'trusting the process' (see Chapter 16).

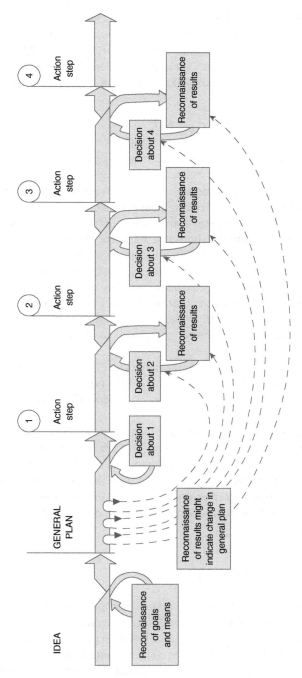

Figure 7.1   Planning, fact-finding and execution, as described by Kurt Lewin (1947)

PAR researchers also use the arts and performance as vehicles for envisioning and promoting change. Two examples are the photo novella (Wang et al., 1996; Lykes, 2001) and PhotoVoice (Haaken and O'Neill, 2014; Vaughan, 2014). Research participants in PhotoVoice take and display photographs with the aim of becoming more reflectively aware and are able to mobilize around personal and local issues. Tucker and Smith (2014) developed a Lewinian approach to the investigation of life situations and a specific example of self-care in a service user's home. A study of accidents in a fishing community used the PAR approach (Murray and Tilley, 2004), as did Gray and his colleagues when they transformed interviews with cancer patients into plays performed to support groups (Gray et al., 2001; Gray and Sinding, 2002).

BETWEEN GROUPS DESIGNS

A **between groups design** allocates matched groups to different treatments. If the measures are taken at one time, this is called a cross-sectional design, in contrast to a longitudinal design where the groups are tested at two or more time points. When we are comparing only treatment groups, a failure to find a difference between them on the outcome measure(s) might be for one of three reasons: they are equally effective; they are equally ineffective; they are equally harmful. For this reason, one of the groups should be a control group that will enable us to discover whether the treatment(s) show a different effect from no treatment.

Ethical issues arise over the use of control groups. Not treating someone in need of treatment is unacceptable. However, if there is genuine uncertainty about what works best, it is better to compare the treatments with a control condition than to continue forever applying a treatment that may be less effective than another. Once it has been determined which therapy is the most effective, this can be offered to the control group and to all future patients (Clark-Carter and Marks, 2004).

The choice of the control condition is important. The group should receive the same amount of attention as those in the treatment condition(s). This type of control is known as a placebo control (see below) as treatment itself could have a non-specific effect to 'please' the client and enhance his/her well-being.

If all of the various groups' responses are measured only after an intervention, then we haven't really measured change. All groups, including the control group, could have changed, but from different starting positions, and failing to find a difference between the groups after the treatment could miss this. We can help to deal with this problem by using a mixed design when we measure all groups before and after the treatment. However, we would be introducing some of the difficulties mentioned above for a cross-over or within-subjects design (Clark-Carter, 1997).

BONFERRONI CORRECTION

It is common in research to make multiple statistical comparisons. At the .05 or 5% significance (α) level with 20 tests there is a 64% chance of observing at least one significant result, even if none is actually significant (a Type I error). In a research project, numerous simultaneous tests may be required and the probability of getting a significant result simply by chance may be very high. The α level must be adjusted in some way, so that the probability of observing at least one significant result due to chance remains below the desired significance level. The Bonferroni correction places the significance cut-off at α/n. For example, with 20 tests and α at .05, you would only reject a null hypothesis if the *p*-value were less than .05/20 = 0.0025.

CASE STUDIES

The term '**case study**' is used to describe a detailed descriptive account of an individual, group or collective. The purpose of case studies is to provide a 'thick description' (Geertz, 1973) of a phenomenon that would not be obtained by the usual quantitative or qualitative approaches. It requires the researcher to be expansive in the types of data collected, with a deliberate aim to link the person with the context, e.g., the sick person in the family. The researcher usually attempts to provide a chronological account of the evolution of the phenomenon from the perspective of the central character.

A challenge for the researcher is in establishing the boundaries of the case. These need to be flexible to ensure that all information relevant to the case under investigation is collected. The major strength of the case study is the integration of actor and context and the developmental perspective. Thus, the phenomenon under investigation is not dissected but rather maintains its integrity or wholeness and it is possible to map its changes over time.

There are several different types of case study. The empirical case study is grounded in the data. The theoretical case is an exemplar for a process that has already been clarified. The researcher can conduct interviews, or repeat interviews and observe the case in different settings. The process of analysis can be considered the process of shaping the case. Thus, the researcher selects certain pieces of information and discards others so as to present a more integrated case. One example is De Visser and Smith's (2006) investigation of the links between masculine identity and social behaviour with a 19-year-old man living in London.

CONFIDENCE INTERVAL

A **confidence interval** (CI) is the interval around the mean of a sample that one can state with a known probability contains the mean of the population. A population parameter is always estimated using a sample. The reliability of the estimate varies according to sample size. A confidence interval specifies a range of values where a parameter is estimated to lie. The narrower the interval, then the more reliable the estimate. Typically, the 95% or 99% CI is stated in the results of a study that has obtained a representative sample of values, e.g., the mean heart rate for a sample might be 75.0 with a 95% CI of 72.6 to 77.4. Confidence intervals are normally reported in tables or graphs, along with point estimates of the parameters, to indicate the reliability of the estimates.

CONFLICTS OF INTEREST

Conflicts of interest (also known as 'competing interests') occur when an investigator is affected by personal, company or institutional bias towards a conclusion that is favourable to a treatment yet unsubstantiated by research findings. Authors are expected to declare any conflicts of interest at the point of publication. One can argue that this may already be too late in the process to trust the findings.

CROSS-OVER OR WITHIN-PARTICIPANTS DESIGNS

The **cross-over or within-participants design** is used when the same people provide measures of a dependent variable at more than one time and differences between the measures at the different times are recorded. An example would be a measure taken before an intervention (pre-treatment) and again after the intervention (post-treatment). Such a design minimizes the effect of individual differences as each person acts as his/her own control.

There are a number of problems with this design. Any change in the measure of the dependent variable may be due to other factors having changed. For example, an intervention designed to improve quality of life among patients in a long-stay ward of a hospital may be accompanied by other changes, such as a new set of menus introduced by the catering department. In addition, the difference may be due to some aspect of the measuring instrument. If the same measure is being taken on both occasions, the fact that it has been taken twice may be the reason that the result has changed.

Failure to find a difference between the two occasions doesn't tell you very much; in a worsening situation, the intervention still might have been effective in preventing things from worsening more than they have already. The counterfactual scenario in which nothing changed is an unknown entity.

CROSS-SECTIONAL DESIGNS

Cross-sectional designs obtain responses from respondents on one occasion only. With appropriate randomized sampling methods, the sample can be assumed to be a representative cross-section of the population under study and it is possible to make comparisons between sub-groups (e.g., males versus females, older versus younger people, etc.). However, cause and effect can never be inferred between one variable and another and it is impossible to say whether the observed associations are caused by a third background variable not measured in the study.

Cross-sectional designs are popular because they are relatively inexpensive in time and resources. However, there are problems of interpretation; not only can we say nothing about causality, but generalizability is also an issue whenever there is doubt about the randomness or representativeness of the samples. Many studies are done with students as participants and we can never be sure that the use of a non-random, non-representative sample of students is methodologically rigorous. The **ecological validity** of the findings is strongly contentious in the sense that they are unlikely to be replicated in a random sample from the general population. Any study with a non-random student sample should be repeated with a representative sample from a known population. Cross-sectional designs are also unsuited to studies of behaviour change and provide weak evidence in the testing of theories.

DIARIES AND BLOGS

Diaries and **diary techniques** have been used frequently as a method for collecting information about temporal changes in health status. These diaries can be prepared by the researcher or participant or both, and can be quantitative or qualitative, or both. They can be compared to the time charts that have been used by health professionals for generations to track changes in the health status of individuals. Blogs also provide a rich source of data on different illnesses and conditions and lay ideas on 'healthy living'.

A summary of the current uses of the diary in health research is reproduced in Table 7.1.

Table 7.1   The applicability of a diary or blog in health psychology research

Type of diary or blog	Description of use	Participant(s)	Reference
Validation of questionnaires	Examining the same behavioural change or psychological characteristics as recorded in diary	Chronic headache sufferers	Stewart et al. (1999)
Reflective understanding	Personal and scholarly reflections on experience of struggling with meaning-making	Cancer sufferer	Willig (2009)
Communication device	Provides a voice for the patient and an insight into how the patient interprets illness and treatment	Patients with longstanding illness	Stensland and Malterud (1999)
Evolving methodology	Provides an opportunity to gain qualitative data that can inform hypothesis generation and testing	ICU patients and families	Berghom et al. (1999)
Developing or testing theories	Constructs from a theoretical model and behaviour are measured	Patients	Ferguson and Chandler (2005)
Tracking/time series	Psychological, behavioural and physiological data can be collected to map changes over time	Non-clinical and clinical samples	Eissa et al. (2001)
Efficacy of treatment	Outcome measure	Behavioural therapy for irritable bowel syndrome	Heymann-Mönnikes et al. (2000)
Bloggers' experiences with disease or condition	Virtual social support and sharing of information	Patients	Miller and Pole (2010)
Personal experiences of health professionals	Virtual social support and sharing of information	Health care professionals	Miller and Pole (2010)
Healthy living blogs	Advice on improving physical and mental health, eating, exercise and self-image	Various	Boepple and Thompson (2014)

Diaries and blogs have benefits for the participant irrespective of the researcher (Murray, 2009). Research by Pennebaker (1995) and others has demonstrated that expressive writing can be psychologically beneficial. A series of studies has provided evidence that journal writing can lead to a reduction in illness symptoms and in the use of health services (e.g., Smyth et al., 1999). There are a number of explanations for this, including the release of emotional energy, cognitive processing and assistance with narrative restructuring. However the effects are small, and not always easy to replicate.

The internet provides a resource for blogs, diaries and forums in which individuals share their experiences, seek information and provide virtual social support. Anonymity may be used by bloggers to foster self-disclosure in describing embarrassing conditions. Chiu and Hsieh (2013), using focus group interviews with 34 cancer patients, explored how cancer patients' writing and reading on the internet play a role in their illness experience. They found that personal blogs enabled cancer patients to reconstruct their life stories, and express closure of life and how they expected to be remembered after death. Reading fellow patients' stories significantly influenced their perceptions and expectations of their illness prognosis, which was sometimes a greater influence than their doctors.

DIRECT OBSERVATION

The simplest kind of study involves directly observing behaviour in a relevant setting, for example patients waiting for treatment in a doctor's surgery or clinic. **Direct observation** may be accompanied by recordings in written, oral, auditory or visual form. Several investigators may observe the same events so that reliability checks can be conducted. Direct observation includes casual observation, formal observation and participant observation. However, ethical issues are raised by planned formal observational study of people who have not given informed consent to such observations.

DISCOURSE ANALYSIS

Discourse analysis is a set of procedures for analysing language as used in speech or texts. It focuses on the language and how it is used to construct versions of 'social reality' and what is gained by constructing events using particular terms. It has links with ethnomethodology, conversation analysis and the study of meaning (semiology). There are two forms of discourse analysis. The first, discursive psychology, evolved from the work of Potter and Wetherell (1987) and is concerned with the discursive strategies people use to further particular actions in social situations, including accounting for their own behaviour or thoughts. This approach has been used to explore the character of patient talk and the character of doctor–patient interactions. There is a particular preference for naturally occurring conversations, e.g., mealtime talk (Wiggins et al., 2001). Locke and Horton-Salway (2010) analysed how class leaders talked to antenatal class members about pregnancy, childbirth and infant care in 'golden age' or 'bad old days' stories variably to contrast the practices of the past with current practices. The second type of discourse analysis, Foucauldian discourse analysis (FDA), was developed by Ian Parker (1997) and others because they criticized the previous approach as evading issues of power and politics. FDA aims to identify the broader discursive resources that people in a particular culture draw upon in their everyday lives. This approach has been used to explore such issues as smoking (Gillies and Willig, 1997) and masculine identity (Tyler and Williams, 2014).

DOUBLE-BLIND CONTROL

A **double-blind control** is used in randomized controlled trials to prevent bias: both the investigator and the participant (subject) are prevented from knowing whether they are in the treatment or control condition. A single-blind is when only the participant is unaware of the condition they have been allocated to.

EFFECT SIZE

An **effect size** is the strength of the association between study variables and outcome as measured by an observed difference or correlation. Cohen's *d* and Person's *r* are the most popular indices of effect size in psychological studies. The effect size is a measure of the importance of an effect rather than its statistical significance. Effect sizes are used in meta-analysis as a means of measuring the magnitude of the results obtained over different studies. Effect size is related to the power of a study to detect a difference that really exists. A weak study cannot detect a real difference because it has samples that are too small relative to the magnitude of the difference that exists, a common problem in psychology. It is estimated that 60–70% of published studies in psychology journals lack sufficient power to obtain statistical significance.

ETHICAL APPROVAL

This is a necessary requirement before any research can be started. Ethics boards and research review panels in all research institutions and universities have been established for this purpose. Any research project must present before a panel of experts on ethical issues, and have the panel's explicit approval of: the full details of the aims, the design, the participants and how they will be chosen; the information provided to the participants; the method of consent used; the methods of data analysis; the nature and timing of debriefing of participants; and the methods of dissemination. Funding and publication are normally contingent on **ethical approval** being obtained.

ETHNOGRAPHIC METHODS

Ethnographic methods seek to build a systematic understanding of a culture from the viewpoint of the insider. Ethnographic methods are multiple attempts to describe the shared beliefs, practices, artefacts, knowledge and behaviours of an intact cultural group. They attempt to represent the totality of a phenomenon in its complete, naturalistic setting. Detailed observation is an important part of ethnographic fieldwork. Ethnography can provide greater ecological validity. The processes of transformation can be observed and documented, including how the culture becomes embodied in participants, alongside the recording of their narratives. It is more labour-intensive, but combining ethnography with narrative interviews can produce richer information than qualitative interviews alone (Paulson, 2011).

The observation can be either overt or covert. In the overt case, the researcher does not attempt to disguise his/her identity, but rather is unobtrusive so that the phenomenon under investigation is not disturbed. In this case, the researcher can take detailed notes, in either a pre-arranged or discursive format. In certain cases, the researcher may decide that his/her presence may disturb the field. In this case, two forms of covert observation may be used. In one form, the focus of observation is not aware at all of the presence of the researcher. An alternative approach is when the person observed may be aware of the researcher's presence but is unaware that he/she is a researcher. In both of these forms the researcher needs to consider whether such covert surveillance is ethically justified. A form of participant observation that is not covert is when the researcher accompanies the person but tries not to interfere with the performance of everyday tasks. Priest (2007) combined grounded theory and ethnography to explore members' experience of a mental health day service walking group, including the psychological benefits of the physical activity, the outdoor environment and the social setting. Stolte and Hodgetts (2015) used ethnographic methods to study the tactics employed by a homeless man in Central Auckland, New Zealand, to maintain his health and help him to gain respite while living on the streets, an unhealthy place.

FOCUS GROUPS

Focus groups comprise one or more group discussions in which participants 'focus' collectively upon a topic or issue that is usually presented to them as a series of questions, although sometimes as a film, a collection of advertisements, cards to sort, a game to play, or a vignette to discuss. The distinctive feature of the focus group method is its generation of interactive data (Wilkinson, 1998). Focus groups were initially used in marketing research. As its title implied, they had a focus that was to clarify the participants' views on a particular product. Thus, from the outset the researcher had set the parameters of the discussion and as it proceeded he/she deliberately guided the discussion so that its focus remained limited. More recent use of the focus group has been much more expansive. In many cases, the term 'discussion group' is preferred to give an indication of this greater latitude. The role of the researcher in the focus group is to act as the moderator for the discussion. The researcher can follow similar guidelines to those for an interview by using a guide, except the discussion should be allowed to flow freely and not be constrained too much by the investigator's agenda. The researcher needs to ensure that all the group participants have an opportunity to express their viewpoints. The method is often combined with interviews and questionnaires.

Although it is usual for the moderator to introduce some themes for discussion, this can be supplemented with a short video extract or pictures relevant to the topic being investigated. As the discussion proceeds, the researcher can often take a background role, while ensuring that the discussion does not deviate too far from the focus of the research and that all the participants have an opportunity to express their views. An assistant can help in completing consent forms, providing name-tags, organizing refreshments, keeping notes on who is talking (this is useful for transcription), and monitoring the recording equipment. The focus group recording should be transcribed as soon as possible afterwards since it is often difficult to distinguish speakers. Here are a few examples: Jones et al. (2014b) carried out a focus group and telephone interviews with patients in rural areas to examine the management of diabetes in a rural area; Liimakka (2014) drew upon focus group discussions to explore how young Finnish university students viewed the cultural ideals of health and appearance; Griffiths et al. (2015) used pre- and post-intervention focus groups to test a website, Realshare, for young oncology patients in the south-west of England; and Bogart (2015) examined the social experiences of 10 adolescents aged 12–17 years with Moebius Syndrome, a rare condition involving congenital facial paralysis.

GROUNDED THEORY ANALYSIS

Grounded theory analysis is a term used to describe a set of guidelines for conducting qualitative data analysis. It was originally developed by Glaser and Strauss (1967) and has subsequently gone through various revisions. In its original form, qualitative researchers were asked to dispense with theoretical assumptions when they began their research. Rather, they were encouraged to adopt a stance of disciplined naïvety. As the research progresses, certain theoretical concepts are discovered and then tested in an iterative fashion. In the case of the qualitative interview, the researcher is encouraged to begin the analysis at a very early stage, even as the interview is progressing. Through a process of abduction, the researcher begins to develop certain theoretical hypotheses. These hypotheses are then integrated into a tentative theoretical model that is tested as more data are collected.

This process follows a series of steps beginning with generating data. At this stage, the researcher may have some general ideas about the topic but this should not restrict the talk of the participant. From the very initial stages the researcher is sifting through the ideas presented and seeking more information about what are considered to be emerging themes. From a more positivist perspective, it is argued that the themes emerge from the data and that the researcher has simply to look for them. This approach is often associated with Glaser (1992). From a more social constructionist perspective, certain theoretical concepts of the researcher will guide both the data collection and the analysis. This approach is more associated with the symbolic inter-actionist tradition (Strauss, 1987; Charmaz, 2003).

Having collected some data, the researcher conducts a detailed coding of it, followed by the generation of bigger categories. Throughout the coding the researcher follows the process of constant comparative analysis. This involves making comparisons of codes within and between interview transcripts. This is followed by the stage of memo-writing, which requires the researcher to begin to expand upon the meaning of the broader conceptual categories. This in turn can lead to further data generation through theoretical sampling. This is the process whereby the researcher deliberately selects certain participants or certain research themes to explore further because of the data already analysed. At this stage, the researcher is both testing and strengthening the emergent theory. At a certain stage in this iterative process the researcher feels that he/she has reached the stage of data saturation – no new concepts are emerging and it is considered fruitless to continue with data collection.

A few examples are as follows: DiMillo et al. (2015) used grounded theory methodology to examine the stigmatization experiences of six BRCA1/2 gene mutation carriers following genetic testing; Searle et al. (2014) studied participants' experiences of facilitated physical activity for the management of depression in primary care; Silva et al. (2013) used the method to study the balancing of motherhood with drug addiction in addicted mothers.

HIERARCHY OF EVIDENCE

In traditional top-down approaches to research, a hierarchy of evidence or research methods is often utilized (Figure 7.2). In this pyramidical hierarchy of methods, meta-analyses and systematic reviews occupy the pinnacle and qualitative methods are at the base. Researchers who prefer the alternative, bottom-up approach are much more likely to employ qualitative and mixed methods. Critical health psychologists dispute the validity of the evidence hierarchy, which tends to be formulaic, restrictive and lacking in innovation.

HISTORICAL ANALYSIS

Health and illness are socially and historically located phenomena. As such, psychologists have much to gain by detailed historical research (**historical analysis**) on the development of health beliefs and practices. They can work closely with medical or health historians to explore the evolution of scientific and popular beliefs about health and illness or they can work independently (see Chapter 6). An example is the work of Herzlich and Pierret (1987). Their work involved the detailed analysis of a variety of textual sources such as scientific medical writings, but also popular autobiographical and fictional accounts of the experience of illness. They noted the particular value of literary works because of their important contribution to shaping public discourse. Such textual analysis needs to be guided by an understanding of the political and philosophical ideas of the period.

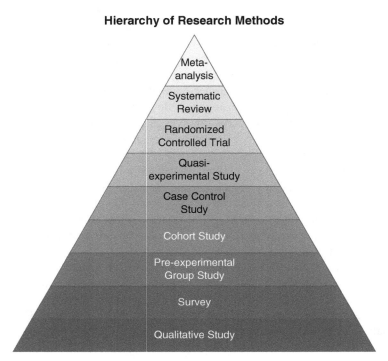

Hierarchy of Research Methods

Figure 7.2   Hierarchy of evidence

Source: Public domain

Health psychologists need also to be reflexive about the history of their own discipline. It arose at a particular historical period sometimes described as late modernity. Initially it was seen as providing a complement to the excessive physical focus of biomedicine. Now some see it as part of the broader lifestyle movement.

There are different approaches to the writing of history. There are those who can be broadly characterized as descriptive and who often provide a list of the growth of the discipline in laudatory terms (e.g., Stone et al., 1987). Conversely, there are those who adopt a more critical approach and attempt to dissect the underlying reasons for the development of the discipline. Within health psychology, this latter approach is still in its early stages (e.g., Stam, 2014).

INTERPRETATIVE PHENOMENOLOGICAL ANALYSIS

Phenomenological research is concerned with exploring the lived experience of health, illness and disability. Its aim is to understand these phenomena from the perspective of the particular participant. This in turn has to be interpreted by the researcher. A technique that addresses this challenge is **interpretative phenomenological analysis (IPA)** (Smith, 2004). IPA focuses on the cognitive processing of the participant. Smith (2004) argues that it accords with the original direction of cognitive psychology that was concerned with exploring meaning-making rather than information-processing. IPA provides a guide to conducting the researcher's making sense or meaning of reported experiences. It begins by accessing the participant's perceptions through the conduct of an interview or series of interviews with a homogeneous sample of individuals. The interview is semi-structured and focuses on the particular issue of concern.

Data analysis in IPA goes through a number of stages. Initially, the researcher reads and re-reads the text and develops a higher order thematic analysis. Having identified the key themes or categories, the researcher then proceeds to look for connections between them by identifying clusters. At this stage, the researcher is drawing upon his/her broader under-standing to make sense of what has been said. Once the researcher has finished the analysis of one case, he/she can proceed to conduct an analysis of the next case in a similar manner. Alternatively, the researcher can begin to apply the analytic scheme developed in the previous case. The challenge is to identify repeating patterns but also to be alert to new patterns. Further details of this form of analysis are available in Smith et al. (1999) and Smith and Osborn (2003).

A few examples are as follows: Conroy and De Visser (2013) studied the importance of authenticity for student non-drinkers; Mackay and Parry (2015) studied two perspectives on autistic behaviours; Burton et al. (2014) used an interpretative phenomenological analysis of sense-making within a dyadic relationship of living together with age-related macular degeneration; Ware et al. (2015) used IPA to study the experience of hepatitis C treatment for people with a history of mental health problems; Levi et al. (2014) investigated phenomenological hope among perceptions of traumatized war veterans.

INTERVENTIONS

Interventions are deliberate attempts to facilitate improvements to health. The idea for the intervention can come from a theory or model, from discussions with those who are knowledgeable about the condition or situation that needs to be changed, or from 'out of the blue'.

A key aspect of designing and/or implementing any intervention is evaluation – attempting to prove whether or not the intervention is effective or efficacious. Furthermore, reports of intervention studies are typically brief, opaque descriptions of what can often be complex interventions.

Reports of behaviour change studies typically provide brief summaries of what in reality may be a highly complex and unique intervention. One problem is that there is no meaningful method of classifying interventions for behaviour change into any single theory or method of description.

There is no meaningful method of relating the practice of behaviour change to any single theory or taxonomy. This means that the researcher does not know how to label what they have done in a way that communicates this in any precise manner to others (Marks, 2009). A key criterion for the reporting of an intervention must be transparency. Can another person or group repeat the study in his/her/their own setting with his/her/their own participants? The need to be concise in publishing studies means that the level of detail required for successful replication may often be missing. It is therefore almost impossible for new investigators to repeat a published intervention with any exactitude in their own settings.

INTERVIEWS (SEMI-STRUCTURED)

Semi-structured interviews are designed to explore the participant's view of things with the minimal amount of assumptions from the interviewer. A semi-structured interview is more open-ended than a structured interview and allows the interviewee to address issues that he/she feels are relevant to the topics raised by the investigator (see Qualitative research methods below). Open-ended questions are useful in this kind of interview. They have several advantages over closed-ended questions. The answers will not be biased by the researcher's preconceptions as much as closed-ended questions can be. The respondents are able to express their opinions, thoughts and feelings freely, using their own words in ways that are less constrained by the particular wordings of the question. The respondents may have responses that the structured interview designer has overlooked. They may have in-depth comments that they wish to make about the study and the topics that it is covering that would not be picked up using the standard questions in a structured interview.

In preparing for the interview the researcher should develop an interview guide. This can include a combination of primary and supplementary questions. Alternatively, the researcher may prefer to have a list of themes to be explored. However, it is important that the researcher does not formally follow these in the same order but rather introduces them at the appropriate time in the interview. Prior to the interview, the researcher should review these themes and order them from the least invasive to the more personal.

INTERVIEWS (STRUCTURED)

A structured interview schedule is a prepared, a standard set of questions that are asked in person, or perhaps by telephone, of a person or group concerning a particular research issue.

LITERATURE SEARCH

An essential skill in any research project is to carry out a **literature search**. Usually this will be best achieved using keywords. The key data in all scholarly publications consist of the title, the abstract, which is a summary of 100 to 250 words, and the keywords that are listed with the data about the article. By inserting keywords into any search engine, it is possible to obtain a comprehensive list of scholarly research reports, dissertations and conference papers, books and monographs. One popular search engine is Google Scholar. Another major database for researchers is the 'ISI Web of Knowledge'. This contains a large selection of peer-reviewed publications from journals with a proven track record of high-quality publications. Examples of the results from searches of the health psychology literature are shown in Figures 7.1 and 7.4.

LONGITUDINAL DESIGNS

Longitudinal designs involve measuring responses of a single sample on more than one occasion. The measurements may be prospective or retrospective. Prospective longitudinal designs allow greater control over the sample, the variables measured and the times when the measurements take place. Such designs are superior to cross-sectional designs because one is better able to investigate hypotheses of causation when the associations between variables are measured over time. Longitudinal designs are among the most powerful designs available for the evaluation of treatments and of theories about human experience and behaviour, but they are also the most expensive in terms of labour, time and money.

META-ANALYSIS

Meta-analysis is the use of statistical techniques to combine the results of primary studies addressing the same question into a single pooled measure of effect size, with a confidence interval. The analysis is often based on the calculation of a weighted mean effect size in which each primary study is weighted according to the number of participants. A meta-analysis follows a series of steps, as follows: (1) develop a research question; (2) identify all relevant studies; (3) select studies on the basis of the issue being addressed and methodological criteria; (4) decide which dependent variables or summary measures are allowed; (5) calculate a summary effect; and (6) reach a conclusion in answer to the original research question.

MIXED METHODS RESEARCH

Methodology that involves collecting, analysing and integrating quantitative and qualitative research. Examples can be found in Creswell and Clark (2007), Johnson et al. (2007), Lucero et al. (2016) and Kuenemund et al. (2016).

NARRATIVE APPROACH

This approach is concerned with the desire to seek insight and meaning about health and illness through the acquisition of data in the form of stories concerning personal experiences. The **narrative approach** assumes that human beings are natural storytellers and that the principal task of the psychologist is to explore the different stories being told (Murray and Ziegler, 2015). The most popular source of material for the narrative researcher is the interview. The focus of the narrative interview is the elicitation of storied accounts from the interviewee. This can take various forms. The life-story interview is the most extended form of interview. As its name implies, the life-story interview seeks to obtain an extended account of the person's life. The primary aim is to make the participant at ease and encourage him/her to tell their story at length.

Narrative analysis (NA) can take various forms. It begins with a repeated reading of the text to identify the story or stories within it. The primary focus is on maintaining the narrative integrity of the account. The researcher may develop a summary of the narrative account that will help identify the structure of the narrative, its tone and the central characters. It may be useful to engage in a certain amount of thematic analysis to identify some underlying themes. But this does not equate with narrative analysis. NA involves trying to see the interconnections between events rather than separating them. Having analysed one case, the researcher can then proceed to the next, identifying similarities and differences in the structure and content of the narratives.

OBSERVATIONAL STUDIES

The term 'observational study' is used to describe research carried out to evaluate the effect of an intervention or treatment that does not have the advantages of a control group. A single group of patients is observed at various points before, during and after the treatment in an attempt to ascertain the changes that occur as a result of the treatment. There are strict limitations on the conclusions that can be reached as a consequence of the lack of a control group (e.g., see Randomized controlled trials below). However, there are occasions when a randomized controlled trial is impossible to carry out because of ethical or operational difficulties.

PARTICIPATORY ACTION RESEARCH

Participatory action research (PAR) is a version of action research (see above) that deliberately seeks to provoke some form of social or community change.

POWER AND POWER ANALYSIS

Power refers to the ability of a study to find a statistically significant effect when a genuine effect exists. The power $(1-\beta)$ of a statistical test is the complement of β, the Type II or beta error probability of falsely retaining an incorrect H_0. Statistical power relies on three parameters: (1) the significance level (i.e., the Type I error probability or α level); (2) the size(s) of the sample(s); and (3) an effect size parameter defining H_1 and thus indicating the degree of deviation from H_0 in the underlying population.

Cohen (1973) found that psychology studies had about a 50% chance of finding a genuine effect owing to their lack of statistical power. The situation has changed in the last 40 years but it remains problematic. This lack of power is caused by study samples being too small to permit definite conclusions. Given the easy availability of free software online, there can be little excuse for not doing a power analysis before embarking on a research project. Funding agencies, ethics boards, research review panels and journal editors normally require a power analysis as a condition of funding, approval and publication.

There are several different types of power analysis, some being more robust than others. In a priori power analyses (Cohen, 1988), sample size N is computed as a function of the required power level $(1-\beta)$, the pre-specified significance level α, and the population effect size to be detected with probability $1-\beta$. Cohen's definitions of small, medium and large effects can be helpful in effect size specifications.

A variety of software is available to expedite rapid power analyses, including G* Power 3 (Faul et al. 2007) and free online software online such as OpenEpi (Dean et al., 2014).

QUALITATIVE RESEARCH METHODS

Qualitative research methods aim to understand the meanings, purposes and intentions of behaviour, not its amount or quantity. A huge variety of methods are available and these are described in this A–Z under the following headings: diaries and blogs; discourse analysis; focus groups; grounded theory; historical analysis; interpretative phenomenological analysis; interviews, especially semi-structured; and narrative approaches. Figure 7.3 shows the rapid growth of qualitative research in health psychology over the last few decades. This trend is expected to continue. A wide variety of software is available to support qualitative and mixed methods research analyses, such as NVivo, MAXQDA and QDA Miner Lite.

QUESTIONNAIRES

Questionnaires in health psychology consist of a standard set of questions with accompanying instructions concerning attitudes, beliefs, perceptions or values concerned with health, illness or health care. Ideally, a questionnaire will have been demonstrated to be a reliable and valid measure of the construct(s) it purports to measure.

Questionnaires vary in objectives, content (especially in their generic versus specific content), question format, the number of items, and sensitivity or responsiveness to change. Questionnaires may be employed in cross-sectional and longitudinal studies. When looking for changes over time, the responsiveness of a questionnaire to clinical and subjective changes is a crucial feature. A questionnaire's content, sensitivity and extent, together with its reliability and validity, influence a questionnaire's selection. Guides are available to advise users on making a choice that contains the appropriate generic measure or domain of interest (e.g., Bowling, 2001, 2004). These guides are useful as they include details on content, scoring, validity and reliability of dozens of questionnaires for measuring all of the major aspects of psychological well-being and quality of life, including disease-specific and domain-specific questionnaires and more generic measures.

The investigator must ask: What is it that I want to know? The answer will dictate the selection of the most relevant and useful questionnaire. The most important aspect of questionnaire selection is therefore to match the objective of the study with the objective of the questionnaire. For example, are you interested in a disease-specific or broad-ranging research question? When this question is settled, you need to decide whether there is anything else that your research objective will require you to know. Usually the researcher needs to develop a specific block of questions that will seek vital information concerning the respondents' socio-demographic characteristics. This block of questions can be placed at the beginning or the end of the main questionnaire.

Questionnaire content may vary from the highly generic (e.g., How has your health been over the last few weeks? Excellent, Good, Fair, Poor, Very Bad) to the highly specific (e.g., Have you had any arguments with people at work in the last two weeks?). Questionnaires vary greatly in the number of items that are used to assess the variable(s) of interest. Single-item measures use a single question, rating or item to measure the concept or variable of interest. For example, the now popular single verbal item to evaluate health status: During the past four weeks how would you rate your health in general? Excellent, Very good, Good, Fair, Poor. Single items have the obvious advantages of being simple, direct and brief.

Questionnaires remain one of the most useful and widely applicable research methods in health psychology. A few questionnaire scales have played a dominant role in health psychology research over the last few decades. Figure 7.4 shows the number of items in the ISI Web of Knowledge database for three of the most popular scales. Over the 20-year period 1990–2009, usage of scales designed to measure health status has been dominated by three front-runners: the McGill Pain Questionnaire (Melzack, 1975), the Hospital Anxiety and Depression Scale

(HADS; Zigmond and Snaith, 1983), and the SF-36 Health Survey (Brazier et al., 2002). The SF-36 is by far the most utilized scale in clinical research, accounting for around 50% of all clinical studies (Figure 7.3).

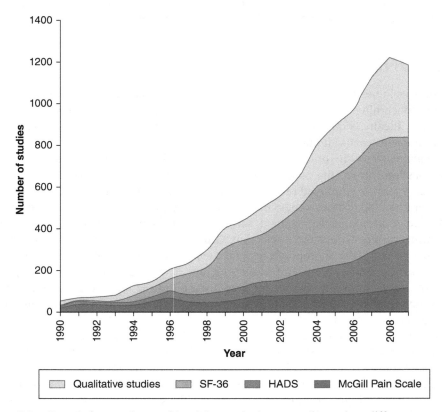

Figure 7.3   Trends in numbers of health psychology studies using different research measures and methods, 1990–2009

Source: Marks (2013)

RANDOMIZED CONTROLLED TRIALS

Randomized controlled trials (RCTs) involve the systematic comparison of interventions using a fully controlled application of one or more 'treatments' with a random allocation of participants to the different treatment groups. The statistical tests that are available have as one of their assumptions that participants have been randomly assigned to conditions. In real-world settings of clinical and health research, the so-called 'gold standard' of the RCT cannot always be achieved in practice, and in fact may not be desirable for ethical reasons.

We are frequently forced to study existing groups that are being treated differently rather than have the luxury of being able to allocate people to conditions. Thus, we may in effect be comparing the health policies and services of a number of different hospitals and clinics. Such 'quasi-experimental designs' are used to compare treatments in as controlled a manner as possible, when, for practical reasons, it is impossible to manipulate the independent variable, the policies, or allocate the participants.

The advantage of an RCT is that differences in the outcome can be attributed with more confidence to the manipulations of the researchers, because individual differences are likely to be spread in a random way between the different treatments. As soon as that basis for allocation of participants is lost, then questions arise over the ability to identify causes of changes or differences between the groups; in other words, the internal validity of the design is in question.

Randomized controlled trials are complex operations to manage and describe, which has led to a difficulty in replication of RCTs. To help solve this problem, the CONSORT guidelines for RCTs published by Moher et al. (2001) and the TREND statement for non-randomized studies (Des Jarlais et al., 2004) were intended to bridge the gap between intervention descriptions and intended replications. These guidelines have driven efforts to enhance the practice of reporting behaviour change intervention studies. Davidson et al. (2003) expanded the CONSORT guidelines in proposing that authors should report: (1) the content or elements of the intervention; (2) the characteristics of those delivering the intervention; (3) the characteristics of the recipients; (4) the setting; (5) the mode of delivery; (6) the intensity; (7) the duration; and (8) adherence to delivery protocols/manuals.

Another issue with RCTs has been bias created by industry sponsorship. Critics claim that research carried out or sponsored by the pharmaceutical industry should be treated with a high degree of suspicion as the investigators may have a hidden bias that can affect their ability to remain independent. Lexchin et al. (2003) carried out a systematic review of the effect of pharmaceutical industry sponsorship on research outcome and quality. They found that pharmaceutically sponsored studies were less likely to be published in peer-reviewed journals. Also, studies sponsored by pharmaceutical companies were more likely to have outcomes favouring the sponsor than were studies with other sponsors (odds ratio 4.05; 95% confidence interval 2.98–5.51). They found a systematic bias favouring products made by the company funding the research.

There have been significant abuses of RCTs in clinical and drug trials. Many trials have not been registered so that there is no record of them having been carried out. Trials showing non-significant effects have been unreported, which distorts the evidence base by suggesting that a drug is better than it actually is. Placebo control conditions have been manipulated to enhance drug effects. The double-blind requirements for RCTs have been broken. Investigators who have received funding from drug companies have written biased or misleading reports. Ghost writers have been employed to write glowing reports. These abuses have led to the wastage of public funds on ineffective drugs and treatments, missed opportunities for improving treatments, and trials being repeated unnecessarily.

The AllTrials movement is campaigning to remove these abuses and to obtain publication of all clinical trials (see www.alltrials.net/).

REPEATABILITY

Reproducibility is one criterion for progress in science. If a study is repeated under similar conditions, then it should be possible to obtain the same findings. However, journal reviewers and editors may not accept a replication or failed replication for publication on the grounds that it is not as 'newsworthy' as an original study. In one landmark study, fewer than half of 100 studies published in 2008 in three top psychology journals could be successfully replicated

(Open Science Collaboration, 2015). Lack of replication indicates that: (1) Study A's results may be false, or (2) Study B's results may be false, or (3) both may be false, or (4) there may be some subtle differences in the way the two studies were conducted – in other words, there were differences in the *context*. The OSC analysis showed that a low *p* value was predictive of which studies could be replicated. Twenty of the 32 original studies with a $p < 0.001$ could be replicated, while only 2 of the 11 papers with a value greater than 0.04 were successfully replicated. The reproducibility of health psychology studies is yet to be fully evaluated.

REPLICATION

Replication is one of the most important research methods in existence. Yet it is hardly used or mentioned in textbooks about research methods. Replication refers to the attempt by an investigator to repeat a study purely to determine whether the original findings can be repeated. Essentially, the researcher wants to know whether the original findings are reliable or whether they have been produced by some combination of chance or spurious factors. If study findings can be replicated, then they can be accepted as reliable and valuable to knowledge and understanding. However, if the findings of a study cannot be replicated, then the findings cannot be accepted as a genuine contribution to knowledge.

Lack of replication has been a bone of contention in many areas of psychology, including health psychology. Traditionally, a low priority has been given to replication of other researchers' results. Perhaps researchers believe that they will not be perceived as sufficiently creative if they replicate somebody else's research. In a similar vein, journal editors do not give replications of research – especially failed replications – the same priority as novel findings. This bias towards new positive results, and away from failed replications, produces a major distortion in the academic literature. Lack of replication before publication is the main reason for the so-called 'Repeatability Crisis' in psychology and other disciplines.

SINGLE CASE EXPERIMENTAL DESIGNS

Single case experimental designs are investigations of a series of experimental manipulations with a single research participant.

SURVEYS

Surveys are systematic methods for determining how a sample of participants respond to a set of standard questions. They attempt to assess their feelings, attitudes, beliefs or knowledge at one or more times. For example, we may want to know how drug users' perceptions of themselves and their families differ from those of non-users, or better understand the experiences of patients receiving specific kinds of treatment, how health and social services are perceived by informal carers of people with dementia, Parkinson's, multiple sclerosis (MS) or other chronic conditions, or learn more about how people recovering from a disease such as coronary heart disease feel about their rehabilitation. The survey method is the method of choice in many of these types of study.

The survey method, whether using interviews, questionnaires, or some combination of the two, is versatile and can be applied equally well to research with individuals, groups, organizations, communities or populations to inform our understanding of a host of very different research issues and questions. Normally, a survey is conducted on a sample of the study population of interest (e.g., people aged 70+, women aged 20–44, teenagers who smoke, carers of people with dementia, etc.). Issues of key importance in conducting a survey are the objective(s), the mode of administration, the method of sampling, the sample size and the preparation of the data for analysis.

As in any research, it is essential to have a clear idea about the objective, why we are doing our study (the theory or policy behind the research), what we are looking for (the research question), where we intend to look (the setting or domain), who will be in the sample (the study sample) and how we use the tools we have at our disposal. The investigator must be cautious that the procedures do not generate any self-fulfilling prophecies. Lack of clarity about the purposes and objectives is one of the main stumbling blocks for the novice investigator to overcome. This is particularly the case when carrying out a survey, especially in a team of investigators who may have varying agendas with regard to the why, what, who, where and how questions that must be answered before the survey can begin.

Modes of administration include face-to-face interview, telephone interview, social media, group self-completion and postal self-completion.

Next, you need to decide who will be the sample for your survey and also where you will carry it out. Which population is your research question about? The sample should represent the study population as closely as possible. In some cases, the sample can consist of the entire study population (e.g., every pupil in a school; every student at a university; every patient in a hospital). More usually, however, the sample is likely to be a random selection of a proportion of the members of a population (e.g., every tenth person in a community, or every fourth patient admitted into a hospital). This method is called simple random sampling (SRS). A variation on SRS is systematic sampling. In this case, the first person in the sampling frame is chosen at random and then every nth person on the list from there on, where n is the sample fraction being used.

In stratified sampling, the population is divided into groups or 'strata' and the groups are randomly sampled, but in different proportions so that the overall sample sizes of the groups can be made equal, even though they are not equal in the population (e.g., the 40–59, 60–79 and 80–99 age groups in a community sample, or men and women in a clinical sample). These groups will therefore be equally represented in the data. Other methods include non-probability sampling of six kinds: convenience samples, most similar/dissimilar samples, typical case samples, critical case samples, snowball samples and quota samples.

All such sampling methods are biased; in fact, there is no perfect method of sampling because there will always be a category of people that any sampling method under-represents. In any survey, it is necessary to maximize the proportion of selected people who are recruited. If a large proportion of people refuse to participate, the sample will not represent the population, but will be biased in unknown ways. As a general principle, surveys that recruit at least 70% of those invited to participate are considered representative. The sample size is a key issue. The variability of scores obtained from the sampling diminishes as the sample size increases, so the larger the sample, the more precise will be the estimates of the population scores, but the more the survey will cost.

SYSTEMATIC REVIEWS

A **systematic review** (SR) is a method of integrating the best evidence about an effect or intervention from all relevant and usable primary sources. What counts as relevant and usable is a matter for debate and judgement. Rules and criteria for selecting studies and for extracting data are agreed in advance by those carrying out the review. Publishing these rules and criteria along with the review enables such reviews to be replicable and transparent. Proponents of the SR therefore see it as a way of integrating research that limits bias. Traditionally, the method has been applied to quantitative data. Recently, researchers have begun to investigate ways and means to synthesize qualitative studies also.

Knowing how to carry out and to critically interpret an SR report are essential skills in all fields of health research. They enable researchers and clinicians to integrate research findings and make improvements in health care.

Systematic reviews act like a sieve, selecting some evidence but rejecting other evidence. To retain the metaphor, the reviewers act as a filter; what they see and report depends on how the selection process is operated. Whenever there is ambiguity, the process may well tend to operate in confirmatory mode, seeking positive support for a position, model or theory rather than disconfirmation. It is essential to be critical and cautious in interpreting and analysing SRs of biomedical and related topics. If we want to implement new practice as a direct consequence of such reviews, we had better make certain that the findings are solid and not a mirage. This is why the study of the method itself is so important. Systematic reviews of the same topic can produce significantly different results, indicating that bias is difficult to control. Like all forms of knowledge, the results of an SR are the consequences of a process of negotiation about rules and criteria, and cannot be accepted without criticism and debate. There are many examples of SRs causing controversy, for example Law et al. (1991), Swales (2000), Marks (2002c), Dixon-Woods et al. (2006), Roseman et al. (2011) and Coyne and Kok (2014).

TAXONOMY FOR INTERVENTION STUDIES

This section describes an idea for a **taxonomy** designed to help solve a variety of issues mentioned elsewhere in this A–Z, namely, the description of interventions, replication and transparency. As noted, lack of replication has been a major issue in psychology. One reason for the failure to replicate is the sheer complexity of different interventions that are available. A vast array of interventions and techniques can be delivered in multitudinous combinations, enabling literally millions of different interventions designed to change behaviour (Marks, 2009).

If interventions are incompletely described, it is not possible to: (1) determine all the necessary attributes of the intervention; (2) classify the intervention into a category or type; (3) compare and contrast interventions across studies; (4) identify which specific intervention component was responsible for efficacy; (5) replicate the intervention in other settings; or (6) advance the science of illness prevention by enabling theory testing in the practice of health care.

One way to put order into the chaos is to use a taxonomic system similar to those used to classify organisms or substances. Taxonomies for living things have been constructed since the time of Aristotle, with the periodic table in chemistry being the best-known example. Some researchers approached this issue by generating 'shopping lists' of interventions used in different studies. For example, Abraham and Michie (2008) described 26 behaviour change interventions, which they claimed provided a 'taxonomy' of generally applicable behaviour change techniques. Michie et al. (2008: Appendix A) also produced a list of 137 heterogeneous techniques. However, these lists are not useful as taxonomies because they do not demonstrate any systematic structure or organization of classification. A list of techniques is no more useful than a list of chemicals. Only when there is an organization like the periodic table do we gain an understanding of the underlying structure and the relationship between the various elements that lie in the table.

Psychology lacks a system for classifying interventions into a single system consisting of all known techniques and sub-techniques. In an effort to fill this gap, one of the authors has described a taxonomic system which includes six nested levels:

1. Paradigms, e.g., individual, community, public health, critical.

2. Domains, e.g., stress, diabetes, hypertension, smoking, weight, exercise, etc.

3. Programmes, e.g., smoking cessation, obesity management, stress management and assertiveness training.

4. Intervention types, e.g., relaxation induction, imagery, planning, cognitive restructuring, imagery, buddy system monitoring.

5. Techniques, e.g., within imagery there are a large number of techniques, such as mental rehearsal, guided imagery, flooding in imagination and systematic sensitization.

6. Sub-techniques, e.g., within guided imagery there exist a variety of sensory modalities (sight, sound, smell, taste, touch, warmth/coldness), scenarios (e.g., beach, forest, garden, air balloon), delivery methods (e.g., spoken instruction, self-administered by reading, listening to audio tapes), settings (e.g., individual, group) and participant positions (e.g., supine, sitting on floor, sitting on chair).

This taxonomic system is capable of including all health psychology paradigms, domains, programmes, intervention types, techniques and sub-techniques, as defined with universal reference in the form of a tree diagram. Any research design that is sufficiently specific can be placed within this taxonomic system to enable any imaginable intervention to be constructed, delivered, evaluated, labelled, reported and replicated in an unambiguous fashion. This system, or something similar, is needed to remove some basic problems that hold back progress in psychology as a discipline.

TOP-DOWN VERSUS BOTTOM-UP RESEARCH APPROACHES

A '*top-down*' research approach is where an executive decision-maker, who may be a theorist, a research director or other influential person within an organization, makes decisions about the nature of a research programme that should be carried out, the objectives of the research, and the methodology, with or without the consultation of an advisory board. This executive decision requires the existence of suitable funding, for example from governmental and/or commercial sources. A hierarchical system with different levels of research personnel responds according to the requirements of the programme. In many instances, the research programme will be carried out across multiple institutions, which compete for the resources by demonstrating their excellence in their commitment to the research question and in their competence to carry it forward.

The top-down research approach mirrors the social hierarchy found in ancient Egypt, wherein the Pharaoh ruled over a hierarchy of social and occupational classes residing at various levels below (Figure 7.4).

A top-down research approach has been the predominant approach across universities, institutes and research organizations. The 'Pharaoh' is normally a leading theoretician, funding body, institute director or professor who sets the goals for the research, organizes the funding and appoints the principal investigators (PIs) who are responsible for implementing the research programme, including the methodology, defining the specific research questions, and selecting personnel qualified to organize recruitment of the participants (or 'subjects') and the data collection. In turn, the PIs are responsible for recruiting assistants to collect data and statisticians to analyse the data from participants, who are normally patients or college students, at the bottom of the research hierarchy. Expert paper writers may consist of the PIs themselves or be especially hired for their ability to write up the study in the most favourable light to the study hypotheses. The 'Pharaoh' rarely, if ever, interacts or communicates with anybody lower in the hierarchy than the PIs, especially the research participants. Typically, 'Pharaohs' prefer quantitative variables that are believed by him/her to be less prone to error and bias, but they may also opt for subjective, self-report measures, which are more prone to confirmation bias in a non-blinded trial (e.g., see White et al., 2011)

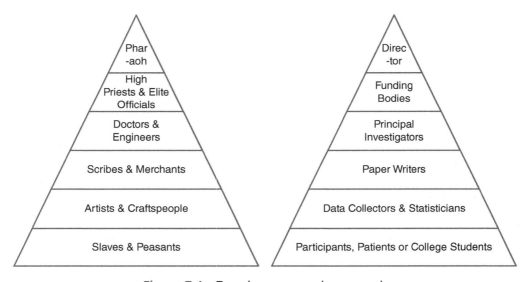

Figure 7.4   Top-down research approach

Some health psychologists, especially those who prefer qualitative methods, disagree with the top-down approach, which imposes a particular theoretical framework or mould on the research and the research participants. They argue that a formulaic, top-down approach tends to produce confirmation biases and group-thinking, which constrain creativity and innovation. Researchers who prefer the reverse approach, the so-called '**bottom-up approach**' (please note that it is 'bottom-up' and *NOT* 'bottoms up', which is the kind of thing people say before downing a stiff drink!) tend to use an open-ended approach using qualitative or mixed methods data to learn about the thoughts, feelings and lived experiences of the research participants to produce a set of findings that are out of the mould. They argue that the voices of patients are crucially important in the production of new theories and therapies.

TRANSPARENCY

A key issue in designing and reporting research studies in health psychology is **transparency**. This refers to the ability to accurately and openly describe in full detail the participants or patient population (P), intervention (I), comparison (C) and outcome (O) ('PICO'). Above, we have mentioned the CONSORT and TREND guidelines that were designed to improve transparency of the descriptions of interventions. Intervention studies are typically designed to compare one, two or, at most, three treatments with a control condition consisting of standard care, a waiting list control, a placebo, or no treatment.

The standard designs are simple because precious resources must be stretched across a large number of trials. Rarely, if ever, does an intervention include only one technique, with practically all trials including two or more techniques in combination. If an intervention domain such as smoking has, say, 500 techniques, then there would be 2.5 million possible two-technique combinations, 124 million three-technique combinations and 62 billion four-technique combinations! These eye-watering figures may help to explain why replication so often fails. Which specific combination is used in any individual case, and in what order, depends on the subjective choices of the practitioner. Only if the 'PICO' description is fully detailed and transparent can an independent investigator have the opportunity to reproduce a replica of the study.

TYPE I ERROR

The probability of falsely rejecting an incorrect H_0, leading to the false conclusion that there is a statistically significant effect (a false positive). A Type I error is detecting an effect that is not present. At the .05 significance level, the probability of a Type I error is .05. When making multiple statistical tests it is necessary to reduce the risk of a Type I error by using a higher level of significance (e.g., .01, .001, or .0001) or by making a correction such as the Bonferroni.

TYPE II ERROR

The probability of falsely retaining an incorrect H_0 (a false negative); failing to detect an effect that is present.

UNCONTROLLED VARIABLE

An **uncontrolled variable** is the *bête noire* of any research study. This is a background variable that, unknown to the investigator, operates within the research environment to affect the outcome in an uncontrolled manner. As a consequence, the study will contain the risk of producing a false set of findings.

FUTURE RESEARCH

1. More studies using qualitative and action research methods will help to broaden the focus on quantitative research in health psychology.

2. More research is needed on the health experiences and behaviour of children, ethnic minority groups, disabled people and older people.

3. The evidence base on the effectiveness of behaviour change interventions needs to be strengthened by larger-scale randomized controlled trials.

4. More extensive collaboration with health economists is needed to carry out cost-effectiveness studies of psychosocial interventions.

SUMMARY

1. The principal research methods of health psychology fall into three categories: quantitative, qualitative and action research.
2. Quantitative research designs emphasize reliable and valid measurement in controlled experiments, trials and surveys.
3. Qualitative methods use interviews, focus groups, narratives, diaries or texts to explore health and illness concepts and experience.
4. Action research enables change processes to feed back into plans for improvement, empowerment and emancipation.
5. A top-down research approach is when a theorist, director or senior professor decides on the nature of the research to be carried out, the research goals, the questions or hypotheses to be investigated, and the methods used. Critics argue that the top-down approach tends to produce confirmation biases and group-thinking, which constrain creativity and innovation.
6. The 'bottom-up approach' uses an open-ended approach with qualitative or mixed methods data to learn about the thoughts, feelings and lived experiences of the research participants. The voices of patients and their families are viewed as crucially important in the production of new theories and therapies.
7. A hierarchy of evidence has been proposed which places meta-analyses and systematic reviews at the top of the hierarchy and qualitative research at the bottom. Multiple sources of evidence may be synthesized in systematic reviews and meta-analyses, which is helpful in appraising the state of knowledge in particular fields. However, qualitative methods about lived experience provide a necessary counterweight to descriptive methods that are purely quantitative in nature.
8. Evaluation research to assess the effectiveness of health psychology interventions has generally been too small-scale and of low quality. There is a need for large-scale studies that are methodologically rigorous to evaluate interventions.
9. Interventions need to describe completely, using a taxonomy, so that we can compare and contrast interventions across studies, replicate the intervention in other settings and advance the science of illness prevention by enabling theory testing in the practice of health care.
10. Health psychology has yet to show its full potential by conducting high-quality research with a full gamut of methods and disseminating the findings across society.

THEORIES, MODELS AND INTERVENTIONS FOR HEALTH BEHAVIOUR CHANGE

In Part 2 we review the theories, models and interventions for health behaviour change that are most relevant to the major causes of illness and premature death. We consider the environmental influences that affect these health-relevant behaviours and the factors that make these behaviours so resistant to change. We review interventions that offer the best opportunities for behaviour change and practical recommendations on how knowledge from health psychology can be applied to improve current systems of health care.

In Chapter 8 we review the principal theories and models of health behaviour. We illustrate their application to sexual health, the topic of our next chapter. Although the models have yielded disappointing results, they continue to dominate the research in the field. Our critique of the approach indicates the need for fresh lines of inquiry.

In Chapter 9, we focus on sexual health, and the prevention of unintended pregnancies and sexually transmitted infections.

In Chapter 10 we examine the part played by food, diets and dieting in the changing patterns of illnesses and deaths associated with the obesity pandemic. The sub-optimal food environment has generated high levels of obesity, diabetes, cardiovascular diseases, cancers, osteoporosis and dental disease.

In Chapter 11 we discuss theories and research concerned with alcohol consumption and the causes, prevention and treatment of drinking problems.

In Chapter 12 we document the extent of smoking, its major health impacts and the factors that help to explain its continued popularity. Three main theories, the biological, psychological and social, are outlined.

In Chapter 13 we review evidence on the increasing prevalence of sedentary behaviour and its potential impact on health. We consider the social and psychological factors associated with participation, the various meanings of different forms of physical activity, and the strategies that have been used to promote greater participation.

THEORIES, MODELS AND INTERVENTIONS FOR HEALTH BEHAVIOUR CHANGE

'A fresh approach is needed, yielding new theories and interventions that work.'

Fine and Feinman (2004)

OUTLINE

We review the principal theories, models and interventions designed to explain, predict and control health behaviour. Most models and theories in health psychology are at the level of the individual and are based on constructs that are purported to be universally applicable. The models and theories have been widely applied for several decades to many health behaviours and scenarios. Self-reported intention to change, rather than actual behaviour, has often been the focus of attention. Unfortunately, the outcomes generally have been disappointing, including the as-yet unsolved problem of the intention–behaviour gap. Our theoretical critique indicates the scope, and hope, for fresh lines of inquiry, including a new Homeostasis Theory of Well-being.

The goal of theories in psychology is to explain and predict **behaviour** which is anything a person says or does in response to internal or external events. In psychology, theorizing of the type described in this chapter is known as '**black box**' theorizing, because processes are represented as boxes with invisible, unknown workings inside. Interventions using this approach are based on preconceived, theoretical ideas. They may be described as '**top-down**' as they are constructed by the theorist, who decides what makes people behave in the way they do. The theorist makes use of internalized concepts and then tests the theory to see if it fits a controlled set of data.

The findings are a 'mixed bag', and in-depth testing has not gone well for many of the models that can, respectfully, be viewed today as 'museum pieces'. Some are still actively admired, are being polished and worked on, and may yet yield results in the field of prevention. However, the flaws in many of the theories and models suggest a need for new approaches grounded in realistic assumptions about emotion, motivation, and the social and economic constraints of contemporary living that exist for the vast majority of people.

THE HEALTH BELIEF MODEL

The **health belief model (HBM)** was developed by Rosenstock (1966) more than 50 years ago. The HBM (see Figure 8.1) contained four central constructs:

1. Perceived susceptibility (an individual's assessment of their risk of getting the condition).

2. Perceived severity (an individual's assessment of the seriousness of the condition and its potential consequences).

3. Perceived barriers (an individual's assessment of the influences that facilitate or discourage adoption of the promoted behaviour).

4. Perceived benefits (an individual's assessment of the positive consequences of adopting the behaviour).

The likelihood of a behaviour is influenced by **cues to action** that are reminders or prompts to take action consistent with an intention. These cues to action can be *internal* (e.g., feeling fatigued) or *external* (e.g., seeing health promotion leaflets/posters or receiving personal communication from health professionals, family members, peers, etc.)

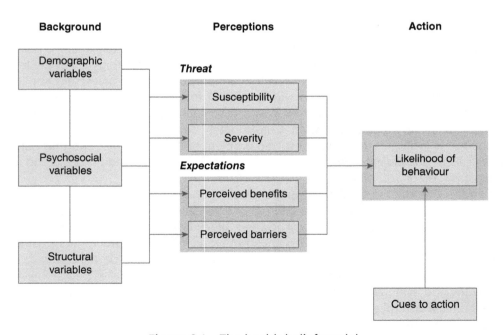

Figure 8.1   The health belief model

The aim of the HBM is to predict the likelihood of implementing health-related behaviour. Additional factors are included in the model: demographic factors (e.g., age, sex and socio-economic background), psychosocial factors (e.g., personality traits, peer influence, family, etc.) and structural factors (e.g., knowledge of the health condition or previous contact with the disease).

The HBM was tested in many studies and used as a theoretical framework for interventions. Jones et al. (2014a) addressed the HBM as the theoretical basis for interventions to improve adherence. Of 18 eligible studies, only 6 used the HBM in its entirety and 5 measured health beliefs as outcomes, not behaviour. The authors' conclusion stated: 'Intervention success appeared to be unrelated to [the] HBM construct addressed, challenging the utility of this model as the theoretical basis for adherence-enhancing interventions' (Jones et al., 2014a: 253). This conclusion is an accurate reflection of the literature across the board. It can be truthfully stated that the HBM died a natural and fairly painless death. Other theories, to be discussed next, have been more resilient.

PROTECTION MOTIVATION THEORY

Protection motivation theory (PMT) was developed by Rogers (1975) to describe coping with a health threat in light of two appraisal processes – threat appraisal and coping appraisal. It introduces a most basic human emotion into health protection: *fear*. Fear is widely used in campaigns and behavioural change interventions, yet empirical support for its use remains unconvincing. According to PMT, the appraisal of the health threat, basically one's fear of the consequences of one's actions, and the possible coping response result in an intention, or 'protection motivation', to perform either an adaptive response or a maladaptive response. According to PMT, behaviour change is best achieved by appealing to an individual's fears. The PMT proposes four constructs, which are said to influence the intention to protect oneself against a health threat:

1. The perceived *severity* of a threatened event (e.g., HIV infection).

2. The perceived probability of the occurrence, or *vulnerability* (e.g., the perceived vulnerability of the person to HIV).

3. The efficacy of the recommended preventive behaviour (i.e., how effective is the wearing of a condom?).

4. The perceived *self-efficacy* (e.g., the person's confidence in putting a condom in place) (see Figure 8.2).

This theory takes account of both the costs and benefits of behaviour in predicting the likelihood of change. PMT assumes that protection motivation is maximized when:

the threat to health is severe;

the individual feels vulnerable;

the adaptive response is believed to be an effective means for averting the threat;

the person is confident in his or her abilities to complete successfully the adaptive response;

the rewards associated with the maladaptive behaviour are small;

the costs associated with the adaptive response are small.

Such factors produce protection motivation and subsequently an adaptive, or coping, response (Figure 8.2).

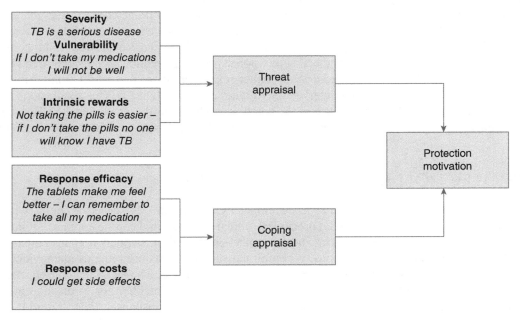

Figure 8.2   The four constructs and the two appraisal processes that result in protection motivation

Source: Adapted from Stroebe (2000)

Bui et al. (2013) carried out a systematic review on protection motivation theory and physical activity in the general population. The authors concluded that 'the PMT shows some promise, however, there are still substantial gaps in the evidence' (Bui et al., 2013: 522).

Ruiter et al. (2014) reviewed six meta-analytic studies on the effectiveness of fear appeals. They concluded that coping information aimed at increasing perceptions of response effectiveness and especially self-efficacy is more important than presenting health information aimed at increasing risk perceptions and fear arousal. Attempts to change behaviour by appealing to fear receive only limited empirical support. The fear approach has fallen into disrepute and faded away. Alternative approaches seem more fruitful.

THEORY OF REASONED ACTION AND THEORY OF PLANNED BEHAVIOUR

The theory of reasoned action (TRA) includes three constructs: behavioural intention, attitude and subjective norm. The TRA is based on the assumption that a person is likely to do what he or she intends to do. It assumes that a person's behavioural intention depends on the person's attitude about the behaviour and subjective norms, and is illustrated in Figure 8.3.

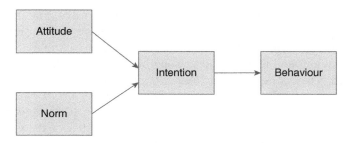

Figure 8.3   The theory of reasoned action

Source: Fishbein and Ajzen (1975)

In spite of efforts to apply the TRA to health behaviour, it fails to capture the complexity of health experience. Like other models reviewed in this chapter, the TRA is based on the assumption of rationality, that human beings ordinarily make systematic and logical use of available information. It also assumes that human behaviour is determined by free choice in a manner that is unrestrained by political or economic factors, neglects the role of emotion and feelings, and does not incorporate self-efficacy and self-esteem. For these reasons, the theory failed to provide an explanatory account of health behaviour. Along came the theory of planned behaviour (TPB).

Behaviour is complex and rarely controlled with as much rationality as the TRA suggested. Sex, smoking, eating, and substance and alcohol use are all examples of behaviour that people have difficulty controlling in a completely rational and voluntary way. Ajzen (1985) added **perceived behavioural control** to produce the TPB (see Figure 8.4). In doing so, Ajzen produced *the most cited theory in the history of psychology*.

Perceived behavioural control refers to one's perception of control over the behaviour, and reflects the obstacles and successes encountered in past experience with this behaviour. The TPB proposes that perceived behavioural control influences intentions and behaviour directly.

For the college student population, attitudes towards safe sex, condom use self-efficacy and beliefs about peer norms have all been shown to predict unsafe sexual activity (Lewis et al., 2009; Hittner and Kryzanowski, 2010). The success of the TPB in predicting safer sexual behaviour was reviewed in a meta-analysis published by Albarracín et al. (2001) (see below).

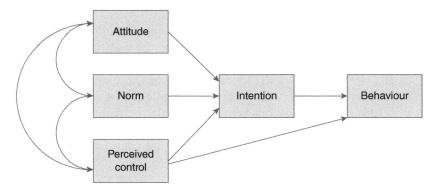

Figure 8.4   The theory of planned behaviour

Source: Ajzen (1991)

However, not all in the TPB garden has the sweet smell of roses. The important factors of moral norms (Godin et al., 2005), culture and religion also have a strong influence on behaviour but are are missing from the TPB. To give one of many examples, Sinha et al. (2007) studied sexual behaviour and relationships among black and minority ethnic (BME) teenagers in East London. They collected data from 126 young people, aged 15–18, mainly using focus groups in three inner-London boroughs. Sexual behaviour was mediated by gender, religion and youth in ways not included in the TPB. A systematic review of 237 independent prospective tests found that the TPB accounted for only 19% of the variability in health behaviour (McEachan et al., 2011). This is typical of many systematic reviews.

Multiple studies concur that the TPB, and its many extensions and adaptations, fail to account for more than 20% of the variability in health behaviour. Thus, 80% of health behaviour variance is unexplained by the TPB. This is not an exciting amount of success. Sniehotta et al. (2014) suggested that it was 'time to retire' the TPB. Unperturbed by the critics, Ajzen (2014) remained steadfastly convinced that the THP is 'alive and well'. Every holy cow needs its guru. Citations rain down like the monsoon, and the theory just will not be washed away.

THE COMMON-SENSE MODEL

The 'common-sense model' (CSM), also known as the 'self-regulatory model' (SRM) or 'Leventhal's model', was developed by Howard Leventhal and colleagues (Leventhal et al., 1980, 2003, 2016). In this approach, the patient is viewed as a problem solver, attempting to make sense of an illness. A key construct within the CSM is the idea of illness representations or 'lay' beliefs about illness. These representations integrate with normative guidelines that people hold to make sense of their symptoms and guide any coping actions. Five components of illness representations in the CSM are: *identity*, *cause*, *time-line*, *consequences* and *curability/controllability*.

A systematic review determined whether people's beliefs about their illness, expressed in CSM terms, prospectively predict adherence to self-management behaviours (e.g., attendance, medication, diet and exercise) in adults with physical illnesses (Aujla et al., 2016). Data from 52 studies were extracted, of which 21 were meta-analysed using correlation coefficients while the remainder were descriptively synthesized. The effect sizes for individual illness belief domains and adherence to self-management behaviours indicated very weak, predictive relationships. The authors concluded that 'Individual illness belief domains, outlined by the CSM, did not predict adherence to self-management behaviours in adults with physical illnesses' (Aujla et al., 2016: 1).

Weinman et al. (1996) developed the Illness Perception Questionnaire (IPQ) to assess the cognitive representation of illness in the CSM. The predictive validity of a brief version of the IPQ was evaluated using correlations between illness perceptions and depression, anxiety, blood glucose levels and quality of life (Broadbent et al., 2015). Findings showed modest but reliable associations with outcome measures (0.25–0.49 for consequences, identity and emotional representations; −0.12 to −0.27 for personal control).

However, psychometric research used **Rasch analysis** to assess the validity of the IPQ–Revised to assess beliefs about diabetes in 470 participants with Type 2 diabetes and 71 participants with Type 1 diabetes (Rees et al., 2015). All IPQ–Revised scales were found to have psychometric issues, including poorly utilized response categories, poor scale precision and multidimensionality. Only four of the eight scales were found to be psycho-metrically adequate (Consequences, Illness coherence, Timeline cyclical and Emotional representations). Rees et al. (2015: 1340) concluded: 'the diabetes-specific version of the Illness Perception Questionnaire–Revised provides suboptimal assessment of beliefs held by patients with diabetes'.

Meta-analyses have found weak relationships between CSM mental representations and adherence (Brandes and Mullan, 2014; Law et al., 2014). One systematic review examined the use of the CSM to develop interventions for improving adherence to health care behaviours (medication and dietary/lifestyle) and assessed intervention effectiveness (Jones et al., 2016). Six of the nine studies (67%) obtained a statistically significant effect of the intervention on improving at least one aspect of adherence.

THE INFORMATION–MOTIVATION–BEHAVIOURAL SKILLS MODEL

The information–motivation–behavioural skills model (IMBS; Fisher and Fisher, 1992, 2000) focuses on (yes, you guessed it) information, motivation and behavioural skills associated with wellness behaviours. According to the IMBS model, the learning of health-related infor-mation is a prerequisite to action in these areas. In the context of sexual health, HIV-related information is likely to include statements about HIV infection (e.g., 'Oral sex is safer than vaginal or anal sex') designed to facilitate preventive behaviour. The IMBS model assumes that having the motivation to practise specific sex-related behaviours is necessary for the pro-duction of problem prevention or wellness promotion. Finally, sexuality-related behavioural skills are a third fundamental determinant of acting effectively to avoid sexual problems and achieving sexual well-being. The behavioural skills construct focuses on the person's self-efficacy in performing sexual problem-prevention or well-being-related behaviours, includ-ing insisting on abstinence from intercourse, discussing and practising contraceptive use, and sexual behaviours that optimize a couple's sexual pleasure. Barak and Fisher (2001) pro-posed an internet-driven approach to sex education based on the IMBS model. An illustration of the IMBS model applied to adherence in using HAART medication for HIV infection is shown in Figure 8.5.

There have been many studies of the IMBS model in different settings. Eggers et al. (2016) tested the IMBS model with 1,066 students from Cape Town, South Africa to assess the hypoth-esized motivational pathways for the prediction of condom use during last sexual intercourse. Knowledge of how to use a condom and how STIs are transmitted directly predicted behaviour as hypothesized by the IMBS model. However, an alternative model had a higher proportion of significant pathways.

THE TRANSTHEORETICAL OR STAGES OF CHANGE MODEL

The transtheoretical model (TTM), otherwise known as the 'Stages of Change Model', was developed by Prochaska and DiClemente (1983). It is a general model that applies across all

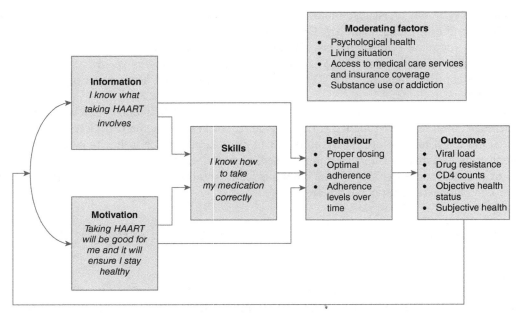

Figure 8.5 The information–motivation–behavioural skills model

Source: Adapted from Fisher et al. (2006)

types of psychological change and which has been highly influential in the research literature. The TTM hypothesizes six discrete stages of change (see Figure 8.6), through which people are alleged to progress in making a change:

Pre-contemplation – a person is not intending to take action in the foreseeable future, usually measured as the next six months.

Contemplation – a person is intending to change in the next six months.

Preparation – a person is intending to take action in the immediate future, usually measured as the next month.

Action – a person has been making specific overt modifications in his/her lifestyle within the past six months.

Maintenance – a person is working to prevent relapse, a stage that is estimated to last from six months to about five years.

Either *termination* – an individual has zero temptation and 100% self-efficacy, or *relapse* – an individual reverts to the original behaviour.

The TTM has been tested in multiple studies with mixed results.

A meta-analysis by Noar et al. (2009) indicated that interventions using the Stages of Change Model were relatively effective. However, critics have suggested that the model contains arbitrary time periods and that the supportive evidence is meagre and inconsistent (e.g., Sutton, 2000a; West, 2005; Armitage, 2009). The TTM has been defended by its advocates (e.g., DiClemente, 2005; Prochaska, 2006), is resilient and remains popular as a model of change.

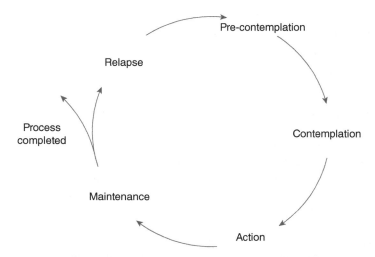

Figure 8.6 The transtheoretical model or Stages of Change Model

Source: Prochaska and DiClementi (1983); Prochaska and Velicer (1997)

Critics have offered nothing that is more valid in its place. If there is a better description than stages of change, what would that description be? For these reasons, it is likely that the TTM will continue to be an active focus for research and interventions.

THE SOCIAL COGNITIVE THEORY OF BANDURA

Bandura's (1986) social cognitive theory (SCT) examines the social origins of behaviour in addition to the cognitive thought processes that influence human behaviour. Bandura's social-cognitive approach proposes that learning can occur through the observation of models in the absence of any overt reinforcement. The acquisition of skill and knowledge has an intrinsic reinforcement value independent of biological drives and needs. Two key planks in the social-cognitive platform are observational learning and self-efficacy.

Observational learning

Bandura observed that people learn by watching or observing others, reading about what people do, and making general observations of the world. This learning may or may not be demonstrated in the form of behaviour. Bandura proposed a four-step conceptual scheme for observational learning:

Step 1: attentional processes, including certain model characteristics that may increase the likelihood of the behaviour being attended to and the observer characteristics, such as sensory capacities, motivation and arousal levels, perceptual set, and past reinforcement.

Step 2: retention processes, including the observer's ability to remember and to make sense of what has been observed.

Step 3: motor reproduction processes, including the capabilities that the observer has to perform the behaviours being observed. Specific factors include physical capabilities and availability of responses.

167

Step 4: motivational processes, including external reinforcement, vicarious reinforcement and self-reinforcement. If a behaviour is to be imitated, an observer must be motivated to perform that behaviour.

Self-efficacy

Bandura (1994: 71) defined the concept of 'perceived self-efficacy' as:

> People's beliefs about their capabilities to produce designated levels of performance that exercise influence over events that affect their lives. Self-efficacy beliefs determine how people feel, think, motivate themselves and behave. Such beliefs produce these diverse effects through four major processes. They include cognitive, motivational, affective and selection processes.

Self-efficacy is a person's belief that they have behavioural competence in a particular situation ('I can do it'). It is related to whether or not an individual will undertake particular goal-directed activities ('I will do it'), the amount of energy that he or she will put into their effort ('I want to do it') and the length of time that the individual will persist in striving to achieve a particular goal ('I need to do it'). Among the sources of self-efficacy are:

performance accomplishments: past experiences of success and failure ('I have already done it');

vicarious experience: witnessing others' successes and failures ('I saw somebody do it');

verbal persuasion: being told by others that one can or cannot competently perform a particular behaviour ('You can do it');

emotional arousal: when engaging in a particular behaviour in a specific situation ('I would love to do it').

The self-efficacy concept has been widely applied in studies and interventions. Models of human health behaviour – the PMT, the HBM, and TPB – include self-efficacy as an important component. Self-efficacy refers to one of the 'truths': believing that we can accomplish what we want to accomplish is 'one of the most important ingredients – perhaps the most important ingredient – in the recipe for success' (Maddux, 2002: 277). Self-efficacy can be viewed as one of the sources of the human meaning of life. Major human needs related to subjective fulfilment include purpose, value, self-efficacy and self-worth (Baumeister and Vohs, 2002).

Bandura has made some extremely important observations about human learning and thought. Observational learning and self-efficacy are invaluable concepts. However, critics argue that the relationship between the concepts is not clear. Others say it's just common sense, written in abstract jargon.

ATTEMPTS AT THEORETICAL INTEGRATION

The great range and variability in theories, models and concepts call for integration. One integrated model is the 'COM-B', which focuses on capability, opportunity and motivation, and the 'Behaviour Change Wheel' (Michie and Wood, 2015). An analysis of 83 theories and frameworks included 1,659 constructs in three dimensions: comprehensiveness, coherence and a clear link to an overarching model of behaviour. The Behaviour Change Wheel has been proposed for physical activity, weight loss, hand hygiene, dental hygiene, diet, smoking, medication adherence, prescribing behaviours, condom use and female genital mutilation.

One critic questioned whether the COM-B and the Behaviour Change Wheel 'can ever be tested' and points out that it remains 'unclear how it can be ever falsified if its constructs remain broad and all encompassing. … And does it promote and facilitate creativity in those that do the thinking?' (Ogden, 2016: 247). An excellent question.

The complex array of theories and models can be a little overwhelming. Theories are often poorly applied and interventions suffer because they lack empirical support. One way of making progress would be to determine a consensus among knowledgeable researchers about what works and what doesn't. Michie et al. (2005) developed a consensus on theoretical constructs, a 'Theoretical Domains Framework' (TDF), in six phases: (1) identifying theoretical constructs; (2) simplifying into domains; (3) evaluating the domains; (4) interdisciplinary evaluation; (5) validating; and (6) piloting interview questions. The contributors were a 'psychological theory' group ($n = 18$), a 'health services research' group ($n = 13$) and a 'health psychology' group ($n = 30$). A total of 12 domains were initially identified, which were later refined to 14 domains: Knowledge, Skills, Social/professional role and identity, Beliefs about capabilities, Optimism, Beliefs about consequences, Reinforcement, Intentions, Goals, Memory, attention and decision processes, Environmental context and resources, Social influences, Emotions and Behavioral regulation (Cane et al., 2012).

A questionnaire was designed to facilitate the use of the TDF in practice change (Huijg et al., 2014). A systematic literature review comparing the original with the refined TDF found that the 'environmental context and resources', 'beliefs about consequences' and 'social influences' were the three domains most frequently cited in the reviewed studies (84%, 74%, and 66%, respectively; Mosavianpour et al., 2016). This finding is consistent with the idea that self-control is constrained, as we stated in a previous chapter: 'what individuals can do to change their lives is not simply a matter of personal choice – choices are constrained biologically, culturally, economically and environmentally'. These constraints are one of the reasons that individual-level black-box models and theories are unable to explain more than 20% of health behaviour.

INTENTIONS VERSUS BEHAVIOUR AND THE 'INTENTION–BEHAVIOUR GAP'

The evidence from studies of the models and theories is that it is relatively easy to predict the self-reported intention to act, but more difficult to predict action itself. It is commonly the case that a person develops an intention to change their health behaviour (e.g., to stop smoking), but they might not take any action (e.g., actually to stop smoking). This discrepancy has been labelled the 'intention–behaviour gap'. What leads to the translation between an intention and an action is reduced in many models to an arrow between two black boxes. However, we need to break down intention into two phases: goal intention and implementation intention (Gollwitzer, 1993, 1999; Gollwitzer and Brandstätter, 1997). Goal intention is a commitment towards a goal ('I intend to achieve the goal X'), while implementation intention is about the necessary action ('I intend to initiate the behaviour Y in situation Z'). This second phase is not addressed in the models but is a key part of the process of performing a behaviour.

We know that unhealthy behaviour is more common among lower SES groups, which helps to create health inequalities. One possibility is that the intention–behaviour gap is wider among the lower SES groups. Vasiljevic et al. (2016) tested this hypothesis using objective and self-report measures of three behaviours, pooling data from five studies. The intention–behaviour gap did not vary with deprivation for diet, physical activity or medication adherence in smoking cessation. However, they did find a larger gap between perceived control over behaviour (self-efficacy) and behaviour in the more deprived. Choices are especially constrained economically and environmentally among lower SES groups, regardless of the good intentions to change towards healthier behaviours.

Interventions to plug the intention–behaviour gap have been employed, such as self affirmation tasks, planning or implementation intentions. These have met with some limited success (Steele, 1988; Gollwitzer, 1993; Gollwitzer and Sheeran, 2006; Epton et al., 2015; Synergy Expert Group, 2016: 814). Another approach has been to catelogue behaviour change techniques with the aim of making interventions repeatable and replicable. As we shall see, the hype has run ahead of the actual results.

BEHAVIOUR CHANGE TECHNIQUES

A **behaviour change technique (BCT)** is a systematic procedure (or a category of procedures) included as an active component of an intervention designed to change behaviour. The defining characteristics of a BCT are that it is:

1. Observable.

2. Replicable.

3. Irreducible.

4. A component of an intervention designed to change behaviour.

5. A postulated active ingredient within the intervention (Michie et al., 2011).

A BCT taxonomy has been employed to code descriptions of intervention content into behaviour change techniques (Michie et al., 2011). The taxonomy aims to code protocols in order to describe transparently the techniques used to change behaviour. If the protocols can be made clearer, then studies can be replicated (Abraham and Michie, 2008; Michie et al., 2011). A taxonomy can also be used to identify which techniques are most effective so that intervention effectiveness can be raised and more people will be able to change their behaviour. Two reviewers independently coded BCTs and then discussed their presence/absence. Fidelity of treatment refers to confirmation that the manipulation of the independent variable occurred as planned. A 30-item Treatment Fidelity Checklist (Borrelli, 2011) was used to assess whether treatment fidelity strategies were in place with regard to study design, interventionist training, treatment delivery, treatment receipt and treatment enactment. Percentage scores for each area were awarded to reflect the proportion of items with evidence of at least one treatment fidelity strategy.

A total of 27 BCTs were identified across 5 interventions with a mean number of BCTs coded per intervention of 10 and a range of 4 to 15. Michie et al. (2011) found that the most frequently occurring BCT was 'problem solving', which occurred in four of the five interventions.

Three BCTs were coded in three out of five interventions: 'information about social and environmental consequences', 'reduce negative emotions' and 'pros and cons'. All studies measured outcomes using self-reports.

The production of a structured list of BCTs provides a 'compendium' of behaviour change methods that helps to map the domain of behaviour change and inform practitioner decision-making. However, it also risks becoming a prescriptive list of ingredients for a 'cookbook' of which therapeutic techniques must be applied to patients presenting with a specific behavioural problem.

Another problem with the compendium approach is that BCTs are not all optimally effective when combined in a 'pick-and-mix' fashion. There needs to be a coherence to the package of BCTs, and the BCTs need to be combined in the right amounts and proportions. This optimum mix of 'ingredients' can only be provided by a theory that offers power and meaning and connects the BCT components into an integrated and coherent combination. To use again the analogy of baking, if you have eggs, flour, baking powder, salt and pepper but no recipe and no chef, the ingredients are useless. If the ingredients fall into the wrong hands and are badly combined, the outcomes could well be disastrous (Figure 8.7). There is a need for a coherent theory and expertise to provide structure and meaning both for the change agent (chef) and the client (diner).

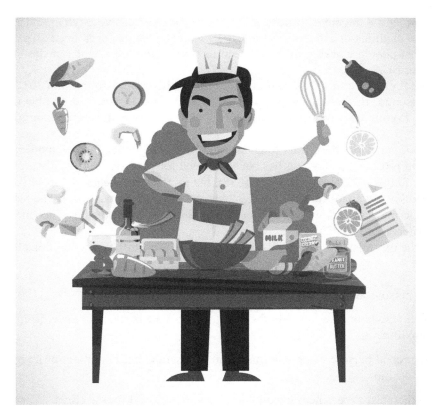

Figure 8.7 I have everything I need except I don't know how to cook

Source: Ngkrit's portfolio, Photo ID: 287581859, acquired via Shutterstock

By way of illustration, consider an intervention for smoking cessation, *Stop Smoking Now* (Marks, 2017a). This integrative therapy is an effective method for clearing the human body of nicotine. The desire to smoke and any satisfaction gained from smoking are abolished using a combination of BCTs consisting mainly of different forms of cognitive behavioural therapy (CBT) and mindfulness meditation. *Stop Smoking Now* includes 30 BCTs integrated within a coherent theory of change based on the concept of homeostasis (Chapter 2). In *Stop Smoking Now*, a structured sequence of BCTs is provided that takes into account the nesting of BCTs such that guided imagery works best in combination with relaxation and both of these work best following enhancement of self-efficacy, which is achieved using self-recording, positive affirmations and counter-conditioning. In a theory of change, the whole is always more than the sum of the parts.

Of equal importance to the necessary theory of change, which is required to integrate the BCTs, is the quality of the change agent.

BEHAVIOUR CHANGE AGENTS

We find it helpful to use an analogy that there is more to baking a cake than the ingredients. Of course, one needs a good set of ingredients (the BCTs), but one also needs a good baker – the behaviour change agent (BCA). The BCA/therapist must be fit for purpose and so fully capable and competent to deliver the BCTs in a persuasive, stylish and professional manner. The qualities of effective therapists have been studied for at least 50 years. It is an oversight that people working on BCTs tend to neglect the importance of the 'baker' – the all-important BCA.

In a recent critique of the cookbook approach, Hilton and Johnston (2017) point out that: 'In essence, the *where, when, why, who* and *how* of practice has been relatively ignored in favour of vague suggestions of *what* practice ingredients might include' (2017: 2).

The role of **empathy**, the ability to understand and share the feelings of another, in therapy, medicine and prosocial behaviour, has been accepted for centuries. Originally a part of 'sympathy' (e.g., Smith, 1759/1976; Darwin, 1888), the English word *empathy* is derived from the Ancient Greek word ἐμπάθεια (*empatheia*, 'physical affection or passion'). The term had been adapted in German as *Einfühlung* ('feeling into'), which was translated by Titchener to become *empathy* (Titchener, 1909/2014).

In 1957 the therapist Carl Rogers listed the necessary and sufficient conditions for constructive change:

- Two persons are in psychological contact.

- The first, whom we shall term the client, is in a state of incongruence, being vulnerable or anxious.

- The second person, whom we shall term the therapist, is congruent or integrated in the relationship.

- The therapist experiences unconditional positive regard for the client.

- The therapist experiences an empathic understanding of the client's internal frame of reference and endeavors to communicate this experience to the client.

- The communication to the client of the therapist's empathic understanding and unconditional positive regard is to a minimal degree achieved.

- No other conditions are necessary. If these six conditions exist, and continue over a period of time, this is sufficient. (Rogers, 1957: 96)

Research over many decades has confirmed the positive role of empathy in medical and psychological practice, along with other characteristics such as warmth (Rollnick et al., 1992; Marshall et al., 2002; Skinner and Spurgeon, 2005; Avenell et al., 2006; Hassed et al., 2009). Therapists' interpersonal style, empathy and communication skills are essential requirements for successful behaviour change (Hagger and Hardcastle, 2014).

In contrast with an almost obsessional effort to categorize BCTs, there has been hardly any research effort in health psychology on specifying the essential characteristics of the successful BCA: empathy, warmth and positivite regard. However, there are some interesting studies on the part played by these characteristics in motivational interviewing (e.g., Miller and Rose, 2009) and mindfulness training (e.g., Birnie et al., 2010). Empirical evidence suggests that empathy is teachable, for example to undergraduate medical students (Batt-Rawden et al., 2013) or physicians (Riess et al., 2012; Kelm et al., 2014). To neglect the key variables of the BCA 'ignores the need for flexibility, variability and change according not to the type of behaviour, or the type of intervention or even the type of patient but how that individual patient happens to feel, think, look, behave or respond at any particular time' (Ogden, 2016). It is essential to explore not only the *what*, but the *where*, *when*, *why*, *who* and *how* of implementation science in putting theory into practice.

CRITIQUE OF INDIVIDUAL-LEVEL THEORIES AND MODELS

In spite of widespread use in health psychology research, the evidence does not justify any confidence in the majority of theories and models reviewed in this chapter. The outcome of meta-analyses of theory testing paints a disappointing picture. The pattern of evidence suggests that current psychological theories and models do not provide a viable foundation for effective interventions. We analyse some of the reasons for this situation in the following paragraphs.

Individualistic bias

Choice and responsibility are internalized as processes within individuals in a similar way to the operating system of a computer. The human 'operating system' is assumed to be universal and rational, following a fixed set of formulae that the models attempt to describe. Yet even within its own terms, the programme of model testing and confirmation is failing to meet the goals it has set.

Lack of ecological validity and questionable statistical methods

Thousands of published studies have used null hypothesis testing with small samples of college students or patients. The power, ecological validity and generalizability of these studies is questionable. We do not really know their true merit because of uncertainties about representativeness, sampling and statistical assumptions. Rarely are alternative approaches to theory testing utilized (e.g., Bayesian statistics and power analyses) to assess the *importance* of the effects rather than their *statistical significance* (Cohen, 1994).

Self-report measures

Most studies use self-reported measures of intention and behaviour rather than objective measures. This always presents a huge problem! It means that the academic studies have little contact with the universe of real-world, objective behaviour.

Neglect of culture, religion and gender

Religion, culture and gender are neglected by most socio-cognitive models. The models aim at universal application, which is unachievable.

Unfalsifiability

Some strident critics have suggested that the models are **tautological** and therefore unfalsifiable (Smedslund, 2000; Ogden, 2003). A tautology is a statement that is necessarily true, e.g., 'Jill will either stop or not stop smoking' or 'the earth is a sphere' (not 'The earth is round ($p < .05$)', as one famous paper would have it! – Cohen, 1995). Whatever data we obtain about Jill's smoking, the statement will always be true; it is a very safe prediction. Smedslund (2000) further deduced that, if tautological theories are disconfirmed or only partially supported by empirical studies, then the studies themselves must be flawed for not 'discovering' what must be the case! Bad models can only be supported by bad research. Others have argued that behavioural beliefs (attitudes) and normative beliefs are basically the same thing. Ogden (2003) analysed empirical articles published between 1997 and 2001 from four health psychology journals that tested or applied at least one social cognition model (the theory of reasoned action, the theory of planned behaviour, the health belief model, and protection motivation theory). Ogden concluded that the models do not enable the generation and testing of hypotheses because their constructs are unspecific. Echoing Smedslund (2000), she suggested that the models focus on analytic truths that must be true by definition.

However, not all theorists agree that social cognition models (SCMs) are tautological and/or unfalsifiable. Trafimow (2009) claimed to have demonstrated that the TRA and TPB are falsifiable because these theories make risky predictions. Furthermore, he claimed to have falsified one of the assumptions of the TPB, namely, that perceived control is a worse predictor of behavioural intentions than perceived difficulty (Trafimow et al., 2002). Yet perceived behavioural control is usually measured by items evaluating control and items evaluating difficulty. If empirical falsification of the TPB has actually occurred then the theory must, *ipso facto*, be falsifiable, and one of the main criticisms has been eliminated.

Unsupported assumptions

The transtheoretical model has received particular criticism. Sutton (2000b) argued that the stage definitions are logically flawed, and that the time periods assigned to each stage are arbitrary. Herzog (2008) suggested that, when applied to smoking cessation, the TTM does not satisfy the criteria required of a valid stage model and that the proposed stages of change 'are not qualitatively distinct categories'.

Procedural issues

French et al. (2007) investigated what people think about when they answer TPB questionnaires using the 'think aloud' technique. They found problems relating to information retrieval and to participants answering different questions from those intended. They concluded that 'The standard procedure for developing TPB questionnaires may systematically produce problematic questions' (French et al., 2007: 672).

Neglect of motivation

Another common complaint about the SCMs is that they do not adequately address the motivational issues about risky behaviours. Surely it is their very riskiness that in part is responsible for their adoption. Willig (2008: 690) questioned the assumption that lies behind behind much of health and sex education 'that psychological health is commensurate with maintaining physical safety, and that risking one's health and physical safety is necessarily a sign of psychopathology'. On the basis of current evidence, grand theories claiming universal application are lacking any empirical support.

Other criticisms

Studies measuring social cognitions rely upon questionnaires that presuppose that cognitions are stable entities residing in people's heads. They do not allow for contextual variables that may influence social cognitions. For example, an individual's attitude towards condom use may well depend upon the sexual partner with whom they anticipate having sexual contact. It may depend upon the time, place, relationship and physiological state (e.g., intoxication) within which sex takes place.

Economics of health care

The ability of health care practitioners to provide face-to-face therapy to change behaviour is far outstripped by need. Attempts to provide distance cost-effective treatments include bibliotherapy (Glasgow and Rosen, 1978; Marrs, 1995) and internet-based self-help treatment with minimal therapist contact (e.g., Carlbring et al., 2006; Riper et al., 2014). Another option is **mobile health or m-health**, the practice of medicine, health psychology and public health supported by mobile devices. The internet, text messaging and social networking enable m-health tools for health promotion and risk reduction. This is an area that is rapidly changing. Current m-health interventions and programmes include: mobile phone text messaging to support patients with diabetes, hypertension, asthma, eating disorders and HIV treatment; mobile text messaging and personal digital assistants (PDAs) as aids to smoking cessation, body weight loss, reducing alcohol consumption, sexually transmitted infection prevention and testing; and PDAs for data collection and to support health education and clinical practice (Phillips et al., 2010). There is great potential for extending the range of application of m-health in low-income countries as access to mobile phones in these regions increases.

Apps are being increasingly used for the delivery of interventions designed to promote health behaviour change. Webb et al. (2010) found that interventions had a small but significant effect on health-related behaviour. Interventions that incorporated more BCTs also tended to have larger effects compared to interventions that incorporated fewer techniques. Effectiveness of internet-based interventions was enhanced by the use of SMS reminders.

As noted above, e- and m-health have become popular approaches for attempting to improve population health. The efficacy of behavioural nutrition interventions using e-health technologies to decrease fat intake and increase fruit and vegetable intake has been demonstrated, with approximately 75% of trials showing positive effects (Olson, 2016). However, objective measures are rarely available and almost total reliance is placed on self-reported measures of behaviour.

THE ELEPHANT IN THE ROOM: THE PERSISTENCE OF ERROR

There is an embarrassing, unanswered question about theories and models in psychology that is screaming to be answered. If the evidence in support of SCMs is so meagre and feeble, how have they survived for such a long time? The scientific method is intended to be a fail-safe procedure for abandoning disconfirmed hypotheses and progressing with improved hypotheses that have not been disconfirmed. The psychologists who dream up these theories and test them claim to be scientists, so what the heck is going on?

One reason why theories and models become semi-permanent features of textbooks and degree programmes is that simple rules at the very heart of science are persistently broken. If a theory is tested and found wanting, then one of two things happens: either (1) the theory is revised and retested or (2) the theory is abandoned. The history of science suggests that (1) is far more frequent than (2). Investigators become attached to the theories and models that they are working with, not to mention their careers, and they invest significant amounts of time, energy and funds in them, and are loath to give them up – a bit like a worn-out but comfortable armchair.

The process of theory or model testing is illustrated in Figure 8.8. The diagram shows how the research process insulates theories and models against negative results, leading to the persistence of error over many decades. Continuous cycles of revisions and extensions following meagre or negative results protect the model from its ultimate abandonment until every possible amendment and extension has been tested and tried and found to be wanting. Several methods of protection are available to investigators in light of 'bad' results: (1) amend the model and test it again, a process that can be repeated indefinitely; (2) test and retest the model, ignoring the 'bad' results until some positive results appear, which can happen purely by chance (a Type II error); (3) carry out some 'statistical wizardry' to concoct a more favourable-looking outcome; (4) do nothing, i.e., do not publish the findings; and/or (5) look for another theory or model to test and start all over again! Beside all of these issues, there is increasing evidence of a lack of replication, the selective publication of positive findings and outright fraud in psychological research, all of which militate against the authentic separation of fact from fantasy (Yong, 2012).

As we have seen, critics of the socio-cognitive approach have suggested that SCMs are tautological and irrefutable (Smedslund, 2000; Ogden, 2003). If this is true, then no matter how many studies are carried out to investigate a social cognitive theory, there will be no genuine progress in understanding. Weinstein (1993: 324) summarized the state of health behaviour research as follows: 'despite a large empirical literature, there is still no consensus that certain models of health behaviour are more accurate than others, that certain variables are more influential than others, or that certain behaviours or situations are understood better than others'. Unfortunately, there has been little improvement since then. The individual-level approach to health interventions focuses on theoretical models, piloting, testing and running randomized controlled trials to demonstrate efficacy. It has been estimated that the time from conception

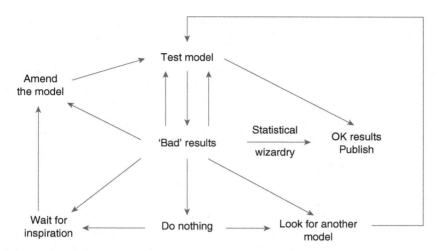

Figure 8.8 Another thing most textbooks don't tell you: the persistence of error – the manner in which a model or theory is 'insulated' against negative results

to funding and completing the process of demonstrated effectiveness can take at least 17 years (Clark, 2008). The meta-analyses, reviewed above, suggest that the 'proof of the pudding' in the form of truly effective individual-level interventions is yet to materialize. Alternative means of creating interventions for at-risk communities and population groups are needed.

HOMEOSTASIS THEORY OF WELL-BEING

A new theory proposes that behaviour and experience follow the principle of homeostasis (Marks, 2015, 2016a, 2018). It is established across multiple fields of natural science that homeostasis is a singular unifying principle for all living beings. In the theory, which extends this well-known principle from Physiology to Psychology, all human behaviour and experience, including health protection and illness prevention, and the regulation of emotion, are under homeostatic control.

Homeostasis operates at all levels of living systems: in molecules, cells, tissues, organs, organisms, societies, ecosystems and the planet as a whole (Lovelock and Margulis, 1974). Tissue homeostasis regulates the birth (mitosis) and death (apoptosis) of cells; many diseases are directly attributable to defective homeostasis, leading to the overproduction or underproduction of new cells relative to cell deletion (Fadeel and Orrenius, 2005). Biochemical and physiological feedback loops regulate billions of cells and thousands of compounds and reactions in the human body to maintain body temperature, metabolism, blood pH, fluid levels, blood glucose and insulin concentrations inside the body (Matthews et al., 1985). A body in good physical health is in biochemical and physiological homeostasis. Severe disruptions of homeostasis cause illnesses or can even be fatal.

A person in good health is in a state of homeostatic balance that operates across systems of biochemical, physiological, psychological and social homeostasis. Outward and inward stability in a living being is only possible with constant accommodation and adaptation. All living beings strive to maintain equilibrium and stability with the surrounding environment through millions of micro-adjustments and adaptations to the continuously changing circumstances.

177

Adjustments and adaptations can be both conscious and unconscious. The majority of fine adjustments are occurring at an unconscious level, hidden from both external observers and the individual actor. The Homeostasis Theory of Well-being utilizes the fact that human beings are natural agents of change who adapt, accommodate and ameliorate under continuously changing conditions, both external and internal, to maximize the stability of physical and mental well-being. The Homeostasis Theory of Well-being (HTW) is illustrated in Figure 8.9.

Well-being is the outcome of a multiplex of continuously changing feedback loops in a system of **psychological homeostasis**, which has four main component processes: **well-being**, cognitive appraisal, **emotion** and action. Homeostasis maintains both physical and psychological equilibrium with the ever-changing external and internal environments, courtesy of an infinitude of micro-feedback-systems that fall within the four main macrosystems defined above. Psychological homeostasis regulates through feedback loops that control thought, emotion and action. Continuously flexible micro-adjustments of activity within feedback loops maintain equilibrium from moment to moment. Psychological homeostasis occurs in response to the infinite variety of circumstances that can affect well-being, including both internal adjustments (e.g., emotional regulation) and external adjustments using deliberate behavioural regulation (e.g., communicating, working, eating and drinking). In synchrony and synergy with all of the body's other homeostatic mechanisms, psychological homeostasis operates throughout life during both waking and sleeping.

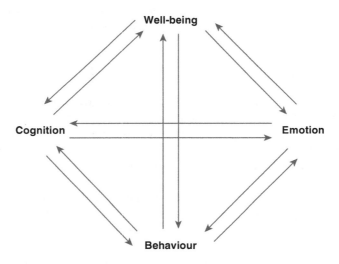

Figure 8.9   The Homeostasis Theory of Well-being

In prevention and treatment of clinical conditions, individuals can help themselves and be helped by external techno aids to monitor and maintain physiological variables using behavioural forms of homeostasis, e.g., in diabetes, metabolic syndrome, hypertension, thyroid problems, skin disorders such as urticaria, or obesity. Biochemical, physiological and psychological homeostasis are of similar complexity. Behavioural forms of homeostasis occur in actions designed to support neural systems of regulation. Social homeostasis in supportive actions by other humans, requested or volunteered, provides another way to support and protect an individual's well-being.

FUTURE RESEARCH

1. People are social and emotional beings, and these features need to be restored into theories and models of behaviour and behaviour change.

2. Future research must look at the potential of m-health as a tool for engaging people of all ages in health promotion and risk reduction.

3. Changing the focus from individuals to communities and populations would also be a sensible decision in maximizing the impact of interventions.

4. The Homeostasis Theory of Well-being needs to be tested in randomized controlled trials and prospective studies to determine its scientific validity and applicability to health care.

SUMMARY

1. Individual-level theories and models are based on universal constructs concerning behavioural adoption, maintenance and change.
2. Thousands of studies and meta-analyses have tested individual-level, social cognitive theories and models with mixed success. Only modest amounts of variation in intentions and behaviour are accounted for using a social cognitive approach.
3. Critics have suggested that individual-level theories and models of social cognition are flawed, unfalsifiable and tautological. On the other hand, others have attempted to integrate theory to produce improved prediction and intervention.
4. A major obstacle has been the 'intention–behaviour gap'. Attempts to bridge the gap, such as the implementation-of-intentions approach, are having some success.
5. Seemingly insulated from the disconfirming results, many theories and models continue to be the main focus for research and interventions. If health psychology is to show its full potential, it will be essential to develop a properly scientific method based on a valid theoretical approach, which to date has not been provided.
6. Another project has been to classify behaviour change techniques into a taxonomy. From this, it is hoped that different techniques can be combined to maximize the chance of successful outcomes. Critics have suggested that creativity, empathy and therapist delivery may be cramped by taxonomic treatments.
7. Another approach is the use of bibliotherapy, m-health and apps for mobile devices. Combined with social networking, apps are a popular approach for engaging people in health promotion and risk reduction, but their potential has yet to be proven.
8. Social support remains indispensable for the maintenance of well-being.
9. The Homeostasis Theory of Well-being applies the core concept of homeostasis from Physiology to behaviour, cognition, emotion and well-being.
10. The Homeostasis Theory of Well-being utilizes the fact that human beings are natural agents of change who adapt, accommodate and ameliorate under continuously changing conditions, both in the external and internal environment, to optimize the stability of physical and mental well-being.

SEXUAL HEALTH

9

'Sexual health is a state of physical, mental and social well-being in relation to sexuality. It requires a positive and respectful approach to sexuality and sexual relationships, as well as the possibility of having pleasurable and safe sexual experiences, free of coercion, discrimination and violence.'

World Health Organization (2002)

OUTLINE

In this chapter, we review some significant aspects of sexual health. In particular, we examine sexual health concerns of men and women, unwanted pregnancy, illness prevention and stigma, victimization, and other issues of current concern. Sexual health issues can have profound and long-lasting impacts on people's lives, their families and communities. There has been progress in reducing teenage births over recent decades. However, sexually transmitted infections are showing increasing prevalence in several areas with high levels of stigma, particularly for the LBGTQ community. Social and health care systems are failing to adequately protect children's sexual safety and well-being. We review key findings and suggest new lines of inquiry.

BOX 9.1

Hypothetical scenario: 'Jack the Lad and Jill the Ladette'*

It is Jack's birthday. He is 18. He's a man! Jack goes out with his mates for a night on the town to celebrate. They hit the city centre and go on a pub crawl. The 'lads' egg Jack on to drink as

(Continued)

much as possible. They are having a great time with many jokes and pranks, as is customary on these occasions all over England (and most other places, one can assume). Suddenly it's 1 a.m., most of the bars are closing, and so they hit a night club, the El Dorado, which stays open until 3 a.m. They smoke a 'spliff' or two in a nearby alley and take a few 'uppers' to keep them going. Inside El Dorado they meet a group of girls on a 'hen night'. They too are feeling 'worse for wear'. Encouraged by his riotous mates, Jack goes to the dance floor with one of the 'hens', Jill. Jill is 17, she is wearing clothes showing generous amounts of her midriff. Jill is all over Jack 'like a rash' and he reciprocates. They dance up close, hands wander and they have a long 'snog'. Jack tells Jill proudly that it's his birthday and says, 'What do I get for my present?' Jill grabs Jack's hand and leads him to the intersex washrooms. Jack and Jill enter a booth, lock the door, and have penetrative vaginal sex ...

As the dishevelled couple re-enter the clubroom, there's a loud cheer and applause from the 'lads' and the 'ladettes'. After a few more cocktails, and a fair amount of gavorting around the dance floor, the lights come on and the patrons are asked to leave by the security staff. The groups head off in their own separate directions. Before they know it, the party is over. No time to exchange contact details.

The next morning Jack remembers very little. Later, he notices a rash on his penis. Over the next few days he finds urination becoming increasingly uncomfortable and a sticky liquid leaks out from his penis. He visits the GUM clinic and is diagnosed with gonorrhoea. With a prescription of antibiotics, the symptoms are quickly gone.

Jill's period was due two weeks after the 'hen night'. This month she misses. Jill waits a few more days and buys a pregnancy kit from the local pharmacy. It's positive. Jill is unsure what to do. She talks to her mother, to her doctor, and to a few close friends. Two of her single friends already have babies. Jill thinks long and hard about having an abortion. At first, she thinks she should have one. Ultimately, however, she decides that she does not want to have one.

Jill and Jack have no way of contacting each other. They don't even remember each other's names.

The baby, Peter, is born. Jill's parents, who are retired, help to look after the baby when Jill is at work. Jill remains single for a few years. Eventually she forms a stable relationship with George and they marry. George has two children from a previous relationship. Jill, George and their three children become a family together.

* We have chosen this vignette because it highlights two key issues for this chapter: unprotected sexual intercourse and unintended teenage pregnancy. For a sociological discussion of 'lads' and 'ladettes', see Jackson (2006).

The vignette of Jack and Jill is hypothetical. However, it is not far removed from scenarios that are replicated all over the world on a frequent basis. Jack-and-Jill encounters of this kind have consequences. The vignette contains a classic mix of biopsychosocial elements:

- in-group conformity
- cultural norms

- alcohol

- drugs

- sex after alcohol

- sex after drugs

- unprotected sexual intercourse

- sexually transmitted infection (STI)

- pregnancy

- childbirth

- single-parent family.

Jack and Jill's story contains significant 'bio', 'psycho' and 'social' elements and illustrates the medium- to long-term consequences that can follow a few minutes of inebriated 'sexual fun'. It is a very human story. What happened can occur in a million different ways. On the medical issue of the STI, Jack and Jill's condition was easily treatable. Other STIs would not be so easily dealt with and could have serious complications, including infertility and disability. In this story Jill will be a single parent, at least for a while. She has the support of her parents, which is likely to be a benefit, but Jack has missed out on fatherhood. Perhaps Jack would have been ill-prepared for this, but so are many fathers or mothers, and he could have been a proud and good father to baby Peter. Before examining some of the issues this story raises in more depth, we outline a few of the pivotal domains that fall under the umbrella of sexual health psychology.

THE SCOPE OF SEXUAL HEALTH PSYCHOLOGY

'Sexual health' can be defined in different ways. In 1994, the United Nations (UN) defined sexual health as 'the enhancement of life and personal relations', and the framing of rights was gender-neutral and cognizant of 'couples and individuals' in terms of rights and responsibilities. The World Health Organization (WHO) defined sexual health as an integral part of overall health. The US Centers for Disease Control and Prevention (CDC) recommended a definition of sexual health in which sexuality is both an intrinsic part of individuals and their overall health and is interwoven with social connections (CDC, 2010). The common elements across the three definitions are that (1) sexuality or relationships with a sexual or romantic component have intrinsic value as a part of health and (2) healthy sexual relationships require positive experiences for individuals *and* their partners (Hogben et al., 2015).

We can see from this last statement that sexual health entails a number of key elements: sexual or romantic relationships are a valuable asset to health; these relationships need to be positive experiences to be healthy. The latter implies that there is choice and enjoyment. The field of sexual health is very broad and encompasses many topics. Examples are:

- the social, cultural and structural determinants of sexual health

- the sexual health of marginalized or oppressed identities (e.g., people with disabilities, transgender persons, refugees)

- living a fulfilling sexual life when living with chronic conditions (e.g., HIV)
- sexual coercion, discrimination and violence
- sexual health and well-being
- sexual health and sexual rights
- critical approaches to sexual health
- the development of new interventions for sexual health
- the evaluation of interventions that improve sexual health.

A special issue of the *Journal of Health Psychology* encompasses the above topics (Rohleder and Flowers, 2018). Box 9.2 lists some commonly cited specific sexual issues that can be perceived as problematic for men and/or women.

BOX 9.2

Typical sexual health concerns of women and men

Many of these concerns share common features for both genders.

Table 9.1   Typical sexual health concerns

Men	Women
Inability to become aroused	Inability to become aroused
Penis and erection problems	Inhibited sexual desire
Penis shape and size anxiety	'Boob and butt' shape and size anxiety
Ejaculation difficulties	Painful intercourse
Ejaculation control/lack of ejaculation	Lack of orgasm (anorgasmia)
Fear of infertility	Fear of infertility
Sexually transmitted infections	Sexually transmitted infections
Pregnancy concerns	Pregnancy concerns
(If applicable) LBGTQ stigma	(If applicable) LBGTQ stigma
Concerns about masculinity	Concerns about femininity

It is impossible to discuss all of these topics in a single chapter. Instead, we highlight a few key topics: 'erectile dysfunction', orgasm and 'anorgasmia', teenage pregnancy, STI prevention, stigmatization, victimization and choice. In our discussion, we observe a tension between traditional biomedical explanations and a more nuanced approach that views sexual experience as a complex of biopsychosocial processes that normally includes the stimulation of anatomical structures.

MASCULINITY, THE PENIS AND ERECTILE DYSFUNCTION

One dominant narrative of masculinity gives primacy to the erect penis. In some ways, contemporary discourse on the penis is similar to ancient fertility cults. Men often perceive their sexual potency as the foundation stone of their identity as a masculine human being. The erect penis has an 'iconic' status as a symbol of virility and masculinity, a qualification of potency in the '*if-a-man-can't-get-a-hard-on, he's-not-fit-to-call-himself-a-man*' school of thought. Having a penis and the ability to have it erect when required are necessary but not sufficient conditions of virility or masculinity, however. There is another preferred condition: the penis should ideally also be large – or even 'huge'.

The penis lends power and potency to male identity, especially if the penis is not small. The media equate a man's penis size with power and masculinity. Some women's magazines convey that a large penis is beneficial to female sexual enjoyment, e.g., '*My best sex ever was ... with a guy who was HUGE*' (*Cosmopolitan* headline, 7 July 2016). Men reporting a larger-than-average penis rate their appearance most favourably, suggesting an effect on male confidence of perceived large penis size (Lever et al., 2006).

A systematic review of studies with up to 15,521 men computed an average penis size of 9.16 cm (3.61 inches) with an SD of 1.57 cm when flaccid and 13.12 cm (5.17 inches) with an SD of 1.66 cm when erect, with an average erect circumference of 11.66 cm (4.59 inches) (Veale et al., 2015). Veale et al. reported a significant positive correlation between men's erect penis length (PL) and their height, which ranged from $r = 0.2$ to 0.6. Above average height with above average PL would thus give a man the best of two worlds.

An internet survey of 52,031 heterosexual men and women by Lever et al. (2006) showed that a majority of men (66%) rated their PL as average, 22% as large and 12% as small. A total of 85% of women were satisfied with their partner's PL, but only 55% of men were satisfied with their PL, with 45% wanting a larger PL and only 0.2% wanting a smaller one. Given its primal role in the psyche, it is important to know in detail the anatomy of the penis and the neighbouring structures.

The penis is the external male organ that serves the dual function of a urinal duct and for the delivery of sperm. The human male urethra passes through the prostate gland, where it is joined by the ejaculatory duct, and then through the penis (Figure 9.1). The urethra traverses the corpus spongiosum, and its opening, the meatus, lies on the tip of the glans penis. It is a passage both for urination and ejaculation of semen.

A major issue in sexual satisfaction is the production of an erection. In so-called 'erectile dysfunction' (ED), this does not happen. ED is defined as the 'inability to achieve or maintain an erection sufficient for satisfactory sexual performance' and it is is estimated to affect as many as 30 million men in the USA (National Institutes of Health, 2017). ED is age-related, with a two- to three-fold increase in prevalence of moderate to severe ED between the ages of 40 and 70 years. It has been estimated that by 2025, the worldwide incidence of ED will approach 322 million, more than double the estimated 1995 incidence rate of approximately 152 million (Newton et al., 2012). When a man ceases to obtain an erection, he will tend to reach out for the little blue pills (Viagra, sildenafil citrate) or the little yellow pills (Cialis, tadalafil). Aids and devices for men with ED are a multibillion dollar industry, giving the hyped obsession with erections and penises in magazines a new meaning.

ED can impact negatively on self-esteem, quality of life and interpersonal relationships in heterosexual (Rosen et al., 1997), gay and bisexual men (Ussher et al., 2016).

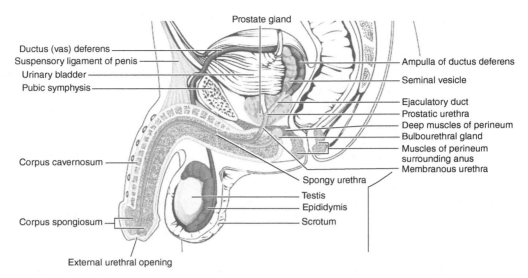

Figure 9.1   Penis and surrounding structures and tissues (lateral cross-section)

Source: Carl Fredrik (2017). Public domain (https://en.wikipedia.org/wiki/Human_penis#/media/
File:Penis_lateral_cross_section.jpg)

Ussher et al. (2016) explored the impact of ED on 46 gay and bisexual men in one-to-one interviews. ED was associated with emotional distress, a negative impact on gay identities, and feelings of sexual disqualification. Other concerns included loss of libido, climacturia, loss of sensitivity or pain during anal sex, non-ejaculatory orgasms and reduced penis size. Such changes can have particular significance to gay sex and gay identities, and can result in feelings of exclusion from a sexual community that can be central to gay or bisexual men's lives. However, Ussher et al. reported that other men were reconciled to their sexual changes, did not experience a challenge to identity, and engaged in sexual re-negotiation.

A variety of medical, psychological and lifestyle factors have been implicated in ED. There is an association between ED and cardiovascular disease, notably coronary heart disease (Shamloul and Ghanem, 2013). Causes of erectile dysfunction include diabetes mellitus and hypertension, and also factors such as limited physical exercise. Lower urinary tract symptoms also have been linked to the development of ED.

The primary treatment for ED has been the **phosphodiesterase type 5 (PDE5) inhibitors** such as Viagra (sildenafil), Cialis (tadalafil) and Levitra (vardenafil). This class of drugs was the first effective oral treatment for ED and has made billions for the companies holding the patents. The PDE5 inhibitors are effective solutions for ED. McCabe and Althof (2014) analysed published findings from randomized controlled trials (RCTs) for (1) the psychosocial outcomes associated with erectile dysfunction (ED) before treatment with a PDE5 inhibitor, and (2) the change in psychosocial outcomes after the use of a PDE5 inhibitor in men with ED. The main outcome measures were scores on psychosocial measures before and after treatment. From a total of 1,714 publications, 40 (32 RCTs) were retained. Before treatment, men reported relatively good quality of life and overall relationships, but poor sexual relationships and sexual satisfaction, diminished confidence, low self-esteem and symptoms of depression. After treatment, there were significant improvements from baseline in most of these measures, except for overall life satisfaction and overall relationship satisfaction. The authors concluded: 'ED and the treatment of ED are associated with substantially broader aspects of a man's life than just erectile functioning. This review demonstrates the importance of evaluating the psychosocial factors associated with ED and its treatment, and the importance of using standardized scales to conduct this evaluation' (McCabe and Althof, 2014: 347).

A narrative review by Schmidt et al. (2014) suggested that psychological intervention combined with a PDE5 inhibitor is more effective than a PDE5 inhibitor alone, although larger-scale RCTs are needed to confirm this finding. Certainly, the PDE5 inhibitors have had a revolutionary impact on improving sexual satisfaction in both men and women.

We turn now to consider the concept and role of the orgasm in human sexual experience.

THE CLITORIS, ORGASM AND ANORGASMIA

If the penis is the epitome of masculinity, then the clitoris must be considered the epitome of female sexuality, and the orgasm the epitome of sexual relations. Fortunately, or unfortunately, depending upon how you look at it and where you're looking from, human sexuality is far more complicated. Sexual behaviour is a complex interaction of biopsychosocial factors involving the central and peripheral nervous systems, modified by emotional, social and physical factors. One of best known classification systems of the human sexual response suggested four phases: desire, excitement, orgasm and resolution (Masters and Johnson, 1966; Kaplan, 1975). Sexual relationship concerns (or 'dysfunctions' according to medical terminology) can stem from psychological and communication issues within a relationship.

Rightly or wrongly, the discourse on this topic focuses on the clitoris. While sexual desire and excitement can be triggered by stimulation of erotogenic areas of the vulva, the clitoris and the anterior wall or outer one-third of the vagina, it can also be triggered by words, thoughts and daydreams (Stock and Geer, 1982; Leitenberg and Henning, 1995). We begin with the 'bio' component of the biopsychosocial approach, focusing on the anatomy and physiology of the female erogenous zones.

How is the clitoris structured and how does it function? The clitoris comprises an external glans and hood, and an internal body, root, crura and bulbs, and is richly supplied with nerve endings (Figure 9.2). The clitoris plays a role in the female orgasm but other factors are also important.

The female orgasm is a complex and contended issue. Although stimulation of the clitoris can trigger orgasm, many factors and theories have been suggested for the female orgasm, clitoral stimulation being only one. The discourse tends to be medicalized. For example, orgasm has been described as 'a sensation of intense pleasure creating an altered consciousness state accompanied by pelvic striated circumvaginal musculature and uterine/anal contractions and myotonia that resolves sexually-induced vasocongestion and induces well-being/contentment' (Meston et al., 2004: 66). Meston et al. (2004) reported a survey of 1,749 randomly sampled US women, of whom 24% reported 'orgasmic dysfunction'. Working within a medical framework, they suggested that **Female orgasmic disorder (FOD)** is the second most frequently reported women's sexual problem (the first being infertility). FOD was defined as 'the persistent or recurrent delay in, or absence of, orgasm following a normal sexual excitement phase that causes marked distress or interpersonal difficulty' (American Psychiatric Association, 2000). Two treatment approaches for FOD have been suggested: cognitive behavioural therapy (CBT) and the pharmacological approach. CBT aims at promoting changes to attitudes and sexually

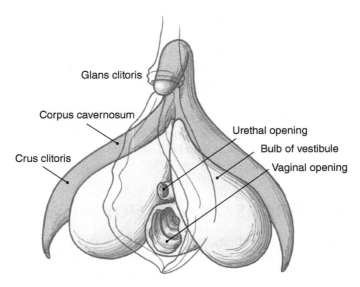

Glans clitoris

Corpus cavernosum

Urethal opening

Bulb of vestibule

Crus clitoris

Vaginal opening

Figure 9.2   The clitoris

Source: Original artwork by Amphis (2007). Public domain

relevant thoughts and anxiety reduction using exercises such as directed masturbation, sensate focus and systematic desensitization, as well as sex education, communication skills training and Kegel exercises (simple clench-and-release exercises that can strengthen the muscles of the pelvic floor).

Risk factors for FOD are classified as psychological, physiological, socio-demographic, hereditary, and with comorbid medical conditions (Cohen and Goldstein, 2016). These authors described multiple psychosocial conditions that can interfere with a woman's ability to reach orgasm, including anxiety, depression, attention deficit disorder, body image, sexual abuse and negative religious views on sex. The relationship with the intimate partner is highly significant. For example, in one study the frequency of penile–vaginal intercourse correlated positively with dimensions of perceived relationship quality: Satisfaction, Intimacy, Trust, Passion, Love (all $r \geq .40$) and Global Relationship Quality ($r = .55$) (Costa and Brody, 2007).

Salisbury and Fisher (2014) explored young adult Canadian heterosexual men's and women's experiences, beliefs and concerns regarding the occurrence or non-occurrence of orgasm during sexual interactions, with an emphasis on the absence of female orgasm during intercourse. Qualitative reports were obtained from five female focus groups ($n = 24$) and five male focus groups ($n = 21$) averaging 19 years of age. The results indicated that the most common concern regarding lack of female orgasm was the negative impact on *the male partner's ego*. Both male and female participants agreed that 'men have the physical responsibility to stimulate their female partner to orgasm, while women have the psychological responsibility of being mentally prepared to experience the orgasm' (Salisbury and Fisher, 2014: 616). Men and women tended to maintain different beliefs, however, regarding clitoral stimulation during intercourse, as well as the importance of female orgasm for a woman's sexual satisfaction in a partnered context.

A qualitative study by Opperman et al. (2014) studied the meanings associated with orgasm and sexual pleasure during sex with a partner, to understand the social patterning of orgasm experience. The sample was 119 sexually experienced British young adults (81% women, mean age 20; 92% heterosexual). The five main themes were: (1) orgasm: the purpose and end of sex; (2) 'it's more about my partner's orgasm'; (3) orgasm: the ultimate pleasure?; (4) orgasm is not a simple physiological response; and (5) faking orgasm is not uncommon. The authors suggested that these themes demonstrate the existence of 'contextualized, complex and contradictory meanings' around orgasm. However, the authors concluded that 'they do resonate strongly with widespread discourses of sexuality which prioritize heterosexual coitus, orgasm, and orgasm-reciprocity' (Opperman et al., 2014: 503). It would appear that, to some degree, medical discourse has seeped into lay discourse about orgasm, in which the orgasm is seen as the 'holy grail' of sexual intercourse such that it will be faked rather than be seen by a partner to be absent. The faking of an orgasm can serve a number of different purposes. To help unravel this complex topic, there is even a scale for measuring female faking of orgasm.

The Faking Orgasm Scale for Women

The Faking Orgasm Scale for Women (FOS) was designed to assess women's self-reported motives for faking orgasm during oral sex and sexual intercourse (Cooper et al., 2014). There are two subscales, one for sexual intercourse and one for oral sex. A factor analysis on the responses of 481 heterosexual undergraduate females (M age = 20.33 years) revealed that the FOS–Sexual Intercourse Subscale was composed of four factors: '(1) Altruistic Deceit, faking orgasm out of concern for a partner's feelings; (2) Fear and Insecurity, faking orgasm to avoid negative emotions associated with the sexual experience; (3) Elevated Arousal, a woman's attempt to increase her own arousal through faking orgasm; and (4) Sexual Adjournment, faking orgasm to end sex' (Cooper et al., 2014: 423). The analysis of the FOS–Oral Sex Subscale also yielded four factors, the first three of which were similar to those for Sexual Intercourse. The fourth was 'Fear of Dysfunction', faking orgasm to cope with concerns of being abnormal. This last factor is a serious indictment of the lack of authenticity in sexual relationships, faking it to appear and feel 'normal'.

The FOS should be helpful to improve understanding of the faking of orgasms and, to complement qualitative studies, provide a method for exploring sexual desire and satisfaction that goes beyond the medicalized discourse about anorgasmia, female sexual dysfunction and FOD. We turn now to consider the issue of female genital mutilation.

Female genital mutilation

Among those who practise it, female genital mutilation (FGM) is believed to be a way of reducing a woman's libido to help her to resist 'illicit' sexual acts. Although the WHO classification of FGM indicates that FGM can involve the complete removal of the clitoris, the clitoris is rarely fully removed, as erectile tissues for sexual arousal, orgasm and pleasure are preserved and normally developed in women with FGM (Okomo et al., 2017). However, any cutting of the clitoris in FGM can impair sexual responsivity and there is trauma with the procedure itself. Impaired sexual function, such as vaginal dryness during intercourse, increased pain, reduction in sexual satisfaction and desire, orgasmic delay and anorgasmia, have been reported among women living with all types of FGM. Scar formation, pain and traumatic memories associated with FGM can also lead to such problems.

Okomo et al. (2017) suggest that orgasmic difficulties may not be seen as a problem if the girl underwent the procedure before becoming sexually active, or if her peers are anorgasmic. Such difficulties are more likely to be reported in groups that undergo the procedure after a period of adolescent sexual activity or before childbirth. Sexual issues for men can be caused by physical discomfort when attempting intercourse with a partner with FGM as well as causing pain for the woman.

FGM has been illegal in the UK since 1985, and since 2003 anyone taking a child out of the UK for FGM faces 14 years in prison. However, enforcement has been lacking and not one successful prosecution of an FGM case had occurred in the UK to the date of this publication.

TEENAGE PREGNANCY

Teenage pregnancy usually refers to cases of unintended pregnancy during adolescence. Approximately 750,000 of 15- to 19-year-olds in the USA become pregnant each year (American Congress of Obstetricians and Gynecologists, 2015). Somewhat bizarrely, teenagers often do not believe that they will get pregnant if they engage in unprotected sexual activity. This fact may seem a little weird, but it possibly stems from the well-established tendency of humans to indulge in unrealistic optimism: the almost universal '*I didn't think this would ever happen to me*' syndrome (Weinstein, 1980). Most people also rarely appreciate the moderate-sized probability that they are themselves the result of an unintended pregnancy. You and me both! Sedgh et al. (2014) reported that 85 million pregnancies, which is 40% of all pregnancies worldwide, were unintended in 2012. Of these, 50% ended in abortion, 13% ended in miscarriage and 38% resulted in an unplanned birth. If reliable, this statistic means that 15.2% of all births in 2012 were unintended.

A large quantity of research has looked for social and psychological predictors of teenage pregnancy and examined the typical outcomes of teen births for babies and mothers. The good news is that teen pregnancy rates have significantly declined over the last few decades in both the UK and the USA (Lindberg et al., 2016; Office for National Statistics, 2016; Figures 9.3 and 9.4). These statistical reductions could possibly be attributed to improved methods of contraception, or teenagers becoming more intelligent (probably not) (Flynn, 2007; Marks, 2010), or, as 'digital natives', teenagers exposing themselves less to pregnancy risk by spending more time on the internet using Facebook, SnapChat and other media and less time experimenting with sex. More research is needed to answer this question.

One of the most commonly cited reasons for teenage pregnancy is **peer pressure**. Teenagers believe that having sex is 'cool'. More than 29% of US pregnant teens reported that they felt pressured to have sex, and 33% of pregnant teens stated that they felt that they were not ready for a sexual relationship, but proceeded anyway because they feared ridicule or rejection (Kaiser Family Foundation, 2016). Another factor is the absence of parents. Teenage girls are more likely to get pregnant if they have received limited or no guidance from parents. If a teenager feels unable to talk to her parents about sex, her only source of guidance will be friends, social media, TV and print publications, resulting in misinformation.

It is often alleged that the movies and media contribute to teen pregnancy by glamorizing it. However, the evidence on glamorization is mixed and some evidence even contradicts the notion. Kearney and Levine (2014) obtained evidence that MTV's *16 and Pregnant* has had a positive effect on reducing teen childbearing in the USA. *16 and Pregnant* is a reality TV series which follows the lives of pregnant teenagers at the end of their pregnancy and in the early days of motherhood. Kearney and Levine (2014) investigated whether the show influenced teens' interest in contraceptive use or abortion, and whether it ultimately altered teen childbearing outcomes. They used data from Google Trends and Twitter to document changes in searches

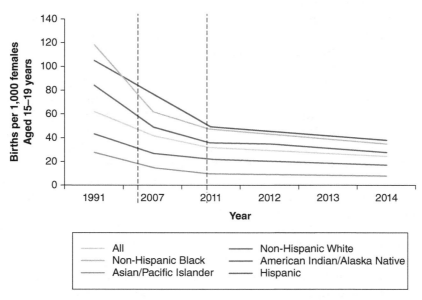

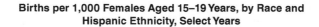

Figure 9.3 Reduction in pregnancy risk among females 15–19 years in the USA from 1991–2014

Source: Martin et al. (2014)

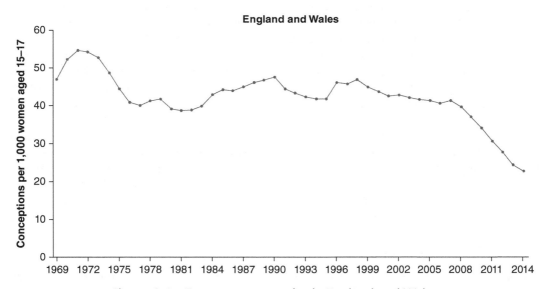

Figure 9.4 Teenage pregnancies in England and Wales

Source: Office for National Statistics (2016)

and tweets resulting from the show, Nielsen ratings data to capture geographic variation in viewership, and Vital Statistics birth data to measure changes in teen birth rates. They found that *16 and Pregnant* led to more searches and tweets regarding birth control and abortion, and ultimately to a 5.7% reduction in teen births in the 18 months following its introduction. The authors claim that this reduction accounted for around one-third of the overall decline in teen births in the USA during that period. If real, this finding would be a progressive step towards the improvement of society.

Around 5% of teens become pregnant as a consequence of rape (Holmes et al., 1996). The Guttmacher Institute (2016) stated that around 50% of teens say that they had been impregnated by an adult male, and two-thirds report that their babies' fathers are as old as 27.

Alcohol drinking is associated with unexpected pregnancy. Drinking lowers a teen's ability to control her impulses, contributing to 75% of pregnancies that occur between the ages 14 and 21. Approximately 91% of pregnant teens reported that although they were drinking at the time, they did not originally plan to have sex when they conceived (Guttmacher Institute, 2016).

The stereotyping of young single mothers has been evident for many decades, going back to the Victorian era. Accepted professional opinion in the 1990s was that adverse birth outcomes with teenage pregnancy are attributable to low socio-economic status, inadequate prenatal care and inadequate weight gain during pregnancy. Empirical research has proved this thinking to be wrong. Chen et al. (2007) studied whether teenage pregnancy is associated with increased adverse birth outcomes independent of known confounding factors. They used a retrospective cohort design with 3.886 M. pregnant women under 25 years of age with a first live singleton birth during 1995 and 2000 in the USA. Chen et al. found all teenage groups were associated with increased risks for pre-term delivery, low birthweight and neonatal mortality. Infants born to teenage mothers aged 17 or younger were at an even higher risk. The sub-sample of white married mothers with an age-appropriate education level and adequate prenatal care, and without smoking and alcohol use during pregnancy, yielded similar results. Chen et al. concluded that 'teenage pregnancy increases the risk of adverse birth outcomes independent of important known confounders. This finding challenged the accepted opinion that adverse birth outcome associated with teenage pregnancy is attributable to low socioeconomic status, inadequate prenatal care and inadequate weight gain during pregnancy' (Chen et al., 2007: 368).

Teenage mothers have been stereotyped and stigmatized in UK media, especially the 'red-top' newspapers, as unmotivated, irresponsible and incompetent (SmithBattle, 2013). Stigmatization is a contributing factor to teenage mothers' difficulties and their health and social disparities. Marginalized youth, unemployed young men and teenage mothers tend to be stereotyped and stigmatized in the UK through labels such as 'chav' and 'pramface' (Nayak and Kehily, 2014). Working-class young men and teenage mothers must learn to manage social class stigma and 'speak back to these markers of abjection' (Nayak and Kehily, 2014: 1330). Stigma and stereotyping are impediments to effective clinical care and contribute to teenage mothers' challenges. Improvements to training with advocacy for services and policies to reduce the stigmatization and marginalization are one way to lessen the negative experiences of teenage mothers.

UNSAFE ABORTION

The World Health Organization defines unsafe abortion as 'a procedure for terminating an unintended pregnancy either by individuals without the necessary skills or in an environment that does not conform to minimum medical standards, or both' (World Health Organization

(WHO), 2011). Unsafe abortion mainly occurs in developing countries where abortion is highly restricted by law and in countries where, although legally permitted, safe abortion is not easily accessible. Women dealing with an unintended pregnancy often self-induce abortions or obtain clandestine abortions from medical practitioners, paramedical workers or traditional healers. The risks of infection and/or incorrect and potentially life-threatening procedures are high.

The WHO (2011) reported that unsafe abortion remains a major public health problem in many countries. It estimated that a woman dies every eighth minute somewhere in a developing country due to complications arising from unsafe abortion. These women were likely to have had little or no money to procure safe services. An estimated 74% of abortions in developing countries, excluding China, were unsafe in 2008, with Africa having a 97% rate of unsafe abortions (Sedgh et al., 2012).

As with HIV infection and AIDS, the disparities between the health of women in developed and developing countries is extreme. Unsafe abortion remains one of the most neglected sexual and reproductive health problems.

PREVENTING STIS: KNOWLEDGE, AWARENESS AND CONDOM USE

Worldwide, the WHO estimated that 499 million new cases of curable STIs occurred in 2008 among 15–49-year-olds globally: 106 million cases of chlamydia, 106 million cases of gonorrhea, 11 million cases of syphilis, and 276 million cases of trichomoniasis (WHO, 2008). More than 30 identified pathogens are known to be transmitted sexually, eight of which have been clearly linked to the greatest amount of morbidity. Three bacterial STIs, *Chlamydia trachomatis* (chlamydia), *Neisseria gonorrhoeae* (gonorrhea) and *Treponema pallidum* (syphilis), and one parasitic STI, *Trichomonas vaginalis* (trichomoniasis), are currently curable. Four viral STIs – HIV, human papillomavirus (HPV), herpes simplex virus (HSV) and hepatitis B virus (HBV) – can be chronic or life-long, although medications can modify disease course or symptoms (Gottlieb et al., 2014).

The Centers for Disease Control and Prevention (CDC, 2016a) reported that there are more than 110 million STIs among men and women across the nation and 20 million new STIs each year in the USA, costing the American health care system nearly $16 billion in direct medical costs alone. The CDC estimated that half of all new STIs in the USA occur among young men and women.

Research on sexual behaviour is procedurally complex. People do not feel comfortable sharing information with strangers carrying clip boards about their intimate experiences. There is an understandable tendency to over-report prudent and wise actions and to under-report casual indulgences, leading to biased data. The reliability and validity of self-report measures of condom use must be questioned because self-reported behaviour is likely to be influenced by self-presentation, social desirability or memory biases. Young people in general often also believe an incorrect and potentially fatal idea: they think that bad things won't happen to them ('**optimistic bias**'; Weinstein, 1980). They are chronic under-reporters of sexual risk taking. There are also gender-based 'double standards' in which males over-report and females under-report sexual activity (e.g., Rudman et al., 2016).

Adolescents have high rates of STIs. Adolescents consuming alcohol and using drugs have markedly greater HIV/STI risk and are a priority for intervention. Recent advances in microbiology, such as the use of less invasive specimen collection for DNA assays, can provide validation of adolescents' self-reported sexual risk behaviour (DiClemente, 2016). However, the majority of studies of adolescents' sexual risk rely solely on self-reports.

Among young adults who use condoms, incomplete condom use (putting a condom on after beginning or taking a condom off before finishing sex) and condom failure (condom breaking or slipping off during sex) are common. Therefore, surveys that only ask whether a condom was used are likely to underestimate the actual prevalence of unprotected sex. Dolezal et al. (2014) used data from 135 sexually active perinatally HIV-infected (PHIV+) youth and perinatally exposed but uninfected (PHIV−) youth aged 13–24. Participants were asked whether they used a condom on their first and their most recent occasion of vaginal sex. Dolezal et al. asked youth who reported using a condom a follow-up question about whether there was any time during that occasion when sex was not protected by a condom. This simple follow-up question identified almost double the proportion who initially said they did not use a condom as having had unprotected sex.

Communication between partners can be another barrier to or a facilitator of safe sexual relations. Lack of communication between partners could help to explain why many adolescents fail to use condoms consistently. Widman et al. (2014) synthesized research linking adolescents' sexual communication to condom use and examined several potential moderators of this association. A total of 41 independent effect sizes from 34 studies with 15,046 adolescent participants were meta-analysed. Their results revealed a modest but statistically significant weighted mean effect size of the sexual communication–condom use relationship of $r = .24$, $p < 2.001$. Communication topic and communication format were statistically significant moderators ($p < 2.001$). Larger effect sizes were found for communication about condom use ($r = .34$) than for communication about sexual history ($r = .15$) or general safer sex topics ($r = .14$). Effect sizes were also larger for communication behaviour formats ($r = .27$) and self-efficacy formats ($r = .28$) than for fear/concern ($r = .18$), future intention ($r = .15$) or communication comfort ($r = −.15$) formats. Widman et al.'s results highlight the need for communication skills, particularly about condom use, in HIV/STI prevention work for youth.

Sheeran et al. (1999) conducted a herculean systematic review of correlates of condom use among heterosexual samples. Altogether, 660 correlations distributed across 44 variables were derived from 121 empirical studies. The findings showed that demographic, personality and labelling stage variables showed small average correlations with condom use. The correlations ranged from −.18 (frequency of intercourse) to .10 (had an HIV test), suggesting that the variables were accounting for only 1–2% of the variability in reported condom usage rates.

Bearing in mind that there were 660 different correlations, then 1 in 20 of the 660 correlations would be significant at the 5% level owing to Type I error. That means there were in the region of 33 $p < .05$ coefficients from Type I errors, i.e., false positives. Applying the Bonferroni correction to the p level requires any individual correlation coefficient to be significant at $p < .05/660$ or $p = .0000757$. For $n = 100$, 200 and 1,000 respectively, r would need to be .37, .27 and .12 to be statistically significant. Table 2 in Sheeran et al. (1999) suggests that few correlations reached the corrected level of significance.

Another factor is publication bias, in which studies reporting statistically significant results and those supporting the investigator's hypotheses are more likely to be published than null or negative findings. Dwan et al. (2013) found strong evidence of an association between significant results and publication. Publications also have been found to be inconsistent with their protocols. Dwan et al. (2013: 1) concluded: 'Researchers need to be aware of the problems of both types of bias and efforts should be concentrated on improving the reporting of trials.'

Sheeran et al. (1999: 90) concluded that their 'findings support a social psychological model of condom use highlighting the importance of behaviour-specific cognitions, social interaction, and preparatory behaviors rather than knowledge and beliefs about the threat of infection'. However, the support offered to the socio-cognitive model of condom use was limited to explaining a maximum of 18.5% in intention to use condoms. Setting aside the slippery problem of good intentions never being carried out, the published figure left 81.5% of the variation in intention to use condoms unaccounted for. Bearing in mind that no corrections were made for publication bias or multiple p values, the 18.5% figure must be assumed to be highly inflated compared to the true figure. Yet this low 18.5% figure is representative for what has been offered as the epitome of the best results offered by socio-cognitive theory. The findings of the best research from health psychology illustrated by the above studies suggest a huge gap between theoretical predictions and real-world sexual behaviour, an issue we highlight in the following in-depth analysis of a recent intervention study.

SOCIAL MEDIA, PORNOGRAPHY AND CYBERSEX

One approach to improving sexual health, awareness and knowledge has been to use digital technology. Information and communications technologies (ICTs) of the internet, text messaging and social networking increasingly are being used in sexual health promotion and risk reduction. Billions of people worldwide actively use social media, yet only a few dozen publications on the use of social media for promoting sexual health could be identified. Gabarron and Wynn (2016) reported that about a quarter identified promising results, and the evidence base is increasing. They concluded there is a need for a theoretical framework and stronger research designs.

Some have suggested the idea of 'internet addiction'. Starcevic and Aboujaoude (2017: 13) find this concept inadequate for several reasons: 'Internet addiction is conceptually too heterogeneous because it pertains to a variety of very different behaviours. Internet addiction should be replaced by terms that refer to the specific behaviours (e.g., gaming, gambling, or sexual activity), regardless of whether these are performed online or offline.'

Unquestionably, access to internet pornography and cybersex are on the rise. In 2008, it was estimated that up to 90% or more of US youth aged between 12 and 18 years had access to pornography on the internet (Sabina et al., 2008). Concerns that such high accessibility may lead to a rise in pornography-seeking among children and adolescents would have implications for adolescent sexual development. Seekers of pornography, online or offline, were in 2008 more likely to be male, with only 5% of self-identified seekers being female. The vast majority (87%) of youth who reported looking for sexual images online were 14 years of age or older.

Accessibility to pornography today is approaching or has already reached 100% of the population. Researchers with both adolescents and adults have suggested evidence of 'pornography addiction', although this idea is controversial. In partial support of the addiction idea, it has been estimated that 17% of individuals who view internet pornography meet criteria for problematic sexual compulsivity (Cooper et al., 2000). One study examined pornography use and well-being, including feelings of addiction, with a cross-sectional sample of 713 adults (Grubbs et al., 2015). A one-year, longitudinal follow-up with a subset of undergraduates found an association over time between perceived addiction to internet pornography and psychological distress.

With increasing use of ICTs across societies worldwide, social, sexual and psychological development of young people is a new focus for health psychology research. The risk of negative sexual experience and victimization online is likely to have real-world consequences for young people. DeMarco et al. (2017) explored adolescent risk-taking online behaviour from a group of young adults in different European countries using a retrospective survey of 18–25-year-olds in higher education. The sample were asked about their online experiences between the ages of 12 and 16. Risky behaviour online and offline, types of victimization (online and offline) and sexual solicitation requests online were analysed together with help-seeking behaviour. Four profiles concerning adolescent risky behaviours were identified using cluster analysis. Two were considered normative (adapted adolescents and inquisitive online) and two high risk (risk-taking aggressive and sexually inquisitive online).

Chang et al. (2014) studied predictors of unwanted exposure to online pornography and sexual solicitation with 2,315 students from 26 high schools in Taiwan. They were assessed in the tenth grade, with follow-up in the eleventh grade using self-administered questionnaires. High levels of online game use, pornography media exposure, internet risk behaviours, depression and cyber-bullying experiences were associated with online sexual solicitation, victimization and perpetration. It may well be the case that frequent and habitual users of online pornography become more risk-averse and bully, victimize or groom unsuspecting 'friends' on Facebook.

The majority of studies in this field are cross-sectional surveys of low quality. Prospective studies are fairly rare, owing to the newness of the field. In spite of the issue of definitions, this field is likely to expand over the next five to ten years.

SEXUAL VIOLENCE AND ABUSE

A substantial proportion of female and male adults report having experienced some form of sexual violence, stalking or intimate partner violence at least once during their lifetime in the USA (Breiding, 2014) and in Europe (Krahé et al., 2015). Both women and men are affected by these types of violence over their lifetime, including sexual violence, stalking and physical violence by an intimate partner.

Children

Over the last decade, media revelations of childhood victimization reached epic levels. Seemingly, there are no boundaries to this problem within the established religious organizations, such as the Roman Catholic Church, media organizations such as the BBC, child protection organizations, and sports clubs in athletics and football. The concern is that the child sexual abuse (CSA) that has surfaced to date is only the tip of a large iceberg. It has been empirically demonstrated since the 1990s that childhood victimization is detrimental to the well-being of victims. Victimization has been shown to be a risk factor for promiscuity, prostitution and teenage pregnancy. However, the CSA area is replete with statistics and moral panic, while theory and explanation are thin on the ground.

The prevalence of child sexual abuse is difficult to estimate exactly because it is often unreported. However, studies in the USA by Finkelhor (1994, 2008) and Finkelhor et al. (2014) show that:

- 1 in 5 girls and 1 in 20 boys is a victim of child sexual abuse;
- 20% of adult females and 5–10% of adult males recall a childhood sexual assault or sexual abuse incident;

- during a one-year period, 16% of youth aged 14–17 had been sexually victimized;
- over the course of their lifetime, 28% of youth aged 14–17 had been sexually victimized;
- children are most vulnerable to CSA between the ages of 7 and 13.

The US Department of Health and Human Services' Children's Bureau (2010) reported that 9.2% of victimized children were sexually assaulted. The National Institute of Justice (2003) statistics suggested that three out of four sexually assaulted adolescents were victimized by someone they knew well. A child who is the victim of prolonged sexual abuse usually develops low self-esteem, a feeling of worthlessness and an abnormal or distorted view of sex. The child may become withdrawn and mistrustful of adults, and can become suicidal. Children who do not live with both parents, as well as children living in homes marked by parental discord, divorce or domestic violence, have a higher risk of being sexually abused. In the vast majority of cases where there is credible evidence that a child has been penetrated, only between 5% and 15% of those children will have genital injuries consistent with sexual abuse. CSA is not restricted to physical contact; it can include exposure, voyeurism and child pornography. Compared to those with no history of sexual abuse, young sexually abused males were five times more likely to cause teen pregnancy, three times more likely to have multiple sexual partners and two times more likely to have unprotected sex (e.g., Beitchman et al., 1992).

Widom and Kuhns (1996) examined the extent to which being abused and/or neglected in childhood increases a person's risk for promiscuity, prostitution and teenage pregnancy. They employed a prospective cohorts design to match age, race, sex and social class in cohorts of abused and/or neglected children from 1967 to 1971. Widom and Kuhns followed participants into young adulthood. Early childhood abuse and/or neglect was a significant predictor of prostitution for females. However, childhood abuse and neglect were not associated with increased risk for promiscuity or teenage pregnancy.

In an open-ended survey question to European 9- to 16-year-olds, some 10,000 children reported a range of risks that concern them on the internet (Livingstone et al., 2014). Pornography (22% of children who mentioned risks), conduct risk such as cyber-bullying (19%), and violent content (18%) were the three main children's concerns. Livingstone et al. observed that many children expressed shock and disgust on witnessing 'violent, aggressive or gory' online content, especially that which graphically depicts realistic violence against vulnerable victims, including from the news. The video-sharing website YouTube was a primary source of violent and pornographic content.

The exploitation and lack of protection of children in both public and private organizations have been a particular weakness of contemporary social, judiciary and systems of care. These systems themselves are in need of radical treatment and reform to reduce harm to children resulting from sexual exploitation.

Adults

Sexual violence is a sexual act committed against someone without that person's freely given consent. The person did not offer their informed consent. Sexual violence can be divided into the following categories:

- Completed or attempted forced penetration of a victim.
- Completed or attempted alcohol/drug-facilitated penetration of a victim.

- Completed or attempted forced acts in which a victim is made to penetrate a perpetrator or someone else.

- Completed or attempted alcohol/drug-facilitated acts in which a victim is made to penetrate a perpetrator or someone else.

- Non-physically forced penetration which occurs after a person is pressured verbally or through intimidation or misuse of authority to consent or acquiesce.

- Unwanted sexual contact.

- Non-contact unwanted sexual experiences. (CDC, 2017c)

Using a definition of rape that includes forced vaginal, oral and anal intercourse, an interview survey of 8,000 women and 8,000 men in the USA found that *one in six women* had experienced an attempted rape or a completed rape (Tjaden and Thoennes, 1998). At the time they were raped 22% were under the age of 12, 54% were under the age of 18 and 83% were under the age of 25. In the same study, *1 in 33 men* had experienced a sexual assault.

A large proportion of rape occurs as intimate partner violence (IPV). In the USA, nearly one in ten women have been raped by an intimate partner, while an estimated 16.9% of women and 8% of men have experienced sexual violence other than rape (Breiding et al., 2014). Women have a higher lifetime prevalence of severe physical violence compared to men, 24.3% and 13.8%, respectively. Almost half of men and women have experienced at least one occurrence of psychologically aggressive behaviour by an intimate partner during their lifetime. Black non-Hispanic women and multiracial non-Hispanic women had significantly higher lifetime prevalence of rape, physical violence and stalking compared to white, non-Hispanic women, while bisexual women had a significantly higher prevalence of lifetime rape, physical violence or stalking by an intimate partner compared to lesbian women.

The poor quality of the processes of law enforcement and the justice system in dealing with rape cases has been widely publicized for decades. Many rape victims suffer secondary victimization after reporting the crime to the authorities. In the USA, for every 100 rape cases reported to law enforcement, 33 on average would be referred to prosecutors, 16 would be charged and moved into the court system, 12 would end in a successful conviction, and seven would end in a prison sentence (Campbell, 2008). Successful prosecution is more likely for those from privileged backgrounds and those who experienced assaults that fit stereotypic notions of what constitutes rape. Younger women, ethnic minority women and women of lower SES are more likely to have their cases rejected by the criminal justice system (Campbell, 2008). Cases of stranger rape (where the suspect was later identified) and rape with the use of a weapon and/or physical injuries to victims are more likely to be prosecuted. Also, alcohol and drug use by the victim significantly increases the likelihood that a case will be dropped.

In a review, 43–52% of victims who had contact with the legal system rated their experience as unhelpful and/or hurtful (Campbell, 2008). Survivors have described their contact with the legal system as a 'dehumanizing' experience, by being interrogated, intimidated and blamed, and many say they would not have reported the rape had they known what the experience would be like (Logan et al., 2005).

Experiences of secondary victimization take a toll on victims' mental health. In self-reports of their psychological health, rape survivors indicated that as a result of their contact with legal system personnel, they felt bad about themselves (87%), depressed (71%), violated (89%), distrustful of others (53%) and reluctant to seek further help (80%) (Campbell, 2008). The harm of secondary victimization is evident in objective measures of PTSD symptoms. Contact with formal help systems, including the police, is likely to result in negative social reactions associated with increased PTSD outcomes (Ullman et al., 2005).

Hogben et al. (2015) reviewed sexual health interventions for adults. They summarized data from 58 studies (1996–2011) by population (adults, parents, sexual minorities, vulnerable populations) across domains. Interventions were found to be predominantly individual and small-group designs that addressed sexual behaviours (72%) and attitudes/norms (55%). Of these interventions, 98% reported a positive finding in at least one domain, while 50% also reported null effects. With vulnerable populations, the results suggested that interventions were more effective in changing sexual behaviour in terms of risk per act than in changing the amount of sexual behaviour. Interventions were found to be successful in increasing contraceptive use, increasing condom use or decreasing the amount of unprotected sex, but only sometimes affected numbers of partners.

The highly positive findings (98% of studies!) in the Hogben et al. (2015) review indicate a very strong publication bias. The bulk of studies focused heavily on heterosexual women and, among LGBT populations, focused heavily on gay men and MSM. Well-controlled, larger-scale studies with more diverse population groups are needed.

Research has explored the psychological correlates of male sexual fantasies about raping women. Bartels et al. (2017) examined the link between imaginal ability and the use of aggressive sexual fantasies, including their link with rape-supportive cognition. They proposed that men who hold hostile beliefs towards women use aggressive sexual fantasies more often if they possess a 'rich fantasy life'. Operationally, they argued that this involves: (1) a proneness to fantasize in general; (2) an ability to vividly envision mental imagery (Marks, 1973); and (3) frequent experiences of dissociation. They hypothesized that a 'Rich Fantasy Life' mediated by 'Hostile Beliefs about Women' influences the use of 'Aggressive Sexual Fantasies'. A sample of 159 community males completed measures of fantasy proneness, dissociation and vividness of mental imagery, along with two measures that assess hostile beliefs about women. Structural equation modelling (along with bootstrapping procedures) indicated that the data had a very good fit with the hypothesized model.

LBGTQ STIGMATIZATION

On 12 June 2016, Omar Mateen, a 29-year-old security guard, killed 49 people and wounded 53 others in an attack/hate crime inside Pulse, a gay nightclub in Orlando, Florida, USA. Mateen was shot and killed by Orlando Police Department (OPD) officers after a three-hour stand-off. This was the most lethal hate crime in the USA since the 2001 September 11 World Trade Center atrocity.

Historically, LBGTQ people typically have hidden their true selves from public view from pure fear of the social stigma that would inevitably follow a 'coming out'. It has been said that Oscar Wilde and Quentin Crisp each performed 'stigma management', deflecting stigma for being gay by projecting the image of a dandy. The stigma attached to being LBGTQ is high.

LBGTQ is an acronym that collectively refers to individuals who are lesbian, gay, bisexual or transgender, with the 'Q' representing queer or questioning. It is sometimes stated as 'GLBT' (gay, lesbian, bi and transgender) or 'LBGT'. Terminology and vernacular change over time. 'Queer' as a descriptor was in common usage in the 1950s and 1960s, as were other terms, such as the 'N word', that today are proscribed, although they still may make occasional appearances as graffiti.

Fear of discrimination is a major concern for LBGTQ people throughout the world. In China, 61% of respondents in an LBGTQ survey reported they were afraid of being treated differently by doctors because of their sexual orientation or gender identity (Love Without Borders Foundation, 2016). Almost half of respondents experienced discrimination from health care workers after disclosing their sexual orientation or gender.

Almeida et al. (2009) evaluated emotional distress among ninth- to twelfth-grade students to examine whether the association between LBGTQ status and emotional distress was mediated by perceptions of having been treated badly or discriminated against because others thought they were gay or lesbian. Data from a school-based survey in Boston, MA, were analysed. In this sample, 10% of a sample of more than 1,000 were LBGTQ, 58% were female and of a 13–19-year age range. About 45% were black, 31% were Hispanic and 14% were white. LBGTQ youth scored significantly higher on depressive symptomatology. They were also more likely than heterosexual, non-transgendered youth to report suicidal ideation (30% versus 6%) and self-harm (5% versus 3%). Perceived discrimination was observed to account for increased depressive symptomatology among LBGTQ males and females, and accounted for an elevated risk of self-harm and suicidal ideation among LBGTQ males.

BOX 9.3

LBGTQ terminology

Asexual: an individual who does not experience sexual attraction.

Assigned sex: the sex that is assigned to an infant at birth based on the child's visible sex organs, including genitalia and other physical characteristics.

Biological sex: anatomical, physiological, genetic or physical attributes that define whether a person is male, female, or intersex. These include genitalia, gonads, hormone levels, hormone receptors, chromosomes, genes and secondary sex characteristics.

Bisexual, or **bi**: a person who experiences romantic, emotional or sexual attraction to the same gender and other genders, whether to equal degrees or to varying degrees.

Closeted: a person who is not open about their sexual orientation or gender identity, or an ally who is not open about their support for people who are LGBTQ.

Gay: the adjective to describe people who are emotionally, romantically or physically attracted to people of the same gender.

Gender: a set of social, psychological or emotional traits, often influenced by societal expectations, that classify an individual as male, female, a mixture of both, or neither.

Gender Nonconforming, or **GNC**: a person whose identified gender is expansive beyond the binary of male or female.

Homophobia: An aversion to lesbian or gay people that often manifests itself in the form of prejudice and bias.

Lesbian: a woman who is emotionally, romantically and/or physically attracted to other women.

Pansexual, or **pan**: a person who experiences romantic, emotional or sexual attraction to persons of all gender identities or sexes.

Transgender, or **trans**: a person whose self-identified gender does not fully align with their physical sex as assigned at birth, and who may choose to take steps to medically alter the gendered features of their body.

Source: PFLAG (2017); www.pflag.org/about

Earnshaw et al. (2016a) noted that bullying of LBGTQ youth is prevalent in the USA, yet multiple studies have shown that bullying undermines the mental, behavioural and physical health of LBGTQ youth, with consequences lasting throughout life. Paediatricians can play a vital role in promoting the well-being of LBGTQ youth by preventing and identifying bullying, offering counselling to youth and their parents, and advocating for programmes and policies.

Issues of masculinity are important to males' self-esteem and to the well-being of boys and young men. The use of anabolic-androgenic steroids is a concern for adolescent boys. Parent and Bradstreet (2017) examined bullying based on being labelled gay/bisexual and steroid use among US adolescent boys, including sexual orientation disparities. They used data from 2,660 boys from the 2015 Youth Behaviour Risk Survey. Among heterosexual boys, Parent and Bradstreet reported that steroid use was higher among those who reported being bullied due to being labelled gay or bisexual. However, no such relationship was observed among non- heterosexual boys.

Meyer (2016) discussed the stigma regarding accessing STI prevention and treatment for the LBGTQ community, which can be a barrier towards accessing services. Meyer found that one in five LBGTQ individuals reported withholding information regarding their sexual history from a health care provider. A survey from the National Coalition for LBGTQ Health cited stigma in health care settings as a top concern. Over half of participants reported stigma and lack of cultural competency in health care.

While there is a tendency of mainstream media to focus on terrorism, drugs and crime, the commonplace existence of stigma and bullying in the everyday lives of millions of people within the LBGTQ community receives far less attention. A cultural change is necessary.

Discussion Topic: 'Live and Let Live'

It is a human right to have freedom of thought, expression and action within the law. If this is true, the scope for health psychology is limited to providing help and advice to those who seek such help and advice. People can choose to smoke, vape, eat unhealthily, have unprotected sex, acquire an STI or HIV infection, and become pregnant in so doing. Is this not their inalienable human right? In what ways can or should the health care professionals/health psychologists intervene?

FUTURE RESEARCH

1. There are several neglected areas of sexual health, such as unsafe abortion, sexual abuse, paedophilia and sexual hate crime, that warrant more research.

2. The campaigns to reduce unwanted teenage pregnancies need to continue with groups and in areas that have not yet been reached.

3. Future sexual health research is needed to cover a greater diversity of population groups, including heterosexual men and a more diverse selection of sexual minorities.

4. The impact of increased access to ICT and the internet on sexual health is likely to be a major theme for research over the next decades.

SUMMARY

1. The incidence and prevalence of sexually transmitted infections is increasing in most regions of the world. Improvements in education and greater access to ICTs may lead to global reductions in both the incidence and prevalence of STIs.
2. The World Health Organization estimates that a woman dies every eighth minute somewhere in a developing country due to complications arising from unsafe abortion.
3. Optimistic bias and lack of preparation contribute to unprotected sex. There is a high probability that the infected person will feel shame, anxiety and stigmatization.
4. Medicalized discourse on topics such as orgasm, erectile dysfunction and female orgasmic dysfunctions indicates physical explanations. This oversimplified discourse is challenged by psychosocial studies of the quality and meaning of sexual relationship s.
5. Sexuality and relationships with a sexual or romantic component have intrinsic value as an aspect of health, and healthy sexual relationships include positive experiences for individuals *and* their partners. Sexual activity is associated with di ding to a rise in pornography-seeking among children and adolescents, with implications for adolescent sexual development. This needs to be monitored.
6. Teenage pregnancy rates have fallen over the last few decades in both the USA and the UK. However, the precise cause of these reductions cannot be unambiguously attributed to improvements in contraception as there may have been a decrease in sexual intercourse among teenagers due to their habitual usage of social media.
7. Studies in the USA show that 1 in 5 girls and 1 in 20 boys are victims of child sexual abuse, with 20% of adult females and 5–10% of adult males recalling a childhood sexual assault or sexual abuse incident.
8. In the USA, one in six women report experiencing an attempted or completed rape. At the time they were raped, 83% were under the age of 25. Only 1 in 33 men experience a sexual assault. Nearly one in ten women have been raped by an intimate partner.
9. Stigma, harassment and bullying are commonly experienced by LBGTQ people.
10. ICTs, text messaging and social media are new tools for sexual health promotion and risk reduction. However, high internet access is leading to a rise in pornography-seeking among children and adolescents, with implications for adolescent sexual development. This needs to be monitored.

FOOD, EATING AND OBESITY

'Obesity does not imply gluttony; gluttons might escape obesity and, conversely, obesity can arise from a perfectly ordinary level of food intake as the long-term result of a near-imperceptible imbalance in homeostatic mechanisms. Blaming the obese for their obesity is rather like blaming the poor for their poverty; they might be able to do something about their condition, but in practice it is often far from easy.'

Gareth Leng (2014: 1101)

OUTLINE

In this chapter, we critically examine the part played by food, diets and dieting in the changing patterns of illnesses and deaths associated with obesity. We review theories, interventions and evidence on effectiveness to explain why the obesity 'pandemic' is so resistant to change. Interventions have commonly used the Energy Surfeit Theory to recommend diets restricting calories of fat. This approach has been unhelpful. More recently, attention has switched to low carbohydrate, vegetarian or vegan diets. There is a need for a scientific approach to obesity prevention rather than the current market-led approach.

Eating and drinking are pleasurable and social activities that provide essential energy to the body. They satisfy hunger and thirst, and are steeped in cultural, moral and symbolic meaning. Food and drink form part of culture itself, a 'food and drink culture' with its own associated beliefs, values and customs. Food consumption consists of a complex set of processes that includes genetic and environmental factors, conditioning and customs. There are many interesting aspects of food, diets and dieting, enough for many volumes. The central issue here is the phenomenon that is today's Public Health Problem Number One: *the global obesity pandemic*.

Here we use 'pandemic' not in a strictly medical sense, but as a descriptor for a highly prevalent condition internationally. In this chapter, we explain why the obesity pandemic is so resilient and the serious errors and false assumptions that are made in current attempts to eliminate it.

Authorities decree that a 'balanced diet' with regular physical activity is of crucial importance to a healthy body. Yet in spite of thousands of studies, hundreds of campaigns, and scores of dedicated institutes and journals, there is not a single validated public health intervention able to achieve sustained long-term weight loss. Some basic questions require answers: *What is causing the obesity pandemic? Why are current attempts to eliminate the pandemic failing? What is the role, if any, for health psychology?*

The obesity pandemic is comparable in importance to the smoking pandemic. It took 50 years of consolidated pressure to reduce the prevalence of smoking-related diseases. It is our contention that there is enough scientific knowledge now to tackle the obesity pandemic. The main obstacle is that our systems of governance are market-led. Food policy and regulation are based as much on economic imperatives as by scientific evidence. If the food chain could be rationally developed on the basis of science rather than profit, the obesity pandemic could be solved right now.

First, let's consider one government report on the subject. The Foresight Report (2007) referred to a 'complex web of societal and biological factors that have, in recent decades, exposed our inherent human vulnerability to weight gain'. The report presented an obesity map with energy balance at its centre *with over 100 variables* directly or indirectly influencing energy balance. This complex mapping was divided into seven cross-cutting themes in four categories, which provides a useful framework for the understanding of overweight and obesity (Figure 10.1).

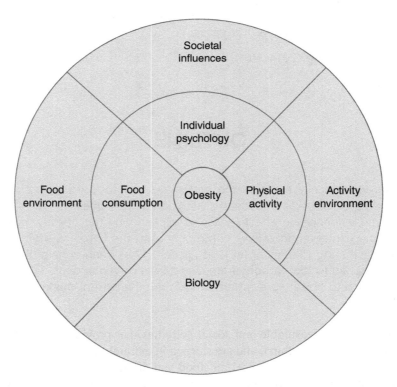

Figure 10.1   Seven influences on overweight and obesity

Source: Foresight Report (2007)

DEFINITION AND PREVALENCE

Obesity has been defined as a chronic, relapsing, neurochemical disease (Bray, 2003). It is manifested by an increase in size and number of fat cells (**adipose tissue**). One definition of obesity uses a measure known as the **body mass index (BMI)**. The BMI is a person's weight in kilograms divided by the square of his/her height in metres (kg/m2). A BMI greater than or equal to 25 is classified as overweight; a BMI greater than or equal to 30 is classified as obesity, and 40+ as extreme obesity.

Another indicator of OAO is **waist circumference**. The correlation between waist circumference and intra-abdominal adipose tissue (IAAT) is 0.8. Abdominal subcutaneous adipose tissue (ASAT), IAAT and the IAAT: ASAT ratio all increase significantly by age and BMI group (Thomas et al., 2012). Belt size may be used as a proxy for waist circumference: >40 inches for males and 35 inches for females indicate excess visceral fat. The body adiposity index (BAI) may also be used: waist circumference as a percentage of height. Another measure, **skin fold thickness**, is obtained using calipers in different bodily areas.

More than one-third (35.7%) of adults are considered to be obese. More than 1 in 20 (6.3%) have extreme obesity. Almost three in four men (74%) are considered to be overweight or obese. The prevalence of obesity is similar for both men and women (about 36%) (National Institute of Diabetes and Digestive and Kidney Diseases, 2017).

By 2050, it is predicted that obesity will affect 60% of adult men, 50% of adult women and 25% of children, making Britain a *mainly obese society* (Butland et al., 2007). Obesity will be the new normal. Similar projections apply to the USA and other European countries. The medical complications of obesity are extensive and lead to higher mortality. Obesity is a marker for insulin resistance, Type 2 diabetes and metabolic syndrome, a collection of cardiovascular risk factors that includes hypertension, dyslipidaemia and insulin resistance (see Figure 10.2).

There have been many hotly debated controversies about food, diets and dieting. Different dietary interventions for obesity have been extensively explored yet interventions have yielded unexciting results. In this chapter, we attempt to address the issue of why this could be. We begin by considering the issue of measuring obesity (Box 10.1) and then review the many different theories of obesity.

Medical diagnosis is based on cut-offs, e.g., BMI > 30 or body fat > 30%. These cut-offs give different outcomes and have low concordance. For accurate measurement, DXA or MRI, in combination with leptin, should be used. Researchers and physicians who use the proxy measure of BMI as the sole basis for classifying OAO are misclassifying obese patients and putting them at risk. For accurate diagnosis of obesity, DXA and MRI should be used as they provide direct images of adiposity throughout the body. Access to these imaging techniques for researchers is currently restricted.

CAUSES OF OBESITY

In considering causation, we need to bear in mind that obesity has multiple causes. We also need to remember that obesity is not itself a disease, but a condition that can increase an individual's risk for disease. We consider here the main biological theories, the environmental theory, social and developmental factors, and psychological explanations.

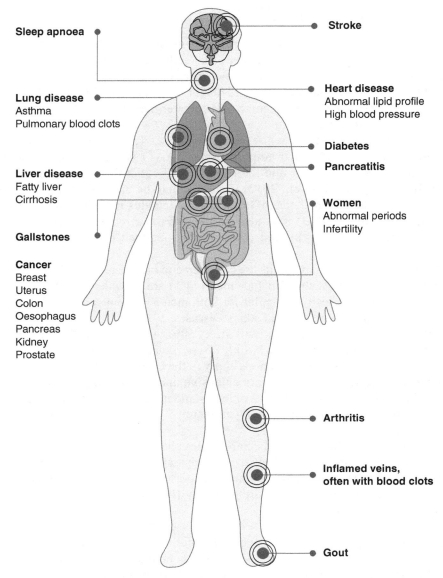

Figure 10.2   The medical complications of obesity

Source: Yale University Rudd Center for Food Policy and Obesity

---

BOX 10.1

How are overweight and obesity measured?

The BMI is a proxy measure of body fat. It does not measure it directly. Because BMI is easy to calculate, shows high test–retest reliability, is inexpensive and correlates with health risk markers and diseases, it is the measurement of choice for researchers. However, it suffers from serious problems.

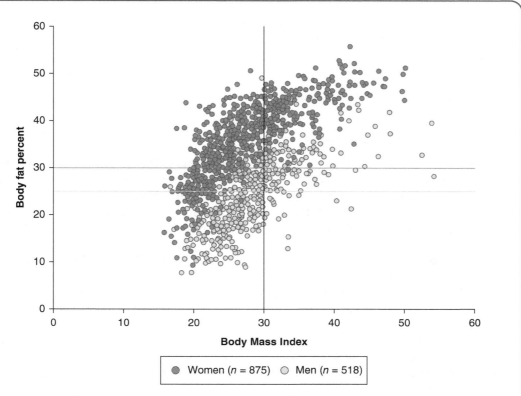

Figure 10.3 BMI versus percentage of body fat in scatterplot

Women who fall above the line are obese according to the American Society of Bariatric Physicians (ASBP) criteria (DXA percent body fat: approx. 30%). Men who fall above the horizontal line are obese according to ASBP criteria (DXA percent body fat: approx. 25%). The upper left quadrant bordered by the horizontal line (30% body fat) and vertical line (BMI = 30) demonstrates the large number of women misclassified as 'non-obese' by BMI yet 'obese' by percent body fat

Source: Shah and Braverman (2012)

The body consists of four compartments: bone, muscle, subcutaneous fat (about 80% of body fat) and visceral fat (about 20% of body fat). The latter consists of fat in organs such as the liver that causes insulin resistance and metabolic syndrome. The BMI does not distinguish between the four bodily compartments. While some people can have a BMI in the obese range and yet have normal levels of visceral fat (e.g., fit gymnasts), approximately 20% of people with normal BMI have clinical levels of visceral fat.

Studies comparing the BMI to measures of body fat yield show plenty or room for error. Shah and Braverman (2012) compared BMI and body fat scores using **dual energy X-ray absorptiometry (DXA)** on 1,393 patients from 1998 to 2009. DXA, originally used to measure bone density and total body composition, can also be used to determine abdominal fat mass. There was agreement for only 60% of the sample, with 39% misclassified as non-obese using BMI. A total of 48% of women and 25% of men were misclassified as non-obese by

(Continued)

BMI, but were obese by percentage body fat scores (Figure 10.3). Other researchers using regression suggested that BMI predicts risk markers in white males as well as skin-fold thickness and DXA (Hariri et al., 2013). Yet the scatterplot in Figure 10.3 shows the huge room for error even when the correlation between BMI and body fat percentage is quite strong.

Evolutionary hypothesis

The genetic make-up of humans is adapted to a nomadic existence of hunting and gathering in which the body stores fat. Early humans have been traced to sites in Africa dating approximately 2.5 million years ago; the tool-making *Homo habilis* ('handy man') lived in the Olduvai Gorge in Tanzania. These Olduvai hominids were hunter-gatherers, killing and processing their food with weapons and tools fashioned from pieces of volcanic obsidian (Lamb and Sington, 1998). Allowing 25 years for each generation, 100,000 generations of humans separate contemporary *Homo sapiens* from *Homo habilis.* In evolutionary terms, this is not long enough for any significant evolutionary change.

Until human beings settled in villages and towns around 10,000 years ago, humans consumed only wild and unprocessed food collected from their environment. They would likely have walked or run 5–10 miles daily searching for their food, drinking only fresh water, yielding a healthful diet of lean protein, poly-unsaturated fats (especially omega-3 fatty acids), mono-unsaturated fats, fibre, vitamins, minerals, antioxidants and other beneficial phytochemicals (O'Keefe and Cordain, 2004). The 'diseases of affluence' of the modern age would have been almost unknown.

For a few million years the capacity to store fat was advantageous. Ice Age hunter-gatherers needed to store fat to survive the winters and long journeys. When the ice retracted and temperatures increased, agriculture developed and foods became more accessible. A metabolic feature to promote survival became a risk factor for diseases.

Genetic pedisposition

Body size, whether large or small, runs in families. This observation has led to many studies of the heritability of excess weight in twins and adoptees. Heritability is the proportion of observed differences in a trait among individuals that is due to genetic differences. Evidence from studies indicates that the tendency to put on weight is inherited and beyond any individual's personal control.

A systematic review explored genetic studies on BMI in pre-adolescence, young adulthood and late adulthood (Nan et al., 2012). Nan et al. searched for studies reporting intra-pair correlations of healthy twin pairs who were raised together, finding data on 8,179 monozygotic (MZ, i.e., identical) and 9,977 dizygotic (DZ, non-identical) twin pairs from 12 studies in addition to data for 629 MZ and 594 DZ pairs from four twin registries. Heritability scores of BMI ranged from 61% to 80% for male and female participants combined, while unique environmental influences increased from 14% to 40% with increasing age.

Genetic predisposition to develop overweight and obesity is a biological fact. However, the human genome has not altered in the last few thousand years and so genetic predisposition is insufficient to explain the increase in obesity over the last few decades.

The fundamental biological process of homeostasis operates to preserve stability and equilibrium within all systems of the organism (Marks, 2015). Homeostasis can be disturbed by any gradual or sudden change in the environment. It is popularly assumed that changes in body weight reflect the choices an individual makes about what food to eat, how much to eat and how much to exercise. *However, the long-term balance between energy intake and energy output is mainly determined by unconscious physiological systems* (Leng, 2014). We turn to discuss how these 'unconscious physiological systems' have been theorized in different approaches to the understanding food, eating and obesity.

The Energy Surfeit Theory

The **Energy Surfeit Theory (EST)** has dominated obesity research over the last 50 years. The EST has been the founding assumption of countless studies, reports and interventions aimed towards breaking the obesity pandemic. All attempts to break the pandemic using the EST concept have been a disastrous failure. In this section, we analyse how this disaster could have happened.

According to the EST, obesity is caused by an imbalance between energy intake and energy expenditure. The **energy balance equation (EBE)** states:

energy intake = internal heat produced + external work + energy stored

Energy is consumed in the diet through intake of three macronutrients: protein, carbohydrate (CHO) and fat. In the presence of excess food, the body will convert and store nutrients as triglycerides in adipose tissue. Translating the EBE in terms of fat, the equation becomes:

rate of change of fat stores in the body = rate of fat intake − rate of fat oxidation

First, consider energy intake. The standard unit of energy, the **calorie**, is defined as the energy needed to increase the temperature of 1 kg of water by 1°C, which is about 4.184 kJ. Fat contributes 9 calories per gram, alcohol 7 calories per gram and carbohydrates 4 calories per gram. The fat content of a food item is the sum of four different fats: saturated, trans- saturated (trans), poly-unsaturated and mono-unsaturated. For sedentary adults, every 22 kcal per day increase in energy intake will increase body weight by roughly 1 kg after several years. Energy can be expended in several ways.

Eating itself expends calories, the 'thermic effect' of food, which is the energy expended in order to consume (bite, chew and swallow) and process (digest, transport, metabolize and store) food. Processing protein, CHO and fat requires 20–35%, 5–15% and 2–3% of energy consumed, respectively. Not only does a gram of fat give you more calories, but a smaller percentage is burned off by the thermic effect.

The majority of diets are based on counting calories. Diet designers assume that diets of equal caloric content result in identical weight change *independent of macronutrient composition*. 'A calorie is a calorie', so the saying goes. This assumption is actually false because it violates the second law of thermodynamics. Feinman and Fine (2004) proposed that a misunderstanding of the second law accounts for the controversy about the role of macronutrients on weight loss: 'Attacking the obesity epidemic will involve giving up many old ideas that have not been productive. "A calorie is a calorie" might be a good place to start' (Feinman and Fine, 2004). All calories are *not* equal. If you eat an equal number of calories of protein, fat and carbohydrates, the metabolic processes are different and calories in the fat are more likely to end up on your waist as fewer calories are burned off by the thermic effect.

Against the energy surfeit model of obesity, recent evidence suggests that increasing energy expenditure may be more effective for reducing body fat than caloric restriction, the most commonly recommended treatment for obesity. This could happen because homeostatic regulation of body weight is more effective when energy intake and expenditure are both high (high energy flux), implying that low energy flux should predict weight gain. Hume et al. (2016) examined whether energy balance or energy flux predicted future weight gain in two independent samples consisting of adolescents (n = 154) and college-aged women (n = 75). Measures of objective doubly labelled water, resting metabolic rate, and percentage of body fat were taken at baseline. Percentage of body fat was measured annually for three years of follow-up for the adolescent sample and for two years of follow-up for the young adult sample. Low energy flux, not energy surfeit, predicted future increases in body fat in both samples. In addition, high energy flux appeared to prevent fat gain in part because it was associated with a higher resting metabolic rate.

Almost all authorities subscribe to the dictum that obesity is caused by an energy surfeit, i.e., eating too many calories (gluttony) and failing to burn off enough calories (sloth). This assumption has been the rationale for thousands of failed interventions and created victim-blaming and stigmatization, which have done little to reduce the incidence of overweight and obesity. There are serious defects with this theory. It is wrong in principle and it doesn't work in practice.

Inactivity

Let's turn to the energy expenditure, the other half of the energy–balance equation. It is alleged by almost all authorities and experts that one of the principal causes of obesity is inactivity/lack of exercise. Energy loss in exercise is measured in joules. One joule in everyday life represents approximately the energy required to lift a small apple (with a mass of approximately 100 g) vertically through 1 metre. Do this a million times and you have used 1 megajoule (MJ) of energy or 239 calories. There are, of course, many quicker ways of burning energy than lifting an apple.

The use of exercise is a recommended part of any weight loss programme. It's almost universally recommended by everybody, but the scientific evidence indicates that exercise interventions actually provide an ineffective procedure for losing weight. The impact of increased activity on body weight is slow-acting and hard to sustain. Simple mathematics suggest that the amount of exercise necessary for significant long-term weight loss maintenance far exceeds the capacity of most people.

Hall et al. (2011) mathematically simulated energy expenditure adaptations during weight loss. A persistent daily energy imbalance between intake and expenditure of about 30 kJ per day underlies the observed average weight gain in the US population. In addition, a heavier person expends more energy to move a certain distance. They calculated that the average increase of energy intake needed to sustain the increased weight (the maintenance energy gap) amounted to about 0.9 MJ per day. To reverse the trend and lose weight, a person would need to burn off at least 0.9 MJ per day, for example 1.0 or 1.2 MJ per day. Let's consider what losing 1.2 MJ per day would actually involve.

A 100 kg man would need to run about 20 km, almost a half-marathon each week, to burn off 1.2 MJ per day in order to reach a weight of around 85 kg. *This would take approximately five years using exercise alone.* To lose 15 kg, a 100 kg person would need to run 5,000 km over five years. It's hardly surprising that obese people find exercise an ineffective method of losing weight, and that attrition rates in exercise programmes are so very high.

There is also a safety issue: harm can result from inappropriate levels of exercise (Cooper et al., 2007; Barg et al., 2011). In spite of all the advice coming from health authorities to exercise more to lose weight, the obesity pandemic would never be reversed by obese individuals increasing their daily amount of exercise. To lose a significant amount of weight, it is necessary for people living with obesity to make major dietary changes.

Dietary change to reduce obesity may require more than calorie reductions. Critics of calorie counting argue that it is not excess calories that cause obesity, but the quantity and quality of carbohydrates consumed (Taubes, 2012). We turn to this theory next.

The insulin theory

The **insulin theory** claims that obesity is caused by a chronic elevation in insulin in a diet that contains too much carbohydrate (Taubes, 2009):

> This alternative hypothesis of obesity constitutes three distinct propositions. First is the basic proposition that obesity is caused by a regulatory defect in fat metabolism, and so a defect in the distribution of energy rather than an imbalance of energy intake and expenditure. The second is that insulin plays a primary role in this fattening process, and the compensatory behaviours of hunger and lethargy. The third is that carbohydrates, and particularly refined carbohydrates – and perhaps the fructose content as well, and thus perhaps the amount of sugars consumed – are the prime suspects in the chronic elevation of insulin; hence, they are the ultimate cause of common obesity. (Taubes, 2009: 359)

CHO is a high **glycaemic index (GI)** food that produces insulin that, in turn, causes the body to store fat. Carbohydrates include starch, which is found in rice, wheat, maize, potatoes and cassava, and all sources of sugar, specifically natural sugars and added sugars and fibre. Sugary beverages including alcohol, sweets, sugary cereals, dried fruits, low-fat crackers, rice cakes, potato crisps, flour, cakes, cookies, jams, preserves, potato products, pickles, sauces, salad dressings and pizzas are all high in carbohydrates.

According to the insulin theory, the CHO content of a person's diet must be rectified to restore health (Taubes, 2012). This is because blood levels of insulin are mainly determined by CHO intake, and insulin regulates fat accumulation. The more digestible the carbohydrates that we eat (i.e., the higher their glycaemic index) and the sweeter they are (the higher their fructose content), the higher our blood insulin level goes and the more fat we accumulate in our bodies.

Food consumption data from the National Health and Nutrition Examination Survey (NHANES) between 1971 and 2004 indicate that the observed increase in energy intake in the USA is accounted for almost completely by increased CHO consumption, with a 67.7 g increase per day in men and a 62.4 g increase per day in women within that time frame (Lim et al., 2010). Meals composed predominantly of high GI foods induce hormonal events that stimulate hunger and cause overeating in adolescents. A high GI diet has been linked with risk for central adiposity, cardiovascular disease and Type 2 diabetes (Ebbeling et al., 2002). Low-CHO diets show a metabolic advantage. An isocaloric diet, which has a fixed number of calories, can be used to compare diets that vary in the percentage of CHO that they contain. If a calorie really was a calorie, then the weight loss obtained in a low-CHO isocaloric diet would be identical to that in a high CHO isocaloric diet. However, in nine out of ten studies, more weight loss occurred in the low-carb diet (Fine and Feinman, 2004). This research led to the conclusion that a good way to take off weight is to switch to a low-carb diet.

Ketosis is a metabolic state in which some of the body's energy supply comes from ketone bodies in the blood. Ketonic diets are very low CHO diets (VLCDs) that restrict the daily intake of carbohydrates but encourage the consumption of fats. Brehm et al. (2013) conducted a randomized controlled trial to determine the effects of a VLCD on body composition and cardiovascular risk factors. A total of 42 healthy, obese female volunteers were randomly allocated to a VLCD or to a calorie-restricted low-fat diet. Women on both diets reduced their calorie consumption by similar amounts at three and six months. However, the VLCD group lost more weight (8.5 ± 1.0 vs. 3.9 ± 1.0 kg) and more body fat (4.8 ± 0.67 vs. 2.0 ± 0.75 kg) than the low-fat diet group.

A systematic review by Gibson et al. (2015) concluded that the true benefit of VLCD is in preventing an increase in appetite, which helps the dieter to severely restrict food intake to achieve substantial weight losses, rather than the absence of hunger altogether. Ketosis provides a plausible explanation for the suppression of appetite during a ketogenic diet.

There can be little doubt that a major contributor to obesity is the consumption of sugar. New guidelines on sugar consumption were proposed by the World Health Organization in 2014 (WHO, 2014a). This was a highly controversial step in the attempt to influence diet by the use of policy and regulation. Box 10.2 summarizes the new WHO guidelines on sugar.

BOX 10.2

WHO guidelines on sugar

The consumption of sugar has grown continuously over the last 200 years and continues to grow. In 2014 the WHO launched a new draft guideline on sugars intake in light of scientific studies on the consumption of sugars and its impact on excess weight gain and tooth decay (World Health Organization, 2014a). Systematic reviews were carried out by Te Morenga et al. (2013), who showed that sugar is a determinant of body weight, and Moynihan and Kelly (2014), who found that 47 of 55 studies reported a positive association between sugars and calories. Yang et al. (2014) examined time trends of added sugar consumption as percentage of daily calories in the USA. They observed a significant relationship between added sugar consumption and increased risk for cardiovascular disease (CVD) mortality. The highest sugar group had a risk of death from a cardiovascular event almost three times higher than those whose sugar consumption was 10% or lower of daily calories.

The WHO's previous recommendation from 2002 was that sugars should make up less than 10% of total energy intake per day. *The new guideline proposes that a reduction to below 5% of total energy intake per day would be beneficial.* A 5% of total energy intake is equivalent to around 25 grams (around 6 teaspoons) of sugar per day for an adult with normal BMI.

Sugar includes monosaccharides (such as glucose or fructose) and disaccharides (such as sucrose or table sugar) that are added by the manufacturer, cook or consumer, and naturally present sugars in honey, syrups, fruit juices and fruit concentrates. Much of the sugars consumed today are 'hidden' in processed foods that are not usually viewed as sweet. For example, 1 tablespoon of ketchup contains around 4 grams (around 1 teaspoon) of sugars. A single can of sugar-sweetened soda contains up to 40 grams (around 10 teaspoons). A Yeo Valley Family Farm 0% Fat Vanilla Yogurt contains 20.9 grams (around 5 teaspoons).

Sugar has become a new watchword, along with fat.

The dangers of sugar were highlighted by John Yudkin in *Pure, White and Deadly* (1972). Following this publication, there should have been a reduction of sugar in the diet. However, Yudkin was ignored. Food consumption and diets do not follow reason or evidence and consumption of sugar-sweetened beverages has risen rapidly ever since.

While a low-CHO diet provides a helpful method of reducing body fat, the insulin hypothesis has not been confirmed in scientific studies (Guyenet, 2012).

Developmental hypothesis

Obesity starts in the womb. The baby is highly sensitive to the environment experienced within the womb. A relationship has been observed between the weight of a mother-to-be and her child. For example, Modi et al. (2011) used MRI to monitor fat levels in 105 unborn babies and found that 30% had more abdominal adipose tissue than expected. The amount of fat was proportional to the mother-to-be's BMI. These findings were reinforced by Schellong et al. (2012), who found that infants with a birthweight in excess of 4 kg were twice as likely to suffer from obesity in later life than normal-weight babies. Preventing *in utero* over-nutrition by avoiding maternal over-nutrition, overweight and/or diabetes during pregnancy would be a promising strategy to prevent overweight and obesity globally. It's a 'chicken-and-egg' problem.

Risk of obesity continues to develop in the crib and accelerates in the first few years of life. A consistent association occurs between faster infant weight gain (from birth to age 1 year) and later overweight or obesity. Druet et al. (2012) assessed the association between infant weight gain and subsequent obesity by meta-analysing individual-level data on 47,661 participants from ten cohort studies. Each unit increase in weight SD scores between 0 and 1 year conferred a two-fold higher risk of childhood obesity and a 23% higher risk of adult obesity (Figure 10.4).

Childhood and adolescence are critical periods for the adoption of a healthy lifestyle. By age 15 many adolescents show consistent behaviour patterns that influence their chances of OAO in later years. Clark et al. (2007) studied how parents' child-feeding behaviours influence child weight. Parents reported using a wide range of child-feeding behaviours, including monitoring, pressure to eat and restriction. Interestingly, a *restriction of children's eating* has most frequently and consistently been associated with child weight gain. The authors found evidence for a causal relationship between parental restriction and childhood overweight, indicating that, inadvertently, parents may promote excess weight gain in childhood by using inappropriate child-feeding behaviours.

Early parental **attachment** plays a critical role in the regulation of emotion and in the formation of drinking habits, substance abuse and food consumption (Marks, 2015; Figure 10.7). Emotion regulation, associated with attachment patterns, plays a critical role in causation of ill health. DeSteno, Gross and Kubzansky (2013) observed that chronic childhood distress at

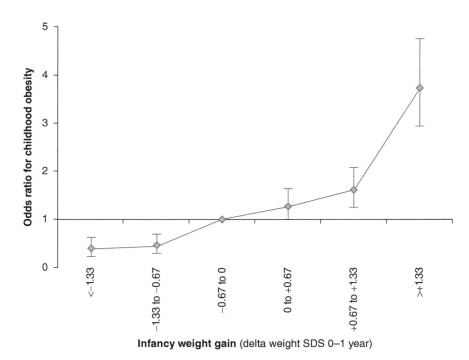

Figure 10.4 Odds ratios for childhood obesity by infant weight gain, 0–1 year, adjusted for sex, age and birthweight

Source: Druet et al. (2012)

age 7 or 8 years is associated with adult physical health outcomes such as obesity, number of physical illnesses and inflammation. Dietary habits from childhood persist into adulthood once formed, and parental influences are internalized and enacted throughout life. Goossens et al. (2012) examined attachment towards mothers and fathers as a predictor of eating pathology and weight gain among 8–11-year-old boys and girls. Insecure attachment to mothers was predictive of increases in dietary restraint, eating concerns, weight concerns and shape concerns, and adjusted BMI in children one year later. Insecure attachments to fathers was predictive of persistence in children's subjective binge eating episodes. Faber and Dubé (2015) investigated the role of caregiver–child attachment quality and its associations with high caloric food consumption in middle socio-economic status children and adults. Data from 213 children and 216 parents showed that an insecure parental attachment, whether actual or recalled, significantly and positively predicted high calorific food consumption in both samples. Faber and Dubé (2015: 521) concluded that: 'From an intervention standpoint, parents-to-be could receive a short information sheet teaching them that responding to a child's attention-seeking does not make the child needy, but rather teaches him or her to become trusting and independent. From a counselling and clinical standpoint, children and parents of children with eating issues could benefit greatly from developing secure and trusting relationships.'

Knowledge about child-feeding is one aspect of parenting and childcare that could benefit from training. Training could be designed to increase provider knowledge and self-efficacy and remove misconceptions as well as educate providers about feeding, nutrition education and family communication.

Sleeping patterns

Another area of concern is children's sleeping patterns. Patel and Hu (2008) found a consistent body of evidence that short sleep duration in childhood is predictive of weight gain. A meta-analysis of cross-sectional studies has shown that there is an almost two-fold higher prevalence of obesity in children and adults who have a short sleep duration (Miller et al., 2014). Padez et al. (2009) studied the association between sleep duration, overweight and body fat in a sample of Portuguese children. Prevalence of overweight decreased with longer night sleep times. Laboratory and epidemiological studies point to short sleep duration and poor sleep quality as factors associated with obesity (Beccuti and Pannain, 2011).

Perhaps there is a simple explanation. **Obstructive sleep apnoea (OSA)**, which is associated with sleep fragmentation, is more common with OAO. Increased visceral adiposity tends to reduce the airway size while lying down. OSA is also known to trigger hypertension, insulin resistance, Type 2 diabetes and, possibly, metabolic syndrome. OSA causes daytime sleepiness and impaired memory and concentration (Dempsey et al., 2010). Sleep deprivation makes a person less attentive and careful in their food choices, reducing their fruit and vegetable consumption but increasing their consumption of fast food (Kruger et al., 2014). In these circumstances, daytime sleepiness and OAO form a vicious circle: OAO — > OSA – > daytime sleepiness – > poor diet – > OAO. This hypothesis warrants further study.

Food reward theory

This theory is based on the fact that food has a reward or reinforcement value that strengthens the desire to eat. The **food reward theory** of obesity argues that the reward value of food influences food intake and body fatness, contributing to the development of obesity (Guyenet, 2012). Cues such as the sight or smell of food stimulate appetite and promote higher consumption. Studies of conditioning carried out by Pavlov and many others show that animals and people learn to associate non-food cues with eating. Exposure to the conditioned stimuli then elicits salivation and changes in blood glucose, and can initiate food intake even in people who are already sated.

To help explain obesity, the food reward theory is paired with the idea that a breakdown can occur in the brain's ability to switch off eating when the stomach is full. As early as 1840, a German physician, Bernard Mohr, suggested that obesity is associated with abnormalities of the basal hypothalamus. The food reward theory hypothesizes that obese people may have impairments in the dopaminergic pathways of their brains that regulate neuronal systems associated with reward sensitivity, conditioning and control (Volkow et al., 2011). Dopamine is involved in reward functions, and is a major regulator of food intake and body fatness. Dopamine signalling in the striatum regulates the motivation to obtain food (wanting), but not the enjoyment or palatability of food (liking). The theory suggests that neuropeptides responsible for regulating energy balance through the hypothalamus also modulate the activity of dopamine cells and their projections into regions involved in the reward process in food intake. Volkow et al. hypothesize that the breakdown of feedback mechanisms and increased resistance to homoeostatic signals in obese people impairs the function of circuits involved in reward sensitivity, conditioning and cognitive control.

Thaler et al. (2012) studied the effect of hypothalamic injury in rodents and humans to look for an association with the development of obesity. MRI was used to image and quantify gliosis, a process leading to scars in the central nervous system, in the brains of 34 young humans undergoing clinical examination. Thaler et al. found evidence of increased gliosis in the medio-basal hypothalamus of obese humans and concluded that, in both humans and rodent models, obesity is associated with neuronal injury in a brain area crucial for body weight control. The food reward theory has implications for obesity prevention and treatment via decreasing the reward value of food and enhancing the reward value of alternative activity.

The obesogenic environment

We all eat what tastes good and is easy to obtain. When human beings started using agriculture and farming instead of hunting and gathering, diets became less varied, fat consumption increased, and activity levels decreased. Today's modern food environment contains large amounts of processed food that has been engineered to maximize food reward. Producers have influenced the palatability of foods by increasing quantities of sugar and salt in combination with fats and flavourings. Consumers buy foods for their palatability, convenience and cost. Such palatable and cheap convenience foods are typically obesogenic, i.e., they contain sufficient sugar and fat to produce overweight and obesity when consumed over months or years.

A summary of overall food intake is the number of calories consumed in the daily diet. Data for the USA on calories consumed and obesity prevalence over the period 1960–2010 show a 17% increase in daily calories over the 50-year period that corresponds almost perfectly with the increase in obesity prevalence. However, as always, it would be a serious mistake to assume causation when all we have is a correlation. But when the environment contains all the necessary 'ingredients' for obesity to happen, then we should not be surprised at the outcome. After all, it is already established that the human body is genetically wired to store fat.

Obesity could well be the inevitable end product of the 'obesogenic' environment. This is an environment engineered by a food and drinks industry that promotes fattening, unhealthful food and drink almost without restriction (Swinburn et al., 1999). Obesity can be classified as a non-communicable disease (NCD), a category that also includes cancer, heart disease, diabetes and dementia. Through the sale of unhealthy commodities – tobacco, alcohol and ultra-processed food and drink – transnational corporations are major drivers of global epidemics of NCDs, of which obesity is just one.

Highly profitable industries and supermarket chains will not curb their activities unless required to do so by legislation. In a capitalist society this simply ain't going to happen. There has been a rise in sales of unhealthy commodities in low-income and middle-income countries compared to high-income countries where sales tended to level off between 1997 and 2009 (Moodie et al., 2013). There is a high concentration in these industries of processed foods and relatively few companies are dominating the market. For example, 75% of world food sales are of processed foods, the largest manufacturers of which control more than a third of the global market.

Common strategies by the transnational corporations deliberately undermine NCD prevention and control. Companies hire doctors to ghost-write scientific papers that cast doubt about findings linking unhealthy products to illness. They also infiltrate governmental committees responsible for regulation. It is evident that *unhealthy commodity industries should not have any role in the formation of national or international NCD policy, yet they are often involved in government advisory bodies on food and drinks policies.* Only public regulation and intervention can be effective in preventing harm caused by obesity and other NCDs that are the direct result of unhealthy commodity industries.

Foods that make us fat

Research on eating behaviour has shown that calorie consumption is higher when meals consist of a variety of foods compared with a single food type, when the food is more palatable, and when it is presented in more energy-dense formulations. More palatable and energy-dense diets result in greater weight gain (Wardle, 2007). Opinions about the optimum macronutrient composition of a healthful diet have been strongly divided. However, three macronutrients have been linked to OAO: fats, sugars and proteins. One of the biggest changes associated with the increase in calories consumed has been the increasing availability of snack and fast foods. These contain high amounts of fat, sugar, protein and salt. In addition to changes in eating habits, portion sizes of main meals have increased substantially. 'Supersizing' increases consumption: doubling of portion size increases consumption by 35% (Zlatevska et al., 2014).

Epidemiological studies show an association between dietary fat and body fat (adiposity). Hooper et al. (2012) reviewed studies that compared lower with usual total fat intake on body fatness. Low-fat diets were associated with lower relative body weight, but the difference in weight was fairly slight – *only 1.6 kg.* Moreover, the prevalence of obesity has greatly increased, despite an apparent decrease in the proportion of total calories consumed as fat in the diet of US children (Ebbeling et al., 2002).

In prospective studies, Mozaffarian et al. (2011) studied data from 120,877 US women and men with follow-up periods from 1986 to 2006. Within each four-year period, participants gained an average of 1.52 kg, which would be 7.60 kg over 20 years. Four-year weight change was most strongly associated with the intake of potato chips (0.76 kg), potatoes (0.58 kg), sugar-sweetened beverages (0.45 kg), unprocessed red meats (0.43 kg) and processed meats (0.42 kg). Weight gain was inversely associated with the intake of vegetables (–0.10 kg), whole grains (–0.17 kg), fruits (–0.22 kg), nuts (–0.26 kg) and yogurt (–0.37). 'Lifestyle' factors associated with weight change included physical activity (–0.80 kg), alcohol use (0.19 kg per drink per day), smoking (new quitters, 2.35 kg; former smokers, 0.06 kg), sleep (more weight gain with < 6 or > 8 hours of sleep) and television watching (0.14 kg per hour per day).

Mozaffarian et al.'s data lead to an interesting inference. If the 'couch potato diet' of red meat, potatoes, chips and cola (+2.31 kg) is replaced by a 'hairy shirt' diet of vegetables, grains, fruits, nuts and yogurt (–1.12) plus some physical activity (–0.80) there could be an average weight reduction of 4.15 kg every four years. That comes to a massive 20.4 kg over 20 years. With this rate of change, the obesity pandemic could be solved. Unfortunately, the human tendency to 'go with the flow' is a more attractive option than to be a lean and restrained spartan. Until the first heart attack, that is.

Food producers have used fats, sugars and salts to tinker with our taste buds while playing havoc with public health. They have experimented with trans fats (a partially hydrogenated oil, PHO), sugars, corn syrup and salt. In 2013, the US Centers for Disease Control and Prevention (CDC, 2013a) estimated that a reduction of trans fat could prevent 7,000 deaths from heart disease and up to 20,000 heart attacks each year in the USA. The high risks associated with PHOs led the Food and Drug Administration (FDA) to suggest that PHOs are no longer 'generally recognized as safe' (GRAS). With the removal of GRAS status, trans fats will all but disappear from the US food chain.

High-fructose corn syrup (HFCS) accounts for 40% of sweeteners used in the USA. The product is in sodas, ketchups and condiments, salad dressings, canned soups, bread, and many other places you possibly don't expect to find it. Consumption of HFCS increased to 27 kg per person per year between 1970 and 2000, a trend mirrored by the figures for obesity. Studies in endocrinology have suggested a causal relationship between sugar intake and weight gain (e.g., Lustig, 2013).

To summarize the obesity story thus far, a complex array of genetic, nutritional, developmental and environmental factors influence overweight and obesity. None 'tells the whole story' on its own. Obesity is a clear case of multiple causation. We need to explain not only *how* obesity can develop in a susceptible individual, but *why some individuals develop it and not others*. We turn now to consider social and psychological explanations for obesity.

Social influences: thin ideal, body dissatisfaction and stigmatization

Society places a high value on the '**thin ideal**', a body image that is slim and slender with a narrow waist and little body fat. Yet for many, the thin ideal is in direct opposition to both a natural predisposition to become obese and to an obesogenic food environment. Psychologist Kelly Brownell (1992) discussed the search for the perfect body as an instance where physiology and culture collide:

> Modern society breeds a search for the perfect body. Today's aesthetic ideal is extremely thin, and now, superimposed on this, is the need to be physically fit. People seek the ideal, not only because of expected health benefits, but because of what the ideal symbolizes in our culture (self-control, success, acceptance). ... Research has shown that biological variables, particularly genetics, are influential in the regulation of body weight and shape. Hence, there are limits to how much a person can change. This places culture in conflict with physiology. In addition, the rewards of being attractive are less than most would expect. There are serious consequences of seeking the ideal and falling short, some psychological and others physiological (e.g. increased health risk for weight cycling). (Brownell, 1992: 1)

The psychological impact of OAO can be measured in terms of the stigma, lowered self-esteem and reduced well-being. The size of the thin ideal is decreasing as the rate of obesity is increasing, making the thin ideal difficult to maintain (Pinhas et al., 1998). Depending on the degree to which the thin body ideal is internalized, the perceived gap between the actual body and the thin ideal can have serious psychological effects (Ahern et al., 2011). Thin ideal internalization is associated with body image and eating disturbances, especially in conjunction with dieting and negative affect (Thompson and Stice, 2001). The thin ideal is a global phenomenon. The influence of the media, especially the representation of the female body on magazine covers, is huge.

Rodgers et al. (2010: 89–95) noted that: 'In Western society, body image concerns are so prevalent among young women they have been called normative, with body dissatisfaction appearing in girls as young as 5 years old.' The thin ideal is 'transmitted' from mother to child. Yamazaki and Omori (2016) asked early adolescents (175 girls and 198 boys) in Japan to complete a questionnaire to assess their drive for thinness and perceptions of mothers' attitudes and behaviours related to body shape. The questionnaire for mothers ($n = 206$) measured mothers' thin ideal internalization. The authors found that mothers' thin ideal internalization was associated with girls' drive for thinness through the perception of mothers' attitudes directed to the girls, and with boys' drive for thinness through observation of their mothers' weight-loss behaviour.

Bojorquez et al. (2013) examined the bodily experiences of Mexican women to investigate their acceptance of the thin ideal and body dissatisfaction. The interviewees accepted the thin body ideal, but experienced their bodies as 'signifiers of motherhood' that protected them from body dissatisfaction. Thus perception of overweight may predict body dissatisfaction and weight loss intentions better than weight status itself.

Fredrickson et al. (2015) examined the association of weight perception and weight satisfaction with body change intentions and weight-related behaviours in 928 overweight adolescents (aged 11–18; 44% female). Accurate perception of weight and dissatisfaction with weight were associated with trying to lose weight, but were negatively associated with some healthy weight-related behaviours. Awareness of overweight and body dissatisfaction may be detrimental to the adoption of healthy weight control behaviours. The authors concluded that interventions with overweight adolescents should encourage body satisfaction. Overweight and obesity are rarely, if ever, a deliberate or conscious choice. Yet the blaming, shaming and stigmatization of people with OAO is very common; it heightens the stress of OAO individuals that, in turn, leads to increased eating. People with OAO are openly stigmatized and often incur more open forms of prejudice and discrimination than other stigmatized social groups (Brochu and Esses, 2011). Obesity is often the butt of jokes and cartoons.

Pearl et al. (2015) investigated the effects of weight bias experiences and internalization on exercise among 177 women with OAO in a cross-sectional study. Participants completed questionnaires assessing exercise behaviour, self-efficacy and motivation, experiences of weight stigmatization, weight bias internalization and weight-stigmatizing attitudes towards others. Pearl et al. found that weight stigma experiences positively correlated with exercise behaviour, but weight bias internalization was negatively associated with all exercise variables.

Seacat et al. (2016) studied daily diaries to assess female weight stigmatization. They recruited 50 overweight/obese women from public weight forums to complete week-long daily diaries. A total of 1,077 weight-stigmatizing events were reported. Results indicated that body mass index, education, age, daily activities and interpersonal interactions all can influence individual levels of stigmatization.

Stigma-based bullying is associated with significant negative mental and physical health outcomes. In a longitudinal study, Rosenthal et al. (2015) used surveys and physical assessments with mostly black and Latino, socio-economically disadvantaged, urban students. Rosenthal et al. reported greater weight- and race-based bullying as being indirectly associated with increased blood pressure and BMI. Bullying was associated with decreased self-rated health across two years.

Public health campaigns designed to prevent or reduce obesity might not be universally helpful and could have detrimental consequences. Simpson et al. (2017) explored the effects of obesity prevention campaigns. Participants viewed either weight-focused or weight-neutral campaigns. Assessments occurred at three time points (pre-, post- and follow-up). Compared with weight-neutral campaigns, weight-focused campaigns were associated with increases in negative perceptions of obesity and decreases in self-efficacy for health behaviour change. People don't like being preached to with scare tactics.

We turn now to consider some of the main psychological processes associated with obesity.

Emotion, personality, body dissatisfaction and depression

One hypothesis to explain obesity has been to attribute overeating to emotionality. People are said to eat to calm themselves, assuage sadness or guilt or reduce feelings of loneliness. In spite of its intuitive appeal, the evidence for this theory is positive but inconsistent.

Rodin (1973) studied the effects of distraction on performance of obese and normal-weight participants. Male undergraduates worked on tasks requiring concentration, while competing; irrelevant material was also used to distract them. Rodin found that overweight students were more disrupted than normal-weight students by interesting, emotionally toned material, while they performed better than normals when there were no distracting events. Rodin suggested that obese people may have a heightened responsiveness to external cues. This finding led to a theory that obese people were not only more responsive to external cues, but also ate more when feeling anxious, bored or depressed (Schachter and Rodin, 1974). This is the theory that obesity is related to emotional eating.

Polivy et al. (1978) compared the emotional responsiveness of dieters and non-dieters in a sample of male college students. Dieters were found to be more extreme emotional responders. When an internal source of arousal (i.e., caffeine) was provided, non-dieters became more emotional and dieters became less emotional.

Lowe and Fisher (1983) compared the emotional reactivity and emotional eating of normal-weight and overweight female college students in a natural environment. Their participants self-monitored food intake and pre-eating mood at each episode of eating for 12 consecutive days. The obese students were more emotionally reactive and more likely to engage in emotional eating than normal-weight individuals with snacks but not with meals. Emotional distress was associated with snack eating, and emotional eating was related to their percentage overweight.

Other studies explored emotional eating and regulation in obese young people from non-student populations and in adults. They have also looked at family and peer relational factors as a source of the emotion and feeling. Vandewalle et al. (2014) explored the association between parental rejection and emotional eating in 110 obese young people aged 10 and 16 years attending a Belgian treatment centre for obesity. Maladaptive emotion regulation strategies mediated the relation between maternal rejection and emotional eating. Paternal rejection itself was not associated with emotion regulation or with emotional eating in the young people.

Personality traits can contribute to unhealthy weight increases and difficulties with weight management. Sutin et al. (2011) studied the association between personality and obesity across the adult lifespan. Their data came from a longitudinal study with 1,988 participants who spanned more than 50 years to investigate personality associations with adiposity and fluctuations in BMI. Participants with higher neuroticism or extraversion or lower conscientiousness had higher BMI, more body fat, and larger waist and hip circumferences. The strongest association was found for impulsivity. Participants who scored in the top 10% of impulsivity weighed, on average, 11 kg more than those in the bottom 10% (Figure 10.5).

Another psychological factor is dietary restraint, the attempt to hold back from eating. Restraint can create a rebound effect in the form of binge eating. In a cross-sectional study, Marcus et al. (1985) determined the prevalence and severity of binge eating among 432 women seeking behavioural treatment for obesity and to assess the relationship between binge eating and dietary restraint; 46% of women reported serious binge eating, especially younger and heavier women, in whom binge-eating severity was related to overall dietary restraint. A prospective study by Johnson and Wardle (2005), however, found no evidence that dietary restraint causes bulimic binge eating. A survey of 1,177 adolescent girls explored whether emotional eating, binge eating, abnormal attitudes to eating and weight, low self-esteem, stress and depression are associated with dietary restraint or body dissatisfaction. Restraint was associated only with more negative attitudes to eating, whereas body dissatisfaction was significantly

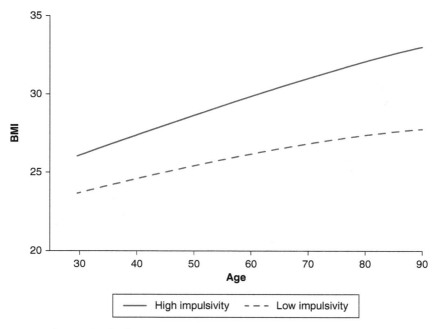

Figure 10.5   Estimated BMI for participants one standard deviation above and below the mean on impulsiveness

Source: Sutin et al. (2011)

associated with all adverse outcomes, casting doubt on the hypothesis that restrained eating is a primary cause of bulimic symptoms and emotional eating. Many studies have shown that body dissatisfaction is associated with depression (e.g., Paxton et al., 2006).

Psychiatric studies indicate a reliable association between depression and obesity both in cross-sectional and prospective studies. Onyike et al. (2003) studied rates of depression in the past month for both men and women as a function of BMI (Figure 10.6). The data came from 9,997 respondents to the National Health and Nutrition Examination Survey (NHANES), an interview survey of the US population.

Obesity was associated with increased rates of depression. Being severely obese (BMI ≥ 40) resulted in markedly higher rates of depression. This study provides no evidence on causation. However, it seems likely from other evidence that causation runs in both directions, which is confirmed in prospective studies.

Luppino et al. (2010) conducted a systematic review and meta-analysis on the longitudinal relationship between depression, overweight and obesity to identify possible influencing factors. They reviewed studies examining the longitudinal relationship between depression and overweight (BMI 25–29.99) or obesity (BMI ≥ 30). Obesity at baseline increased the risk of onset of depression at follow-up by 55%. Overweight also increased the risk of onset of depression at follow-up by 27%. Depression increased the odds for developing obesity by 58%. Luppino et al. (2010: 220) concluded that the meta-analysis confirmed a reciprocal link between depression and obesity.

The evidence on the psychological influences on obesity suggests a homeostatic system, a 'circle of discontent' (Figure 10.7). Empirical evidence of this 'vicious circle' in adolescents

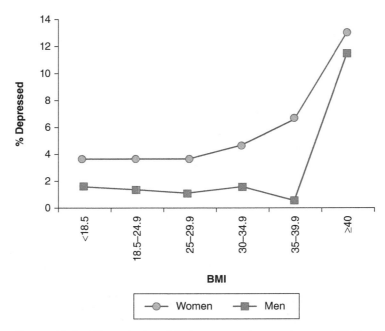

Figure 10.6   The relationship between depression and BMI

Source: Onyike et al. (2003)

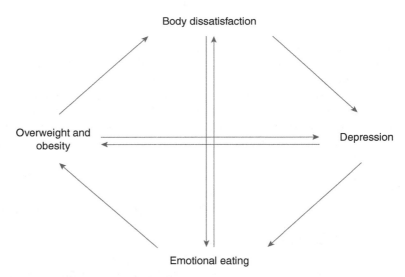

Figure 10.7   A theory linking body dissatisfaction, depression, emotional eating, and overweight and obesity

Source: Marks (2015)

and obese women is present in the literature (e.g., Wardle et al., 2001; Chaiton et al., 2009; Goldfield et al., 2010; Sonneville et al., 2012). This 'circle of discontent' requires systematic investigation using prospective studies (Marks, 2015).

INTERVENTIONS

Dietary guidelines

One of the main strategies for preventing obesity and overweight at a societal or population level is the publication of dietary guidelines. The *Dietary Guidelines for Americans* (DGA) is updated every five years as a blueprint for nutrition policies such as School Lunch. The guidelines are intended to reduce coronary heart disease (CHD) mortality by reducing dietary fat intake. On 7 January 2016, the US Department of Health and Human Services and the Department of Agriculture released the DGA 2015–2020. What if those guidelines are wrong? Evidence from epidemiology suggests that they probably are. The controversy surrounding the 2015 DGA was unprecedented. Critics claimed the DGA was not based on a comprehensive review of the most rigorous and recent science (Teicholz, 2015). The research ignored in the DGA included recent findings on saturated fats and low CHO diets.

Attempts by health authorities to promote healthy eating through guidelines has sometimes led to public anger and confusion about portion sizes, dietary fat, percentage energy and certain nutrients. Nutritional messages in public health and commercial sources are perceived as conflicting and food guides are used minimally by consumers (Boylan et al., 2013). To be usefully applied as a guide to eating behaviour, guidelines need to clearly and consistently inform people what, when and where to eat, not only how much they should consume. De Ridder et al. (2013) argued that people's ability to regulate their eating is compromised by a lack of clear, shared standards that guide eating behaviour.

Harcombe et al. (2016) carried out a systematic review to examine the epidemiological evidence concerning the dietary guideline to reduce the consumption of fat. They found no support for the recommendations to restrict dietary fat. The epidemiological evidence suggested no significant association between CHD mortality and total fat or saturated fat intake and thus does not support the present dietary fat guidelines.

Guidelines that are unreliable and based on dogma will not be trusted and we should not be surprised if people choose not to follow them.

Vegetarianism and veganism

One underutilized intervention for overweight and obesity is a vegetarian or vegan diet. **Vegetarian** diets include eggs and/or dairy but no other foods derived from animal sources. **Vegan** diets exclude all animal-based foods. Such diets can be motivated by ethical beliefs against animal cruelty, by concerns for the environment or by an interest in improved health, including the desire to lose weight. Total consumption of meat and dairy by meat eaters is striking. Each year a US meat eater consumes 130 shellfish, 40 fish, 26 chickens, 1 turkey, nearly half a pig and a little more than a tenth of a cow. That's nearly 200 animals a year or 16,000 animals over a lifetime (Mohr, 2012). Ruminants (cattle, water buffalo, sheep and goats) use 86% of the world's agricultural land and consume 71% of its total biomass, yet produce only 8% of its food (Smith et al., 2013).

Key et al. (1998) compared the mortality rates of vegetarians and non-vegetarians among 76,000 men and women who had participated in five prospective studies. This meta-analysis collated the entire body of evidence collected in prospective studies in Western countries from 1960 to 1981. The original studies were conducted in California (2), Britain (2) and Germany (1) and provided data concerning 16–89-year-olds for whom diet and smoking status information was available. Vegetarians were defined as those who did not eat any meat or fish (*n* = 27,808).

Participants were followed for an average of 10.6 years when 8,330 deaths occurred. The results showed that vegetarians as a group contained a lower proportion of smokers and current alcohol drinkers but a higher proportion of high exercisers, and had a consistently lower BMI. The death-rate ratio for ischaemic heart disease for vegetarians versus non-vegetarians across the five studies was 0.76 (95% CI 0.62–0.94). The all-cause mortality ratio was 0.95 (95% CI 0.82–1.11). When non-vegetarians were subdivided into regular meat eaters and semi-vegetarians who ate fish only or ate meat less than once a week, there was evidence of a significant dose-response. The death-rate ratio for ischaemic heart disease, caused by a narrowing of the arteries, for semi-vegetarians and vegetarians compared to regular meat eaters was 0.78 and 0.66 respectively. Vegetarians have a lower risk of dying from ischaemic heart disease than non-vegetarians.

A meta-analysis with over 120,000 participants reported a 29% lower risk of death from cardiovascular disease in vegetarians (those eating meat or fish less than once a week) and an 18% lower incidence of cancer overall in vegetarians (Huang et al., 2012). Vegetarians have a lower risk of hospitalization or death from ischaemic heart disease (Crowe et al., 2013); lower blood pressure and a lower risk of having hypertension (Pettersen et al., 2012; Yokoyama et al., 2014); lower risk of developing metabolic syndrome (Rizzo et al., 2011); and a lower risk of some cancers than do meat eaters. Vegetarians and fish eaters had a lower risk of cancer compared to meat eaters (Key et al., 2009). They have a lower risk of diverticular disease compared to meat eaters or fish eaters; vegans have an even lower risk (Crowe et al., 2011). Vegetarians, especially vegans, have a lower risk of developing Type 2 diabetes (Tonstad et al., 2009, 2013). However, vegans require dietary supplements of vitamin B12, B6, D and iodine.

A neglected factor has been fibre. The Seven Countries study found fibre intake was inversely related to body weight (Menotti et al., 1989). Large-scale studies by the European Prospective Investigation into Cancer and Nutrition (EPIC) produced data that could be applied to the study of obesity. For example, Fogelholm et al. (2012) examined the role of dietary macronutrient composition, food consumption and dietary patterns in predicting weight or waist circumference change, with and without prior weight reduction. The results show that dietary fibre, especially cereal fibre, fruit/vegetable intake and the Mediterranean dietary pattern, were inversely associated with weight or waist change. A mechanism for the protective effect of fibre was elucidated in 2014 (De Vadder et al., 2014). It involves the intestinal flora and the ability of the intestine to produce glucose between meals.

Vegetarian and vegan diets are affordable and environmentally friendly. One UK study has shown that changing from a non-vegetarian to a vegetarian or vegan diet could reduce greenhouse gas emissions by 22% and 26%, respectively. Any of these changes would be less expensive than the average diet in the UK and would have adequate protein (Berners-Lee et al., 2012). On current evidence, vegetarian and vegan diets provide a sustainable and effective means for achieving healthful levels of nutrition and body weight.

Drug therapies and bariatric surgery

Long-term safety concerns limit the use of drugs to bring about weight loss. Five major drugs have been withdrawn owing to safety concerns.

An average weight loss of 5% is regarded as the minimum threshold for approval guidelines issued by regulatory authorities, yet the majority of patients will often set much higher targets of 10–15%. Modest efficacy is offered by current drug therapies for obesity, but a history of poor tolerability and a lack of safety, a paucity of novel therapies, and a lack of reimbursement have substantially constrained developers of new drugs for obesity (Wong et al., 2012).

In 2014, it was estimated that at least 25% of people in the UK were obese, yet only 1.3% (2.1% of females, 0.6% of males) received anti-obesity medication (Patterson et al., 2014). The relationship between medication rates and age differs by gender, with prescriptions higher in younger females and older males. While the prevalence of obesity worsens with age, younger females are more likely to be prescribed anti-obesity medication, suggesting an element of patient demand.

Medication gives patients an imperfect solution to OAO while perpetuating feelings of learned helplessness. Hollywood and Ogden (2014), using thematic analysis, studied ten participants' experiences of gaining weight after taking orlistat. They found that the participants attributed their failure to lose weight to the medication and emphasized a medical model of obesity. Their weight gain was fatalistically considered an inevitable part of their self-identity, that of a perpetual dieter.

Bariatric surgical procedures forcibly induce a drastic lifestyle change and can elicit up to 20% weight loss, but carry inherent medical risks and high cost. Bariatric surgery is the most effective treatment for the severely obese but it does not work for everyone (Husted and Ogden, 2014). MackSense (2014) reported a huge jump in the number of NHS-funded bariatric procedures in England, from 261 in 2000–2001 to 8,087 in 2010–2011. It estimated that for 2001–2011 less than 1% of people eligible for bariatric surgery received the treatment, i.e., 5,000–10,000 (MackSense, 2014). In the USA, the incidence of bariatric surgery plateaued by 2010 at approximately 113,000 cases per year (Livingston, 2010). Complication rates fell from 10.5% in 1993 to 7.6% of cases in 2006. Bariatric surgery costs the health economy at least $1.5 billion annually.

Another study suggests that a significant variable in predicting the success of bariatric surgery is a person's investment in the operation – i.e., the extent to which they are committed and also their undertaking, in time, finance, emotion, or physical and behavioural effort. In an RCT, Husted and Ogden (2014) found that success following surgery was related to individuals' sense of investment in the surgery, with failure being linked to hedonic motivation to consume food and greater susceptibility to food in the environment. The intervention raised the salience of personal investment in having weight-loss surgery by reducing automatic hedonic thoughts about food to aid weight loss. After three months, the intervention group had a mean weight loss of 6.77 kg compared to 0.91 kg for the control participants. This simple, cost-effective psychological intervention facilitated weight loss and changed hedonic thoughts about food in bariatric patients.

Jumbe et al. (2017) discuss the literature on the psychological impact of bariatric surgery, exploring whether the procedure addresses underlying psychological conditions that can lead to morbid obesity and the effect on eating behaviour postoperatively. Their findings show that this literature suggests some persisting disorder in psychological outcomes like depression and body image for patients at longer-term follow-up, compared to control groups. The authors state that understanding the reasons behind these findings is limited due to a lack of postoperative psychological monitoring and theoretical mapping. Jumbe et al. (2017: 71) conclude that 'Reframing of bariatric approaches to morbid obesity to incorporate psychological experience postoperatively would facilitate understanding of psychological aspects of bariatric surgery and how this surgical treatment maps onto the disease trajectory of obesity'.

Behavioural interventions and the raising of false hopes

A variety of interventions have been tried at the individual level of influence. The quality of the research used to evaluate the interventions is of varied quality but mostly poor. Sample sizes are small, power analyses are rarely if ever carried out, and designs are poor overall. Systematic reviews on effectiveness will briefly illustrate the crisis situation that exists in dealing with obesity using behavioural methods.

Traditional approaches have used diets and exercise. Behavioural programmes have produced weight losses of 10 kg on average at the end of six months (Wing, 2004). Adherence to such programmes is low and attrition high. Those most in need of reducing weight show least adherence. For example, there is an association between waist circumference percentile and non-adherence. Long-term follow-up shows gradual weight regain such that four years after treatment only a modest amount of weight loss remains ($M = 1.8$ kg) (Perri et al., 2004).

The use of temporary diets and activity programmes produce only temporary effects. People who wish to maintain a lower weight over their entire lifetime need to commit to permanent lifestyle change. Only a small percentage of people are willing to make such a commitment. There is no magic bullet.

Lifestyle modifications remain the safest means of prevention and treatment of OAO but they are also the least effective. The Energy Surfeit Theory and dietary guidelines have proven to be a poor basis for interventions.

The basis for dietary interventions often appears to be the existing dietary guidelines themselves. Hafekost et al. (2013) suggested that reliance on dietary guidelines to inform interventions may be holding back progress as few interventions are testing alternative models. They point out that alternative interventions, such as CHO restricted, low glycaemic index and low fructose, have a more plausible rationale than energy balance.

Hafekost et al. (2013) questioned whether 'the public health message' matches scientific knowledge of obesity. They examined the models of energy balance underpinning current research about weight-loss intervention from the field of public health, and determined whether they are consistent with the model provided by basic science. Most public health interventions were based on the energy balance theory, and attempted to reduce caloric consumption and/or increase physical activity in order to create a negative energy balance. Hafekost et al. (2013: 41) concluded that: 'Public health weight-loss interventions seem to be based on an outdated understanding of the science. ... Instead of asking why people persist in eating too much and exercising too little, the key questions of obesity research should address those factors (environmental, behavioural or otherwise) that lead to dysregulation of the homeostatic mechanism.'

They also raise an important ethical point: Is it right to offer interventions that have not worked in the past?

> Despite the extensive literature on their long-term ineffectiveness, interventions based on this simplistic understanding of energy balance continue to be advocated under the assumption that previous interventions have not been pursued sufficiently vigorously or that participants have failed to follow the prescriptions of the intervention. ... Continuing to promote a model that is unlikely to be successful in the longer term, and may result in individuals becoming discouraged, is both unproductive and wasteful of resources that could be better spent on investigating more plausible alternatives to improving weight control. (Hafekost et al., 2013: 41)

The evidence of effectiveness of behavioural interventions is so weak, we can only hope the old dictum 'prevention is better than cure' will one day be acted on. This requires legislation to make healthful foods more affordable and fatty foods and sugary drinks less attractive (Marks, 2015).

FUTURE RESEARCH

1. There is an urgent need for the design of science-based dietary guidelines without any interference from industry to provide effective guidance of eating behaviour.

2. Research is needed into finding ways of making food labelling accessible, clear, transparent, usable and accurate.

3. Research is needed for methods of facilitating long-term dietary change towards reduced consumption of sugars, processed foods and red meats.

4. The insulin theory claims that obesity is caused by a chronic elevation of insulin in a diet that contains too much CHO. The homeostasis theory explains obesity as one unwanted outcome of a 'circle of discontent'. Further research is required to enable these theories to be empirically evaluated.

SUMMARY

1. Human beings are endowed by evolution to store excess food energy as fat. This natural endowment has led to an evolutionary 'hiccough' called the obesity pandemic.
2. The food and drinks industries, with the tacit approval of state bodies, have successfully promoted a large variety of cheap, popular and unhealthy products consisting of snacks, ready meals, junk food and fizzy drinks, together creating an 'obesogenic' environment with excessive sugars, salt and fats.
3. Obesity is an excessive increase in the size and number of fat cells. By 2050, it is predicted that the majority of adults and 25% of children will be obese.
4. According to the Energy Surfeit Theory (EST), obesity is caused by an excess of calories. Interventions based on the EST have failed to break the epidemic and have led to a 'blame and shame' culture in which victims are blamed for their condition and, in some places, health services are withdrawn.
5. Lack of progress and stagnation with the EST approach requires new evidence-based approaches to tackle obesity.
6. Obesity begins in the womb, develops in the crib and accelerates in early life. Attachment patterns, body dissatisfaction and negative affect influence eating and food preferences in early adolescence and these patterns continue into adulthood.
7. In spite of high prevalences of overweight and obesity almost everywhere, the 'thin ideal' pervades popular culture with narratives and images of thinness. This influence can have nothing but a negative effect on both young and adult people the world over.
8. Diets that are low in carbohydrates and plant-based diets containing low amounts of sugar, little or no red meat and the minimum of fats promote weight loss and help prevent obesity, diabetes, metabolic syndrome, coronary heart disease and cancer.
9. Drug therapies have poor outcomes. The most effective treatment, bariatric surgery, is costly and inaccessible to the majority of people who would benefit from it. There also can be unwanted, long-term effects from surgery.
10. Governmental actions, guidelines and programmes *independent of corporate interests* are required at all levels of society to reduce the prevalence of obesity and other chronic, diet-based conditions.

ALCOHOL AND DRINKING

11

'I would not put a thief in my mouth to steal my brains.'

William Shakespeare, *Othello*

OUTLINE

In this chapter, we discuss theories and research about alcohol consumption and the causes, prevention and treatment of drinking problems. Ambivalent attitudes to alcohol have characterized many cultures from the distant past to the present day. A description of the physical and psychosocial dangers of drinking is followed by an examination of contrasting theories about the causes of excessive drinking. We conclude with a critical discussion of recent approaches to the prevention and treatment of drinking problems.

THE BLESSING AND CURSE OF ALCOHOL: PAST AND PRESENT ATTITUDES

The oldest solid evidence of an alcoholic (ethanol) beverage comes from Jiahu, China, where in 7,000 BC farmers fermented rice, grapes, hawthorn berries and honey in clay jars (Curry, 2017). Ethanol's intoxicating power has made it an object of concern – and sometimes outright prohibition. Most societies have felt an ambivalence, trying to strike a balance between moderate drinking for happy relaxation and drinking to get drunk.

The regular use of alcohol by many eminent artists, composers and writers is well documented. Fyodor Dostoyevsky, Henri de Toulouse-Lautrec, Pyotr Ilyich Tchaikovsky, Ernest Hemingway, F. Scott Fitzgerald, William Faulkner, Edgar Allan Poe, John Cheever, Truman

Capote, Dylan Thomas, Jack London, Marguerite Duras and Dorothy Parker are all known to have been frequent users of alcohol. Alcohol's role in artistic and literary work is undeniable, but there are also the 'downsides' to consider, such as depression and suicide.

One important reason for drinking alcohol is the effect that it has on feelings and emotions. Sayette (2017) reviewed the effects of alcohol on emotion in social drinkers. It is alleged that masculine gender norms in some Western cultures tend to constrain expressions of emotion, especially warmth and affiliation among men. Men appear to benefit more than women from drinking alcohol, which helps them to 'loosen up', smile, share feelings and interact socially. In other cultures, these abilities occur freely among both men and women without any need for alcohol.

Since the early nineteenth century popular beliefs about the dangers of alcohol have been shaped by **temperance societies**. Beginning with the American Temperance Society in 1826 and then spreading to other countries, their influence has been enormous in bringing about the era of American prohibition from 1920 to 1934 and also in helping to establish the standard medical opinion, especially in the USA, that alcoholics can never return to moderate drinking but can only be cured by remaining abstinent for the rest of their lives. A range of views can be found among different temperance societies, some simply preaching moderation and the avoidance of excess, some taking the view that spirits are intrinsically dangerous while weaker alcoholic drinks are harmless, some believing that alcohol is highly addictive for everyone, others that it only presents dangers for a small minority of individuals with a predisposition to become addicted. Of particular historical importance were the Washingtonians in the USA in the 1840s. These were self-help associations running regular meetings along the lines of religious revivalist groups with an emphasis on the confessions of the repentant sinner and an appeal to a 'Higher Power' for support. This particular tradition remains strong today in Alcoholics Anonymous, which has branches in almost every North American and British town of any size and in many other countries.

With the exception of some countries with majority Muslim populations, alcohol is legally obtainable in most regions of the world. The predominant view is that it is 'alright in moderation, harmful in excess'. We review the evidence for this view in the next section. Here we focus on the undisputed harm that occurs as a consequence of regular heavy drinking and of 'binge drinking', both now seen as major problems in many countries. The WHO reported that 3.3 million deaths in 2012 were due to harmful use of alcohol (World Health Organization, 2014d). The report drew attention to the fact that alcohol increases people's risk of developing more than 200 diseases, including liver cirrhosis and some cancers. In addition, harmful drinking can lead to violence and injuries, and can make people more susceptible to infectious diseases such as tuberculosis and pneumonia. Overall, 5.1% of the global burden of disease and injury is attributable to alcohol, as measured in disability-adjusted life years (DALYs).

Alcohol problems and approaches to prevention and treatment vary greatly from country to country due to the specific cultural and historical circumstances. In Britain, one source of concern has been binge drinking among young men and women. Many city centres on weekend evenings are notorious for the large numbers of extremely drunk and disorderly young people (Raistrick, 2005; Plant and Plant, 2006). Another concerning issue has been drinking among pre-teens. The UK Millennium Cohort Study found 1.2% of 11-year-olds reported having been drunk and 0.6% reported having had five or more drinks in a single episode (Kelly et al., 2016). The British government has been much criticized for contributing to increased drinking among youth by liberalizing the drinking laws under the influence of the Portman Group, a drinks industry public relations organization, while ignoring medical and other professional opinion opposed to liberalization.

Babor and Winstanley (2008) reviewed papers on the alcohol experiences of 18 countries in a study commissioned for the journal *Addiction* from 2004 to 2007. One problem is the high level of consumption prevalent in the former socialist countries. In Russia, during the Gorbachev era from 1985, public health initiatives led to a 25% reduction in consumption, which was followed by dramatic increases in male life expectancy. These reforms were subsequently abandoned and consumption increased again with concomitant increases in health problems (Zaridze et al., 2014). A problem confronting many countries wishing to address alcohol problems is the powerful influence of international drinks companies. Babor and Winstanley (2008) noted that potentially expanding markets, such as India, Nigeria, China and Brazil, are being targeted with 'highly sophisticated western marketing techniques'. At the same time, the papers which they review mention specifically that the drinks industry is an obstacle to an effective alcohol policy in India, Nigeria, the UK, Thailand, South Africa and Mexico. The alcohol industry resists regulation of marketing, claiming that the industry is responsible and that self-regulation is effective, mirroring the tobacco industry (Savell et al., 2016).

There is a strong relationship between age at first use of alcohol and the prevalence of lifetime alcohol abuse and alcohol dependence. The younger the age at onset of drinking, the higher the likelihood of adult dependency (Grant and Dawson, 1997). The rates of lifetime dependence declined from more than 40% among individuals who started drinking at ages 14 or younger to roughly 10% among those who started drinking at ages 20 and older. Before looking at interventions, we need to understand the impacts of alcohol on physical and mental health.

THE DANGERS AND POSSIBLE HEALTH BENEFITS OF DRINKING ALCOHOL

In this section, we consider evidence of the health risks associated with the consumption of alcohol as well as the possible health benefits. A brief summary of the major risk factors is given in Box 11.1.

BOX 11.1

Risks of alcohol consumption

Risks from any single occasion of heavy drinking:

Driving, industrial and household accidents: falls, fires, drowning.

Domestic and other forms of violence as perpetrator.

Domestic and other forms of violence as victim.

Unwanted pregnancies; HIV or other sexually transmitted diseases following unprotected sexual exposure.

Risks from regular heavy drinking:

Death from liver cirrhosis and acute pancreatitis.

(Continued)

Increased risk of cardiovascular disease and certain cancers.

Problems caused by alcohol dependence.

Exacerbation of pre-existing difficulties such as depression and family problems.

Loss of employment; reduced career prospects.

Risks to women who drink during pregnancy:

Foetal alcohol syndrome.

Miscarriages and premature babies.

Cognitive and behavioural problems of the developing child.

An analysis of the research findings on the health hazards of drinking is considerably more complicated than is the case for smoking. Whereas smoking is dangerous even for low levels of consumption, and increasingly so for heavy smokers, the dangers to health of alcohol consumption are not always found for light and moderate drinkers, who may even experience health benefits compared with non-drinkers. We therefore examine the evidence for risk associated with heavy drinking, and go on to consider the possible benefits of light and moderate drinking.

To begin with, it is necessary to define 'light', 'moderate' and 'heavy' drinking. We adopt the British system in which one 'unit' is assumed to equal 8 g of alcohol or one glass of wine of average strength, half a pint (250 cc) of normal strength beer, and a single measure (25 ml) of spirits. Strong wines and beers may contain up to twice this amount of alcohol. Moderate drinking is an average level of 3/2 units a day for men/women, respectively; less than half of that level can be regarded as light drinking and anything over 7/5 regular daily units can be regarded as heavy drinking.

Liver cirrhosis and acute pancreatitis

Prolonged heavy drinking is known to be the main cause of liver cirrhosis, a serious condition that frequently results in death. Using figures provided by the British Department of Health, the Academy of Medical Sciences (2004) noted a four- to five-fold increase in deaths from chronic liver disease in the UK from 1970 to 2000, with over nine-fold increases among young men and women. Using more recent figures, the UK Office for National Statistics estimated that mortality from liver disease had doubled from 1991 to 2007 (Office for National Statistics, 2009). While some of these changes are attributable to increased rates of hepatitis C infection, effects that are themselves exacerbated by alcohol consumption, the main reason for the changes are increases in levels of heavy drinking. Although it receives much less publicity than liver cirrhosis, acute pancreatitis is another frequently fatal disease that is often caused by heavy drinking. Goldacre and Roberts (2004) surveyed hospital admissions for this disease in England from 1963 to 1998, noting that they had more than doubled over the 35-year period, with particularly large increases among the younger age groups. These changes closely parallel the patterns of increased alcohol consumption over this period of time.

Cancer

The evidence linking alcohol consumption to cancer has been reviewed in various studies. In a study of 109,118 men and 254,870 women from eight European countries, Schütze et al. (2011) estimated that 10% of all cancer cases in men and 3% of cases in women are attributable to alcohol consumption. The most strongly associated are those of the upper aerodigestive tract (44% and 25% of male and female cases respectively), liver (33% and 18%) and colorectum (17% and 4%). The association with breast cancer is weaker, but of particular importance because this is one of the most common causes of premature death in women. Schütze et al. estimated that 5% of cases are attributable to alcohol. This corresponds closely to an earlier estimate by Hamajima et al. (2002), who conducted a detailed re-analysis of data from 53 studies with a total sample size of over 150,000. They found that there was a clear relationship with risk increasing steadily from teetotallers through to those drinking more than five units a day. They concluded that alcohol could be the cause of about 4% of deaths from breast cancer. A similar finding of a small increase in risk at low levels of consumption was reported by Chen et al. (2011) in a 28-year follow-up of 105,986 US nurses. However, the increase in risk was quite modest and, as Hamajima et al. (2002) pointed out, it needs to be interpreted in the context of the possible beneficial effects of moderate alcohol consumption, which is discussed later in this chapter.

A significant proportion of regular alcohol-using males are also smokers. Survey data indicate that approximately 7% of 15–54-year-olds in the USA are co-dependent on alcohol and tobacco (Anthony and Echeagaray-Wagner, 2013). Since 1957 it has been established that the effect of joint exposure to high amounts of alcohol and tobacco on risk of oral cancers confers an excess risk of major proportions, with one estimate being an excess risk of 18.4:1 (Rothman and Keller, 1972). The effects of alcohol and tobacco on excess risk of cancer are not simply additive: they actually multiply. A meta-analysis showed that there is a positive synergistic (multiplicative) effect of alcohol and tobacco use for cancer of the oesophagus (Prabhu et al., 2014). The observed combined effect of alcohol and tobacco was almost double the effect that would be expected if synergy did not happen.

Drinking during pregnancy

This has been the subject of much controversy in recent years. US medical authorities invariably recommend that pregnant women should avoid alcohol completely, while in many other countries the usual advice is that low levels of consumption do no harm. Very heavy drinking is the cause of **foetal alcohol syndrome**, in which the child suffers from a particular type of facial abnormality as well as mental impairment and stunted growth. It has also been established that heavy drinking is associated with miscarriages, premature births, low birthweight and a variety of cognitive and behavioural problems in the developing child. While it may seem tempting to infer from this that there must be some increase in risk even for light drinking, there is in fact surprisingly little evidence that this is the case.

In a useful and challenging review of research findings on many dos and don'ts for pregnant women, Oster (2013) notes that there has been much research but few findings of harmful effects of low to moderate levels of alcohol consumption. In a large-scale Australian study, Robinson et al. (2010) obtained data on weekly alcohol consumption at 18 and 34 weeks for 2,900 women with follow-up testing for child behavioural problems when the children were aged 2, 5, 8, 10 and 14. They found no evidence of an increase in behavioural problems when mothers drank up to 10 units a week as compared with those who were abstinent. In a Danish study of 1,628 women and their children, Skogerbø et al. (2012) found that low to moderate alcohol consumption in early pregnancy had no statistically significant associations with assessments of cognitive functioning of the children at age 5. Similarly, Kelly et al. (2013) carried out a seven-year follow-up of 10,534 children born in the UK between 2000 and 2002 and found no evidence of unfavourable cognitive or behavioural effects on children whose mothers were light drinkers during pregnancy compared with abstainers. In fact, the children of light drinkers performed slightly better on a number of measures.

In contrast to these studies, which may be regarded as good news for women wishing to drink lightly or moderately during pregnancy, two studies indicate that light drinking, especially in the first trimester, is associated with some negative birth outcomes. Andersen et al. (2012) investigated outcomes for 92,719 Danish women and reported that light drinkers, as compared with abstainers, showed an increased risk of miscarriage during weeks 13–16, but no increase later in the pregnancy. Nykjaer et al. (2014) investigated outcomes for 1,303 UK women and found that light drinkers in the first trimester were more likely than abstainers to have premature and low birthweight babies. Given the importance of the issue and the current state of uncertainty about the evidence, women would probably be best advised to adopt the cautious approach of abstinence, at least in the first trimester of their pregnancy.

Health benefits of drinking

The possible benefits of light to moderate drinking have been the subject of a great deal of research and considerable controversy over more than 50 years. The main focus of attention has been cardiovascular disease (CVD), where most studies have reported a U- or J-shaped function, with light and moderate drinkers being at substantially lower risk than both abstainers and heavy drinkers. In a detailed review of publications from 1950 to 2009, Ronksley et al. (2011) found the evidence supporting the protective effect of light to moderate drinking to be compelling. Overall, the relative risk for alcohol drinkers for CVD mortality was 25% lower than for non-drinkers, with the lowest risk for light drinkers with consumption levels between 7 and 14 units a week. In the case of mortality from strokes, there was relatively little indication of a protective effect for light drinkers and a very pronounced negative effect for heavy drinkers. In a review of papers published from 1980 to 2010, Roerecke and Rehm (2012) found that light drinking was associated with a reduced risk of ischaemic heart disease incidence and mortality, but they were cautious in their interpretation of this finding, pointing out that there was considerable variation in the extent of the apparent protective effects reported in different studies.

In addition to an association with reduced risk of CVD, there is also some evidence that light drinking is associated with a reduced risk of death from cancer when compared with abstainers. This is surprising in view of the evidence which we have already noted, that cases of some types of cancer are more frequent among light drinkers. However, in a meta-analysis combining data from 18 studies published up to April 2012, Jin et al. (2013) found that light drinkers (up to 11 units a week) had a 9% reduction in all-cancer mortality, while heavy drinkers (over 44 units a week) had a 31% increase when compared with non-/occasional drinkers.

After considering the costs and benefits of alcohol consumption in relation to different diseases, the natural question to ask is, how is consumption related to all-cause mortality? In addition to their analysis for CVD, Ronksley et al. (2011) also examined this evidence. Of the 84 studies that provided data for CVD, 31 also provided data for all-cause mortality, indicating that there was a J-shaped relationship, with light drinkers having a 13% reduction in mortality compared with abstainers, and heavy drinkers a 30% increase.

The results of these and other studies are not entirely consistent with each other, especially for the purpose of establishing upper limits for safe drinking, but they are at least consistent with the statement that men and women in good health who drink moderately are not taking any significant risk with their physical health. The additional claim that light to moderate drinking is actually beneficial to health is more open to doubt. Although non-drinkers do have higher mortality rates than drinkers, this may be only because the category of non-drinkers includes a substantial number of individuals who have given up drinking because of poor health. This is a useful illustration of the statistician's dictum that 'correlation does not entail causation'. It could be that not drinking is a cause of poorer health but, equally well, it could be that poor health is a cause of not drinking. The latter view was first analysed in detail by Shaper et al. (1988), using data from 7,000 middle-aged men, confirming that those who suffered from health problems cut down or abstained from drinking. The argument was subsequently developed by a number of other critics, notably Fillmore and her associates (Fillmore et al., 2007). An alternative possibility is that a third, 'background' variable could be the cause of both good health and moderate drinking. An example of such a background variable might be having an optimistic style of personality. We discuss the links between personality and health in Chapter 18.

Recent reviews have gone some way towards meeting these criticisms, by dividing abstainers into ex-drinkers and life-long abstainers, and still finding a protective effect for light drinkers. However, a range of further criticisms of this interpretation have been put forward by Fekjær (2013). He points out that light drinking has been shown by various studies to have an apparent protective effect not only against CVD but also against a wide range of diseases, many of which have no obvious physiological connection with alcohol consumption. Thus while plausible biological mechanisms have been proposed for protective effects against CVD (Brien et al., 2011), it is difficult to imagine that this could also be done for such diverse conditions as asthma, gallstones, osteoporosis, hearing loss and Alzheimer's disease. Since the peak protective effects always seem to occur at very similar levels of light drinking, there are grounds for suspecting that we are not dealing with a panacea so much as a flaw in research design. Fekjær argues that the latter is the case. He points out that most studies have been conducted in countries where light or moderate alcohol consumption is very much the prevailing norm, and statistically associated with high social status, while non-drinkers are on average of lower social status and education with less healthy diets and levels of exercise, and many other characteristics which are correlated with poor health. As discussed in Chapters 4 and 5, social inequalities are strongly associated with health.

THE EFFECTS OF ALCOHOL AND CAUSES OF ALCOHOL DEPENDENCE

To understand the motivation for drinking and problems of dependence it is best to begin by considering the psychological effects of alcohol. These effects are much influenced by culture and by people's expectations about potential benefits, including enjoyment, stress reduction and increased sociability (Anderson and Baumberg, 2006). This explains why it is consumed in social gatherings, such as parties and weddings, when people wish to interact in a much more relaxed and informal way than they might otherwise, and also why heavy drinking is common among people with psychological problems. Alcohol dependence is widespread among people suffering from anxiety disorders, and the use of alcohol to induce sleep is also known to aggravate sleep disorders because it leads to increased wakefulness and arousal a few hours later (Anderson and Baumberg, 2006).

Let us now look more closely at the question of why some people develop drinking problems while others do not. Here a number of contrasting theoretical perspectives need to be considered. They are not mutually exclusive in the sense that this can sometimes be said of theories in the natural sciences. The discerning reader will notice various ways in which elements of each can be consistent with elements of the others. They are best thought of as reference points that are useful aids to thinking about the issues. A brief summary of the main theoretical views is given in Table 11.1.

Genetic theories

Genetic theories propose that some people have an inherited predisposition to develop drinking problems. Those who are convinced of the overwhelming importance of heredity believe that certain people are 'born alcoholics', destined to succumb to alcoholism almost as soon as they take their first drink. Perhaps surprisingly, this 'biological determinist' view is also attractive to manufacturers of alcoholic drinks. They can argue that the born alcoholic is bound to have a drink and become an alcoholic sooner or later, however much the availability of drink is restricted. The rest of us can drink as we wish without running the risk of becoming alcoholics.

Table 11.1 Theories of problem drinking

Type of theory	Causes of problem drinking
Genetic theories	DNA variations, possibly associated with the metabolism of alcohol, mean that certain individuals are much more likely than most to develop alcohol problems if they drink
Addiction, disease and dependence theories	Individuals who drink heavily may develop a physiological addiction and psychological dependence, which can only be effectively treated by life-long abstinence
Learning theories	Mechanisms of conditioning and social learning can explain the development of excessive consumption and the phenomena of dependence, craving, increased tolerance and withdrawal symptoms

While it is certainly true that alcohol problems tend to run in families, this is not in itself enough to prove the existence of genetic influences. Drinking habits can be passed on from parents to children as the result of upbringing and imitation just as much as they may be passed on through genes. The most widely cited evidence for genetic influences comes from twin and adoption studies. Twin studies are based on comparisons of the concordance rates for drinking patterns in *monozygotic* (MZ, identical) and *dizygotic* (DZ, fraternal) twins. The theory behind this is that both types of twin grow up in the same family environment, so that a greater concordance for the 100% genetically similar MZ twins than for the 50% similar DZ twins is evidence of genetic effects. Adoption studies examine whether adopted children grow up to acquire similar drinking habits to their biological parents, or whether they are more influenced by their adopting parents.

Twin and adoption studies have been used to estimate 'heritability', a statistical assessment of the relative importance of hereditary and environmental influences which can take values from 100% for fully inherited characteristics to 0% for those which are purely environmentally determined. In practice, heritability estimates for drinking patterns have varied greatly from study to study, partly as the result of methodological problems that are difficult to overcome, and partly because the estimates vary as a function of what is measured. The highest estimates have sometimes been found for 'chronic alcoholism' and sometimes for 'teetotalism'; some have found greater heritability for males than females, and some the exact opposite (see, e.g., Heather and Robertson, 1997). In so far as generalizations have been made about the heritability of alcohol problems, figures of 50–60% have sometimes been suggested (Anderson and Baumberg, 2006). However, Walters (2002) carried out a meta-analysis of 50 studies and concluded that heritability was quite low, unlikely to be higher than 30–36%. Verhulst et al. (2015) suggest the figure is close to 50%.

Given the increasing popularity of DNA-based research, it is not surprising that there have been a number of attempts to demonstrate specific genetic loci for alcohol problems, but these have only met with modest success (Cook and Gurling, 2001; Anderson and Baumberg, 2006). As with other forms of human behaviour, there are likely to be a multitude of complex genetic routes that may make some individuals more likely than others to become problem drinkers (Palmer et al., 2012). For example, there may be inheritable differences in the way that alcohol is metabolized, so that some people find its effects pleasant, others unpleasant, some find it takes more alcohol, others less, to achieve the same effect. There may be differences in genetic predisposition to experience anxiety, so that some are predisposed to drink more than others on discovering that it temporarily suppresses anxiety.

On the basis of existing research evidence, there is certainly no reason to suppose that some people are 'born alcoholics'. Although there is enough evidence to show that there is some degree of genetic predisposition towards different patterns of drinking, it seems unlikely that this is as important an influence as environmental factors. To appreciate what this means, take as an analogy the fact that some people may have an inherited proneness to develop heart disease, but whether or not they will do so still depends on whether they smoke, eat fatty foods, avoid exercise, and so on. The risks are just greater for some people than for others. Similarly, there could be many environmental reasons why drinking problems develop in those who have an inherited predisposition and also in those who do not.

Addiction, disease and dependence theories

The history of these theories has been examined in a broad social and historical context by Thom (2001). **Addiction theories** can be traced back to the classic works of Benjamin Rush of Philadelphia and Thomas Trotter of Edinburgh, published respectively in 1785 and 1804. Rush and Trotter replaced the traditional view of habitual drunkards as moral degenerates by one in which they are victims of an addiction. Once the addiction is established, the victims lose all voluntary control over their drinking. They have become incapable of resisting their craving for the 'demon drink'. Rush and Trotter succeeded in popularizing their belief that alcohol is a highly addictive substance 70 years before the case was made for opium.

Later **disease theories** focused increasingly on the at-risk individual who has a predisposition to become alcoholic once he or she starts drinking. Although a predisposition to become alcoholic does not have to be hereditary (we have already mentioned that it may be the result of upbringing), nevertheless the concept of the born alcoholic proved attractive to disease theorists. In common with earlier addiction theories, disease theories emphasized craving and loss of control. The difference was that, for the later disease theorists, alcohol is only highly addictive for a small number of people. The rest of us can drink with impunity. This change of emphasis proved attractive, especially to a North American society that had abandoned prohibition, embraced personal liberty and responsibility and has a powerful drinks industry.

From the mid-1970s, the disease theory was being revised and extended, notably by Griffith Edwards and Milton Gross, to become the **alcohol dependence syndrome**. In this new conceptualization, the sharp distinction that had previously been made between physical addiction and psychological dependence was abolished and the syndrome was viewed instead as a psychophysiological disorder. The descriptions given by Edwards and Gross are not always very clear and tend to change from one publication to another. Box 11.2 lists the main aspects of Edwards' more recent accounts as summarized by Sayette (2007).

The concept of the alcohol dependence syndrome has been much criticized, originally by Shaw (1979), who pointed out that much woolly thinking lies behind it. Most people, on reading the list of symptoms in Box 11.2, would conclude that anyone who drinks regularly would exhibit one or more of them to some degree. As a list, it seems consistent with the idea that, rather than being a disease, alcohol dependence is an arbitrary point that can be chosen on a continuum from the light social drinker to the homeless street drinker. Yet proponents of the syndrome insist that it is a clinical entity, admittedly with somewhat varying symptoms, which only applies to a relatively small number out of all the people who drink heavily.

BOX 11.2

Symptoms of alcohol dependence syndrome

According to Griffith Edwards, this includes some or all of the following symptoms:

tolerance (a diminished effect of alcohol, usually accompanied by increased consumption);

withdrawal symptoms following reduced consumption;

consumption of larger amounts or for a longer time period than was intended;

persistent desire or unsuccessful efforts to cut down or control drinking;

excessive time spent obtaining, consuming or recovering from the effects of alcohol;

reduction of important activities due to drinking; and

continued drinking despite knowing that it is causing or exacerbating a physical or psychological problem.

Source: Sayette (2007)

One should not, of course, 'throw out the baby with the bath water'. No theory of alcohol use can afford to neglect the phenomenon of physical dependence associated with prolonged heavy drinking and most clearly manifested in the spectacular withdrawal symptoms that can occur following sudden abstinence. These include some of the most unpleasant to be found among all types of drug withdrawal, including tremors ('the shakes'), sweating, nausea, vomiting, hallucinations ('pink elephants') and convulsions. Indeed, Lerner and Fallon (1985) noted that, in a significant number of cases, sudden withdrawal can actually prove fatal. The phenomenon of psychological dependence also needs to be addressed by any theory of alcohol use. While alcohol dependence syndrome may be poorly defined as a clinical entity, the psychological problems that are often associated with heavy drinking certainly need to be explained.

Learning theories

Learning theorists consider drinking problems to develop as a result of the same learning mechanisms that are at work in establishing patterns of 'normal drinking'. They argue that the reasons why some people become problem drinkers and others do not lie in their particular personal histories of learning to drink, their present social environment in so far as it provides opportunities and encouragement to drink, and in physiological variables that may make the effects of alcohol more pleasurable or positively reinforcing for some people than others.

Operant conditioning is the type of learning that occurs when animals are trained to respond in a particular way to a stimulus by providing rewards after they make the appropriate response. In the classic experiment, hungry rats were confined in small boxes and trained to press a bar in order to obtain food pellets. This phenomenon, which was of course well known to animal trainers, pet owners and the parents of small children long before it was 'discovered' by psychologists, has some applicability to the understanding of problem drinking. Of particular importance is the **gradient of reinforcement**, the fact that reinforcement which occurs rapidly after the response is much more effective in producing learning than delayed reinforcement. In the case of drinking alcohol, a small amount of positive reinforcement, such as reduced anxiety, that occurs fairly soon after drinking, may cause a strong habit to develop in spite of the counterbalancing effect of a large amount of punishment (hangover, divorce, loss of employment) that occurs much later.

Drinking, eating, smoking, and drug and sexual addictions all have the 'irrational' characteristic that the total amount of pleasure gained from the addiction seems much less than the suffering caused by it. According to learning theorists, the reason for this lies in the nature of the gradient of reinforcement. Addictive behaviours are typically those in which pleasurable effects occur rapidly, while unpleasant consequences occur after a delay. The simple mechanism of operant conditioning and the gradient of reinforcement functions, as it were, to overpower the mind's capacity for rational calculation.

Classical conditioning refers to the process whereby a response that occurs as a natural reflex to a particular stimulus can be conditioned to occur to a new stimulus. In Pavlov's early experiments a bell was rung shortly before food was placed in a dog's mouth, thereby eliciting salivation as a physiological reflex. After a number of pairings of bell and food, Pavlov found that the dog salivated when the bell was rung unaccompanied by food.

A number of interesting models have been developed by applying classical conditioning principles to addictions, and Drummond et al. (1995) provided a useful survey of this now highly technical subject. One application to explain the phenomena of drug dependence, tolerance and withdrawal is the **compensatory conditioned response model**. Initially, when a drug is taken, a physiological 'homeostatic' mechanism comes into operation to counteract its effects. In the case of alcohol, which has a depressing effect, the homeostatic mechanism activates the nervous system in order to maintain the normal level of activation. In the regular drinker, this gradually produces tolerance so that increasingly large quantities of alcohol are required to produce the same effect. Furthermore, the homeostatic response of nervous activation may become conditioned to stimuli normally associated with drinking, such as situations where drinking has frequently taken place in the past. If conditioned drinkers avoid alcohol in these situations, the conditioned response of nervous activation will not be balanced by the effects of alcohol, and the resultant unpleasant state of excessive activation is what is known as a withdrawal state. In this way classical conditioning can account for the close connection observed between the phenomena of tolerance and withdrawal. The compensatory conditioned response model has considerable intuitive plausibility but there is a lack of convincing evidence for its applicability to problem drinking.

Social learning theorists argue that classical and operant conditioning provide incomplete explanations of human learning, which also frequently depends on observation and imitation. Bandura (1977) has been particularly influential in emphasizing the importance of learning by imitation and linking it to his concept of **self-efficacy**, a personality trait consisting of having confidence in one's ability to carry out one's plans successfully. People with low self-efficacy are much more likely to imitate undesirable behaviour than those with high self-efficacy. Collins and Bradizza (2001) reviewed applications of social learning theory to drinking, noting that the evidence points to parents having the strongest influence on the initiation of adolescent alcohol use, while peers are most influential in determining subsequent frequency of use.

PREVENTION AND TREATMENT OF ALCOHOL PROBLEMS

Prevention

Approaches to the prevention of alcohol problems have been the subject of intense controversy in recent years. On the one hand, specialists in this field are generally in favour of measures to reduce overall levels of consumption by increasing prices and imposing restrictions on advertising, promotions and general availability. On the other hand, the drinks industry campaigns against all these approaches and in favour of educational initiatives and self-regulation. The main issues are summarized in Box 11.3.

Probably the most effective measure for reducing population levels of consumption is increased taxation. This is a policy that requires careful analysis and attention to the specific conditions of individual countries, particularly poor countries where large increases in taxation may lead to increases in the production of illicit and potentially lethal distilled liquor. But in relatively wealthy countries, increases in taxation generally lead to proportionate decreases in consumption. The WHO (2007) noted that young people's drinking is particularly sensitive to increases in price, which can therefore reduce underage drinking as well as the extent of binge drinking among teenagers. Furthermore, and contrary to widespread belief, price increases have also been shown to have an impact on the amount consumed among older frequent and heavy drinkers.

BOX 11.3

Population-based prevention: expert opinion versus the drinks industry

Specialists on the prevention of alcohol problems are almost unanimous in their support for the population-based approach, which incorporates the principle that the most effective

---

policies for reducing alcohol problems are those which reduce overall levels of consumption. These policies include higher levels of taxation on alcoholic drinks, restrictions on advertising and sponsorship, limiting opening hours for bars and imposing tight controls on which shops can sell alcohol and the hours during which they can do so.

The population-based approach is opposed by the drinks industry because reduced overall consumption means smaller profits. They propose that 'sensible drinking' can be encouraged by self-regulation of the drinks industry and educational initiatives. They argue that the population-based approach penalizes the majority of sensible drinkers in order to discourage the minority of irresponsible drinkers.

Critics of the drinks industry suggest that the drinks industry claims are disingenuous because it has been clearly shown that educational initiatives are ineffective at curbing heavy drinking, and also because the drinks industry makes most of its profit from the minority of drinkers who consume well above recommended limits.

In many countries the drinks industry has been much more successful than the alcohol experts at influencing government policies. This may be because governments do not wish to risk unpopularity by adopting population-based policies.

Sources: Babor et al. (2003); Academy of Medical Sciences (2004); Anderson and Baumberg (2006); WHO (2007)

Each of the reports referred to in Box 11.3 note that the global drinks industry is deploying sophisticated modern marketing techniques aimed at young people, including lifestyle advertising, promotions involving sporting teams and events, rock concerts and festivals, fashion shows and carnivals, as well as the development of new products specifically aimed at young people, such as 'alcopops' and 'pre-mix cocktails'. An approach, deeply unpopular with the drinks industry, is the introduction of bans on advertising and sponsorship. Although earlier research had indicated that bans have little or no effect on overall consumption, Saffer and Dave (2002) argued that this research is flawed. They use an economic model to analyse pooled data from 20 countries over 26 years and conclude that advertising and sponsorship bans can reduce overall consumption by 5–8%. They note that increases in levels of consumption often stimulate the introduction of bans, but that reductions in consumption often lead to the rescinding of bans, as has happened in recent years in Canada, Denmark, New Zealand and Finland.

One area of legislation to control the dangers of alcohol use, which more and more countries are adopting, is strictly enforced drink-driving laws, with severe penalties for offenders. It is now almost universally agreed that this has played an important role in reducing traffic fatalities. It even commands the support of the drinks industry, which, in view of the high level of public support for the laws, would be foolish to oppose it.

The other main preventive measures that have been much analysed are health education initiatives with the aim of preventing alcohol misuse. Unfortunately, the evidence here indicates that they are not very effective. Health education generally appears to improve knowledge about the effects of alcohol and attitudes to it, but has no effect on the amounts actually consumed.

The ineffectiveness of educational campaigns designed to encourage sensible drinking perhaps explains why the drinks industry is happy to support them and even participate in them.

Although this may seem an unnecessarily cynical view, there are some reasons for taking it seriously. Heather and Robertson (1997) pointed out that the drinks industry derives a good part of its profits from very heavy drinkers. In a 1978 survey of Scottish drinking habits, it was estimated that 3% of the population were responsible for 30% of total alcohol consumption. The loss of this source of profits would be crippling to the drinks industry. Hence the continued profitability of the industry requires the existence of a substantial percentage of very heavy drinkers. This provides another salient example of a conflict of interest between good public health and profits in industry.

In considering international perspectives at the beginning of this chapter we noted that the drinks industry is often mentioned as an obstacle to effective alcohol policy. A good example is provided by the UK in recent years. Heather and Robertson (1997) described attempts by the Portman Group, an organization funded by the British drinks industry, to influence academic debate on alcohol policy by financial offers to academics to encourage them to mount critiques of research supporting the population-based approach. The Institute of Alcohol Studies (2003) commented on the influence of the Portman Group on a decision of the British government to extend permitted drinking hours in England and Wales. The Portman Group was also a key influence on the British government's 2004 alcohol harm reduction strategy (Plant, 2004). This document is replete with positive references to the drinks industry and the Portman Group, emphasizing the value of educational programmes and other drinks industry initiatives, while rejecting any increases in taxation or legislation to control advertising and availability. In 2006 the Portman Group set up a sister organization, Drinkaware, apparently with some government support, and whose activities, like those of its parent organization, seem designed to 'divert attention away from population-level strategies that limit the availability, price and promotion of alcohol, and thus threaten corporate profits, towards those focused on individual responsibility' (McCambridge et al., 2014). The authors also note that these organizations are continuing to enjoy success in countering the one government policy that is most feared by the drinks industry: the introduction of minimum unit pricing.

Paralleling the activities of the Portman Group in the UK, Jernigan (2012) analysed the activities of the International Center for Alcohol Policies (ICAP), funded by the international drinks industry and established in the USA in 1995. Jernigan argued that much of the material published by ICAP appears to be a direct attempt to counter the publications being put out concurrently by the World Health Organization. While superficially mirroring the WHO publications, those of ICAP were heavily dependent on research involving collaborations with the drinks industry and highly selective literature reviews which typically arrive at conclusions either supporting the position of the drinks industry or at least emphasizing high levels of disagreement among researchers. The ICAP publications frequently recommend alcohol policies that are known to be ineffective.

Treatment

A brief synopsis of alternative approaches to treatment is given in Table 11.2. These range from rehabilitation centres offering in-patient treatment over several weeks or months to brief interventions offered by doctors, nurses or other professionals. One area receiving a lot of media hype is the increasing use of 'talking cures'. These are therapies involving one-to-one or one-to-many face-to-face or self-help techniques designed to change experience and behaviour. There are many such therapies, but the most popular over recent decades have been cognitive behavioural therapy, motivational interviewing, mindfulness-based relapse prevention, and Acceptance and Commitment Therapy (ACT).

Table 11.2 Alternative treatment approaches to problem drinking

Type of treatment	Approach to treatment
In-patient treatment	'Drying out' or 'rehab' centres and private clinics focus on the alleviation of withdrawal symptoms followed by counselling and therapy to maintain abstinence following discharge.
Alcoholics Anonymous	Self-help groups run by ex-alcoholics using the '12-step facilitation programme' to maintain life-long abstinence. May receive individuals on discharge from in-patient treatments.
Cognitive behavioural therapy (CBT)	Originally developed by Aaron Beck and Albert Ellis, based on learning and cognitive theories, CBT is concerned with the connections among thinking, emotion and behaviour. Changes in any one of these processes tends to bring about changes in the others. Thus changing the way we interpret or see things can change the way we respond. People learn methods and ways to change old thinking patterns and habits. Some effective techniques are: self-recording behaviour; slowing down to discover what is going on; stopping automatic negative thinking or rationalization; learning rational and helpful self-statements; imaging new ways of being and behaving.
Motivational interviewing (MI)	Motivational interviewing is a 'counselling style' that uses empathic listening to understand the client's perspective and minimize their resistance. Strategies and techniques are used to explore the person's values and goals in relation to the addictive problem, and to elicit motivation for change. Confronting the client with contradictions causes discomfiture that increases the probability of change (Rollnick and Miller, 1995).
Mindfulness-based relapse prevention (MBRR)	Being mindful is a state of active, open attention to the experiences that are present. Mindfulness means living in the present and awakening to one's current experience. It strengthens the idea that life is something to be lived in the present and the things that you do should not always be judged. To quote Shakespeare: *There is nothing either good or bad, but thinking makes it so.* MBRR uses a simple form of meditation that is practised sitting with eyes closed, on a cushion or on a chair.
Acceptance and Commitment Therapy (ACT)	ACT aims to increase a person's willingness to experience physical cravings, emotions and thoughts while committing to values-guided behaviour changes. 'Acceptance' refers to making room for intense physical sensations (e.g., urges), emotions (e.g., sadness) and thoughts (e.g., 'I really need a drink right now') that trigger drinking while allowing them to come and go. 'Commitment' refers to articulating meaningful values to motivate and guide action plans (e.g., stopping drinking) (Hayes et al., 2006).
Brief interventions	Advice on reducing consumption given by general practitioners and other health professionals, including 'opportunistic interventions' given to individuals who have attended for other reasons, such as screening.

None of the treatments outlined in Table 11.2 is a panacea. Reviewing the literature to determine the truth about the effectiveness of particular approaches is no easy task. It is necessary to cut through the hype that frequently accompanies study findings. More frequently than ever, authors of studies, sponsors and journals are using positive spin and exaggerated claims to promote findings in the media and increase altmetric scores. Miller and Wilbourne (2002) provided an extensive review of the amount and quality of the evidence concerning the efficacy of different treatment programmes. They examined studies of 48 different types of treatment, rating each study for its methodological adequacy and then placing the treatments in rank order. Alcohol brief interventions (ABIs) of advice given by general practitioners, nurses and at hospital emergency departments are well supported by the evidence. Whitlock et al. (2004) noted that reductions in amount consumed, and in the proportion of participants who reduced their drinking to moderate or safe levels, were maintained up to four years after the interventions. Bertholet et al. (2005) reviewed brief interventions, brief treatments given at primary care facilities to individuals attending for reasons other than alcohol-related problems. After examining 19 trials that included 5,639 individuals, they concluded that these interventions were effective in reducing alcohol consumption measured at 6 and 12 months after the interventions.

Because ABIs are effective as well as being much less expensive than other forms of treatment, they have become increasingly popular. The main problem that has been identified by researchers is the difficulty that has been experienced in persuading general practitioners to undertake them. Roche and Freeman (2004) proposed that practice nurses could take over the function. Platt et al. (2016) reviewed 52 trials with 29,891 individuals. ABIs reduced the quantity of alcohol consumed by an average of 0.15 of one standard deviation. Neither the setting nor the content significantly moderated intervention effectiveness, but interventions delivered by nurses had the most effect in reducing quantity ($d = -0.23$) but not frequency of alcohol consumption. Brief advice was found to be the most effective in reducing quantity consumed ($d = -0.20$). However, let's be clear that the average effect of ABIs on consumption is modest: only 0.15 of one SD. *That represents a reduction of only one or, at most, two drinks from the drinker's daily consumption of alcohol.* Hardly a cure!

Of the other types of treatment reviewed by Miller and Wilbourne, there is evidence for the effectiveness of **motivational interviewing**. None of the remaining 46 types of treatment considered by Miller and Wilbourne received much support from outcome studies, although **cognitive behavioural therapy (CBT)** appeared to be more effective than psychotherapeutic approaches. Furthermore, and in spite of its enduring popularity, there are few good quality studies that provide support for the approach of Alcoholics Anonymous and their abstinence-based '12-step facilitation programme'. However, the AA's perfectly reasonable insistence on anonymity and the associated difficulty of forming properly randomized control groups make it difficult to scientifically evaluate.

Another approach under the umbrella of **mindfulness-based relapse prevention (MBRP)** has been receiving publicity over recent decades. This technique has been applied to problem drinking as well as other substance use disorders (Witkiewitz et al., 2005). Meditation itself is an ancient mental discipline from the Buddhist tradition, which surfaced in the West as a technique for producing relaxation in the 1960s and 1970s. Early studies claimed a specific and reliable psychophysiological effect that could act as a therapeutic aid for drug abuse and alcoholism (Wallace et al., 1971; Benson and Wallace, 1972). Many Western people tried using meditation to reduce psychological stress and stress-related health problems.

Findings have been mixed, although many studies have produced positive results. Bowen et al. (2014) reported a trial in which 286 participants were randomly assigned to one of three groups: traditional 12-step facilitation, cognitive behavioural relapse prevention and MBRP. At six-month follow-up the CBT and MBRP groups both had lower relapse rates than the 12-step group, and after 12 months MBRP was outperforming both of the other groups.

Goyal et al. (2014) carried out a systematic review to determine the efficacy of meditation in improving stress-related outcomes (anxiety, depression, stress/distress, positive mood, mental health-related quality of life, attention, substance use, eating habits, sleep, pain and weight) in adult clinical populations. Results were unimpressive overall. Mindfulness meditation showed moderate evidence of improved anxiety at eight weeks and at three to six months, depression at eight weeks and at three to six months, and pain, and low evidence of improved stress/distress and mental health-related quality of life. However, Goyal et al. (2014) found low or no evidence of any effect of meditation on positive mood, attention, substance use, eating habits, sleep and weight. They also found no evidence that meditation was better than any active treatment such as drugs, exercise and other behavioural therapies.

There is a need for large-scale, well-controlled clinical trials to evaluate new treatments and therapies. None invented to date is a panacea, and the prospect of finding one is a remote possibility. There is too much profit in the drinks industry to conceive of prohibition or sustained tax increases, the only measures that could effectively reduce the prevalence of alcohol-related illnesses and deaths. So if you like a 'tipple', drink on dear reader, make merry, and hope for the best!

FUTURE RESEARCH

1. Clarification of the health risks and possible benefits of light to moderate drinking, including heart disease and risks to the unborn child.

2. Studies to examine the role of learning processes, including classical and operant conditioning and social learning in the development of alcohol dependence and problem drinking.

3. Investigations to establish the physiological and psychological mechanisms of dependence, tolerance and withdrawal symptoms.

4. Evaluation of the relative effectiveness of different approaches to the treatment of problem drinking, including brief and opportunistic interventions, motivational interviewing, mindfulness-based relapse prevention and self-help organizations.

SUMMARY

1. Most cultures both past and present have an ambivalent view of the use of alcohol. This ambivalence is often associated with the view that alcohol is harmless, possibly beneficial in moderation, but harmful in excess.
2. There is a sharp conflict between addiction and disease models of alcoholism, which are particularly prevalent in North America where life-long abstinence is considered to be the only cure for the alcoholic, and psychological models, which are more common in Europe, where drinking in moderation is sometimes considered to be a viable objective.
3. Drinking has been shown to cause liver cirrhosis, pancreatitis, strokes, various cancers and, in the case of drinking during pregnancy, damage to the unborn child. Most of these physical health risks are confined to the heavy drinker.

(Continued)

4. Hereditary and environmental factors both make a substantial contribution to alcohol consumption.
5. The nature of physical and psychological dependence on alcohol is not well understood; at present, conditioning and learning models represent the most promising approach.
6. The most effective methods for preventing alcohol problems include high taxation, advertising bans and restricted availability. The drinks industry is a powerful lobby against these measures and few political leaders would dare to risk unpopularity by introducing them.
7. Brief interventions from general practitioners, including 'opportunistic interventions', have modest effectiveness in producing reductions in consumption.
8. For individuals seeking treatment for alcohol problems, motivational interviewing and mindfulness-based relapse prevention may be helpful. However, evaluations have not been conclusive and none of the treatments invented to date is a panacea.

TOBACCO AND SMOKING

'Tobacco is the only legal drug that kills many of its users when used exactly as intended by manufacturers.'

World Health Organization (2015c)

OUTLINE

This chapter examines the extent of smoking, its major health impacts, explanations of smoking and interventions to help smokers to quit. Smoking prevalence is increasing throughout the developing world and many people continue to smoke in the industrialized world. Measures to reduce smoking prevalence have met with substantial success, in spite of deceitful practices and disinformation from the tobacco industry. The primary methods to assist smokers to stop are reviewed, together with research on electronic cigarettes.

BRIEF HISTORY OF TOBACCO AND SMOKING

Among recreational drugs, tobacco is by far the biggest killer and nicotine the most addictive substance. Yet tobacco has been in use for millennia and, in spite of the certain knowledge that it can kill, it is used by around 2 billion people, 6 million of whom die each year. If discovered for the first time today, tobacco would definitely be banned. According to the Centers for Disease Control and Prevention (CDC), in the US in 2015 22,073 people died of alcohol, 12,113 died of AIDS, 43,664 died of car accidents, 38,396 died of drug use – legal and illegal – 18,573 died of murder and 33,300 died of suicide. That brings us to a total of 168,119 deaths, far less than the 480,000 who die from smoking annually (CDC, 2016a).

How did the fatal attraction to tobacco begin?

In the first century BC the Mayans in Central America are alleged to have smoked the tobacco in religious ceremonies. The Aztecs took the smoking custom from the Mayans, who later settled in the Mississippi Valley, and smoking was adopted by neighbouring tribes (Figure 12.1). Amazonian Indians also used tobacco in their religious rituals. This group colonized the Bahamas, later discovered by Columbus in 1492.

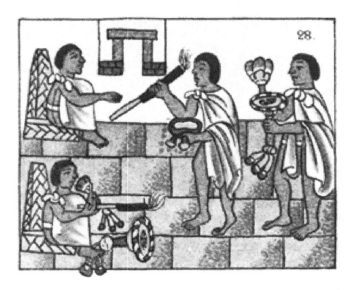

Figure 12.1 Aztec guests being presented with a tobacco tube and a sunflower

Source: The Florentine Codex

The English adventurer Sir Walter Raleigh is alleged to have introduced both potatoes and tobacco to England. Raleigh's public health legacy of tobacco and potato (when cooked as chips or fries) would be hard to rival. Raleigh popularized tobacco at court, and apparently believed that it was a good cure for coughs so he often smoked a pipe. Indeed, it is alleged that Raleigh's final request before his beheading by James I at the Tower of London in 1618 was a smoke of tobacco, a legacy to all subsequent prisoners facing execution.

FREEDOM AND CHOICE

The freedom to smoke or to vape is a basic human right. Each individual has freedom of choice. The main goal of health care interventions must be to facilitate informed choice. This involves offering people information about the possible health consequences of smoking and/or vaping, explanations about the addictive properties of nicotine, methods that could be helpful in stopping the habit, and support while going through the process of cessation. The health psychologist can play a significant role in these activities.

PREVALENCE AND DISTRIBUTION

Although tobacco was popular during the nineteenth century, it was largely smoked by men with pipes. The development of cigarettes towards the end of the nineteenth century led to a rapid increase in tobacco consumption. In the first half of the twentieth century, cigarette smoking became hugely popular, especially among men. In the USA, cigarette consumption doubled in the 1920s and again in the 1930s, peaking at about 67% in the 1940s and 1950s. However, between 1965 and 2004, cigarette smoking among adults aged 18 and older declined by half from 42% to 21%, and rates declined to 20% in 2007. In 2015, about 15% or 36.5 million US adults aged 18 years or older currently smoked cigarettes (CDC, 2016a). More than 16 million Americans are living with a smoking-related disease and there are 480,000 deaths every year, or one in every five deaths (CDC, 2016a). In recent years smoking prevalence has been highest in China.

In Britain, it was estimated that the prevalence among men reached almost 80% during the 1940s and 1950s (Wald et al., 1988). Since then, the prevalence has declined overall, with sex, social class, regional and other differences. There are about 10 million adult cigarette smokers in Great Britain and about 15 million ex-smokers. Since 1990 there has been a steady increase in the number of smokers using mainly hand-rolled tobacco. In 1990, 18% of male smokers and 2% of female smokers said they smoked mainly hand-rolled cigarettes, but by 2011 this had risen to 40% and 26%, respectively.

The 2012 Opinions and Lifestyle Survey found that 38% of men and 24% of women smoked hand-rolled cigarettes (Action on Smoking and Health, 2014). Much of the tobacco used by hand-rollers is smuggled across borders duty free.

The World Health Organization (2013) estimated that tobacco kills approximately 6 million people and causes more than half a trillion dollars of economic damage each year. The WHO report in 2013 estimated that tobacco will kill as many as 1 billion people this century if the WHO Framework Convention on Tobacco Control is not implemented rapidly. Prevalence in developing countries is rising dramatically where there is extensive promotion of smoking by Big Tobacco.

Although fewer women than men are smokers, there have been dramatic increases in smoking among women and the gap in smoking rates between men and women is narrowing in most places. In Europe, there was a consistent decline in the prevalence of smoking among men, from about 70–90% to about 30–50% between 1950 and 1990. However, among women the same period saw a rise in the prevalence of smoking followed by a slow decline, reaching 20–40% in 1990. The initial rise in prevalence was led by women from professional backgrounds, but they have also led the decline such that today smoking is more common among women from poorer backgrounds.

National surveys have established a growing link between smoking and various indicators of social deprivation. In Britain, a national survey of health and lifestyles found that smoking is more prevalent among people on low incomes, the unemployed and those who are divorced or separated.

HEALTH EFFECTS OF SMOKING

The health effects of smoking have been studied for over 100 years. There is hardly a single organ in the body that is not deleteriously influenced by tobacco smoking.

Effects on active smokers

Cigarette smoking accounts for more than 480,000 deaths each year in the USA and 120,000 deaths in the UK, nearly one in every five deaths. The risk of dying from lung cancer is at least

22 times higher among men who smoke, and about 12 times higher among women who smoke, compared with those who have never smoked.

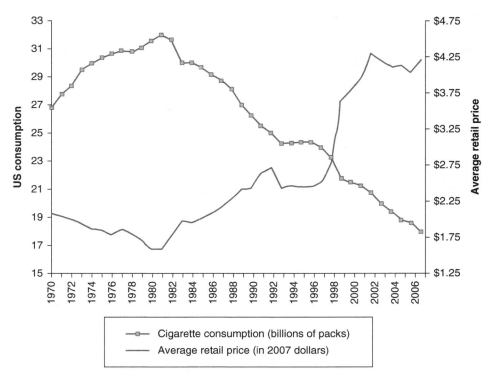

Figure 12.2   Tobacco consumption by price in the USA, 1970–2007

Source: www.tobaccofreekids.org/research/factsheets/pdf/0146.pdf

Chemicals and radiation that are capable of triggering the development of cancer are called 'carcinogens'. Carcinogens initiate a series of genetic alterations ('mutations') that stimulate cells to proliferate uncontrollably. A delay of several decades occurs between exposure to carcinogens in tobacco smoke and the onset of cancer. People exposed to carcinogens from smoking cigarettes generally will not develop cancer for 20 to 30 years.

The 2004 US Surgeon General's report on smoking and health revealed that smoking causes diseases in nearly every organ of the body (US Department of Health and Human Services, 2004). Published 40 years after the Surgeon General's first report on smoking – which had concluded that smoking was a definite cause of three serious diseases – the 2004 report found that cigarette smoking is conclusively linked to leukaemia, cataracts, pneumonia as well as cancers of the cervix, kidney, pancreas and stomach. On average, men who smoke cut their lives short by 13.2 years and female smokers lose 14.5 years. Statistics indicate that more than 12 million Americans have died from smoking since the first (1964) Surgeon General's report, and another 25 million Americans alive today are likely to die of a smoking- related illness. The report concluded that quitting smoking has immediate and long-term benefits, reducing risks for diseases caused by smoking and improving health in general. Quitting smoking at age 65 or older reduces by nearly 50% a person's risk of dying of a smoking-related disease.

Effects on passive smokers

For obvious reasons, tobacco smoke does most damage to the person who is actively inhaling. However, those consistently breathing second-hand smoke (SHS) also have a higher risk of cancer, heart disease and respiratory disease, as well as sensory irritation. The Surgeon General estimated that exposure to SHS killed more than 3,000 adult non-smokers from lung cancer each year, approximately 46,000 from coronary heart disease, and an estimated 430 newborns from sudden infant death syndrome. In addition, SHS causes other respiratory problems in non-smokers, such as coughing, phlegm and reduced lung function. Passive smoking causes the premature death of thousands of non-smokers worldwide.

Big Tobacco campaign of disinformation

Big Tobacco carried out a disinformation campaign over several decades. The campaign deliberately sought to create doubt in the minds of legislators and the public about the effects of smoking. However, through litigation and the action of whistleblowers, and with the release of thousands of tobacco industry documents, the details of the disinformation campaign were revealed. The anti-tobacco organization Action on Smoking and Health (ASH) carried out a survey of the documents, extracted 1,200 relevant quotes, and grouped these under common themes (Action on Smoking and Health, 2010) (see Box 12.1).

BOX 12.1

Tricks of the tobacco trade

Big Tobacco routinely denied that tobacco is addictive, yet it has known this since the 1960s. The idea of nicotine addiction destroyed the industry's stance that smoking is a matter of personal choice, e.g., 'the entire matter of addiction is the most potent weapon a prosecuting attorney can have in a lung cancer/cigarette case. We can't defend continued smoking as "free choice" if the person was "addicted"' (The Tobacco Institute, 1980, cited by Action on Smoking and Health, 2010).

The companies deny that they target the young. Yet company documents revealed the companies' preoccupation with teenagers and younger children and methods to influence smoking behaviour in these age groups, e.g., 'If the last ten years have taught us anything, it is that the industry is dominated by the companies who respond most to the needs of younger smokers' (Imperial Tobacco, Canada, cited by Action on Smoking and Health, 2010).

The industry maintains that advertising is used only to fight for brand share, not to increase total consumption, while academic research shows otherwise, e.g., 'I am always amused by the suggestion that advertising, a function that has been shown to increase consumption of virtually every other product, somehow miraculously fails to work for tobacco products' (Emerson Foote, former Chairman of McCann-Erickson, which handled US$20 million tobacco industry accounts, cited by Action on Smoking and Health, 2010).

The industry promoted 'low-tar' cigarettes knowing that they were lacking any health benefits, or even made cigarettes more dangerous, e.g., 'Are smokers entitled to expect

(Continued)

---

that cigarettes shown as lower delivery in league tables will in fact deliver less to their lungs than cigarettes shown higher?' (BAT in 1977, cited by Action on Smoking and Health, 2010).

The industry refused to accept the evidence of the harm caused by SHS, e.g., 'All allegations that passive smoking is injurious to the health of non-smokers, in respect of the social cost of smoking as well as unreasonable demands for no smoking areas in public places, should be countered strongly' (BAT in 1982, cited by Action on Smoking and Health, 2010).

'Emerging markets'

With reducing smoking levels in the West, the companies moved aggressively into developing countries and Eastern Europe, e.g., 'They have to find a way to feed the monsters they've built. Just about the only way will be to increase sales to the developing world' (ex-tobacco company employee, R. Morelli, cited by Action on Smoking and Health, 2010).

Source: Action on Smoking and Health (2010)

Balbach et al. (2006) argued that the health belief model (see Chapter 8) helped Big Tobacco through its theoretical stance regarding individual choice and 'information'. Balbach et al. analysed trial and deposition testimony of 14 high-level tobacco industry executives from six companies plus the Tobacco Institute to determine how they used the concepts of 'information' and 'choice' in relation to theoretical models of health behaviour change. They concluded that tobacco industry executives deployed the concept of 'information' to shift full moral responsibility for the harms caused by tobacco products to consumers.

Discourses about smoking have a powerful influence on attributions of responsibility, whether the consumer or the provider is ultimately to blame. Our 'blame culture' can easily swing in either direction.

Tobacco promotion to children and 'Third World'

Big Tobacco spends billions worldwide on advertising and promoting tobacco products. The US Federal Trade Commission (2016) reported that the major tobacco companies now spend $9.1 billion per year – nearly $25 million every day – on promoting tobacco products, and much of this activity is directed towards children. Research shows that tobacco advertising encourages children to start smoking and reinforces the social acceptability of the habit among adults. The US Surgeon General (1989) stated that tobacco advertising increases consumption by:

- encouraging children or young adults to experiment with tobacco and thereby slip into regular use;

- encouraging smokers to increase consumption;

- reducing smokers' motivation to quit;

- encouraging former smokers to resume;

- discouraging full and open discussion of the hazards of smoking as a result of media dependence on advertising revenues;

- muting opposition to controls on tobacco as a result of the dependence of organizations receiving sponsorship from tobacco companies;

- creating, through the ubiquity of advertising and sponsorship, an environment in which tobacco use is seen as familiar and acceptable and the warnings about its health are undermined.

Econometric studies find that increased advertising expenditure increases demand for cigarettes, while banning advertising leads to a reduction in tobacco consumption. In 1991, a meta-analysis of 48 econometric studies found that tobacco advertising significantly increased tobacco sales. The UK Department of Health's Chief Economic Adviser found that there was a drop in tobacco consumption of between 4% and 16% in countries that had implemented a tobacco-advertising ban (Smee et al., 1992). Given the huge numbers of people who die from smoking-related diseases, it seems illogical that tobacco companies are allowed legally to advertise their harmful products. However, many issues are intertwined and the abolition of tobacco advertising has not been as simple and straightforward as it might first appear.

First, Big Tobacco argues that there is a lack of evidence to suggest that tobacco advertising significantly influences smoking behaviour. The 'magical potency' of tobacco advertising could be questioned since most advertisements are directed at target audiences who already use the product. Researchers claimed that econometric studies have found either no overall relationship between advertising and sales or a small, statistically significant positive relationship. However, this view can be contested and the results of such studies are equivocal, as much depends on who supplies data for the studies: Big Tobacco or the public health authorities.

The issue of banning tobacco advertising is further tangled when politics are included. The epitome of this can be seen within the European Union, which on the one hand has supported and finances Big Tobacco through the Common Agricultural Policy, and on the other hand recognizes the health effects of tobacco in funding its 'Europe Against Cancer' campaign. However, in financial terms, the former greatly exceeds the latter. Despite this, attempts have been made to persuade tobacco growers to change their crops. Yet the fact remains that in 2000 the EU provided €984.5 million in tobacco subsidies and a mere €64 million to the 'Europe Against Cancer' campaign. The 15-fold greater expenditure on tobacco subsidies surely cancelled out any benefit from the anti-cancer campaign. Crazy!

THEORIES OF SMOKING

Smokers' resistance to large-scale anti-smoking campaigns led to research to explain the popularity of smoking. Smoking is an extremely complex practice involving a mixture of processes. The 'biopsychosocial model' (BPS model) suggested three interrelated influences on health that are mirrored in theories of smoking: the biological, the psychological and the social theories of smoking (Table 12.1).

Table 12.1 The three main theoretical approaches to the understanding of smoking

Theory	Main elements of the theory
Biological	1. Tobacco contains nicotine, an addictive substance 2. Nicotine activates brain circuits that regulate feelings of pleasure, the 'reward pathways' of the brain 3. Nicotine increases the amounts of the neurotransmitter dopamine 4. The acute effects of nicotine disappear in a few minutes, causing the smoker to repeat the dose of nicotine 5. Smoking is an addiction that is repeatedly and immediately reinforced with each new intake of nicotine
Psychological	1. Smoking is a learned habit, which becomes an automatic response to stimuli following repeated reinforcement – a conditioned response 2. The pleasant associations of smoking generalize to a range of settings and situations 3. The smoker learns to discriminate between those situations in which smoking is rewarded and those in which it is punished 4. The smoker develops responses to a number of conditioned stimuli (internal and external 'triggers') that elicit smoking 5. Smoking is an escape/avoidance response to certain aversive states. The smoker will light up a cigarette to escape or avoid an uncomfortable situation
Social	1. Initially, smoking is physically unpleasant but this is overruled because of social reinforcement from peers 2. Smoking is a social activity in which the smoker identifies with others who smoke. There is a rebellious feeling associated with the activity 3. The social identity of the smoker is changed once he/she forms the habit 4. Smokers group together socially and share their experiences, which smokers find pleasurable and empowering. The in-group feeling is heightened by social norms and health advice to quit 5. The strong associations between social identity, in-group feelings and a smoking sub-culture are difficult to change

Biological theory

Nicotine, the main active ingredient in tobacco smoke, is a substance that if taken in large quantities can be toxic and even fatal. However, delivered in small amounts via cigarette smoke it has a range of psychophysiological effects, including tranquilization, weight loss, decreased irritability, increased alertness and improved cognitive functioning. However, tolerance to the effects of nicotine develops such that there is less evidence of performance improvements among regular smokers (Jarvis, 2004). Over time the smoker develops a physical dependence on nicotine.

Nicotine is addictive because it activates brain circuits that regulate feelings of pleasure, the 'reward pathways' of the brain. A key chemical involved is the neurotransmitter dopamine that nicotine increases. The acute effects of nicotine disappear in a few minutes, causing the smoker to repeat the dose of nicotine to maintain the drug's pleasurable effects and prevent withdrawal symptoms.

The cigarette is an efficient and highly engineered drug-delivery system. By inhaling, the smoker can get nicotine to the brain rapidly with each and every puff. A typical smoker will take ten puffs on a cigarette over a period of five minutes that the cigarette is lit. Thus, a person who smokes 30 cigarettes daily gets 300 'hits' of nicotine every day. That is over 100,000 hits a year or one million every ten years! This is why cigarette smoking is so highly addictive. Smoking behaviour is rewarded and reinforced hundreds of thousands or millions of times over the smoker's lifetime. An enzyme called monoamineoxidase (MAO) shows a marked decrease during smoking. MAO is responsible for breaking down dopamine. An ingredient other than nicotine causes the change in MAO, since it is known that nicotine does not dramatically alter MAO levels. Smokers may be increasing central dopamine levels by reducing monoamineoxidase inhibitor activity, reinforcing smoking by keeping high satisfaction levels through repeated tobacco use.

There is evidence that tobacco is a highly addictive drug. More than 30% of people who try tobacco for the first time develop a dependency on tobacco, while for other drugs, this percentage is generally lower. However, there are variations in the speed and strength of addiction to nicotine among smokers. One obvious way to explain individual differences in smoking is our genetic makeup. Twin studies have produced evidence that genetic factors may play a role in several aspects of nicotine addiction, from the tendency to begin smoking to the chances of quitting (Heath and Madden, 1995; True et al., 1997).

Psychological theory

The most frequently used model of smoking is based on learning theory. It argues that people become smokers because of the positive reinforcement they obtain from smoking. The mechanisms are similar to those described in Chapter 11 in reference to alcohol drinking. Initially, smoking is physically unpleasant but this is overruled because of the social reinforcement from peers. The pleasant associations of smoking then generalize to a range of settings. In addition, the smoker learns to discriminate between those situations in which smoking is rewarded and those in which it is punished. The smoker also develops responses to conditioned stimuli (both internal and external) that elicit smoking. Smoking can be conceptualized as an escape/avoidance response to certain aversive states (Pomerlau, 1979). The smoker lights up a cigarette to escape or avoid an uncomfortable situation.

In 1966, Tomkins proposed his 'affect management model' of smoking that was subsequently revised and extended by Ikard et al. (1969), who conducted a survey of a national (US) probability sample. In a factor analysis of the responses, they identified six smoking motivation factors: reduction of negative affect, habit, addiction, pleasure, stimulation and sensorimotor manipulation. Subsequent surveys produced similar factors. Women more than men reported that they smoked for reduction of negative affect and pleasure. In their study of smoking among young adults, Murray et al. (1988) added two additional reasons: boredom and nothing to do.

According to Zuckerman (1979), individuals engage in sensation seeking so as to maintain a certain level of physiological arousal. More specifically, Zuckerman emphasized that sensation seeking was designed to maintain an optimal level of catecholaminergic activity. In a French sample, smokers scored higher on a measure of sensation seeking, in particular on disinhibition, experience seeking and boredom susceptibility sub-scales. From a physiological perspective, these sensation seekers have a low level of tonic arousal and seek exciting, novel or intense stimulation to raise the level of cortical arousal. This argument is similar to that of Eysenck et al. (1960), who found that smokers scored higher on measures of extraversion. This personality dimension is also supposed to reflect a lower level of cortical arousal that can be raised by engaging in risky activities, such as smoking.

A variety of different types of study have found that stress is associated with smoking. For example, among smokers, consumption is higher in experimental, stressful laboratory situations. In surveys, people with higher self-reports of stress are more likely to be heavy smokers. In a study of nurses' smoking practices, Murray et al. (1983) found that those who reported the most stress were more likely to smoke. This relationship remained after controlling for the effect of family and friends' smoking practices. Finally, in a macro-social study, US states that have the highest levels of stress, as measured by a range of social indicators, also have the highest levels of smoking and of smoking-related diseases.

Other researchers have looked for evidence of personality differences between people who smoke and non-smokers. Sensation seeking, neuroticism and psychoticism are all correlated with smoking (Marks, 1998). However, the relationships are fairly weak and it can be concluded that anybody has the potential to become addicted to nicotine.

Across almost all theories, a key concept has been craving, or having the urge to smoke. Urges and cravings are subjective, emotional-motivational states that are normally followed immediately with overt smoking, or within a few minutes. Urges and cravings are normally attributed to drug withdrawal or the positive reinforcing effects of drugs. Tiffany (1990) hypothesized that drug use in the addict is controlled by automatized action schemata. Automatized behaviour is stimulus bound, stereotyped, effortless, difficult to control and regulated largely outside awareness. This theory helps to explain why stopping smoking is so difficult. Interventions that focus on the automatic nature of smoking behaviour invite the smoker to actively become aware or be mindful of the automatic nature of smoking (Marks, 2017a).

Social theory

Smoking is a social activity. Even when the smoker smokes alone, he/she still smokes in a society where cigarettes are widely available and promoted. A number of qualitative studies have considered the social meaning of smoking. Murray et al. (1988) conducted detailed interviews with a sample of young adults from the English Midlands. These suggested that smoking had different meanings in different settings. For example, at work going for a cigarette provided an opportunity to escape from the everyday routine. For these workers, to have a cigarette meant to have a break and, conversely, not to have a cigarette meant not to have a break. The cigarette was a marker, a means to regulating their work routine.

Outside work, smoking was perceived as a means of reaffirming social relationships. For those young people who went to the pub, the sharing of cigarettes was a means of initiating, maintaining and strengthening social bonds. Those who did not share cigarettes were frowned upon.

Graham's (1976) series of qualitative studies has provided a detailed understanding of the meaning of smoking to working-class women. In one of her studies, she asked a group of low-income mothers to complete a 24-hour diary detailing their everyday activities. Like the young workers in the study by Murray et al. (1988), smoking was used as a means of organizing these women's daily routine. Further, for these women smoking was not just a means of resting after completing certain household tasks, but also a means of coping when there was a sort of breakdown in normal household routines. This was especially apparent when the demands of childcare became excessive. Graham describes smoking as 'not simply a way of structuring caring: it is also part of the way smokers re-impose structure when it breaks down' (Graham, 1987: 54).

Smoking is embedded not only in the immediate material circumstances in which the smoker lives, but also in the wider social and cultural context within which smoking is widely promoted. Admittedly, in most Western societies there are considerable restrictions on the sale and promotion of cigarettes. Despite these, tobacco manufacturers continue to find ways to promote their products, e.g., through the sponsorship of sporting and cultural activities. Big Tobacco is a powerful lobby group that has considerable influence on government and policy-making.

INTEGRATIVE THEORY OF HOMEOSTASIS

The three main drivers of addiction are integrated into a single theory of homeostasis (Marks, 2016a). In an addicted smoker, the act of smoking is a restorative behaviour in which the body's nicotine level is increased to produce a feeling of satisfaction (Figure 12.3). With each puff on a cigarette, the habit strength is reinforced by the pleasure received from the nicotine. Thus, a system of homeostasis is established wherein the habit is reinforced by the restoration of nicotine in the body.

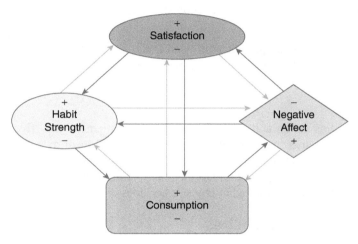

Figure 12.3   Homeostasis theory of smoking

Source: Marks (2016)

SMOKING CESSATION

In the last 20 years smoking has been driven downwards in the majority of countries (World Health Organization, 2015c). Yet millions are still being harmed by tobacco, and to an increasing extent in developing countries, deepening health inequalities. This has led to attempts to develop a more sophisticated understanding of the process of giving up smoking. There is more clarity today about the best ways to help individual smokers.

The majority of smokers spend a considerable portion of their lives wishing they could quit. When they do quit, the vast majority do so on their own, without professional help, and they quit using 'cold finally turkey', i.e., by abrupt withdrawal ('cold turkey'). The American Cancer Society (2009) reported that 91.4% of former smokers quit 'cold turkey' or by slowly decreasing the amount smoked. Doran et al. (2006) surveyed adult patients attending Australian general practitioners in 2002 and 2003. Over a quarter of patients were former smokers and one in five were current smokers. Doran et al. reported that 92% of former and 80% of current smokers used only one method in their last quit attempt, 'cold turkey' being the most common method used by both former (88%) and current (62%) smokers.

For those who seek help, guidelines such as those of the Surgeon General can be followed (Fiore, 2008). For smokers who are willing to quit, the 'five As' are a useful framework:

Ask about tobacco use: Identify and document tobacco use status for every patient at every visit.

Advise to quit: In a clear, strong and personalized manner, urge every tobacco user to quit.

Assess willingness to make a quit attempt: Is the tobacco user willing to make a quit attempt at this time?

Assist in quit attempt: For the patient willing to make a quit attempt, offer medication and provide or refer for counselling or additional treatment to help the patient quit. For patients unwilling to quit at the time, provide interventions designed to increase future quit attempts.

Arrange follow-up: For the patient willing to make a quit attempt, arrange for follow-up contacts, beginning within the first week after the quit date. For patients unwilling to make a quit attempt at the time, address tobacco dependence and willingness to quit at next clinic visit.

For smokers unwilling to quit, it is recommended to implement the 'five Rs': explain the Relevance, Risks, Rewards, run over the Roadblocks, and Repeat at every available opportunity. In the following sections we review the three main approaches to smoking cessation, which are available singly or in combination: pharmacological, psychological and social. It should always be remembered that what any smoker does is their own free choice.

Pharmacological approaches

The first paragraph to read in any paper reporting a drug study is the 'Declaration of Interests'. Some authors are paid lucrative sponsorship deals by the pharmacological industry which should be declared in this section. Frequently, the reader will find that the authors have received honoraria (= money) from companies such as Pfizer®, Novartis®, GlaxoSmith – Kline®, AstraZeneca® and Roche®, and that they act as speakers, undertake consultancy and research, receive travel funds and hospitality from manufacturers of medications, or receive an unrestricted research grant (= more money) from one or more companies. These financial relationships between corporations and researchers are not conducive to unbiased, impartial science. It has been shown that pharmaceutical industry sponsorship of drug studies is associated with findings that are favourable to the sponsor's product (Lexchin et al., 2003; Bero, 2013).

Pharmacological approaches aim to minimize the unpleasant symptoms of withdrawal, i.e., the irritability, difficulty concentrating, anxiety, restlessness, increased hunger, depressed mood and a craving for tobacco that accompanies cessation. These withdrawal symptoms are relieved by the administration of nicotine, but not of placebo. There are three kinds of pharmacological treatment for nicotine withdrawal that aim to raise the chances of cessation.

Nicotine replacement therapy (NRT) reduces symptoms of nicotine withdrawal, thereby, in theory, increasing the likelihood of cessation. Six forms are available: gum, patch, nasal spray, inhaler, tablet and lozenge. Evidence from clinical trials has been interpreted as demonstrating that NRT is effective (e.g., Stolerman and Jarvis, 1995). NRT company websites, and 'independent' sites that are viewed as authoritative, proclaim that the nicotine patch, available over the counter, 'doubles the chances of quitting'. Such sites are unreliable – sadly, even those by government departments. For example, the NHS Smokefree website makes the unsupported claim that: 'If you also use medicines such as patches or gum to manage your cravings, you are up to four times more likely to successfully go smokefree!' (National Health Service, 2010).

Methodological problems exist within many RCTs that compare NRT to placebos. This is because smokers in the placebo condition can detect that they are not receiving any nicotine (Mooney et al., 2004; Polito, 2008). Dar et al. (2005) found that control group members were 3.3 times more likely to correctly guess that they had received placebo than to incorrectly guess that they had received nicotine (54.5% versus 16.4%). If the trials in an RCT are not double blind, the findings give a misleading picture of treatment effectiveness. Cochrane Reviews, which assess the quality of trials from the written reports (e.g., Cahill et al., 2013), have no way of checking whether double blind requirements have been broken. This fact may help to explain why real-world results for NRT are worse than those obtained in RCTs.

Another issue concerning NRT is lack of safety. In 2005 the Medicines and Healthcare Products Regulatory Agency (MHRA) relaxed the restrictions on NRT use, allowing the combined use of patches and gum, and permission for its use by pregnant and young smokers, smokers with cardiovascular disease and smokers who want to reduce their smoking. However, a critical review concluded that NRT use by pregnant women and children would pose a significant risk to neurological development in infants and children (Ginzel et al., 2007). That NRT is used so widely in health care systems in spite of the poor outcomes, and lack of safety is profitable for the pharmaceutical industry but a poor return for taxpayers and smokers. This review suggests that a therapeutic strategy for smoking should look beyond a purely medical model. A psychosocial model would yield a radically different approach. Efficacy and cost-effectiveness will be higher when treatment strategies address the causes, not the symptoms.

Psychological approaches

Quitting smoking or, if that is impossible, reducing cigarette consumption, are both viable targets for a smoking cessation programme. In order to achieve these aims, it is necessary for smokers to control their physical and psychological dependency on smoking. The US Surgeon General's (2008) guidelines on 'Treating Tobacco Use and Dependence' recommended the use of individual, group and telephone counselling (Fiore, 2008). The report concluded that two components of counselling are especially effective: practical counselling concerning problem solving and skills training, and social support. The results of the meta-analysis are shown in Table 12.2. While counselling and medication are effective alone, a combination of counselling and medication is the most effective. The report found a strong association between the number of sessions of counselling, when combined with medication, and smoking abstinence. The best abstinence rate was obtained with more than eight sessions of counselling and behaviour therapy plus medication, giving an odds ratio of 1.7 and an abstinence rate of 32.5%.

BOX 12.2

CASE STUDY: The National Health Service (NHS) in England's Smoking Cessation Service

Pharmacologically mediated cessation, primarily NRT, has been promoted through guidelines that have a questionable evidence base. The English NHS smoking cessation service is based on pharmacotherapy in combination with counselling support. The claims for high efficacy and cost-effectiveness of NRT have not been substantiated in real-world effectiveness studies (e.g., Pierce and Gilpin, 2002; Ferguson et al., 2005; Doran et al., 2006). Pierce and Gilpin (2002: 1260) stated: 'Since becoming available over the counter, NRT appears no longer effective in increasing long-term successful cessation.' Efficacy studies, using randomized controlled trials, do not transfer well to real-world effectiveness. Bauld et al. (2009) reviewed 20 studies of the effectiveness of intensive NHS treatments for smoking cessation published between 1990 and 2007. Quit rates showed a dramatic decrease between four weeks and one year. A quit rate of 53% at four weeks fell to only 15% at one year. Younger smokers, females, pregnant smokers and more deprived smokers had lower quit rates than other groups.

The NHS evaluation data prove that NRT produces poorer outcomes than non-pharmacological methods (Health and Social Care Information Centre, Lifestyles Statistics, 2008). In 2007–2008, 680,000 people set a quit date and 88% of these had received pharmacotherapy at a cost of £61 million. Of these, 49% successfully quit for four weeks compared to 55% of people who had received no pharmacotherapy. Smokers who used NRT had a lower quit rate than those who did not use NRT. The NRT system needs to be replaced by a more effective system.

The guidelines give specific recommendations about particular behavioural and social elements to include in smoking treatments (see Table 12.3). There has been increasing interest in the use of cognitive behavioural therapy (CBT) for the control of smoking and other health-related behaviours. These therapies can be delivered as a brief intervention in one or more sessions to groups of smokers who are at the action stage.

Stop Smoking Now (SSN) is a psychological programme that integrates multiple behavioural techniques (SSN; Marks, 2017a). Based on the earlier Quit For Life Programme (Sulzberger and Marks, 1977; Marks, 1993), SSN uses cognitive behavioural therapy with elements of mindfulness and meditation. SSN encourages a steady reduction of cigarette consumption over seven to ten days followed by complete abstinence. The aim of SSN is the elimination of nicotine addiction without nicotine replacement or pharmaceuticals. SSN methods are listed in Table 12.3. A preliminary observational study with an earlier version indicated that the therapy could be particularly effective when delivered to groups of self-referring smokers (Marks, 1992). Randomized controlled trials later suggested the SSN programme delivered good quit rates at relatively low cost among lower SES smokers with only one intensive session (Sykes and Marks, 2001; Marks and Sykes, 2002).

Table 12.2 Meta-analysis of the effectiveness of and estimated abstinence rates for various types of counselling and behavioural therapies (*n* = 64 studies)

Type of counselling and behavioural therapy	Number of arms	Estimated odds ratio (95% CI)	Estimated abstinence rate (95% CI)
No counselling/behavioural therapy	35	1.0	11.2
Relaxation/breathing	31	1.0 (0.7, 1.3)	10.8 (7.9, 13.8)
Contingency contracting	22	1.0 (0.7, 1.4)	11.2 (7.8, 14.6)
Weight/diet	19	1.0 (0.8, 1.3)	11.2 (8.5, 14.0)
Cigarette fading	25	1.1 (0.8, 1.5)	11.8 (8.4, 15.3)
Negative affect	8	1.2 (0.8, 1.9)	13.6 (8.7, 18.5)
Intra-treatment social support	50	1.3 (1.1, 1.6)	14.4 (12.3, 16.5)
Extra-treatment social support	19	1.5 (1.1, 2.1)	16.2 (11.8, 20.6)
Other aversive smoking	19	1.7 (1.04, 2.8)	17.7 (11.2, 24.9)
Rapid smoking	19	2.0 (1.1, 3.5)	19.9 (11.2, 29.0)

Source: US Surgeon General (2008)

Table 12.3 Elements of problem-solving and skills training recommended in the Surgeon General's (2008) guidelines that are included in *Stop Smoking Now* (Marks, 2017a)

Practical counselling (problem-solving/ skills training) treatment component	Examples
Recognize danger situations – identify events, internal states or activities that increase the risk of smoking or relapse	Negative affect and stress
	Being around other tobacco users
	Drinking alcohol
	Experiencing urges
	Smoking cues and availability of cigarettes
Develop coping skills – identify and practise coping or problem-solving skills. Typically, these skills are intended to cope with danger situations	Learning to anticipate and avoid temptation and trigger situations
	Learning cognitive strategies that will reduce negative moods
	Accomplishing lifestyle changes that reduce stress, improve quality of life and reduce exposure to smoking cues
	Learning cognitive and behavioural activities to cope with smoking urges (e.g., distracting attention, changing routines)
Provide basic information about smoking and successful quitting	The fact that any smoking (even a single puff) increases the likelihood of a full relapse
	Withdrawal symptoms typically peak within one to two weeks after quitting but may persist for months. These symptoms include negative mood, urges to smoke and difficulty concentrating
	The addictive nature of smoking

SOCIAL APPROACHES

Smoking is deeply embedded in everyday social activities. Today, smoking has become almost taboo, and smokers are seen as 'outsiders'. Cessation attempts must take these aspects into consideration, including the increasing social gradient in smoking prevalence. Smoking cessation efforts not only need to provide social support but also attempt to enhance people's sense of control and mastery through changing their social conditions. Smoking cessation interventions may thus form part of a general community intervention to promote empowerment and health advocacy (see Chapter 16).

Many group treatment programmes use the 'buddy system', in which smokers are paired up to provide mutual support. A variety of organizations also offer group support for quitters. These are organized at a local level by health care providers and charities. The NHS Stop Smoking Services offer free local group sessions, which start a week or two before the official quit date. The group then meets weekly for four weeks to give advice and motivation. Some people prefer to talk one-to-one with a professional adviser, but many find the group support helpful. Many support systems are provided by hospitals and clinics.

Another social intervention is to invite smokers to quit on a particular national day. Two examples are the 'Great American Smokeout' (GASO) in the USA and 'National No-Smoking Day' in the UK. Every year, on the third Thursday of November, smokers in the USA are invited to take part in GASO. An evaluation explored quitting rates from the Great American Smokeout and New Year's Day (Gritz et al., 1989). The rate of non-smoking declined from 34% at one month to 25% at one year; 21% of participants never stopped smoking, and 68% of those who quit had relapsed by one year.

Another evaluation observed cessation-related news reports, Twitter postings and cessation-related help seeking via Google, Wikipedia and government-sponsored quitlines (Ayers et al., 2016). Time trends (2009–2014) were analysed to isolate spikes during the GASO compared to a control day – a 'simulated counterfactual had the GASO not occurred'. Cessation-related news increased by 61% and tweets by 13% during the GASO day compared with what was expected had the GASO not occurred. Cessation-related Google searches increased by 25%, Wikipedia page visits by 22% and quitline calls by 42%. Cessation-related news media positively coincided with cessation tweets, internet searches and Wikipedia visits; a 50% increase in news for any year predicted a 28% increase in tweets for the same year. Increases on the day of the GASO rivalled about two-thirds of a typical New Year's Day – the day presumed to have the greatest increase in cessation-related activity. There were about 61,000 more instances of help seeking on Google, Wikipedia or quitlines on GASO each year than would normally be expected. Good news for population health; bad news for tobacco sales!

Quitting without help: cold turkey

The most popular method of smoking cessation remains 'cold turkey', i.e., abrupt cessation without any outside help.

The Australian study by Doran et al. (2006) reported success rates among 2,207 former smokers and 928 current smokers as follows: cold turkey 77.2%; nicotine patch 35.9%; nicotine gum 35.9%; nicotine inhaler 35.3%; and bupropion 22.8%. According to these data, NRT and bupropion reduced the odds of quitting when considered across the whole population of quitters. Health care professionals tend to see only those smokers who have the most difficulty quitting by themselves. It is therefore likely that, as the smoking population shrinks over time, those who seek help will become harder to treat.

As is the case with problem drinking, gambling and narcotics use, studies show that at least 90% of smokers who permanently stop smoking do so without any form of assistance (Chapman and MacKenzie, 2010). In 2003, 20 years after the introduction of NRT, smokers trying to stop unaided were twice as numerous as those using pharmaceutical methods, and only 8.8% of US quit attempters used a behavioural treatment. Yet the most common method used by people who successfully stopped smoking is unassisted cessation (cold turkey or reducing before quitting). Great gains could be made if public health authorities highlighted this fact rather than emphasizing NRT and e-cigarettes as methods of smoking cessation.

Electronic cigarettes

Electronic cigarettes or e-cigarettes are a commonly used method for cutting down or eliminating conventional smoking. They were first developed in China in 2003. Users are called 'vapers'. E-cigarettes are battery-operated cylindrical devices designed to replicate smoking without combustion of tobacco. Some look like conventional cigarettes, while others with larger tanks are more clunky. They use heat to vaporize a liquid-based solution containing nicotine and flavouring into an aerosol mist, and have been proposed as a way to help smokers quit the habit. They are actively promoted as a smokeless and safer way to inhale nicotine without being exposed to tar and the many other toxic components of standard cigarettes, and as an aid to smoking cessation.

The industry started on the internet and at shopping-mall kiosks, and sales have rocketed. An ASH Fact Sheet published in May 2016 reported that:

1. An estimated 2.8 million adults in Great Britain were currently using electronic cigarettes.

2. Users were fairly evenly divided between smokers (1.4 million) and ex-smokers (1.3 million).

3. The proportion of ex-smokers had increased; in 2014 two-thirds of current vapers were smokers and one-third ex-smokers.

4. The main reason given by ex-smokers who are currently vaping is to help them stop smoking, while for current smokers the main reason is to reduce the amount they smoke.

5. Perceptions of harm from electronic cigarettes have grown, with only 15% of the public accurately believing in 2016 that electronic cigarettes are a lot less harmful than smoking.

Endorsement by celebrities on social media exert a strong influence on e-cigarette uptake. Phua et al. (2017) examined the effects of endorser type (celebrities, non-celebrities, products only) in e-cigarette brand Instagram advertisements on e-cigarette attitudes and smoking intentions. Celebrity endorsers significantly increased positive attitudes towards e-cigarettes and smoking intentions, compared to non-celebrities or products only. Celebrity endorsers rated significantly higher on trustworthiness, expertise, goodwill and attractiveness compared to non-celebrities. Hence the use of celebrity endorsement by companies.

E-cigarettes are subject to limited regulation and are not licensed as a medicine in the UK. In 2014, under regulations by the Food and Drug Administration, the US federal government banned sales of electronic cigarettes to minors and required approval for new products and health warning labels. Researchers are still unsure how effective e-cigarettes are as a quitting aid in comparison to other therapies, such as nicotine patches.

Glynn (2014) summarized current concerns about e-cigarettes. There is a lack of sufficient scientific data about their long-term safety, not only for users, but for infants and children. For example, Bassett et al. (2014) reported nicotine poisoning in an infant who consumed a quantity of e-cigarette liquid. Other areas of uncertainty are: their effectiveness as smoking cessation aids; their ability to deliver enough nicotine to satisfy withdrawal effects; the potential for e-cigarette use to reverse the decades-long public health effort to 'denormalize' combusted cigarette use; the effects of second-hand vapour from e-cigarettes, as well as the desire of most people to avoid being exposed to this vapour in public places such as restaurants, movie theatres and aeroplanes, whether proven to be a health hazard or not; whether the use of e-cigarettes encourages smokers who might have otherwise quit to continue smoking and only use e-cigarettes when they are in no-smoking environments (i.e., the 'dual use' concern); and whether young people may use e-cigarettes as an introduction to smoking regular combusted cigarettes. Until we have answers to these questions, it would be wrong to assume that e-cigarettes are the panacea that producers and users like to assume. The jury is still out.

FUTURE RESEARCH

1. There is a need for increased understanding of the social, ethnic and gender variations in smoking among young people and the impact of tobacco advertising on different groups.

2. Much of the research to date on smoking cessation has been biased by industrial interests. Research is necessary by independent investigators on effective methods of smoking prevention and cessation.

3. More real-world research is needed on e-cigarettes as a potential gateway to smoking, on the dual use of e-cigarettes with conventional cigarettes, and on the long-term effects of vaping on nicotine addiction, to clarify the impact of vaping on human health.

4. More evaluation is needed of non-pharmaceutical methods of smoking cessation that aim at nicotine abstinence rather than substitution by vaping or NRT.

SUMMARY

1. Smoking prevalence varies according to sex, social class and ethnicity.
2. A biopsychosocial model focuses on the experience of smoking, its motivation, and its emotional and social associations. Biological, psychological and social factors contribute to the smoking epidemic.
3. Effective tobacco control requires a multi-level approach, including economic, political, social and psychological interventions.
4. Most smokers report difficulty in quitting the habit. However, significant progress has been made in understanding smoking cessation from a psychological perspective.

5. Efficacy and cost-effectiveness are higher when treatment strategies address the causes and not the symptoms.
6. Smokers wishing to quit are helped using the 'five As': Ask about tobacco use; Advise to quit; Assess willingness to make a quit attempt; Assist in quit attempt; Arrange follow-up.
7. Smokers unwilling to quit are helped using the 'five Rs': explain the Relevance; Risks; Rewards; run over the Roadblocks; and Repeat at every available opportunity.
8. Health care systems in Western countries have been compromised by experts working with the pharmaceutical industry to promote treatments such as nicotine replacement therapy that are less effective than other available interventions.
9. Evaluation studies using real-world observation have produced outcomes that are significantly less favourable to products such as NRT than randomized controlled trials.
10. The vast majority of smokers who stop smoking have done so without outside help. Self-quitting to become nicotine free is safer than vaping and using nicotine replacement. The self-help route needs to be promoted as a viable alternative to pharmaceutical interventions.

PHYSICAL ACTIVITY AND EXERCISE

'By equating certain types of behaviour with virtue and others with vice, the secular moralists ... threaten to undermine the critical task of educating the public in general ... to the very real dangers lurking behind everyday behavioural choices.'

Leichter (1997: 360–1)

OUTLINE

Recent years have seen an increased official concern about the apparent widespread decline in the participation of people in all types of physical activity. In this chapter, we review evidence on the increasing prevalence of sedentary behaviour and its potential impact on health. We consider the social and psychological factors associated with participation, the varying meanings of different forms of physical activity, and strategies that have been used to promote greater participation.

EXTENT OF PHYSICAL ACTIVITY

Evidence from a variety of social surveys has confirmed the increasingly sedentary lifestyle of modern society. A summary of physical activity statistics in the UK (Townsend et al., 2015) found that in 2012 67% of men in England and Scotland met recommended levels of physical activity. Women were less active than men, with 55% reporting meeting recommended levels.

According to a survey of types of physical activity which adults engage in in England (Craig and Mindell, 2013), men spent only 2.7 hours per week walking and 2.1 hours per week in sports/exercise. The comparable figures for women were 2.5 and 1.2 hours.

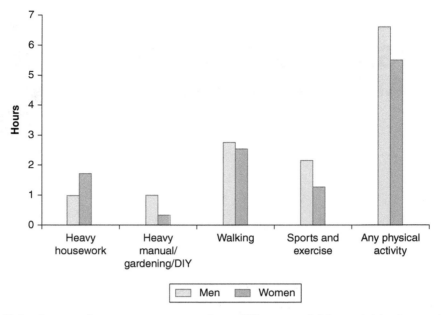

Figure 13.1   Average hours spent per week on different activities outside the workplace, by gender, England 2012

Data from Europe suggest that the main reasons people give for engaging in sport or physical activity are to improve health, to improve fitness and to relax (European Commission, 2014). To have fun comes fourth in the list of reasons (Figure 13.2).

VARIATION IN PARTICIPATION

Evidence from national surveys in England (Craig and Mindell, 2013) confirm that physical activity is related to household income, with 76% of men in the highest income quintile reaching recommended activity levels compared with only 55% of men in the lowest quintile. It was also related to age, with only 30% of men in England over 75 years meeting recommended activity levels. These figures concealed the large amount of time that adults spend engaging in no physical activity. A total of 59% of men and 54% of women in England reported spending five plus hours a day sitting or standing (see Figure 13.3).

There are also substantial international variations, with evidence that adults in the UK are much less likely to engage in physical activity. For example, whereas 44% of adults in the Netherlands engage in physical activity outside sport, the comparable figure for the UK was 14%. One problem with many of the estimates of participation of physical activity is that they often focus on leisure time activity, especially organized sports. Attempts to measure the extent of physical activity at work and at home are more limited. The study by Cochrane et al. (2009) used the International Physical Ability Questionnaire, which requires participants to complete a daily record for seven days of activity in four domains: work related, active transport, gardening and domestic, and leisure. It is then possible to obtain a measure of energy in each of these domains. In the survey of a sample of residents of an English Midlands city, they found that work accounted for 44% of reports of physical activity, compared to 32% for garden and domestic activity, and 12% for both active transport (walking and cycling) and leisure. However, the median level of physical activity at work was zero for both men and women and zero for leisure activity for women. This would suggest that many people have very sedentary working styles and most women participate little in leisure-time physical activity.

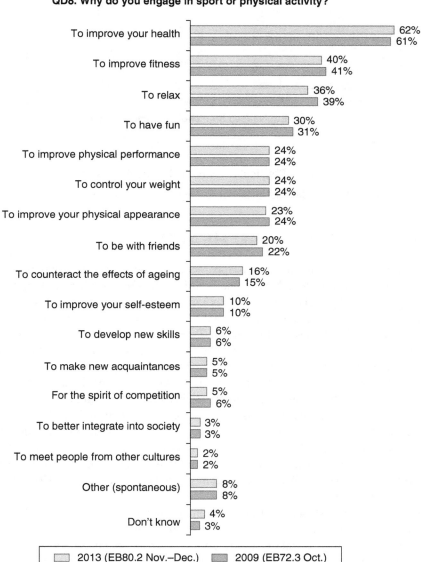

QD8. Why do you engage in sport or physical activity?

	2013 (EB80.2 Nov.–Dec.)	2009 (EB72.3 Oct.)
To improve your health	62%	61%
To improve fitness	40%	41%
To relax	36%	39%
To have fun	30%	31%
To improve physical performance	24%	24%
To control your weight	24%	24%
To improve your physical appearance	23%	24%
To be with friends	20%	22%
To counteract the effects of ageing	16%	15%
To improve your self-esteem	10%	10%
To develop new skills	6%	6%
To make new acquaintances	5%	5%
For the spirit of competition	5%	6%
To better integrate into society	3%	3%
To meet people from other cultures	2%	2%
Other (spontaneous)	8%	8%
Don't know	4%	3%

Figure 13.2   Data from the Eurobarometer on motivation for sport and physical activity

Source: European Commission (2014)

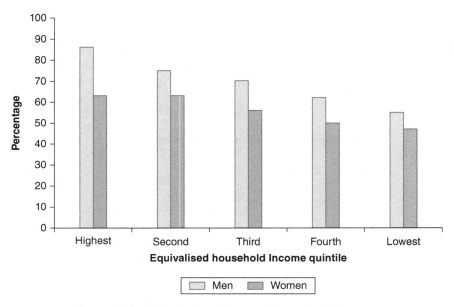

Figure 13.3   Physical activity and household income

Source: Data based on Health Survey for England - 2012, December 18, 2013

PHYSICAL ACTIVITY AND HEALTH

The reason for governmental interest in this apparent decline in physical activity is the increasing evidence of the negative impact on health. The World Health Organization (2004b) has identified the decreasing level of physical activity as a major cause of death and chronic disease worldwide. Rates of the following diseases have been found to be associated with higher rates of physical inactivity: cardiovascular disease, colon cancer, Type 2 diabetes, stroke and breast cancer. The WHO also highlighted the dose–response character of this activity–disease relationship with the greater amounts of physical activity being associated with greater levels of health.

A result of inactivity has been the increase in levels of obesity in the population. Since increased levels of obesity are due to an imbalance between energy intake and energy expenditure it is not surprising that evidence of a decrease in physical activity has been followed by evidence of an increase in rates of obesity. According to Public Health England (Health and Social Care Information, 2014), approximately one in four adults in the country are now classified as obese. International comparisons show that while the USA has the highest rates of obesity, other industrialized nations are catching up. (For further discussion of the obesity pandemic, see Chapter 10.)

This evidence has led to a series of governmental reports recommending increased participation in physical activity. However, these reports can adopt a victim-blaming stance to those who participate little in physical activity and ignore the broad social context.

Much psychological research in this field is far removed from 'rocket science'. Typically, it is based on very basic models and simple variables, and often the findings are self-evident and no more than 'common sense'. Because of the shortcomings and lack of sophistication in models and theories, our ability to provide a satisfactory account of the bigger issues remains limited. It is important to consider in a more nuanced fashion how social, environmental and psychological processes work together in explaining participation in physical activities. Of key importance is the meaning of exercise, not its actual amount.

CONTEXT OF PHYSICAL ACTIVITY

Socio-cultural context

As noted, an understanding of the variations in the extent of participation in physical activities requires attention to the socio-cultural and political context within which they have meaning and which promote or discourage involvement in such pursuits. We discussed in Chapter 10 the evidence that human beings traditionally required considerable energy expenditure for survival. In ancient times hunter-gatherers needed to expend substantial energy on a regular basis to ensure access to food and shelter. This need to expend significant amounts of energy remained well into the twentieth century and continues in much of the developing world. However, the rapid increase in technology in industrialized societies over the past generation has led to a much more sedentary lifestyle. This decline in physical activity is a consequence of the reduced need for energy expenditure in all spheres of human life, including work, transportation and home maintenance (Eaton and Eaton, 2003). Technological developments in entertainment have reduced the role of physical activity in leisure time (King, 1994).

Increasing attention has been paid to the influence of neoliberalism on everyday lives. One concept that has gained interest is **affluenza**, a combination of the concepts influenza and affluence. In modern consumer society, we are constantly persuaded that the key to success is greater consumption of commodities. Everything is offered for sale, including a certain lifestyle and a certain body shape. According to James (2007), the growth of 'affluenza' is one of the symptoms of the broader move towards increasing social inequality. He defined 'affluenza' as the increasing value placed on money, possessions and appearance. Part of this is the trend towards a more passive consumerist lifestyle and the belief that it is possible to purchase physical health through health supplements and membership of sports clubs. However, increasing social inequality has placed many of these products outside the reach of an increasing number of people who initially bought into this dream. Nowadays there is more evidence that people are increasingly resisting the myths peddled by advertisers (Hamilton and Denniss, 2010). While more empirical research is needed on this concept, it highlights the importance of the broader socio-cultural context.

Physical activities are also conducted within a cultural context that promotes different ideals about physicality. For example, the muscular physique is presented as the ideal male form in Western societies. As Luschen et al. (1996: 201) noted, the emergence of bodybuilding exercises aimed at building muscular strength and fitness 'reflects a bodily culture that is in line with American values of masculine prowess'. They continued: 'activities like American football, weightlifting, and boxing set a premium on brute physical force and place much less emphasis on endurance and relaxation' (Luschen et al., 1996: 202). The ability to attain this physical shape is promised to those who participate in various fitness gyms. However, access to these somewhat elite facilities is often restricted to those with money. In addition, aggressive sporting activities are also promoted among the middle class as a training ground for developing an aggressive business attitude, not to mention the making of useful social contacts. This begins at an early age, as is illustrated in studies of school sporting activities (Wright et al., 2003).

An important aspect of culture is religion. Different religions have different concepts of the body (see Chapter 6). For example, certain forms of Christianity traditionally held a negative view of excessive concern about the body. It has been suggested that this is a reason for the poorer performance of athletes from more Catholic countries in sporting events (Curtis and White, 1992). Conversely, in more Protestant or secular societies, concern with body shape and performance is promoted. Indeed, Turner (1984) has argued that contemporary concern for the body could be described as the 'new Protestant ethic'. As health psychologists, we need to engage with research into these broad socio-cultural processes.

Environmental context

Environmental psychologists emphasize the importance of considering the **behavioural setting**, or the physical and social context within which the behaviour occurs (Stokols, 1992). This includes the built environment, the buildings in which we live and work, and the communities in which we reside. The contemporary urban environment is 'passivogenic'. Modern buildings certainly are not designed with increasing physical activity in mind. Architects have created environments that foster inactivity and obesification (see Chapter 10). For example, stairways are often more difficult to access than either escalators or elevators. Airports use 'travelators' that allow people to stand still while being moved from A to B. Suburban bus services take shoppers directly from a nearby bus stop to superstores. Huge shopping malls have replaced high streets. Communities often have poor play facilities and unaffordable fitness centres, which is especially the case in low-income neighbourhoods. The most common means of transport is cars; cycling and walking are discouraged or dangerous (Sallis et al., 1998). In a city such as London there is a high rate of fatalities among cyclists, who still have to navigate their way on the same roads as heavy goods vehicles (HGVs). In this respect, countries such as Germany and the Netherlands are more progressive.

An Australian study by Salmon et al. (2003) found that personal barriers, such as lack of time, other priorities, work and family commitments, predicted the extent of involvement in physical activities more than environmental barriers such as weather, cost and safety. It is worth noting that these immediate personal barriers reflect broader social demands. Another Australian study by Giles-Corti and Donovan (2002) also found that individual and social environmental factors were more important than physical environmental factors in predicting exercise participation. They found that the most important predictors of participation in recreational physical activity were perceived behavioural control, behavioural intention, habit and exercising peers. The most important environmental predictor was accessibility to recreational facilities.

In the USA, Wilson et al. (2007) conducted a telephone survey of physical activity among residents of South Carolina. They found that those residents who reported that they lived in a pleasant neighbourhood were trusting of their neighbours and had sidewalks in their neighbourhood were less likely to report being physically inactive. A study in Chicago found that residents of suburbs and those who had elevated levels of fear about their neighbourhoods were less likely to walk (Ross, 2000).

Humpel et al. (2002) conducted a review of 19 studies that looked at the relationship between physical activity and objectively determined physical environments. They found that physical activity was greater where there was evidence of accessibility, opportunities and aesthetic features of the neighbourhood, including safety. While these studies demonstrate the importance of environmental factors, it is important to consider the limited activity-friendly features and the greater exposure to various environmental threats for residents of disadvantaged neighbourhoods.

PSYCHOLOGICAL MODELS

Various social cognition models (SCMs) of health behaviour have been used to account for variations in the extent of participation in physical activity among adults. The four that have attracted most research interest are the theory of reasoned action/theory of planned behaviour, the social cognitive model, the self-determination theory and the transtheoretical model. We provided further details of these models in Chapter 8. Here we illustrate the application of the models to exercise behaviour.

Theories of reasoned action and planned behaviour

The theory of reasoned action (TRA) was developed by Ajzen and Fishbein (1980). As described in Chapter 8, this theory proposes that behaviour such as physical activity and exercise is predicted by intention to engage in such behaviour, which in turn is predicted by the individual's attitude towards exercise and the perceived social norm. The attitudinal component is a function of the perceived consequences of participating and a personal evaluation of those consequences, while the perceived norm is a function of the perceived expectations to participate and the motivation to comply with those expectations.

The theory of planned behaviour (TPB) developed by Ajzen (1985) introduced *perceived behavioural control* into the basic TRA theory and suggested that, besides the attitudinal and social norm components, whether someone intended to behave in a certain way depended upon the extent to which they believed they had control over a particular behaviour. There have been several meta-analytic studies that have used the TPB to account for involvement in physical activity. In a review of more than 30 studies, Hausenblas et al. (1997) found that there were significant mean correlations between exercise intention and attitude, subjective norm and perceived behavioural control. A subsequent review by Hagger et al. (2002) also found significant but lower correlations. However, a substantial proportion of the variance in studies of physical activity remains unaccounted for.

Hamilton and White (2010) explored the role of salient behavioural, normative and control beliefs among mothers and fathers of young children, drawing on the TPB framework. Interview data were analysed using thematic content analysis. Hamilton and White identified a range of advantages (e.g., improves parenting practices), disadvantages (e.g., interferes with commitments), barriers (e.g., time) and facilitators (e.g., social support) to performing physical activity, and normative pressures.

Extensions of the TPB have investigated the role of a range of other psychological factors, such as moral norms, affect, self-efficacy and past behaviour (Conner and Armitage, 1998). An example of the use of an extended TPB is a study by Abraham and Sheeran (2004). This found that **anticipated regret** accounted for an additional proportion of the variance in exercise intentions besides the core TPB variables.

Social cognitive theory

Bandura's (1986, 2001) social cognitive theory has been used extensively to account for participation in physical activity. Bandura's argument that self-efficacy is the common cognitive mechanism that mediates behavioural responses has been applied. It is argued that whether a person persists in a behaviour in different circumstances depends upon his/her perception of individual mastery over the behaviour. This sense of self-efficacy develops through personal experiences of success, but also from verbal support from others and the perceived level of physiological arousal. This theory is bidirectional such that not only can self-efficacy contribute to increased behavioural effort, but also success in the behaviour can contribute to increased self-efficacy.

In physical activity and exercise research, it has been found that self-efficacy predicts greater involvement (e.g., McAuley and Jacobson, 1991). Variants of self-efficacy have been found to predict involvement. These include *barrier self-efficacy,* or the confidence in one's ability to overcome barriers to regular exercise attendance (Brawley et al., 1998), *scheduling self- efficacy* (DuCharme and Brawley, 1995) and *exercise self-efficacy* (Poag-DuCharme and Brawley, 1993). Some studies have found a negative relationship such that lower levels of self-efficacy statistically predicted more physical activity. Rimal (2001), in a longitudinal study, found evidence of this and suggested that those with lower self-efficacy improved their self-efficacy over time which, in turn, led to greater exercise behaviour. Together these findings would confirm the interactive nature of self-efficacy beliefs and physical activity.

However, there remains concern about the value of self-efficacy as an explanation of the extent of involvement in physical activity. In his critical review of the evidence, French (2013) identified limitations with previous research, including the issue of generalizability from small studies. A crucial factor is whether such concepts as self-efficacy are relevant to all population groups. In a meta-analysis of studies of physical activity, Vasilijevic et al. (2016) found that the gap between self-efficacy and behaviour was greater among participants with low SES and who resided in deprived neighbourhoods. This would confirm that the ability to exert control over our behaviour is dependent upon circumstances.

Bandura distinguished between three forms of agency or efficacy: personal, collective and proxy. *Proxy efficacy* is the belief in the role of others in aiding the achievement of desired outcomes. Although at first this might seem to be the converse of self-efficacy, evidence suggests that it can be an important complement. The proxy is someone who will provide assistance and help a person to achieve his/her goals. A study of participants in a fitness class found that *fitness instructor efficacy* as well as self-efficacy beliefs were predictive of class attendance for initiates (Bray et al., 2001). However, Bandura (1997) cautioned that an over-reliance on the proxy may reduce the cultivation of personal competencies. In a study to test this possible negative effect, Shields and Brawley (2007) conducted a questionnaire study of participants in an exercise class. They found an interactive effect such that those participants who preferred proxy assistance expressed lower self-regulatory and task self-efficacy when faced with a class without a proxy. To promote sustainability of exercise behaviour, they concluded that proxy-agents (exercise instructors) should balance between helping participants and encouraging greater self-regulation.

Self-determination theory

A related factor to self-efficacy is **self-determination**. According to Deci and Ryan's (1985) self-determination theory (SDT), people will engage in many activities simply because of pure enjoyment or *intrinsic motivation*. A study in Wales (Ingledew et al., 1998) found that participants in the initial stages of exercising attributed participation more to extrinsic motives (e.g., appearance/weight management), whereas in the later stages they referred to intrinsic motives, such as enjoyment. It was concluded that intrinsic motives are important for progression to and maintenance of the exercise.

The self-determination theory also argues that there are basic psychological needs for autonomy, competence and relatedness. It is the satisfaction of these needs that leads to feelings of well-being. Teixeira et al. (2012) conducted a systematic review of studies which explored the value of self-determination theory for explaining participation in exercise and physical activity. They found that autonomous forms of motivation were strong predictors of exercise participation over time. More specifically, they found that internalized extrinsic regulation (e.g., valuing the outcomes of exercise) was an important initial motivator, while intrinsic motivation (e.g., valuing the experience of exercise) predicted long-term adoption of exercise.

Another related factor is the extent to which people predict that some activity will make them happy. Ruby et al. (2011) found that people underestimated how much they would enjoy participating in an exercise class. This was especially so on beginning an exercise programme, suggesting that getting over that initial apprehension about the programme is crucial to promoting greater activity. Kwan et al. (2017) found in an experimental study that encouraging participants to focus on the positive outcomes of exercise contributed to a more positive affective experience but no change in actual behaviour.

Transtheoretical model

The transtheoretical model (TTM) was developed by Prochaska and DiClemente (1983) to explain why anti-smoking messages were more successful for some people than others. According to the TTM, people adopting a new behaviour move through a series of stages of change within which they utilize different processes to support the changes. These stages are described in Chapter 8. Movement across the stages is dependent on *decisional balance* and *perceived self-efficacy*. *Decisional balance* is a cognitive assessment of the relative merits of the pros and cons of the exercise behaviour while *self-efficacy* is the belief in one's ability to perform the exercise. This model has been applied to physical activity by many researchers to describe the so-called five stages of exercise behaviour change (Marcus et al., 1992):

Pre-contemplation: sedentary, no intention of becoming active within six months.

Contemplation: still sedentary but does not accept the value/need for physical activity.

Preparation: person is intending to become more active in the very near future.

Action: person is physically active but only in the last six months.

Maintenance: person has been active for more than six months.

In addition to these five stages, an integral part of the TTM is the processes of change that describe movement from one stage to the next. Box 13.1 describes the character of the five experiential and the five behavioural processes of exercise behaviour change. Marcus et al. (1992) found that the five experiential change processes were more important in predicting progress in the initial stages of exercise behaviour change, while the five behavioural processes were more important in the later stages.

BOX 13.1

Processes of exercise behaviour change

Cognitive

Consciousness raising: gathering information about the benefits of exercise.

Dramatic relief: feelings about inactivity and its consequences.

Environmental re-evaluation: consideration of the consequences of inactivity on others.

Self re-evaluation: reconsidering the consequences of physical activity for self.

Social liberation: awareness of social norms.

Behavioural

Counter-conditioning: substituting alternatives to sedentary behaviours.

Helping relationships: support of others in becoming physically active.

Reinforcement management: rewards for physical activity.

Self-liberation: commitment to physical activity.

Stimulus control: avoiding environmental stimuli associated with physical activity.

Source: Derived from Marcus et al. (1992)

Moving across the stages is said to depend on '**decisional balance**', the balance of pros and cons. In a study that compared reasons for and against participation in exercise in groups of non-exercisers and regular exercisers, Cropley et al. (2003) found that the pre-contemplators provided relatively more *con* reasons while the maintainers provided relatively more *pro* reasons. It was concluded that one reason why people do not exercise is that they cannot think of good reasons to do so.

Evidence of the importance of self-efficacy was provided by Marcus et al. (1992), who found that those who were regularly participating in physical activity (action or maintenance stages) scored higher on this measure. They concluded that this suggests that those who are at the early stages (pre-contemplation and contemplation) have little confidence in their ability to exercise.

A comprehensive review of literature using the TTM to explain exercise found lots of inconsistencies (Spencer et al., 2006). It found that much of the research was conducted on white, middle-class female populations, which raised questions about the generalizability. Second, it found that specific research projects often did not assess all the components of the TTM.

Besides these operational criticisms of the TTM there have also been more conceptual criticisms. Sutton (2000a) argued that the TTM is not really a theoretical model at all but merely a description of 'pseudo stages' that are really arbitrary steps on a continuum of motivation. Armitage (2009) is sympathetic to this critique and suggests an alternative two-stage motivational–volitional model. However, he also argued that the focus of the critique on the stages of change has diverted attention away from the more interesting processes of change. West (2005) suggested moving on to develop a more theoretically coherent approach.

Self-concept

Recent social cognition modellers have suggested introducing a variety of additional psychological variables. Hagger et al. (2003) suggested introducing *perceived competence* (like self-efficacy) and self-concept. There is evidence that there is a positive relationship between physical self-concept and participation in physical activity. It is supposed that a person who feels positively about him- or herself in one domain (physical) is more likely to perform well in that domain. Marsh (1990) argued that this relationship is reciprocal such that prior self-concept affects subsequent physical activity and vice versa. Marsh et al. (2006) confirmed this reciprocal relationship and found that physical self-concept had an independent effect in the prediction of exercise intention beyond perceived control. In a study of American students, Brudzynski and Ebben (2010) found that most of them reported that the amount they exercised was related to how they felt about their body. Those who felt overweight or unattractive reported more exercise participation. In a study in Israel (Korn et al., 2013) it was found that among students, engagement in physical exercise enhanced self-reported body image. Interestingly, they concluded that future efforts to promote health promotion (including exercise) should reflect a collectivist rather than an individualistic ethos. Thus, the college health policy should promote greater opportunity for all students to engage in physical activities.

Comments

Health psychologists have tended to focus their attention on SCMs, such as those described above, as the prime determinants of physical activity. These models continue to attract substantial research interest. As noted in Chapter 8, these models have attracted criticism of their methodological and theoretical shortcomings (Sniehotta et al., 2014). Detailed meta-analyses of studies which have considered their predictive power have identified their weaknesses. For example, Rhodes and de Bruyn (2013) found that only 42% of intenders (from the TRA) successfully engaged in physical activity subsequently. From a conceptual level, cognitive models are insufficient because they rely on a restrictive individualistic and rationalistic view of humans (e.g., Marks, 1996; Mielewczyk and Willig, 2007; Murray, 2014b). They locate thinking in the head of the individual rather than as something that unfolds in interaction with others, leading to an individualistic focus in health promotion. There have been attempts to move beyond the focus on intrapsychic processes. For example, Ranby and Aiken (2016) identified the importance of the husband's role on wives' physical activity. Molloy et al. (2010) found that lower levels of social support for physical activity were associated with less activity, but only for women. This effect was partly mediated by perceived behavioural control and coping with planning.

Integrating psychological and environmental models

There have been increasing attempts to develop a more integrative ecological view of physical activity that combines environmental and psychosocial factors. For example, in a Canadian study, it was found that access to recreational facilities was associated with enhanced physical activity among those with elevated levels of intention to be active (Rhodes et al., 2007). In a US study, it was found that a combination of psychosocial factors (perceived social support, perceived barriers and self-efficacy) and environmental supports (walkability, aesthetics and walking facilities) was the best predictor of physical activity among older adults (Carlson et al., 2012).

In an extensive three-country study (Belgium, the USA and Australia), Van Dyck et al. (2014) examined the interaction of psychosocial and environmental factors in predicting the extent of walking and leisure time physical activity. They found that perceived social support from friends and perceived barriers were the strongest psychosocial correlates of these activities. They also found that the role of perceived social support from family was more important for women. However, even after controlling for the psychosocial attributes, environmental factors emerged as important. These included perceptions of residential density, proximity of destinations and aesthetics.

A social interactionist views the individual as part of a group and of a society. The individual's behaviour, thoughts and beliefs can be considered as unfolding in interaction with the groups and society as a means of adapting to changing circumstances. The person's decision to become involved in physical activity is the result of an ongoing engagement with his/her immediate social world.

Further criticisms of SCMs can be found in Chapter 8 and in Murray and Chamberlain (2015). There is increasing critical and qualitative research that considers the various meanings of physical activity and considers these within varying social and cultural contexts.

MEANINGS OF PHYSICAL ACTIVITY AMONG ADULTS

Understanding the extent of participation in physical activity requires an understanding of the different meanings of physical activity. This depends upon the character of everyday social experience.

Social class

People from diverse social backgrounds perceive physical activity differently. Calnan and Williams (1991) conducted detailed interviews with a sample of middle-aged men and women from south-east England. The participants were from different social backgrounds. They found clear social class differences in perceptions of exercise. Those from working-class backgrounds perceived exercise in relation to everyday tasks, activities and duties at home and at work. They adopted a functional definition of health and fitness. For them, their ability to 'exercise' their everyday tasks both confirmed and reaffirmed their health. For example, one farm worker said: 'I get enough exercise when I am working on the farm shovelling corn all day, you get enough exercise. In the garden out there, I take the dog for a walk, yet I get enough exercise' (Calnan and Williams, 1991: 518). They tended to be satisfied with their physical health, which they could enhance during their everyday activities.

Middle-class people tended to perceive exercise as not being part of their everyday activities. They preferred to define it with reference to recreational or leisure activities that they sometimes felt they could not engage in because of lack of time. Fitness for these individuals was defined in terms of athleticism, not in ability to perform everyday tasks. This group also made more reference to the health-promoting effects of exercise in terms of 'well-being' and relief from routine daily obligations. In discussing these class differences in perceptions of exercise, Calnan and Williams (1991) referred to the work of Bourdieu (1984: 214), who suggested that whereas working-class people express an instrumental relation to their bodily practices, middle-class people engage in health practices that are 'entirely opposed to (such) total, practically oriented movements'.

In a large-scale survey of young people's physical activity in Norway, Oygard and Anderssen (1998) also considered the importance of the meaning of exercise and the physical body. In discussing the relationship between social class and exercise, they also referred to the work of Bourdieu (1984), who suggested that this relationship derives from social class differences in attitude towards the body. In our society, the legitimized body emphasizes both inner and outer characteristics. While the former is concerned with the healthy body, the latter refers to the fit and slim body. The middle and upper classes are more able to produce this legitimized body since it requires investment in time and money. Working-class people, who have less free time, from necessity have a more instrumental view of their body and view concern with exercise and fitness as pretentious. Conversely, middle-class people with more leisure time and resources to expend promote a cult of health and a concern with physical appearance.

Gender

Men and women perceive physical activity differently depending upon their social and cultural background. In their survey, Oygard and Anderssen (1998) found that level of education was positively associated with extent of participation in physical activity among females, but not among males. In reviewing this finding, they referred to the suggestion that concern with the body is more common among those belonging to the cultural elite, who are more anxious about their appearance and their 'body for others' (Bourdieu, 1984: 213). Oygard and Anderssen (1998: 65) concluded: 'For females in higher social positions, it may be of importance to show others who they are by developing healthy and "delicate" bodies, i.e., they are more concerned with the inner and outer body than females in lower social positions.' However, they also added more prosaically that the lesser involvement of less educated females in physical activity may be due to them having limited access to leisure facilities. They found little evidence of a relationship between education and physical activity among males and suggest that this may reflect the greater promotion of male sporting activities and the greater integration of physical activity into male culture.

Age

It is well established that participation in physical activity declines steadily with age. This may reflect a variety of factors, including limited socialization into physical activity among that generation to perceived social exclusion. A study in New Zealand found that older people who participated in sporting activities reported that they were often confronted by a discouraging stance from younger people (Grant, 2001). This negative social value regarding seniors and sports would seem to be internalized such that many elderly people report limited participation for fear that they might incur an injury (O'Brien Cousins, 2000). Hardy and Grogan (2009) investigated older adults' influences and motivations to engage in physical activity in 48 52–87-year-old participants. Preventing disability through exercise was a key factor in determining physical activity participation. Other influences included enjoyment of exercise, having support from others as motivators to exercise and a perception of a limited appreciation for older people's needs.

Ethnicity

People from ethnic minorities participate less in various physical activities. This is due both to the social and environmental constraints and differences in the perceived nature of physical activity. Henderson and Ainsworth (2003) conducted interviews with African-American and American-Indian women about their perception of physical activity. These women emphasized not only the physiological but also the spiritual benefits of physical activity. As one woman said: 'I love being outside. Mostly I love taking walks. I love the quietness with that' (Henderson and Ainsworth, 2003: 317). Despite this positive view of physical activity, these women identified various obstacles to participation. This included perceived lack of time, job demands, tiredness, illness, family needs and safety issues. These constraints are not peculiar to women from ethnic minorities. Other studies (e.g., Verhoef Vézina-Im et al., 1992) have identified similar constraints as being common among other groups of women.

Culture

In an intensive qualitative study of adults from the Netherlands, the USA and Korea, Lim et al. (2011) explored the importance of both individual and structural factors in sports participation and how this differed between countries. In the US sample, the participants reported involvement in team sports while at school, but this declined as they moved into adulthood. Those who continued with sports tended to be involved in more individualistic activities, such as running, working-out or golf. They recalled fondly the social aspects of youth sports (e.g., 'Probably the thing I loved most about childhood sports was [that] "the neighbourhood" played whatever sport was in season'). However, they felt that this was less obvious among modern young people ('This is long gone in today's culture for most children and certainly for most adults'; Lim et al., 2011: 212). Among US adults the predominant form of sport experience was passive – they watched sports on television and perhaps at a stadium. This was an opportunity for social interaction since it was easier to find people who had shared fanship rather than shared sports involvement. In the Netherlands sample, there was evidence of greater continuity of sports participation from youth to adulthood. There was less evidence of the passive participation evident in the US sample. Conversely, the Korean sample was more like the US sample. Together, this cross-country comparison reveals the cultural variation in sports participation, with passive sporting participation being more extensive in the USA and Korea.

In terms of individual motivations for sports participation, there was also evidence of cultural variations. The Korean adults referred to social, business, health and entertainment factors. While the American adults also referred to the importance of social and health reasons, they referred to competition as well. In addition, they detailed more reasons for non-participation, such as career and family commitments and lack of time. This need for justifying non-participation could perhaps be interpreted as evidence of personal conflict with a great cultural expectation of participation.

Body image

There is growing interest in the concept of 'body image' or, more precisely, 'body imaging', and its relationship with physical activity. The term 'body image' is defined by Grogan (2006: 524) as 'a person's perceptions, feelings and thoughts about his or her body'. There has been extensive research exploring the relationship between exercise participation and body image. In an extensive review of over 100 studies, Hausenblas and Fallon (2006) concluded that exercise participation was associated with a more positively perceived body image. In addition, this relationship was apparent not only in correlational studies, but also in intervention studies such that those who participated in physical exercise programmes reported an enhanced body image following the programme. This led Hausenblas and Fallon (2006) to conclude that exercise programmes may be an effective intervention for people with poor body image. However, they also caution that there may be a negative effect with some sub-groups. For example, Slater and Tiggemann (2006) found that women who exercise a lot have higher levels of body dissatisfaction and a great drive for thinness. This follows the general critique of modern representations of women equating beauty with slimness. Not surprisingly, it has been found that women and girls who weigh more are more dissatisfied with their body (Healey, 2006), although this relationship depends upon various social and cultural factors.

There is less research on male body image. Most studies have investigated the dimensions of adiposity and muscularity. As expected, males have reported a greater desire than females to become more muscular (Grogan and Richards, 2002). The covers of men's health magazines show a globalized obsession with muscularity.

Campbell and Hausenblas (2009) conducted a meta-analysis of the research on the effects of exercise interventions on body image. They identified 57 interventions with pre-and post-data for the exercise and control groups. There was a small random effect, indicating that exercise interventions had improved body image compared to control conditions.

In our view, body imaging is not a fixed and static, intra-psychic phenomenon; like beliefs more generally, it develops in interaction and conversation with others and is embedded within a specific socio-cultural context (for more discussion of beliefs, see Chapter 6). As Gleeson and Frith (2006: 88) emphasize, 'it is more useful to consider body imaging as a process, an activity, rather than a product'. This re-orientation away from a static definition of body image emphasizes the need for more sophisticated qualitative work to explore the connection between the evolution of body imaging and physical activity.

EXERCISE AMONG CHILDREN

In the UK, it has been estimated that among 2–15-year-olds, four out of ten boys and six out of ten girls are not participating sufficiently in physical activity (Prescott-Clarke and Primatesta, 1998). As with adults, the extent of participation varies substantially. In Norway, Oygard and Anderssen (1998) found that teenage girls with higher levels of education were more physically active, whereas among boys there was less evidence of a relationship with level of education.

Physical activity levels established in childhood are maintained to some degree across the lifespan. Friedman et al. (2008) extracted data from the American Terman Life-Cycle Study, which began in 1922 and collected data on participants at regular intervals in subsequent decades. People with high active levels in childhood tended to report greater participation in physical activity in adulthood. This was especially the case for males. The longevity of activity levels added to governmental concern at the evidence of a decline in recent decades of the involvement of children in physical activity and exercise.

Several studies have confirmed the importance of family and friends. Coleman et al. (2008) found that parents and siblings served as prominent role models for children's physical activity. Wheeler (2012) found that this socialization of activity occurs through direct and indirect strategies and practices. Direct strategies include telling the child about the benefits of physical activity, while indirect strategies include parents' modelling physical activity. Downward et al.

(2014) found a gender linkage in these relationships, in particular for boys. In a longitudinal study, Bunke et al. (2013) identified the importance of social support from outside the family, including involvement in sports clubs and schools' informal connections.

Several psychosocial factors have been associated with participation, including physical competence, social acceptance and enjoyment. One can't help thinking that *joy* or *fun* must be *the* key element in participation in physical activities and exercise for people of all ages. The opportunity to enhance competence and skill level were identified by Weiss and Williams (2004) as other factors in maintaining involvement in sports. Conversely, factors that deterred involvement included expense, travel, limited choice of activity, experience, adult support, familiarity with the environment and knowledge of activities (Girginov and Hills, 2008). Factors predicting drop-out included negative experiences, such as *lack of fun*, coach conflicts and lack of playing time (Fraser-Thomas et al., 2008).

A decline in participation in physical activities occurs as children enter adolescence. This is particularly pronounced among girls. Not to put too fine a point upon it, looking 'cool' isn't easy in a sweaty T-shirt, lycra shorts and trainers with your hair in a mess and your makeup all smudged! It just isn't cool for adolescent girls to do sport (Slater and Tiggemann, 2006). The Scottish Health Survey 2012 (Rutherford et al., 2013) found that while eight out of ten 5–7-year-old children met the physical activity guideline, by 13–15 years this had dropped to 55%. The drop was most pronounced between 11–12 years (68%) and 13–15 years (55%), especially among girls, who showed a 21% drop in participation between these age groups from 66% to 45%. Reasons for a growing disinterest in physical activity among girls included perceptions of their femininity, fears about looking stupid and fears about safety (Dwyer et al., 2006).

During adolescence girls become particularly concerned with their body image. A large study of over 50,000 Australians found that concern among females about body image increased from 28% of 11–14-year-olds to 33% of 15–19-year-olds to 40% of 20–24-year-olds (Mission Australia, 2010). A survey of teenage girls by Symons et al. (2013) found that body dissatisfaction was associated with low physical activity levels and higher extrinsic motivation for physical activity. They concluded that education programmes should emphasize both the diversity of body shapes and intrinsic motivations for physical activity. Related to this is the extent that young people believe that their body shape can be changed. Lyons et al. (2015) found in a survey of female students that those who agreed with an incremental theory of the body (one that can change) were more likely to engage in physical activity than those who endorsed an entity theory of the body (one that is fixed).

MEANING OF PHYSICAL ACTIVITY FOR YOUNG PEOPLE

An increasing number of qualitative studies have begun to clarify the changing experiences of physical activity among young people. Kunesh et al. (1992) investigated school play activities of 11–12-year-old girls in central USA. In interviews, the girls reported that they found physically active games at home and at school enjoyable. However, in the school playground the girls preferred to stand in a group and talk while the boys participated in various games. When the girls did participate in games often they were criticized by the boys for their supposed inferior performance. To avoid this negative treatment, the girls excluded themselves. The girls reported that when playing at school they felt nervous and embarrassed. These findings suggest that while at an early age boys and girls both enjoy physical activities, by the time they reach puberty the girls feel that they are being excluded or they exclude themselves for other reasons.

Qualitative studies have investigated gender and social class factors associated with different forms of participation of children in various forms of physical activity. In a study of the images in teenage girls' magazines, Cockburn and Clarke (2002) found two polarized female images: one actively involved in romantic activities versus the aberrant female involved in physical activity. The teenage girls in her study resented these stereotypical images and felt that it did not accord with the everyday conflicts they experienced. However, they also voiced concern at the increasing social restraints on their involvement in sporting activities. For example, one girl said: 'when I was at primary school I just used to go out there and I'd do anything ... I wouldn't care what other people thought, I'd just go out and enjoy it ... now it's more, "Oh my god can I do this?" And you know, like everybody's looking at you ... I hate it.'

Together, these studies confirm the importance of the various meanings associated with physical activity among children and young people. For teenagers, being cool and looking cool is the main issue.

PROMOTING PHYSICAL ACTIVITY

With the growing evidence on the health benefits of physical activity and exercise, governments and health authorities have become keen to promote greater participation. For example, in the UK, the Department of Health requires all health authorities to contribute to local programmes designed to promote greater physical activity (Department of Health, 2011). These have included population-, community-, school- and clinic-based interventions.

Population-based strategies

Population-based strategies are designed to promote more widespread participation in physical activity in society. The strategies range from ones with an environmental focus, such as the introduction of cycle lanes in cities and reducing traffic speed, to mass media campaigns. The impact of these interventions varies. An evaluation of an intervention designed to promote physical activity (Sallis et al., 2007) found that it had a greater impact among women in the area who reported no unattended dogs and low crime in their neighbourhood, and among men who reported often seeing people being active in their neighbourhood.

However, these environmental supports for physical activity are not equally distributed in society. In a review of the literature, Taylor et al. (2006) identified the strong inverse relationship between what they termed physical activity-friendly environments and low-income and ethnic minority groups. To promote an activity-friendly environment requires an 'environmental' or 'social justice' approach that aims to redress social inequalities in exposure to environmental hazards. We covered this issue in detail in Chapter 5.

In public buildings, physical strategies have been employed to promote greater physical activity. It isn't rocket science: simply displaying posters near stairwells promotes greater usage. A variant of this is the positioning of health promotion messages on the actual stair rises. A study of a shopping centre in England found that such an initiative more than doubled stair usage (Kerr et al., 2001). While these cheap and simple measures are important, the many occupational hazards in the workplace, which are again unfairly distributed, cannot be ignored.

The third population-based strategy is mass media campaigns. A survey of European countries found that residents of those countries who perceived that public policy was promoting physical activity were more likely to report participating in such activity (Von Lengerke et al., 2004). However, moves to promote exercise through healthy public policy must be distinguished from the further promotion of the ideology of individualistic self-control (Marks, 1996). Although middle-class adults may be attracted to this message, many people from working-class and more deprived backgrounds may treat it with cynicism (Crossley, 2003). Often, there seems to be a disconnection between healthy public policies and the material circumstances of people's everyday lives (Murray and Campbell, 2003) and it invites the same 'victim-blaming' criticism as traditional health education (Crawford, 1980). An inactive and obese person might well feel that they are to blame, and feel more than their fair share of stigma and shame.

Community-based strategies

Interventions that have attempted to increase participation in communities have often been based upon social cognition models (SCMs), especially the TTM. Marcus et al. (1992) designed an exercise intervention for volunteers recruited from a community. The character of the intervention was matched to the initial stage of change of the volunteers. On follow-up, there was evidence of a significant increase in involvement in exercise commensurate with the initial stage. In a subsequent randomized controlled trial, Marcus et al. (1994) found further supportive evidence. At three-month follow-up the participants in the stage-matched group showed stage progression (i.e., greater interest or involvement in exercise), while those in the standard group showed stage stability or regression.

Clarke and Eves (1997) found partial support for the TTM in describing the willingness of sedentary adults to participate in an exercise programme prescribed by their family doctor. They classified the participants into the pre-contemplation, contemplation and preparation stages, reflecting the fact that at this stage they had not begun the programme. As predicted, the cons of participation in the exercise programme decreased across the stages, although there was slight change in the pros. The barriers to participation identified were lack of support, lack of facilities, dislike of exercise and lack of time. The importance of dislike of exercise declined across the stages, while the importance of lack of facilities increased. The finding that lack of time was used as frequently by those in the pre-contemplation as those in the preparation stage was interpreted as evidence that it is more a justification for lack of participation rather than a convincing reason.

Other studies have expanded the basic TTM to consider the importance of *outcome expectancies* (Williams et al., 2005). For example, Dunton and Vaughan (2008) investigated the role of anticipated positive and negative emotions. This study was a three-month follow-up of a sample of healthy, community-dwelling adults who agreed to participate in an exercise programme. Dunton and Vaughan found that anticipated emotions interacted with stage of behaviour change in predicting activity adoption and maintenance. At baseline, they found that anticipated positive emotions of success were lowest in those classed in the pre-contemplation stage, while anticipated negative emotions of failure were highest in those classed in the maintenance stage. Further, anticipated positive emotions of success predicted physical activity adoption and maintenance.

Hutchison et al. (2013) presented an alternative to the dominant SCMs of physical activity promotion derived from in-depth interviews with a sample of previously sedentary adults who had successfully completed a physical activity course. This alternative model consists of cues, leading to certain cognitions and action determinants and then to behavioural responses (physical activity). Underlying this model were intervening core values that were the key to behaviour change. The most important values that were associated with uptake of physical activity were social orientation (importance of close interpersonal relations), competence orientation (importance of personal success or competence), control orientation (importance of independence of action) and health orientation (importance of health). It is argued that the derivation of this model from detailed interviews provided ecological validity. However, absent from their model is the broader socio-cultural and political context within which the values draw meaning.

A related cognitive intervention that has attracted attention is that based on control theory (Carver and Scheier, 1982). This theory argues that people self-monitor their behaviour against certain standards. When their performance drops below the standard, they attempt to rectify this by increasing their activity. Based upon this theory, attempts to promote greater physical activity should promote self-monitoring, goal-setting and provide feedback. In an experimental study, Prestwich et al. (2016) examined individuals who were encouraged to self-monitor their planned physical activity and to set goals as regards their level of physical activity. Those individuals assigned to the group which promoted self-monitoring, goal-setting and received feedback reported greater physical activity.

However, these cognitive interventions continue to focus on the individual. More recent community-based approaches adopt a more critical approach, emphasizing various forms of community mobilization. For example, Campbell (2014) emphasizes the need to consider broader political issues and the power relationships. As she argues, the focus should be on developing social interventions to 'reduce power inequalities (e.g., between rich and poor) that undermine people's opportunities to be healthy' (Campbell, 2014: 46).

School-based activities

Since children and young people spend much of their daily lives at schools or colleges, they have become the focus in promoting physical activity. The two main opportunities for children to participate in physical activity at school are during less-supervised breaks and during physical education classes.

Some research has focused on the less-organized physical activity that occurs during break times. It has been found that the larger the schoolyard, the more physical activity takes place. Also, if there are playground markings indicative of sporting/play activities, children are more likely to engage in physical activity (Escalante et al., 2012).

There is a long history of physical education (PE) in schools. This tradition, especially in British schools, has been based upon a nineteenth-century model of teaching children to perform a range of very masculinist and militaristic physical exercises where discipline and stoicism are key features (Paechter, 2003). Perhaps girls and less 'macho' or 'sporty' boys are rather more reluctant to give their all to too many of these exercises. In their study of teenage girls, Cockburn and Clarke (2002: 654) noted that: 'Many of these traditional and stereotypical rituals in PE contradict the notion of acceptable/desirable "appearance" within the teenage feminine culture and cause conflict for girls.' Indeed, this conflict with the dominant image of femininity can lead to a clash between what Cockburn and Clarke describe as two polarized identities. A girl can identify herself as a masculinized 'doer' of PE (a 'tomboy') or a feminized ('girlie') 'non-doer' of sport and physical activity. It is highly unlikely that girls can achieve both physically active and (heterosexually) desirable, so they are obliged to choose between these images (Cockburn and Clarke, 2002: 661). Further, in her study Paechter (2003) found that some girls demonstrate their femininity through deliberate resistance to PE.

Boys who are poor at school sporting activities also often attract ridicule from their more athletic peers. This is especially the case in those schools that emphasize the more physical sports. These games in which the boys are expected to demonstrate their strength have many similarities with military exploits (Paechter, 2003).

In a study of PE in Australian schools, Wright et al. (2003) showed how its character was clearly related to social class. Boys, especially those from affluent backgrounds, participated in organized team sports from an early age. For these boys, participation in sports was a very important part of the school ethos and identity. This led Wright et al. (2003: 25) to describe the social practices around sport as 'powerful disciplinary technologies (Foucault, 1980) whereby particular kinds of citizens, forms of masculinity and ways of interacting with physical activity are shaped'. In this setting, the young people are being trained to strongly identify with their school team and to act in a particularly aggressive way towards others. Sport thus becomes part of the training for a form of officer class and, indeed, competitions between teams representing schools, colleges or even nations take on some of the characteristics of battle or warfare.

In an Australian study of participation in sports and physical activity by rural teenage girls, Casey et al. (2009) found that the girls reported that they were more keen to participate if the activities were fun, involved being with their friends, and were supported by family and friends through role modelling and feedback.

Finally, in a comprehensive review of school-based physical activity programmes, Erwin et al. (2012) drew attention to the many difficulties involved in conducting comparative evaluations. They highlight the many difficulties of integrating physical activities into the school day, especially with the increasing attention to improving academic performance.

Clinic-based physical activity programmes

Exercise interventions are often targeted at certain sub-groups of the population, including people who are overweight, the elderly or those who suffer from particular health problems. The evaluations of these programmes have often been quantitative in design and have identified a limited number of social cognition variables that predict adherence to the programmes. In a review of the impact of exercise programmes for coronary heart disease, Woodgate and Brawley (2008) identified the importance of personal efficacy. They distinguished between task self-efficacy and self-regulatory efficacy.

A frequent problem with exercise programmes is that while many people sign up for such programmes, it has been estimated that 50% or more drop out after a brief period of participation (Dishman, 1986). In an exercise intervention study with older adults by Neupert et al. (2009), it was found that those who had greater self-efficacy and control beliefs at six months were more likely to continue exercise after one year. Somewhat similar findings were reported in a qualitative study of older adults in south-west England (Beck et al., 2010). This study found that all the older people interviewed searched for purpose in their lives, and for those older people who were physically active having an exercise schedule contributed to this sense of purpose. In addition, the physical activity offered a personal challenge to the older exercisers.

A wide range of techniques have been used to promote greater involvement in physical activity. Abraham and Michie (2008) identified 26 behaviour change techniques (BCTs), ranging from providing information about the behaviour–health link to providing information on others' approval. These reflected a range of different theoretical techniques: the theory of planned behaviour, social-cognitive theory and control theory. There has also been substantial intervention work exploring the value of interventions based upon various social cognitive models of physical activity. However, these have met with limited success. For example, in their meta-analysis of interventions based on the theory of planned behaviour, Rhodes and Dickau (2012) found limited impact on intention and behaviour. A more detailed meta-analysis by McDermott et al. (2016) found some behaviour change techniques had a positive impact on physical activity, although those based more on social cognitive theory (especially self-efficacy) had a more positive effect on intention than those based on the theory of planned behaviour.

Most of the interventions targeted at enhancing physical activity have used quantitative assessments. This restricts the opportunity to clarify what the participants feel about the various interventions. Several evaluations that have used qualitative methods have emphasized the importance of perceived enjoyment. A study by Daley et al. (2008) included a qualitative study within the larger randomized controlled trial of an exercise intervention for obese adolescents. This revealed that the participants expressed a variety of feelings, including feeling more energetic and pleased about potential weight loss.

In an intensive study of an exercise programme with older people, Hudson et al. (2015) found two comparative narratives. The first involved a narrative of 'decelerated decline' where, although the exercise programme was integrated into the current life narrative of the older person, there was limited personal meaning of the exercise. Conversely, the second narrative involved a re-storying of the personal narrative such that instead of the inevitable decline there was the prospect of challenging the so-called narrative foreclosure (Freeman, 2000). These two emergent narratives may depend upon the previous life-histories of the individuals.

Another qualitative study (Graham et al., 2008) explored the experiences of people with chronic illness and disability who participated in a physical exercise programme. Analysis of the interviews identified three polarized themes, which are summarized in Box 13.2. In reviewing these themes, it is apparent that the intervention is effective not just through improving physical ability. On a more social and psychological level the activity intervention also had value in enhancing mood, social connections and identity.

BOX 13.2

Reactions to participating in an exercise programme for disabled people

Passive distress vs. active mood management: whereas disability can contribute to a passive inactive lifestyle, participation can enhance mood and reduce patterns of rumination. For example: 'My energy wasn't great. I would get into the house and just sit down and say, "I can't be bothered", I was doing nothing at all. I was just going home, watching TV all day. I don't do that now because I think of the exercises. … I imagine myself within the group and I do a few [exercises] at home. I'm sort of motivated now.'

(Continued)

> *Identity erosion vs. identity renewal*: whereas disability and chronic illness can lead to feelings of identity loss, participation in physical activity contributed to a new identity of physical competence. For example, 'From being an outgoing, physical sort of person you were bedridden. That was mind-blowing. Terrible. Shattered. Suddenly this residual bit of fitness I had all my life was going out the window.' The exercise programme stopped that slide into inactivity.
>
> *Detachment vs. connection*: while disability can lead to detachment from familiar valued aspects of everyday life, such as friends and familiar bodily functioning, the intervention provided new connections. For example, 'Since getting so unwell I have lost contact with a lot of people I would have met when I was out and about. Now I don't have those kinds of contacts because I'm inside most of the time. I meet people here [day centre]. It's a bit like being exiled or being cast out – you think I'd leprosy sometimes! [laughs] Maybe I'll get a bell to warn people off.'
>
> *Source*: Graham et al. (2008). Reproduced by permission

Further, these strategies are largely focused at the individual level. They ignore the social context and the social meaning of exercise and physical activity. Social approaches attempt to widen the traditional individual change approach to include 'changes in social networks and structures, organizational norms, regulatory policies, and the physical environment as a means of enhancing long-term maintenance of the target behavior' (King, 1994: 1406).

ALTERNATIVE FORMS OF PHYSICAL ACTIVITY

There is increasing challenge to the dominance of the functional approaches to promoting physical activity with its attendant emphasis on physical health. Alternative strategies consider such issues as the more social, emotional and aesthetic aspects of physical activity. Three such alternative forms are dance, walking groups and lifestyle sports.

Dance

There has been a recent growth of interest in the health benefits of dance. It is considered a very non-intrusive means of promoting participation in physical activity and is attractive to men and women from different social backgrounds. For example, Baker (2002: 18) notes that, especially for younger people, dance is an important way of playing being sexual in which 'they try a more sexual presence on for size'. Among older people, it is a very enjoyable means of developing social interaction (Paulson, 2005).

Walking groups

Walking, especially in natural, semi-rural or rural settings, can be both physically and mentally exhilarating. Priest (2007) investigated what she termed the 'healing balm effect' of using a walking group to feel better. Priest combined methods from grounded theory and ethnography to explore members' experience of a mental-health day-service walking group. An overall model, the healing balm effect, integrated seven categories to describe the 'healing' properties of the experience: Closer to what is more natural; Feeling safe; Being part; Striving; Getting away; Being me; and Finding meaning. Several of the features reported by Priest would not be present, or would only be partially present, walking in towns or cities. The most beneficial urban walking places are likely to be commons or parks.

Kassavou et al. (2015) studied environmental factors that influence walking in groups using a walk-along interview procedure with ten leaders of walking groups. The leaders took groups to parks, city centres or did laps. Kassavou et al. identified the characteristics of place that influenced the type of walking that people do in groups and the processes used by walkers to find meaning in the places they walk. They found that the walking places were 'nodes' where people formed social networks. They were not restricted to the specific place (e.g., the park during walks), but expanded beyond that to other places for socializing. Walking alone would seemingly serve a different function, that of reflection, problem solving and creative thinking.

Lifestyle sports

Over the past 10–20 years a counter-establishment form of sporting activity has grown in popularity. A report by Tomlinson et al. (2005) collectively termed these activities as 'lifestyle sports'. They are also frequently termed *extreme sports* and include such activities as bungee jumping, white-water rafting, rock-climbing and surfing. These activities are especially popular among young people.

There is a growing body of research on who participates in these activities and the perceived character of the experience. Willig (2008) analysed detailed interviews with a small sample of eight extreme sports practitioners. The interviews were phenomenological in orientation and sought to grasp the meaning of the sports to the practitioners.

Unlike populist characterizations of these activities as reckless or sensation-seeking, it was apparent from these interviews that the participants carefully considered them. Willig suggested that participation in these activities enabled the participants to attain a state of being comparable to what Csikszentmihalyi (1997) has termed 'flow'. This is the experience of a sort of unity of the self, world and activity in which the more mundane, everyday worries and concerns become less important. As such, it could be argued that participation in these sports is a reaction to broader cultural demands on young people in our consumer society, which provides limited opportunity for such experiences. However, the individualistic nature of such activities can pose potential threats. For example, Willig cautions that while participation in these activities may be therapeutic, it may also lead to dependency.

AFTER ALL THAT

The past generation has seen the promotion within Western societies of a neoliberal philosophy promoting greater individual responsibility and minimal government intervention together with market fundamentalism (Ayo, 2012). This is particularly apparent within the physical activity arena. Harrington and Fullagar (2013) detailed how the promotion of the active living agenda by many Western governments positions the individual as responsible and ignores the other social and material constraints on participation. They note that 'the decline of the welfare state and the rise of liberal notions of responsibility have occurred alongside an increased reliance on market forces and voluntary organizations with stretched resources to provide opportunities for active leisure and sport' (Harrington and Fullagar, 2013: 141). In their study of Australian sport and recreation workers, they found that, while the workers were very committed to promoting enhanced participation, they were unsure of their impact in the light of limited resources. Instead people from disadvantaged backgrounds found it difficult to engage with these activities. This led to the victim-blaming of those such as overweight women, migrants, low-income families, older people, and those with disabilities, who found it difficult to participate in organized physical activities.

Ayo (2012) noted the pervasiveness of the active living agenda within Western societies. This ranges from the marketing of membership of sports clubs to sportswear. This promotion of an active health agenda contributes to what Galvin (2002) has termed a 'consumerist frenzy'. People join sports clubs and wear sports clothes but do not participate in sporting activities. Membership of elite sports clubs and purchase of expensive sportswear form part of a process of gaining enhanced social status and reinforcing social inequalities. A similar critique has been made of the 'active ageing' agenda (e.g., Timonen, 2015). There is a need to develop a more sophisticated approach to promoting physical activity.

FUTURE RESEARCH

1. Public participation in physical activity is continuing to decline, including participation of children and young people. We need to know more about why.

2. There is still a need to explore the specific impact of exercise interventions on the health of different population groups to demonstrate that increased activity improves health.

3. Research is needed to develop our understanding of the different meanings for different subgroups of the population.

4. Participatory action research offers an opportunity to increase our understanding of different perceptions of several types of physical activity programme.

SUMMARY

1. Interest in exercise has waxed and waned over the years. The past generation has witnessed increasing interest in the health benefits of exercise.
2. A substantial proportion of the populations of Western societies is sedentary.
3. Results of several comprehensive surveys indicate that moderate degrees of physical activity have both physical and psychological benefits.
4. There is some evidence to suggest that excessive exercise can have negative health effects. It may even prove fatal.
5. The degree of participation declines during adolescence, especially among girls.

6. In adulthood, there is less participation among females, those from poorer social positions and those from ethnic minorities.

7. Various psychological factors have been found to be associated with participation in both childhood and adulthood.

8. The meaning of exercise is linked to the varying social contexts. For young people, if it isn't perceived as 'cool' or as 'fun', they are unlikely to do it.

9. Exercise participation programmes can be either population based or aimed at high-risk groups. The main problem with both forms of programme is adherence, which is generally low.

10. Alternative methods of activity, such as dance, group walking and lifestyle sports, are capable of evoking joy, excitement and pleasure, which means that the activity is more likely to be repeated.

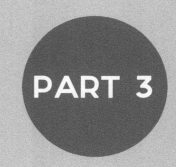

PART 3

HEALTH PROMOTION AND DISEASE PREVENTION

In Part 3 we introduce the key concepts, theories and approaches to health promotion and disease prevention. An ounce of prevention is worth a pound of cure, so the saying goes. The trouble is that the huge costs of medical and surgical treatments in health care leave only bread crumbs for health and illness prevention. The full potential for health psychologists in these fields is yet to be reached, but we review here some of the more valuable lines of inquiry.

In Chapter 14 we discuss the key roles provided by health information, communication and health literacy. We introduce communication theory and the e-health revolution and consider how health literacy can influence people's ability to access, understand and use health information.

In Chapter 15 we consider two forms of disease prevention within health care systems: screening and immunization. Both programmes have the objective of controlling and reducing risk. We discuss various social and psychological processes that are involved in explaining these processes of risk management.

In Chapter 16 we focus on the psychological dimensions of health promotion. We describe two contrasting approaches to health promotion: the behaviour change approach and the community development approach.

INFORMATION, COMMUNICATION AND HEALTH LITERACY

'The problem with communication is the illusion that it has been accomplished.'

George Bernard Shaw

OUTLINE

Here we discuss health information, communication and the role of health literacy. We begin with an introduction to communication theory and discuss the e-health revolution, research about health care professional–patient communication and health message framing. We consider how health literacy can influence people's ability to access, understand and use health information. Finally, we examine strategies to make health communication more effective by enhancing the skills of health care providers and service users, simplifying the health care system and promoting health-sustaining environments.

WHAT IS HEALTH COMMUNICATION?

Health communication refers to all interpersonal, organizational or mass communication that concerns health. It can occur in various *contexts* (e.g., doctor–patient communication, public health campaigns); be applied in a variety of *settings* (e.g., clinics, schools, workplaces, online communities); use a variety of *channels* (e.g., face-to-face communication, posters, social media); deliver a variety of *messages* (e.g., healthy eating, smoking cessation, safe sex); and serve a variety of *purposes* (e.g., risk assessment, communication of diagnosis, service awareness, advocacy). To understand the nature of health communication, first we need to understand what is meant by the term 'communication'.

Communication refers to the exchange of information between one person, or 'entity', and one or more others. There is a magic to excellent communication that can be instantly recognized, but precisely how this 'magic' is achieved is slightly mysterious. To describe how messages are transmitted in the communication process, Shannon and Weaver (1949) proposed one of the best-known (and longest lasting) models of communication. As we have seen, most models have a shelf life of about 15 or 20 years, but this model has been mentioned in dispatches for 65 years and is about to draw its pension. The model has five basic components:

- *Source* – where the message is coming from.
- *Transmitter* – something that 'encodes' the message into signals.
- *Channel* – where encoded signals are transmitted.
- *Receiver* – something that 'decodes' the signal back into the message.
- *Destination* – where the message goes.

As an example, writing and reading this book form part of a communication process. As authors (source), we have a message to communicate to you, our reader (destination). We transmit this message through printed text (transmitter) using this book (channel). You read the book with your eyes and then decode the message with your brain (receiver). Hopefully the message will reach you as we originally intended! However, *noise* can also interfere in the communication process. Noise can be translated literally as *physical noise* (e.g., a crackly phone line or loud music in the background), *cognitive noise* (e.g., being distracted by other concerns such as remembering to telephone a friend, feed the cat or water the pot plants), *affective noise* (e.g., you may be feeling anxious about a forthcoming meeting with your instructor), or *socio-cultural noise* (e.g., we write 'cool' as in 'temperature' and you read 'sick' as in 'awesome'). Considering these factors, it is important that all forms of noise are minimized.

Originally developed in a technical report for a telephone company, Shannon and Weaver's model evolved over time and is the simplest and most influential model of communication. As a receiver of health information, it is important to consider the *message* and its *source*. This is a useful descriptive model that serves a didactic function but precious little more. What is the message being communicated? How reliable and accurate is the source? For health information providers, it is important to consider the *purpose* of communication and the target *destination* – who are they trying to reach and why? How will they effectively reach their audience considering personal backgrounds, capabilities, and socio-cultural contexts in which they operate? What would be the best mode of communication to transmit information? How can distortions (noise) be minimized and clarity in understanding maximized? What are the factors that compete for the recipients' attention and what strategies can be used to ensure that the communication aims are achieved? These are some questions health communication researchers look into.

In this chapter, we discuss health care professional–patient communication, health-message framing, e-health and m-health. We also consider how health literacy influences effective health communication and the strategies that can be used to promote it.

HEALTH CARE PROFESSIONAL–PATIENT COMMUNICATION

Effective communication between health care professionals (HCPs) and patients is integral to health promotion, disease prevention and treatment, and is an essential skill that can greatly improve the quality and efficiency of care. The way HCPs relate to and communicate with service users can have a profound impact on their psychosocial adjustment, decision-making, treatment compliance and satisfaction (Rodin et al., 2009). As shown in Figure 14.1, there are direct and indirect pathways that link effective communication with health outcomes (Street et al., 2009). The direct path highlights benefits related to improved survival and remission rates, enhanced emotional well-being, pain control, functional ability, vitality and reduced suffering. Good communication may also facilitate better HCP–patient relationships, which can improve intermediate outcomes, such as access to care, treatment adherence, self-management, support and trust in the health care system.

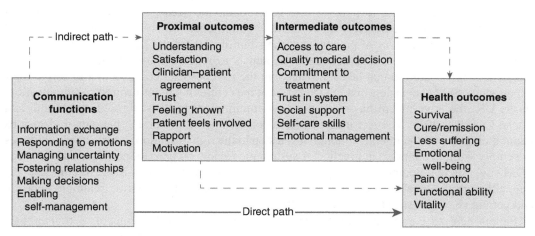

Figure 14.1 Communication and health outcomes

Source: Adapted from Street et al. (2009)

In a 'classic' study, Byrne and Long (1976) identified different doctors' styles of communicating with patients. They analysed audiotape interactions from 71 GPs and about 2,500 patients. They identified four diagnostic styles and seven prescriptive styles used by the doctors. These styles constituted a continuum from 'patient-centred' to 'doctor-centred' styles. A **patient-centred communication style** makes use of the patient's knowledge and experience through techniques such as silence, listening and reflection, whereas a **doctor-centred communication style** makes use of the doctor's knowledge and skill with minimal input from the patient. Using leadership theory, Huynh and Sweeny (2013) updated these communication styles and outlined three patterned approaches to patient care among clinicians: (1) *laissez-faire* (negligent and unsympathetic towards patients); (2) *transactional* (sets health goals and provides patients with instructions, feedback and reinforcement to pursue these behaviour goals); and (3) *transformational* (provides health goals, inspires and motivates patients to be personally engaged in those goals). Using patient-reported data and observer ratings, it has been suggested that the transformational patient care style is the best predictor of patient satisfaction and health expectations compared to other communication styles (Huynh et al., 2016).

Since the 1970s there has been a movement towards a consumerist model of health care that places patients to the fore. While doctors and HCPs were once viewed as figures of authority, patient empowerment has become a trend that encourages service users to question authority, demand more from practitioners and be more proactive in their own health care. The major criticism of doctors' traditional communication style was that it was characterized by working to rigid agendas and little listening to patients' accounts and discussion of treatment options. Thus, a more patient-centred approach has been called for and, to varying degrees across different settings, this has been received.

PATIENT-CENTRED COMMUNICATION

Patient-centred communication (PCC) refers to communication among HCPs, service users and their families that is intended to promote patient-centred care. Patient-centred care is 'compassionate, empathetic and responsive care that reflects the needs, values and preferences of patients' (Institute of Medicine, 2001). PCC is a communication style that aims to elicit and understand the perspectives of patients and their families about the patient's particular health condition, its management and treatment. Its aim is to reach a shared understanding of the patient's health condition that takes into account the psychosocial contexts that underpin their experiences. Shared decision-making (SDM) is at the centre of patient-centred communication. In the UK, the government has made a strong commitment to SDM through the Health and Social Care Act 2012. The Act incorporates a commitment to involving patients in decisions about their care and treatment. Although it is a step in the right direction, policy-level initiatives are empty without adoption in practice. A systematic review on practitioners' attitudes towards SDM suggests that doctors generally express positive attitudes towards SDM in clinical practice, although the level of support can vary according to clinical scenario, treatment decision and patient characteristics (Pollard et al., 2015).

Patient-centred communication has strong associations with the concept of **therapeutic alliance,** a term used to describe the relationship between mental health practitioners and their clients. While this term has often been confined to psychological interventions, the changing dynamics in HCP–patient interactions has led to the emergence of the idea of therapeutic relationships between HCPs and patients with physical illnesses. When HCPs listen to what patients have to say, ask questions and show sensitivity to their emotional concerns, the therapeutic alliance is reinforced. Evidence from a systematic review suggests that having a good therapeutic alliance between HCPs and patients can positively influence treatment outcomes through improvements in symptoms and general health status (Hall et al., 2010). While there were mixed findings concerning the impact of PCC on clinical outcomes, it was shown that this style of communication can facilitate patient satisfaction and self-management (Rathert et al., 2013). It has also been shown that tailoring communication for patients can improve medicine adherence (Linn et al., 2016). Furthermore, taking time for reciprocal discussion and alleviating patient anxiety has also been shown to promote greater referral for cardiovascular rehabilitation (Pourhabib et al., 2016).

Although the rhetoric around PCC can be used to signify patient participation and autonomy, it also implies greater personal responsibility for health. Therefore, caution is necessary when promoting discourses of patient-centred care to avoid disproportionate burdens of care and responsibility being placed on patients and families. A balance must be reached between patient empowerment and responsibility, while leaving HCPs accountable.

E-HEALTH AND M-HEALTH

With the arrival of the World Wide Web, individuals were able to gain instant access to almost *any* information from any source at their fingertips. This amazing technical achievement created the **e-health** and **m-health (mobile health)** revolution. E-health is a general term referring to the application of digital technology (e.g., the internet, digital gaming, virtual reality and robotics) to health promotion, treatment and care, whereas m-health refers to the use of mobile and wireless applications (e.g., SMS, apps, wearable devices, remote sensing and use of social media, such as Facebook, Twitter and Instagram) to health-related purposes. The health care world is experiencing a paradigm shift like no other as a consequence of a virtual 'explosion' in digital technology.

The internet is bringing a shift in the patient role from that of a *passive recipient* to an *active consumer* of information. In fact, many patients are far more than *consumers*; they are among the most innovative *creators* of information and *critics* of health care provision through their personal websites, social media, blogging, forums, noticeboards and chat rooms. There has never existed such a powerful and sophisticated technology to boost and foster patient empowerment and engagement in health care. The aphorism 'knowledge is power' has never been more apt. As internet access expands to an even broader spectrum of society, and a greater proportion of people globally become computer-literate, there is almost limitless potential for e-health and telemedicine.

Online interventions are also being developed for health-related purposes. Hou et al. (2014) conducted a systematic review of internet-based health-related interventions in the USA published between January 2005 and December 2013. A total of 38 articles met assessment criteria. Targeted health behaviour interventions included: smoking (5), alcohol (4), weight loss (7), physical activity (7), diet (2), exercise and diet combined (5), HIV or sexual health (4), and chronic diseases (4). Interventions ranged from 1 session to 24 weeks and included strategies such as the use of web-based information, tailored feedback, weekly e-mails, goal setting and self-assessment. Social cognitive theory and the transtheoretical model were commonly used to develop these interventions. Most papers reported positive outcomes, except for smoking interventions. Recent studies have also shown how internet-based physical activity can improve self-efficacy to exercise (Hartman et al., 2015) and reduce the likelihood of indoor tanning use among women (Stapleton et al., 2017).

Innovative mobile apps are also being developed to support self-management of chronic conditions. For example, de la Vega et al. (2016) developed Fibroline, which is a mobile app with a self-administered cognitive behavioural treatment (CBT) to improve the quality of life of young people with fibromyalgia. It includes various modules and four task bars which allow the user to access resources (i.e., presentations, videos and audios), assessment (i.e., to record user's sleep quality, pain intensity, mood, anxiety and fatigue), notes (i.e., to annotate treatment objectives) and reminders (i.e., including a 'to do' list and reminders regarding medication and appointments). The app also includes a 'Progress' section so that the user can monitor his/her development (i.e., levels of pain, sleep, anxiety and physical activity). Qualitative feedback was collected. It suggests that users liked the app and found it easy to use. The app is available to download on iTunes.

Examining the impact of m-health on chronic disease management, treatment adherence and patient outcomes, Hamine et al. (2015) found that of the 107 studies included in their systematic review, the short message service was the most commonly used m-health tool (40.2%). Acceptability and patient preferences were assessed in 57.9% of the studies and were found to be generally high. Of the 27 studies that used RCTs to assess adherence behaviours, 56% showed significant improvements. Furthermore, of the 41 RCTs that assessed disease-specific outcomes, only 39% reported significant improvements.

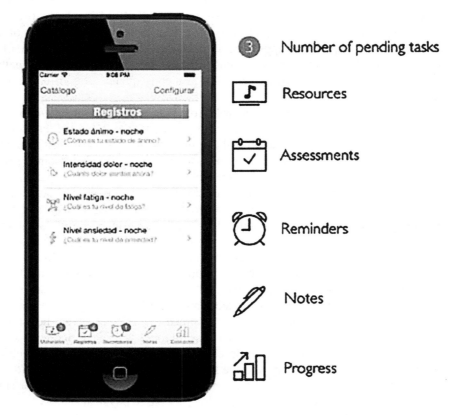

Figure 14.2   The Fibroline app

Source: de la Vega et al. (2016). Reproduced with permission

Online platforms are widely used to share health data. There is a wide variety of available platforms, including social media, Facebook, Twitter, wikis, forums, blogs, virtual communities and conferencing technology. In a qualitative study of an internet forum for patients with systemic lupus erythematosus, Mazzoni and Cicognani (2014) found that participants post messages online to start new relationships, seek information, receive emotional support and contribute to discussions. An example of such an online group is *Realshare*, which is an online support group for teenagers and young adults with cancer that was developed by Griffiths et al. (2015). It includes a forum whereby users can share general and regional information and interact with each other, and there is a page with details of charities and other support groups.

The website was developed using a participatory action research approach and is available to teenagers and young adults with cancer in south-west England.

Participating in online health support groups can be empowering and can help to facilitate self-management. Chiu and Hsieh (2013) found that writing online blogs also enabled cancer patients to reconstruct their life story, express closure of life and their hope that they will be remembered after their death. Reading other patients' stories also influenced their own experiences of living with cancer. Sometimes other patients influenced their perceptions of their prognosis more than their doctors did. In a qualitative systematic review, Kingod et al. (2017) suggested that online peer-to-peer communities can help to strengthen both online and offline social ties (e.g., with physicians and health care providers) by enabling users to reflect and gain knowledge on illness-specific concerns. By facilitating discussion around positive experiences, online communities also foster social support and interactive discussion, which in turn helps to sustain active participation in the group (Wang and Willis, 2016).

The proliferation of health-related online blogs and discussion groups also provides new opportunities for health research. For example, blogs have been used to explore positive outcomes after burn injuries (see Garbett et al., 2016). Hall et al. (2016) used an online forum to analyse the construction of bodybuilders' accounts of synthol use in an online forum. Discourse analysis of posts suggests that users draw upon a medical and pharmaceutical discourse to legitimate its use. They also build trust and rapport with new users through positive personal narratives, and thereby gain credibility as experts in this area. Similarly, Thompson et al. (2016) analysed an online discussion board used by teenagers and young adults with cancer. They found significant differences between discussions stemming from online and face-to-face support groups. Online users were more likely to use words related to friends and sex than those in face-to-face groups. They were also more likely to use the future tense and emotion words (e.g., anger and sadness) than in face-to-face groups. This implies that online platforms can encourage users to discuss future goals more and to share their thoughts and emotions more openly with others than when in a face-to-face context.

The e-health and m-health revolution has many profound implications for health care systems. For example, a systematic review showed that mobile phone messaging reminders can improve attendance in health care appointments (Gurol-Urganci et al., 2013). Health information can also be stored electronically, which has implications for how patient records are shared and stored. A systematic review by Rathert et al. (2017) showed that although the use of electronic health records can improve documentation and sharing of biomedical information, it may interfere with doctor–patient communication and the collection of psychosocial information. However, allowing patients to access electronic health records can potentially improve doctor–patient communication, patient empowerment, participation and self-care. HCPs need to acknowledge that patients generally want to be fully informed about their concerns, illnesses, treatments and prognoses, and this information, whether reliable or not, will be available, searched for and accessed by patients online. **Patient informatics** is becoming an increasingly useful addition to the training of HCPs by first, increasing their own awareness, knowledge and skills through access to the internet, and second, learning how best to engage with the growing use of online health information by increasingly sophisticated service users. However, while the use of e-health and m-health interventions can promote positive health literacy outcomes in a variety of contexts, for a number of chronic conditions and among diverse populations (Jacobs et al., 2016) there is a risk of widening social and health inequalities if care is not taken. Since those with limited health literacy skills tend to have limited access to the internet, these groups may become even more marginalized as health and social care services become more digitized (Estacio et al., 2017).

MESSAGE FRAMING

The way messages are framed influences people's intentions and willingness to change their behaviour (Rothman and Salovey, 1997). Tversky and Kahneman's (1981) **prospect theory** proposed that people consider their 'prospects' (i.e., potential gains and losses) when making decisions and therefore people's preferences are sensitive to the framing of information. People tend to avoid risks when considering potential gains, but will be willing to take risks when considering potential losses. Gain- or loss-framed messages can be tailored to specific behaviours to maximize message effectiveness. **Gain-framed messages** give information about a health behaviour that emphasizes the benefits of taking action, whereas **loss-framed messages** give information that emphasizes the costs of failing to take action (see Figure 14.3).

Research into message framing has grown dramatically over recent years. Studies have been carried out to examine the effectiveness of health-message framing on improving cervical screening uptake (Adonis et al., 2016), reducing heavy drinking among college students (Kingsbury et al., 2015), promoting condom use (Garcia-Retamero and Cokely, 2011) and encouraging maternal influenza immunization (Frew et al., 2014). While findings from a meta-analytic review by Gallagher and Updegraff (2012) showed no significant differences in screening behaviours between loss-framed and gain-framed messages, gain-framed messages were more likely than loss-framed messages to encourage prevention behaviours such as smoking cessation and physical activity. Subsequently, Updegraff and Rothman (2013) identified two major approaches in message framing research: (1) exploring the perceived risks and uncertainties of the health behaviour; and (2) exploring the motivational orientation of the recipient.

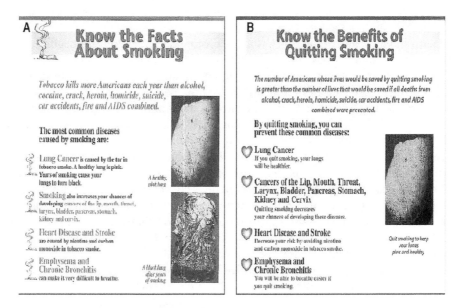

Figure 14.3   Examples of loss-framed (A) and gain-framed (B) messages
for smoking cessation

Source: Benjamin Toll, www.yalescientific.org/2011/04/smoking-cessation-a-gain-framed-counseling-approach

Both the perceived effectiveness of behaviour and perceived susceptibility to and severity of health risks can moderate the effects of message framing. For example, Hwang et al. (2012) examined how perceived effectiveness of sun safety behaviours and perceived susceptibility to skin cancer can moderate message-framing effects. Loss-framed messages were more effective when perceived effectiveness was low, whereas gain-framed messages were more effective when perceived effectiveness was high. Intention to use sunscreen and to wear long trousers to prevent skin cancer were also moderated by perceived susceptibility to skin cancer (i.e., loss-framed messages were more effective when perceived susceptibility was high). This was consistent with Bassett-Gunter et al.'s (2013) study, which found loss-framed messages to be more effective in promoting physical activity beliefs and intentions than gain-framed messages.

Culturally targeted messages and perceived racism can also influence message-framing effects. Lucas et al. (2016) examined the effect of gain- versus loss-framed messages on African Americans' receptivity to colorectal cancer screening and its association with perceived racism. African Americans ($n = 132$) and white Americans ($n = 50$) who were non-compliant with the recommended screening completed online modules on colorectal cancer which were either loss- or gain-framed. Half of the African-American sample was also exposed to a culturally targeted self-control message. Receptivity to the message and perceived racism were measured as outcomes. Findings suggest that white Americans were more receptive to a loss-framed message, whereas African Americans were more receptive to a gain-framed message. This difference was mediated by an increase in perceived racism. However, adding a culturally targeted prevention message appeared to mitigate the impact of a loss-framed message for the African-American participants.

While message-framing research has focused on efforts to promote specific health behaviours, practitioners frequently face the challenge of encouraging people to perform a series of behaviours and sustain such actions. The majority of research on message framing has been quantitative in nature. There is a need to adopt new methods to progress message-framing research and practice (van't Riet et al., 2016). It would also be useful for future research to explore people's subjective experience of message framing using qualitative approaches.

HEALTH LITERACY

What is health literacy?

There is no universal definition of **health literacy**. Early definitions focused on the application of *literacy skills* (e.g., reading and numeracy) to *understand* and *use* information to enable individuals to *function* in the health care setting (Kirsch et al., 1993). Later definitions expanded the concept to include *social skills* and the application of these skills to include the ability to *access* information to *promote* and *maintain* health (Nutbeam, 1998). More recent definitions incorporate ideas from health promotion and patient empowerment to include evaluation and communication skills to enable people to make informed decisions, increase control and take responsibility for health in various contexts (Kickbusch et al., 2005; Murray, 2007; Rootman and Gordon-El-Bihbety, 2008; Sorensen et al., 2012). For the purposes of this chapter, we draw upon the World Health Organization (2015b) definition: 'the personal characteristics and social resources needed for individuals and communities to access, understand, appraise and use information and services to make decisions about health'.

Health literacy may be categorized into three levels (Nutbeam, 2000):

- *Functional health literacy* refers to the basic reading, writing and numeracy skills that enable individuals to function effectively in health care. Activities associated with this level of health literacy often involve communication of health information to improve patient knowledge, e.g., leaflets, websites and other available media.

- *Interactive health literacy* refers to the development of personal skills to improve personal capacity to act independently based on knowledge. It focuses on improving motivation and self-confidence to act upon the advice received, i.e., self-efficacy. Examples include tailored health communication, community self-help and social support groups.

- *Critical health literacy* refers to the ability to critically evaluate and use information to actively participate in health care. Activities include cognitive and social skills development and capacity-building to influence the wider, social health determinants.

Health literacy skills are not limited to functional reading and numeracy skills. People need a skill-set that enables them to handle the complex nature of promoting and maintaining health. Table 14.1 lists the skills and tasks required for health promotion and management. Standardized tests measuring health literacy are beginning to acknowledge the dynamic and complex nature of health literacy. In a systematic review, Altin et al. (2014) found 17 articles detailing the development and validation of 17 health literacy standardized measures from 2009 to 2014. The majority of these instruments were based on a multi-dimensional construct of health literacy.

Table 14.1   Skills and tasks relevant to health promotion and management

Skills	Examples of tasks relevant to health promotion and management
Reading and comprehension	Understanding written health information materials Making sense of doctor's prescription, food labels, health-risk precautions Understanding policies on patients' rights
Listening and comprehension	Understanding spoken medical advice Making sense of significant others' health concerns Listening to specific health issues relevant to the community
Speaking	Reporting health status to health professional Asking for clarifications regarding health condition or treatment Communicating health information with others Providing patient perspectives on how to improve health care
Writing	Keeping personal records of medication intake Communicating with health professional by email Writing a petition to improve equal access to health care for all
Numeracy	Timing and applying appropriate dosage for prescribed medications Budgeting personal finances to accommodate 'healthy living' Interpreting relevance of statistical information concerning a public health issue

Skills	Examples of tasks relevant to health promotion and management
Analytical	Making sense of medical test results Evaluating credibility and accuracy of health information Assessing implications of public issues on health
Decision-making	Providing informed consent for treatment procedures Working as partners in the design, implementation and evaluation of health programmes Voting on organizational or government policies affecting health
Navigation	Locating health facilities Navigating oneself through the health care system Scheduling doctor's appointments
Negotiation	Negotiating treatment options Negotiating ways to improve personal and public health
Awareness	Being aware of physical symptoms and personal health status Recognizing social barriers and opportunities to promote health Recognizing shared social beliefs to around the social determinants of health
Advocacy	Obtaining information and resources needed to promote health Mobilization of action to address public health issues

Why is health literacy important?

The National Assessment of Adult Literacy in 2003 showed that 77 million people in the USA had basic or below-basic health literacy – more than one-third of the population. Europeans have similar levels of health illiteracy. The European Health Literacy Survey (HLS-EU) showed that 12% of the population had inadequate health literacy and 35% had problematic health literacy (Figure 14.4). These are worrying findings, considering that inadequate levels of health literacy can have damaging repercussions.

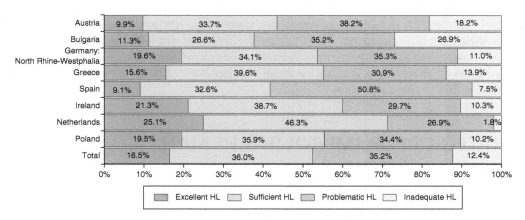

Figure 14.4   Health literacy (HL) levels in eight European nations

Source: HLS-EU Consortium (2012). Reproduced with permission

Protheroe et al. (2016) found that limited literacy is associated with demographic factors such as older age, lower educational level, lower income, perceived poor health and lack of access to the internet. A systematic review has also shown that older age is strongly associated with limited health literacy when it is measured as reading comprehension, reasoning and numeracy skills. By contrast, there is a weak association between older age and limited health literacy when it is measured as medical vocabulary. This implies that while functional health literacy skills can decline with age, vocabulary-based health literacy skills are more stable. There is limited evidence on the mediating role of cognitive function between ageing and functional health literacy (Kobayashi et al., 2016).

The associations between health literacy, access to health care and health outcomes are well established. Berkman et al. (2011) showed how poor health literacy was consistently associated with higher hospitalization rates, greater use of emergency care and poorer access to immunization and screening services. People with inadequate health literacy were less able to take medications appropriately and interpret labels. Among elderly persons, limited health literacy was associated with poorer overall health and higher mortality. Even after adjusting for SES and health status, people with limited health literacy make fewer visits to their doctors, prefer emergency care, and have more preventable hospital admissions than those with adequate literacy skills (Schumacher et al., 2013). Systematic reviews have also shown that adequate health literacy is associated with higher knowledge about salt and cardiac failure (Cajita et al., 2016), better reproductive health knowledge and adoption of health-related behaviours such as prenatal vitamin use and breastfeeding (Kilfoyle et al., 2016), and cervical screening uptake (Kim and Han, 2016).

Health literacy can also mediate self-rated health status across racial/ethnic and educational disparities (Mantwill et al., 2015). In a qualitative study, Vamos et al. (2016) explored narratives of women living in a Hispanic migrant farmworker community following abnormal pap test results. Using health literacy as a conceptual framework, the research explored how women obtained information about getting a pap test, how they understood their results, how they felt and talked about it, how they received social support, and what they did afterwards. The narratives highlighted the diversity of patient reactions and experiences.

A review by McCaffery et al. (2013) showed that limited health literacy was not only linked with poorer health knowledge, but also associated with less desire for involvement, less question-asking and less patient-centred communication with their doctors. When patients with limited health literacy did engage in health decisions, they were more likely to report higher decisional uncertainty and regret. While patient decision aids can help, this review found that very few studies had explicitly acknowledged the needs of patients with limited health literacy. Interventions on shared decision-making must consider health literacy as a potential limiting influence in health communication.

STRATEGIES FOR IMPROVING HEALTH COMMUNICATION

In spite of the increasing availability and sophistication of ICT, the weak link in any communication system remains the human being. There are diverse ways to improve health communication, which is hardly ever perfect, but effective communication is not 'rocket science' either. Unless human HCPs are replaced by robots in some future universe (which seems to us highly unlikely), people will always play a crucial role in the delivery of health care. In a study in two clinics in Dallas, Texas, Gutierrez et al. (2014) observed that, regardless of health literacy, patients relied on their HCPs to obtain health information.

HCPs everywhere need to take into account the *messenger*, the *receiver*, the *message* and the *context*. Interventions that aim to promote effective health communication must consider the best ways to: (1) improve HCP communication skills; (2) promote individual and community capabilities; and (3) simplify and clarify all health care information.

IMPROVING HCP COMMUNICATION SKILLS

HCPs and patients often have very different perceptions of how well an episode of HCP–patient communication actually went. Probably this is true of the majority of human beings. Dickens et al. (2013) found that nurses tend to overestimate patients' health literacy skills. HCPs also have a tendency to overestimate the clarity of their own oral communication skills. Similarly, in a study comparing self-reported and actual use of clear verbal communication among medical residents, Howard et al. (2013) found that although the majority of the medical residents reported using plain language when communicating with patients (88%), on average, while completing a standardized low-literacy patient encounter, they used *two jargon terms per minute*. Similarly, while 48% reported using the *teach-back technique* (i.e., confirming that the delivered information was understood by asking patients to repeat or demonstrate what they had been told), only 22% used it in the standardized encounter. They failed to translate their training into everyday practice.

To enable patients to make informed choices, HCPs need to take steps to communicate in a manner that patients can understand. Protheroe and Rowlands (2013) argue that HCPs need to adapt their communication techniques to take into account the patients' different levels of health literacy. To promote effective interactions with patients, HCPs need to improve their communication skills and be aware of the varying levels of health literacy that exists across patients. It has been shown that communication training for clinicians can improve patient satisfaction, especially in reducing pain and disability in primary care and rehabilitation (Oliveira et al., 2015). The following strategies can be considered to improve communication:

- *Slow down.* Spend some time talking with patients using plain language. In a study by Sadeghi et al. (2013), it was found that time constraints and use of medical jargon are the main barriers that impede HCP–patient communication. It is important for HCPs to speak slowly and use language that is easy to understand.

- *Show or draw pictures.* Visual aids can help to enhance understanding and recall. Simple line drawings and cartoons will suffice. As an example, Mohan et al. (2013) have shown how illustrated medication instructions can be used to improve medication management among Latino patients with diabetes in the USA.

- *Limit the amount of information provided and repeat it.* This is particularly important for patients with limited literacy skills since health literacy can significantly influence people's ability to remember verbal instructions and to recall information (Miller et al., 2013). Information is easier to understand and to remember when given in small doses. Repeating and highlighting key tasks can help enhance recall.

- *Create a shame-free environment.* Some patients may feel embarrassed to share their literacy difficulties because of stigma (see Box 14.1). It is important for HCPs to promote a culture of helpfulness in their everyday practice by encouraging patients to ask questions. The *Ask Me 3*™ programme can be a useful guide for patients and HCPs. In this programme, patients are encouraged to ask HCPs three questions:

  1. What is my problem?

  2. What do I need to do?

  3. Why is it important for me to do this?

There is sufficient evidence to support the effectiveness of communication skills training courses to improve communication styles and attitudes among HCPs (Barth and Lannen, 2011). In particular, programmes that last for at least a day, are learner-centred, focus on practising skills, and include activities such as role-play, feedback and small group discussions, are shown to be most effective for training communication skills among GPs (Berkhof et al., 2011).

BOX 14.1

KEY STUDY: Stigma of low literacy and spoken interactions between patients and HCPs

Aim

This qualitative study explored how limited literacy could influence access to health care, self-management and health outcomes.

Method

Participants were recruited from a community-based adult learning centre in Dundee, Scotland. Participants (*n* = 29) were working-age adults who had English as a first language and had sought support for literacy difficulties. Using interviews, researchers explored personal experiences of literacy, health care (including self-care) and self-reported health outcomes. The interviews were supplemented with focus group discussions to further explore ideas about how health services could be improved to support people with literacy difficulties. The interviews and focus groups were transcribed and analysed using framework analysis.

Findings

Participants explained that limited literacy skills impaired their interactions with HCPs. These difficulties were expressed in terms of understanding written information, complex explanations and instructions that subsequently ripple onto their broader health care experiences and ability to self-care. For some, interactions with HCPs were so bad that they described these scenarios as all 'gobbledygook' to them. Some participants also felt that HCPs did not make any effort to help them to understand what was being said. This is reflected in the quote below:

... and he [hospital consultant] was 'blah blah blah' and he knew fine I didn't have the foggiest idea what he was talking about. (Harry, male, 40s, quoted in Easton et al., 2013: 6)

Findings also suggest that some of the communication difficulties experienced by patients were further exacerbated by the stigma associated with limited literacy. The participants' narratives revealed how they had tried to conceal their limited literacy from their HCPs and in other social contexts. Some participants felt the need to hide their literacy difficulties because of the negative experiences they had had in the past. In fear of revealing their limited literacy skills, some participants would refrain from engaging in the process, as reflected in the quote below:

I couldn't spell it. I just went, 'You know what, I'm going to have to go. I'm not feeling very good. I'll come back, I will come back' and I grabbed it [the form] and ran out. (Barbara, female, 50s, quoted in Easton et al., 2013: 7)

Conclusion

Limited literacy can seriously impair interactions between HCPs and their patients. However, it is not only the difficulties associated with reading and understanding information that can interfere with the process. The stigma associated with limited literacy often exacerbates problems when patients try to hide the difficulties they experience to avoid embarrassment. Complex processes and HCP communication styles that are littered with medical jargon often can drive some patients to avoid these interactions to prevent exposing their literacy difficulties in public. It is important for HCPs to recognize the needs of people with limited literacy skills by communicating effectively (without jargon) and by creating a shame-free and non-judgemental environment.

Source: Easton et al. (2013)

Promoting individual and community capabilities

Health promotion requires the development of skills that are necessary to enable individuals and communities to take control over the determinants of health. Chervin et al. (2012) worked in partnership with adult education centres to incorporate health literacy into the curriculum. Six adult education centres that served ethnic minority, immigrant and low-income learners in a small north-eastern state in the USA received a grant to deliver health literacy sessions as part of their curriculum. Quantitative and qualitative methods were used to assess its processes and outcomes. Health literacy instruction was found to have a positive impact on the learners' knowledge and understanding of health issues, the health care system, medical terminology and patient rights and responsibilities. Furthermore, the centres reported that learners were able to apply the health literacy skills they had developed in practice, such as healthier eating, scheduling doctor's appointments, communicating effectively with HCPs and following medical instructions. Levels of self-efficacy had also increased. Towards the end of the project, nearly three-quarters of the centres included health literacy sessions in the curriculum, with almost half of the teachers continuing to attend professional development activities for health literacy. Over the course of the project, each centre also developed partnerships with health care providers that established the infrastructure for further knowledge and opportunities for teachers and learners.

Health literacy interventions, however, do not need to be isolated within the education setting. Considering that difficulties associated with limited health literacy are often exacerbated by social, cultural and historical contexts, it is important that interventions consider alternative environments to ensure that these are appropriate and relevant to the target audience.

A word of caution, however – promoting health literacy does not necessarily lead to patient empowerment. As Schulz and Nakamoto (2013) argue, although health literacy and empowerment may be related, they are distinct concepts, and one may not necessarily lead to the other. Presuming this to be the case can lead to deleterious consequences. As shown in Figure 14.5, high levels of health literacy without improving patient empowerment can lead patients to become overly dependent on HCPs. On the other hand, improving patient empowerment without corresponding improvements in health literacy potentially can lead to dangerous self-management among patients. When aiming to help patients become effective self-managers of health, interventions need to encompass methods for improving *both health literacy and empowerment.* Only these two in combination can ensure patients have the knowledge, skills and confidence to use appropriate resources effectively to promote and maintain their health.

One way to improve health literacy, build capacity and promote empowerment is by actively engaging participants themselves in the intervention process. **Participatory action research (PAR)** (Chapters 7 and 16) is one approach that can help to develop skills and raise critical consciousness at the same time.

Simplifying and clarifying health information and the wider health care system

Using text-based materials containing lengthy, complex information can be difficult for people with limited literacy skills. It is important that information materials are clear and easy to understand. However, simplifying health information is not just about improving its readability by using shorter words. Designing effective health information needs to consider the materials' cultural appropriateness, relevance and context to narrow the gap between the health message, the messenger and its intended recipients (Zarcadoolas, 2011). It is also important to consider what information patients actually need, based on their goals and circumstances. For example, Hingle et al. (2013) piloted text messages for young people to influence their knowledge, attitudes and behaviour towards nutrition and physical activity. Based within youth programmes in Arizona, nine focus groups, four classroom discussions and an eight-week pilot study were conducted over a 12-month period to engage young people in discussing the content, format, origin and delivery of the text messages. By engaging young people in the process, more than 300 text messages that were relevant, acceptable and suitable to this target group were developed and tested.

Kennedy et al. (2014) evaluated a series of self-management guidebooks using cartoons for people with inflammatory bowel disease, irritable bowel syndrome, diabetes, chronic obstructive pulmonary disease and chronic kidney disease. The content was informed by qualitative research to obtain lay views and experiences. In general, the cartoons depicted common patient situations and dilemmas, decision-making choices and uncertainties associated

Empowerment		
	Low	High

| Health literacy | | Low | 'High-needs patient' | 'Dangerous self-manager' |
| | High | 'Needlessly dependent patient' | 'Effective self-manager' |

Figure 14.5   Health literacy, empowerment and patient behaviour

Source: Schulz and Nakamoto (2013)

with these conditions. After the guidebooks had been piloted, in-depth interviews and 'think-aloud' methods were used to evaluate them. The cartoons invoked amusement, recognition and reflection and helped provide clarity and understanding that otherwise may have been impossible.

Research has shown that publicly available health information may not necessarily suit people's existing knowledge and health literacy skills (Protheroe et al., 2015; Damman et al., 2016). It is important that information pamphlets are a clear and appropriate match to the needs and skills of end-users. In England, for example, the Information Standard is used to ensure that the quality of health and social care information is clear, accurate, impartial, evidence-based and up to date. The Information Standard is an independent certification programme commissioned by NHS England and run by Capita on their behalf. Any organization producing evidence-based health and social care information for the public across England can apply for a mark. Organizations that pass this rigorous assessment are awarded the Information Standard Quality Mark.

Individual HCPs – health psychologists included – may be small cogs in a huge wheel, but, without effective cogs, the huge wheel quickly grinds to a halt. Improving communication skills is by far the best and most cost-efficient way to 'oil the cogs', keeping this marvellous 'wheel' of the health care system moving in a positive direction – providing patients with the best possible care.

FUTURE RESEARCH

1. How to use health-message framing to promote the initiation and maintenance of health behaviours, including qualitative explorations of people's subjective experiences of behaviour change.

2. How health literacy can be incorporated into the design of patient decision aids to foster better shared decision-making.

(Continued)

3. More participatory action research projects to develop interventions to narrow social inequities in health information.

4. Robust evaluation of processes and outcomes to examine its effectiveness and impact on health service users' and providers' experiences.

SUMMARY

1. Health communication refers to all interpersonal, organizational or mass communication that concerns health. It can occur in various contexts, settings and channels, and deliver a variety of messages for a variety of reasons.
2. Shannon and Weaver's telephone model of communication considers six key components to communication: (1) source, (2) transmitter, (3) channel, (4) receiver, (5) destination and (6) noise. This is a basic descriptive model that serves a didactic function and little more.
3. Good communication between HCPs and patients is essential to health promotion, disease prevention and treatment, and serves as the foundation for an effective HCP–patient partnership.
4. Message framing can be used to influence people's motivation to undertake specific health behaviours.
5. E-health and m-health are growing rapidly as internet access widens. The role of the patient is shifting from a 'passive consumer' to an 'active consumer of information' who is able to access an almost unlimited amount of health information and support, free at the point of delivery, online.
6. Health literacy refers to the capacity to access, understand, appraise and apply health information and services to make appropriate health decisions to promote and maintain health. It has three general levels: (1) functional, (2) interactive and (3) critical.
7. There are a number of skills concerning health literacy that are relevant to health promotion. These skills include reading, writing, numeracy, analysis, decision-making, navigation, negotiation, awareness and advocacy.
8. Low literacy has been associated with poor health outcomes, including knowledge, intermediate disease markers, measures of morbidity, general health status and use of health resources. Patients with low literacy may also be reluctant to seek assistance due to the stigma and shame attached to it.
9. HCPs need to be aware of health literacy levels when communicating information to ensure effective interactions with patients.
10. Building HCPs' and patients' skills and simplifying the health care system are useful ways to improve health communication.

SCREENING AND IMMUNIZATION

'We are living in a world that is beyond controllability.'

Ulrich Beck

OUTLINE

We consider two forms of disease prevention available within health care systems: screening and immunization. These programmes are premised on the basis of controlling risk. Screening programmes are designed to identify individuals who, because of certain personal characteristics, are considered at risk of developing a certain disease. Immunization programmes are designed to vaccinate people who are at risk because of their exposure to environmental pathogens. Various social and psychological processes are involved in explaining these processes of risk management.

RISK AND RISK CONTROL

According to various sociologists, we live in a 'risk society' (Beck, 1992), by which is meant that people feel that they are under threat from an increasing range of hazards. The role of the state in this later modern era is promoted as being to identify and bring under control these many hazards. Joffe (1999: 4) argued that while risk in general is defined in the language of science, behind it is a 'more moralistic endeavour, one that routes dangers back to those responsible for them'. This follows the well-trodden blame and shame path of personal responsibility.

The control of risk is a central theme in contemporary health care. Once again, the dominant language of science conceals a more moralistic message about personal responsibility. Preventive health care has been predicated upon epidemiological research that has estimated the statistical importance of various so-called 'risk factors'. According to these statistical models, individuals or groups who are exposed to certain pathogens, either internally or externally, or who behave in a certain manner are at higher risk of developing a particular health problem. The task of preventive health programmes then becomes one of identifying individual risks for particular health problems and bringing these risks under control. A central challenge is the extent to which people are willing to participate in these programmes.

Health psychologists have contributed to attempts to explore this issue by investigating cognitive and other psychological processes that can help clarify risk control actions. Research on preventive health services, such as screening and immunization, has been dominated by the cognitive approach, which focuses on the information-processing model of the single individual, in contrast to a more socio-cultural approach, which considers the interaction between the individual and the socio-cultural context. Both approaches are considered below.

SCREENING

One of the main forms of health risk management is the early detection of disease through screening. This is the procedure whereby those sections of the population that are considered statistically more at risk of developing a particular disease are examined to see whether they have any early indications of that disease. The rationale behind this strategy is that the earlier the disease is identified and treated, the less likely it is to develop into its full-blown form. Within public health circles there has been sustained debate about the value of this strategy. A variety of criteria have been identified for deciding to implement screening (Wilson and Jungner, 1968). These include the character of the evidence regarding its effectiveness, benefits, harms and costs.

In Western countries, there have been several attempts to introduce mass screening for a limited number of conditions that satisfy all or most of these criteria. However, despite the supposed benefits of these programmes, there has been a variety of problems in their implementation. It was generally assumed by their proponents that the major problem would be the introduction of the programmes. However, the challenge has been not a technical one of implementing the programme, but rather a human one concerned with the reluctance of at least a proportion of the targeted population to make use of these programmes and the unexpected negative side effects of participation. In addition, there continues to be debate about the effectiveness of forms of screening.

SCREENING FOR CANCER

Over the past decade there has been a concerted effort in most industrialized societies to introduce screening programmes for breast cancer. The reason for this was that it is a common health problem and there was evidence that those detected and treated at an early stage had better survival prospects. It is currently one of the most prevalent forms of female cancer in Western society. It is estimated that one in nine women will develop breast cancer at some point in their lives.

Partly in response to the epidemiological and medical evidence about the widespread prevalence of the disease and the association between stage of identification and success of treatment, there has been a demand not only from health authorities but also from women's organizations for the introduction of breast cancer screening programmes. Initially, the method favoured was breast self-examination (BSE), but due to debate about the accuracy of this procedure most health authorities now favour mammography coupled (sometimes) with clinical breast examination by a health professional. In most industrialized countries mammography programmes have been targeted at all women aged 50 to 69 years, who are invited on a 2–3-year basis to undergo the procedure.

Although mammography is widely promoted by health authorities, evaluations of its effectiveness have not been conclusive. The Cochrane Collaboration review estimated that the breast cancer mortality reduction due to mammography was 15% rather than the 29% previously reported (Gøtzsche and Jørgensen, 2013). They concluded that while screening reduces breast cancer mortality by 15%, they estimated that overdiagnosis and overtreatment occurs in 30% of cases. They argue that these women will experience psychological distress for years after because of this false positive finding.

The authors refer to a range of harmful consequences of mammography that have often been ignored in evaluations, including heightened levels of distress among the women, harmful effects of radiation, and overdiagnosis (i.e., cases that would never become clinically detectable or pose a threat to health without screening) leading to surgery and other forms of treatment. Another commentary noted that 'it seems likely that little of the decline in breast cancer mortality since 1990 is due to mammography screening, and nearly all to improved therapy of breast cancer' (Miller et al., 2008: 785).

A review of 11 randomized trials concluded that the relative risk of breast cancer mortality for women invited to screening compared with controls was 0.80 (95% CI 0.73–0.89), which is a relative risk reduction of 20% (Marmot, Altman, Cameron et al., 2013). Marmot et al. concluded that 20% was still a reasonable estimate of the relative risk reduction. A Danish study (Njor et al., 2015) found similar evidence of reduced mortality among women targeted for breast cancer screening. However, in a review of mammography screening among 39–49-year-olds in the USA, Magnus et al. (2011) issued some cautions about the evidence and advised that women of this age group be advised of both the negative and positive aspects of screening.

Despite widespread support for mammography, there is concern that some of the evidence on the effectiveness of alternative approaches to detection, such as BSE, may be underestimated. Kearney and Murray (2009) highlighted the limitations of previous evaluative research, suggesting that BSE was of limited benefit in reducing mortality on the grounds that the evidence was drawn from trials of BSE education, not of BSE practice. It has been discouraged because BSE would also lead to heightened anxiety among women and unnecessary visits to the family doctor. However, there is little evidence for the latter. Rather, there is evidence that the majority of breast cancer tumours are discovered by the women themselves.

Cervical cancer is a much less prevalent condition. In 2011, over 3,000 new cases of cervical cancer were diagnosed in the UK, making it the twelfth most common cancer in women and accounting for around 2% of all female cancers (Cancer Research UK, 2013). The incidence rate for cervical cancer is highest for those aged 30–40, reaching around 17 per 100,000 women. In 2011, there were 972 deaths from cervical cancer in the UK. It has been established that the human papillomavirus (HPV) is the main risk factor and a necessary cause of cervical cancer. This virus is spread particularly through sexual activity. There is evidence that the pre- cancerous stage of the disease can be detected at an early stage using a simple cervical smear test (pap test). Most Western countries have introduced campaigns to encourage women to attend for regular smear tests, usually at least once every three to five years. Another prevention strategy has been the introduction of HPV vaccination. In many countries, an HPV immunization programme has been introduced into schools for teenage girls (see later).

Evidence from several countries suggests that a substantial proportion of women do not use cancer screening programmes. Approximately 2.75 million women aged 50–70 were invited for breast cancer screening in 2009–2010 in the UK. Of these, approximately 2.02 million were screened and 16,500 cancers and tumours were detected (Cancer Research UK, 2013). The cervical smear test has been around for a longer period but it also has encountered reluctance of a substantial proportion of targeted women to participate. More recently, there have been attempts to introduce screening for other forms of cancer. There has been interest in developing screening for colorectal cancer, which is the second major cause of cancer in Western society and affects both men and women. However, the uptake of the test has not been high.

HEALTH BELIEFS AND CANCER SCREENING

The dominant approach used by health psychologists to explain participation in screening programmes has been underpinned by social cognition models (SCMs), especially the health belief model (HBM), with the focus on barriers to and benefits of screening, and the theory of reasoned action (TRA), with the focus on intentions to participate and attitudes towards screening. (For further details, please see Chapter 6.)

In the case of breast cancer screening, most of the studies have considered participation in mammography programmes and fewer have considered BSE. The most frequently cited predictors of participation in both are perceived susceptibility and perceived barriers. A meta-analysis of many US studies (McCaul et al., 1996) found a strong relationship between family history (actual risk) and mammography utilization, but also a moderate relationship between perceived vulnerability (perceived risk) and use of mammography. In a reanalysis of the data from two studies of the effects of testimonials in health messages about colon cancer screening, Dillard et al. (2012) found that feelings of risk were predictive of intentions and attitudes about screening.

Various barriers to attendance for mammography, both physical and psychological, have been reported. Rimer et al. (1989) found in their survey of women in the USA that those who did not attend for mammography had a stronger belief that screening was not necessary in the absence of symptoms, preferred not to think about it and worried about the effect of radiation. Murray and McMillan (1993) found that perceived barriers were the most important predictor of attendance for a smear test. The barriers they considered included dislike of the health service, fear of the examination and fear of the result. Moore et al. (1998) found that the main barriers to both breast and testicular self-examination were embarrassment, perceived unpleasantness and difficulty, reliability concerns and concerns about the findings.

McCaul et al. (1996) found that women who worry about breast cancer are more likely to engage in self-protective actions such as BSE and attendance for mammography. Sutton et al. (1994) found a non-linear relationship, with the highest attendance among women who were 'a bit worried', while those at the two extremes of worry were less likely to attend. They concluded that health promotion campaigns must balance advice to women on perceived risk with the negative impact of excessive worry. Other barriers reported include belief that a mammogram is appropriate only when there are symptoms, as well as concern about radiation exposure, cost and access-related factors (Slenker and Grant, 1989).

With respect to benefits, several studies have indicated that the most frequently given reason for non-participation in cancer screening is that the women do not feel it necessary – they were healthy so they did not feel it was necessary to use it. It was thought that it was only necessary to have mammograms when one was sick. Potvin et al. (1995) found that perceiving one's health as good was inversely associated with recent mammography. Harlan et al. (1991) found that the most frequently given reason for not having a cervical smear was not believing it necessary.

A criticism of many of these studies of breast cancer screening is that they used a cross-sectional design. One study that used a longitudinal design (Norman and Brain, 2005) found that previous experience of BSE was the best predictor of the practice. Among the HBM factors considered to be the best predictors were perceived emotional barriers (e.g., 'Finding breast cancer is emotionally distressing') and perceived self-efficacy barriers (e.g., 'I am confident that I can examine my own breasts regularly'). This would suggest that the barriers dimension should be considered in more detail. In addition, this study found that those women who scored low on perceived self-efficacy barriers and high on breast cancer worries and perceived severity of cancer were more likely to conduct BSE excessively. It was suggested that these women may carry out more frequent but less thorough BSE.

Studies of screening for other cancers have confirmed the importance of perceived risk. In a survey of a large sample of Scottish residents invited to participate in colorectal cancer screening, Wardle et al. (2004) found that interest in participating in screening was predicted by higher perceived risk, worry and benefits, and lower perceived barriers, fears and fatalism. They also found that those from lower SES backgrounds perceived the benefits of screening less and the barriers to it more. Although their study was not formally based on the HBM, it does agree with other studies of cancer screening. The TRA and TPB have met with some success in predicting cancer screening behaviour. Cooke and French (2008) conducted a large meta-analysis of 33 studies that used this approach. They found that attitudes had a large-sized relationship with intention to participate in screening, while subjective norms and perceived behavioural control had medium-sized relationships. Intention had a medium-sized relationship with participation. They also considered the role of moderator variables and identified (1) type of screening, (2) location of recruitment, (3) screening cost and (4) invitation to screen as important.

Several researchers have used the transtheoretical model (TTM) of change (Prochaska and DiClemente, 1983, 1992) to explore the extent of participation in screening programmes. Rakowski et al. (1992) found that women who were classified as pre-contemplators (i.e., those who had never had a mammogram and did not plan to have one) scored higher on a measure of negative beliefs, including the beliefs that mammograms lead to unnecessary surgery and that they are only advisable if you have some breast symptoms. Skinner et al. (1997) found that action/maintainers were less likely to agree with the psychological and physical barriers to screening.

Social variations in participation

The growth of research on health gradients (see Chapter 4) has confirmed that not only do people from poorer backgrounds experience worse health, but also they make less use of preventive health services such as screening. The US Centers for Disease Control and Prevention (2012) reported on a National Health Interview Survey on colorectal screening in 2000, 2003, 2005, 2008 and 2010 with a civilian non-institutionalized population aged 50–75. The data showed that the overall percentage of adults aged 50–75 who reported receiving colorectal cancer screening significantly increased from 34% in 2000 to 59% in 2010 and that rates increased among all racial and income groups. However, in all years except 2008, Asians were less likely to receive colorectal cancer screening than whites. Since 2005, blacks have also been less likely than whites to receive screening. In all years, poor, low-income and middle-income adults were less likely to receive colorectal cancer screening than high-income adults.

A framework for integrating the psychological evidence on the relationship between SES and use of screening has been developed by von Wagner et al. (2011). Box 15.1 shows that this framework classified the evidence into two broad categories: corollaries of SES and attitudinal mediators. In the former category, they group a mixture of social stressors that they argue reduce the perceived importance of preventive health behaviours. It also includes educational opportunities that contribute to health literacy and the ability to access and process information about preventive and other health services.

The third social corollary is illness experience. It is suggested that this corollary is associated with lower use of cancer prevention services via three pathways. The first is cancer fatalism. A study by Wardle et al. (2004) found that people of lower SES were more likely to agree with the statement 'It's not worth having the test because "what will be will be"'. The second illness experience pathway was characterized by a lack of confidence in dealing with the medical system. It is known that people of lower SES have less confidence and express greater dissatisfaction with the medical system. Low rates of participation in screening are more common among those who express dissatisfaction with health care (Ackerson and Preston, 2009). The third proposed pathway was low perceived personal value of cancer screening. Since people of lower SES have lower life expectancies and have what Barrett (2003) described as 'older identities', they are more sceptical of the benefits of preventive health care such as screening.

In reviewing the evidence for the psychosocial mediators, von Wagner et al. (2011) expressed surprise that despite the large amount of research on social cognitive processes, a limited amount of research had connected these processes with details of the SES status of the study participants. Despite these limitations they suggested three broad blocks of attitudinal mediators. These were the perceived threat of unpleasant or invasive medical procedures, self-efficacy for participating in cancer screening, and response efficacy for screening to detect cancer early, prolong life or minimize treatment. These attitudinal mediators are then hypothesized to contribute to the low uptake of cancer screening among low SES adults through inadequate information processing (e.g., lack of information seeking) and limited goal setting (e.g., prioritization of alternative activities).

Although the von Wagner et al. framework integrated a large amount of empirical work, there is still a tendency to adopt a *deficit model* to explain non-participation in screening. Those who do not use the service tend to be characterized as lacking in knowledge and concern about their health. An alternative perspective is to view this non-attendance within its socio-cultural context and as a form of *resistance* to what is perceived as an unnecessary interference in their lives or even as something that could increase the likelihood of cancer.

BOX 15.1

Social corollaries and psychosocial mediators of cancer screening

COROLLARIES OF SOCIOECONOMIC STATUS

Stressors and resources for change
- Levels of unemployment, crime
- Quality of housing and of medical, educational, occupational, and recreational facilities

Educational opportunities
- Experience of reward and achievement
- Perseverance and goal setting
- Lifelong learning and skill attainment

Illness experiences
- Vicarious experience of cancer
- Life expectancy
- Experience with the medical system

ATTITUDINAL MEDIATORS (THREAT AND EFFICACY BELIEFS)

Perceived threat of unpleasant/invasive medical procedures and cancer diagnosis

- Negative expectations: negative beliefs about screening procedures and consequences of a cancer diagnosis

- Lack of knowledge: screening procedures and consequences of diagnosis

- Cancer fatalism

Self-efficacy for participating in cancer screening

- Reactive responding
- Learned helplessness: lack of personal control
- Prohibitive social influences: social support

- Lack of confidence in ability to understand, persevere, and succeed

- Lack of confidence in dealing with the medical system

Response efficacy for screening to detect cancer early, prolong life, or minimize treatment

- Learned helplessness: belief in chance
- Prohibitive social influences: social norms

- Low consideration of future consequences
- Lack of knowledge: benefits of cancer screening and early detection

- Negative beliefs about benefits of medical intervention
- Low personal value of screening given lower life expectancy

Information processing
- Lack of information seeking and engagement
- Poor comprehension of information
- Message rejection

Goal-setting and behavioral translation
- Prioritization of alternative activities
- Forgetting appointments and ignoring reminders
- Patient errors (e.g., failure to prepare for screening/administer tests)

NONPARTICIPATION IN CANCER SCREENING

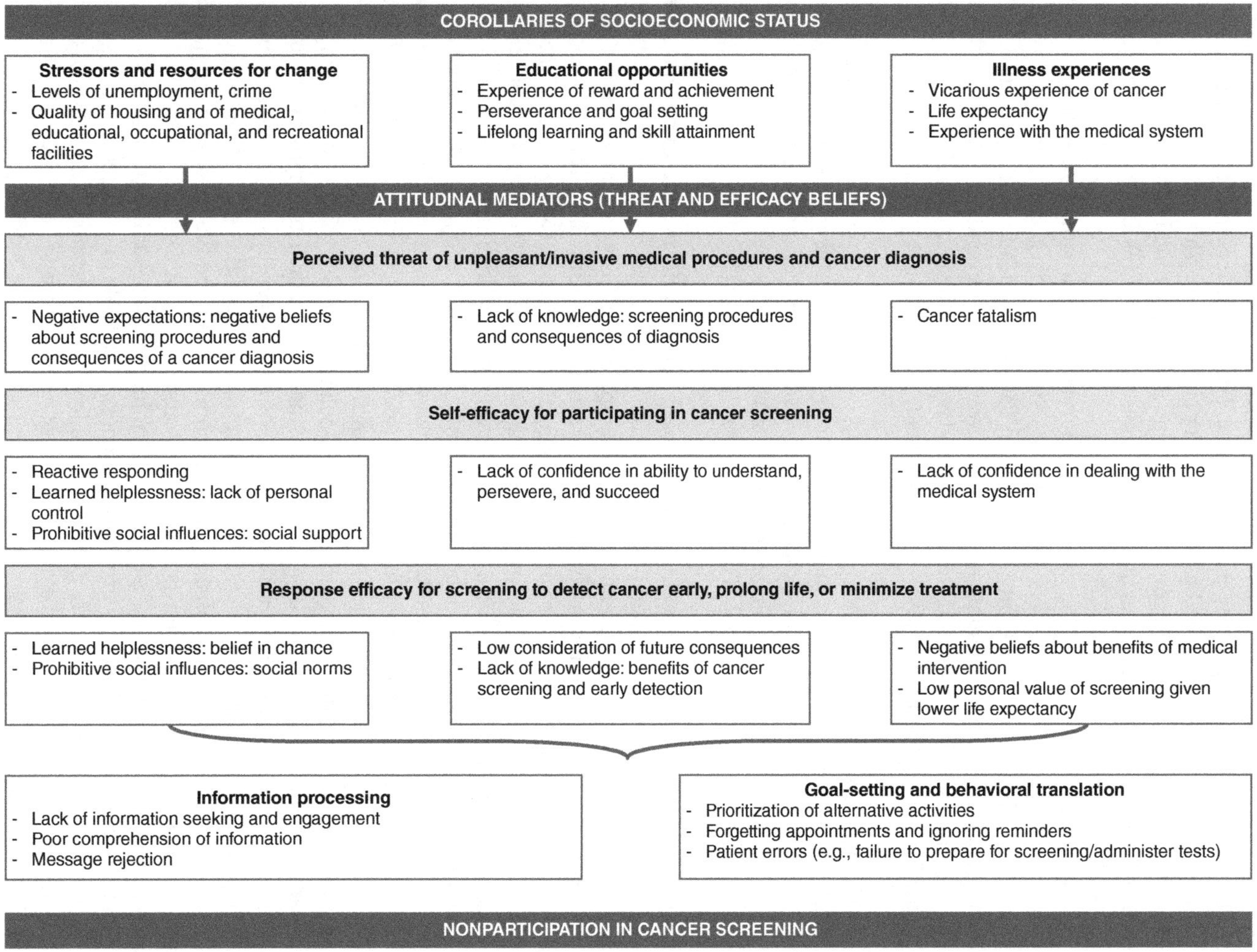

Figure 15.1   A framework to explain socioeconomic status differences in psychosocial predictors of cancer screening.

Source: Adapted from von Wagner et al. (2011)

MEANING OF CANCER AND CANCER SCREENING

Despite the advances in the treatment of cancer, or indeed partly due to the character of these advances, cancer remains the most feared disease. Murray and McMillan (1993) conducted a survey of a random sample of adults resident in Northern Ireland. They found that cancer was the most feared disease, especially among women. The reason for this fear was because cancer was perceived as incurable and as leading to a painful death. Slenker and Spreitzer (1988) conducted a survey of a random sample of adults in Ohio. They found that not only was cancer the most feared disease, but approximately half the respondents felt there was little you could do about the disease.

Gregg and Curry (1994) conducted detailed interviews with a sample of African-American low-income women on their beliefs about cancer. Not surprisingly, they had a very negative image of the disease. They not only believed that cancer was deadly, but also felt that if the cancer could be detected by mammography then it was already beyond cure. An example of this attitude is the case of a 62-year-old woman who had received a negative result from her pap test. Her reaction was a refusal to obtain a follow-up test:

> My last pap didn't come back good and they want me to go over to Grady, but I didn't go because I'm afraid they're going to tell me that I've got cancer. I've just had so much experience with cancer, and I know that if they operate on me it's going to get worse. So, I'm just going to prolong it as much as I can. ... We all going to die anyway. ... It's too late now. (Gregg and Curry, 1994: 524)

Balshem (1991) linked these negative beliefs about cancer with the life experiences of the women. She conducted an ethnographic study of a working-class community in Philadelphia that seemed very resistant to a health promotion campaign aimed at encouraging healthier lifestyles, including attendance for breast cancer screening. When she interviewed these women, Balshem found that the health promotion message was counter to their experience. They believed that fate determined who got cancer and who survived. To look for cancer was to tempt fate; it was 'looking for trouble'. To quote Balshem: 'Challenging fate is a risky business. Cancer inspires not challenge but taboo.' Thus, the women preferred not to think about cancer.

Other qualitative work suggests that some women would prefer to conduct self-examination rather than attend a medical centre for investigation. For example, Tessaro et al. (1994) interviewed a sample of older African-American women and found that they did not think it necessary to use the health service since after self-examination they had found no lumps.

Kearney (2006) conducted focus groups with women about their perceptions of cancer and cancer screening. This study used action research with the two groups of women meeting regularly to discuss the issues over several weeks. Over the course of this study the women became more critical of the medical establishment. One woman described the promotion of mammography as the preferred method for breast cancer screening as an example of 'boys with toys' and as reflecting the masculine preference for technology within health care in general. Another woman described as 'chilling' her growing awareness of the role of medical technology.

The women in these studies were generally from lower socio-economic backgrounds or from ethnic minorities, who tend to have a higher rate of cancer but a lower uptake of mammography. Rather than acquiescing with scientific medical advice, these women protected themselves from the threat of cancer either by refusing to discuss it, by associating it with other people, or by characterizing cancer screening as a potential cause of the disease itself. This accords with

Joffe's (1999: 10) argument that 'people are motivated to represent the risks that they face in a way that protects them, and the groups with which they identify, from threat. They make meaning of the threat in line with self-protective motivations rather than with rational dictums'.

Another screening programme within the UK NHS is screening for bowel cancer using a faecal occult blood test that people carry out in their own homes using cardboard spatulas and sending samples through the post. Uptake is relatively low, ranging from 35% in the most deprived areas to 61% in the least deprived areas. Palmer et al. (2014) used focus groups to explore reasons for this low uptake. Participants described sampling faeces and storing faecal samples as crossing a cultural taboo, and causing shame. Having to complete the test kit within the home rather than a formal health setting was felt to be unsettling and reduced the perceived importance of the test.

Not knowing the screening results was reported to be preferable to the implications of a positive screening result. Feeling well was associated with low perceived relevance of screening, and talking about bowel cancer screening with family and peers emerged as the key to subsequent participation in screening after receiving the test kit through the post. Palmer et al. (2014: 1705) concluded that 'Initiatives to normalise discussion about bowel cancer screening, to link the (screening) to general practice, and to simplify the test itself may lead to increased uptake across all social groups'.

EXPERIENCE OF CANCER SCREENING

Most of the research on cancer screening has concentrated on describing those factors associated with initial attendance for mammography. However, according to current guidelines, women are expected to attend not once but on a regular basis. Fewer studies have examined this process of re-attendance, although the evidence does suggest that rate of attendance for follow-up is lower than for initial examination (Sutton et al., 1994). One key factor in re-attendance is the woman's reaction to the initial test. Evidence suggests that this is not always positive.

Women often find mammography screening painful. Keefe et al. (1994) reviewed studies on the experience of pain during mammography and found that the percentage of women reporting pain varied widely across studies, with a range of 1–62%. Admittedly, four of the eight studies reviewed by Keefe et al. (1994) found that at least one-third of the women reported some degree of pain during mammography. Admittedly, many accept the pain and discomfort since it is of short-term duration and has long-term benefits. However, some are less accepting and indeed feel that the pain may increase their risk of cancer. Whelehan et al. (2013) found in a review of 20 studies that 25–46% of women who had not re-attended cited pain as a reason.

There is also evidence that cervical screening can be uncomfortable for some women. Schwartz et al. (1989) found in her survey of women in the East End of London that 54% rated having a smear test as painful or uncomfortable and 46% found it embarrassing. Similarly, in a qualitative study (Waller et al., 2012) it was found that the women often talked about the test in terms of embarrassment, violation or pain. Again, such experiences would not be expected to encourage re-attendance.

In her study in the East Midlands of England, Armstrong (2007) contrasted the official discourse on cervical screening with that of the women. Whereas the former presented the smear test as a simple, painless and non-intrusive procedure, the women characterized it as invasive and very uncomfortable. Armstrong, using Foucauldian discourse analysis, referred to three resources on which the women drew to challenge the official discourse. The first of these was their emotional experiences through which the women could explain their feelings. For example, one woman said:

> It's just something that I just hate, I think it's, you know I don't know what it is and I know to the nurse it's nothing but I think it's just, perhaps because I'm such a private person. (Armstrong, 2007: 77)

In this case, the woman is emphasizing her 'private' nature that led to her feeling particularly uncomfortable about the test. A second resource was the actual physical experiences in that the women drew attention to their physical experiences. For example, one woman said:

> every time uncomfortable and painful, they're just horrible … apparently, erm, I've got a funny shape so when the instrument is put in it goes in to open your cervix up it doesn't always go properly because of the shape. (Armstrong, 2007: 79)

The third resource was the changing body that was an extension to the physical experiences. In talking about the smear test, these women were not trying to find a way to avoid attending for the test, but rather were challenging the official medical discourse of the smear test as routine.

PSYCHOLOGICAL CONSEQUENCES OF CANCER SCREENING

In the initial haste to establish screening programmes, the psychological cost in terms of increased anxiety was overlooked. There are obvious adverse psychological consequences for women from being recalled following screening, even if they are subsequently cleared. In the UK, about 5% of women who undergo breast cancer screening are called back for further tests. This is termed a 'false positive' diagnosis. Although recalled women may be given the 'all-clear' following the further tests, they often still harbour uncertainty and anxiety.

The false positive result is followed by further anxiety-provoking investigation that will include clinical examination and possibly surgery. In a ten-year follow-up, Elmore et al. (1998) found that as many as one-third of women who obtained positive results were required to undergo additional investigations, including biopsies, even though it turned out that they did not have breast cancer.

In a large Danish study, women who underwent screening for breast cancer were surveyed at baseline, then at 1, 6, 18 and 36 months (Brodersen and Siersma, 2013). The women were classified into three groups – those with a diagnosis of breast cancer, the false positives and those with a normal result. Those with the diagnosis of breast cancer had the most psychological disruption, followed by those with the false positive diagnosis. Even at 36 months after they had been given the all-clear, the women who had been false-positively diagnosed still reported substantial psychological disruption. An earlier UK study found similar findings. Women who had initially been falsely diagnosed but then were cleared of having breast cancer were found still to be suffering psychological symptoms three years later (Brett and Austoker, 2001). Further, those women who had undergone the most additional tests experienced greater anxiety.

In a qualitative study of the impact of a false-positive mammography result Bond et al. (2015) found that the reaction ranged from nonchalance to extreme fear. The former group of women claimed that when they received the initial letter they were not overly concerned, but rather curious or surprised. Conversely, the latter group of women described the intense anxiety they felt on receiving the recall letter. For them, it opened the prospect of cancer and death. This anxiety increased when they attended the assessment clinic. This is when they became acutely aware of the potential implications if the diagnosis was confirmed. After they were cleared, some of the women reported intense emotional reactions. However, some of the women reported continuing anxiety, which was related to how the result was communicated by the physician. Some of the women reported that this anxiety continued for many years after they were given the all-clear. For them, there still lingered the fear of developing breast cancer.

Moving beyond false positives are those women who are diagnosed and treated for cancer and found not to have it. The term 'overdiagnosis' is used to describe the diagnosis of cancer at screening that would not have been clinically apparent in the woman's lifetime. There is debate about the extent of such overdiagnosis, with most estimates around 19–35%. An independent UK panel (Marmot et al., 2013) reviewed the evidence and concluded that for every 10,000 UK women aged 50 years invited for screening over the next 20 years, a total of 43 deaths would be prevented while 129 cases would be overdiagnosed, i.e., one breast cancer death prevented for every three overdiagnosed cases. A focus group study of women concluded that the benefits still outweighed the risks. The Panel concluded that information should be made available in a transparent and objective way to women invited to screening so that they can make informed decisions.

HEALTH SERVICE ORGANIZATION FOR CANCER SCREENING

Several studies have found that the most influential factor in explaining variation in participation is the extent to which the woman's doctor recommends participation (National Cancer Institute, 1990). Further, Lurie et al. (1993) found that women are more likely to undergo screening with pap smears or mammograms if they see female rather than male physicians. There is evidence to suggest that some physicians are reluctant to advise mammography for a variety of reasons, including scepticism about its effectiveness in general or for certain groups of women and fear of the effect of radiation.

A further reason for the hesitancy among some physicians in the USA as to recommending screening is fear of litigation. It has been suggested in the USA that many physicians may be reluctant to talk about screening with their patients because of the public controversy about screening guidelines (Leitch, 1995). This could lead to anxiety among some physicians, bearing in mind that delayed diagnosis of breast cancer is one of the most common causes of malpractice complaint. In the USA, women who have developed cervical or uterine cancer after smear tests have won legal cases because of inappropriate treatment.

More countries and regions are now establishing dedicated cancer screening programmes with postal invitations to women to attend on a regular basis. Despite these moves, a proportion of women are still reluctant to participate in screening. Similarly, some women do not participate even when they are personally encouraged to attend by their physician (May et al., 1999). Sharp et al. (1996) found that a personal invitation by a woman's family doctor was as effective as a home visit from a nurse conveying the same message.

It has been shown that campaigns designed to increase awareness of breast cancer contribute to increased uptake of both breast self-examination and mammography screening (Anastasi and Lusher, 2017). The type of message seems to be important, with narrative messages about screening being more effective than statistical messages for women with low levels of education (Perrier and Martin Ginis, 2017).

MEN AND CANCER SCREENING

Most of the research on psychological aspects of cancer screening has been on women and their use of breast and cervical cancer screening programmes. Since there are no similar programmes for men it is not surprising that there is less research. However, there is increasing discussion about the potential value of screening for both colorectal and prostate cancers among men. The limited psychological research has often been from a social cognition framework. These studies have referred to the importance of such factors as attitude, perceived behavioural control and perceived social norms as important predictors of intention to participate in such screening (e.g., Sieverding et al., 2010).

Several studies have confirmed the lower rates of uptake of screening programmes among men from low SES and ethnic minority backgrounds (e.g., von Wagner et al., 2011). In a study of US Hispanic males, Goodman et al. (2006) identified a series of perceived barriers to participation in screening for colorectal cancer. These included low levels of knowledge and awareness, lack of understanding of the screening test, and language and communication challenges.

The importance of the cultural context was identified in a qualitative study of New Mexico Hispanic men and women (Getrich et al., 2012) that considered the meaning of machismo – or the 'tough guy' attitude. They found that it was particularly important among the Mexicans interviewed. One woman said: 'Yes, machismo's a problem. I think that [men] are all the same. They feel that they are not sick – they say, "Nothing hurts me!"' Conversely, this was less evident among the Hispanos interviewed. For example, one man said: 'Macho is gone, those days are gone. It's a lot different than it was before ... people get together and talk.' A qualitative study of Latino men's views of prostate cancer screening (Rivera-Ramos and Buki, 2011) also identified the importance of machismo as a deterrent to participation. The men interviewed in this study frequently referred to the digital rectal examination that is part of the prostate cancer screening as being a threat to their masculinity. As one participant said: 'It's almost the worst thing that can happen to a man.'

Similarly, a qualitative study of UK males found apprehension about screening for prostate cancer (Grogan et al., 2017). Analysis of interviews with a sample of middle-aged men identified limited understanding of the screening test. Most of the men expressed discomfort at the idea of an anal examination. Whether they sought support for any possible prostate symptoms would depend upon how medical professionals communicated with them. A large survey study of men facing diagnosis for prostate cancer reported higher levels of anxiety which increased as they came nearer to finding out (Dillard et al., 2017). The anxiety level was higher among those with limited knowledge of the cancer. This would confirm the importance of providing education to men receiving a biopsy.

GENETIC SCREENING

The rapid advances in genetic research now hold out the prospect of genetic screening for different diseases. This can take various forms (see Lerman, 1997). Carrier testing investigates people who are likely to be carriers of the genes for such diseases as cystic fibrosis or Tay–Sachs disease. This form of testing is usually conducted in the context of reproductive decision-making. Presymptomatic testing allows the identification of a disease before the symptoms develop. This form of testing is used to determine the person's risk of developing such late-onset diseases as Huntington's disease. Susceptibility testing is designed to test for a person's susceptibility to develop a disease, although whether that disease develops depends upon a variety of environmental and nutritional factors partly outside the person's control.

Although the general principles underlying genetic screening are like those of other forms of screening, there are certain unique features. Lerman (1997) described several distinguishing features that need to be taken into consideration when investigating the psychological aspects (see Box 15.2). These factors need to be accounted for in exploring the development of these services.

An extension of cancer screening programmes has been genetic testing for cancer. This is still not a very common procedure but has attracted substantial interest among certain population sub-groups. In a study in New Zealand, Cameron and Reeve (2006) found that worry about cancer was associated with interest in obtaining such a test, although perceived risk was not. It was suggested that this may be due to perceived risk leading to more cautious appraisals of the benefits of genetic testing.

The importance of the patients' assessment of the benefit of the test was shown in a qualitative study of patients, patient group representatives and health professionals involved in clinical genetic services (McAllister et al., 2008a). This study found that a common integrating theme in the patients' accounts was perceived *empowerment*. By this was meant that participating in the genetic testing enhanced the patients' feelings of control over their disease. As one patient group representative said:

> Information is power, [you're] powerless if you don't have information and that's one of the problems that we've come across. Families feel isolated, they have anxiety because they have no information therefore they have no power … I mean power to make the right decisions. (McAllister et al., 2008b: 898)

BOX 15.2

Features of genetic screening

Type of information

Genetic information is probabilistic and uncertain. In some cases you can say with certainty that a person will develop a disease, but *when* is less clear (e.g., Huntington's disease). In other cases, it is unclear whether the person will develop the disease at all (e.g., cancer).

Medical value

Control over disease onset is limited for certain diseases (e.g., cancer) and non-existent for others (e.g., Huntington's disease).

(Continued)

> ### Timescale
>
> The timescale is variable in that the results of genetic testing concern events that may occur far in the future.
>
> ### Impact of results
>
> The results affect not only the individual but also the family, since genetic susceptibility is transmitted within families.
>
> *Source*: Lerman (1997: 4)

PSYCHOLOGICAL CONSEQUENCES OF GENETIC SCREENING

Unlike cancer screening, genetic testing is often initiated by individuals when they suspect that because of family history they may be carriers. Thus, they would be expected to be in a heightened state of anxiety. Several studies have found a reduction in such anxiety following testing (e.g., Tibben et al., 1993). However, some studies have reported evidence of subsequent psychological distress. Lawson et al. (1996) found that of 95 individuals receiving the results of a test for Huntington's disease, two made plans for suicide and seven had clinical depression. Interestingly, there was no difference between those who tested positive and those who tested negative. Tibben et al. (1993) found that carriers tended to minimize the impact of the test results on their futures.

In a large systematic literature review, Broadstock et al. (2000) found no evidence of increased distress (general and situational distress, anxiety and depression) in carriers or non-carriers within 12 months after testing. Rather, both carriers and non-carriers showed decreased distress after testing; this was greater and more rapid among non-carriers. However, they point out that the studies were on self-selected populations who had agreed to participate in psychological assessment and that there was a need for further research.

There is some evidence that the positive effect of screening may only be short term. At six-month follow-up Tibben et al. (1993) found that one-quarter of the carriers exhibited signs of psychopathology. They continued to follow the group for three years (Tibben et al., 1997) and found that for the first six months there was a rise in avoidant thoughts and a decrease in intrusive feelings. This was followed by a reversal of this pattern. It was suggested that this was evidence of a coping strategy whereby the carriers 'dose themselves' with tolerable levels of intrusive thoughts as they begin to process and accept the test results.

Genetic screening can also have a dramatic impact on the family of the carrier. Hans and Koeppen (1989) found that partners often reacted with disbelief and denial. However, this turned to resentment and hostility as they became aware of the threat of transmission to their children. The partners can play a key role in helping the carrier cope with the diagnosis (Tibben et al., 1993).

The prospect of widespread genetic screening has provoked sustained debate about the ethical issues. Harper (1997) voiced concern that the needs of individuals and families are being made subservient to broader eugenic goals. Stone and Stewart (1996) claimed that the voice of the public is rarely heard in this debate. They argue that the advocates of genetic screening often falsely claim that their programmes are based on the public's right to know. Yet there is little evidence that the public wants to know. Stone and Stewart also raised a variety of other questions about genetic screening, such as the ability of lay people to interpret genetic information, the competence of health personnel in explaining aspects of genetic screening and the use made of genetic information.

In a review of the social impact and ethical implications of genetic testing, Davison et al. (1994) identified three areas of popular perception that have implications for predictive testing for Huntington's disease:

1. Both positive and negative results can lead to personal and family anguish. While the former is expected, there is also evidence that those who are cleared suffer from survivor guilt and a feeling they do not belong to their family.

2. Some families who inherit the gene have developed ways of deciding who in the family will be sufferers. This lay procedure is undermined by medical investigation.

3. Knowing about possible futures may decrease the quality of a person's life. Davison et al. (1994: 354) note that this finding 'is not easily accommodated within the essentially rationalist or utilitarian philosophy underlying the idea of screening'.

One aspect of remaining ignorant is that it allows the maintenance of hope. Many lay people are happy to tolerate uncertainty because of the hope that they will survive.

The premise of much genetic testing is that people understand the basic principles of inheritance. However, this may not always be the case. In an interview study of members of families at risk of familial adenomatous polyposis (FAP), which geneticists consider to be almost 100% genetic, Michie et al. (1996b) found that many referred to what they considered to be the vital role of the environment. Many of the family members also minimized the threat posed by the disease. While advising these people that they are at risk may be formally correct, it has immense implications for the future quality of their lives.

Riley et al. (2012) present recommendations on the essential elements of genetic cancer risk assessment, counselling and testing on behalf of the National Society of Genetic Counsellors in the USA. They argue that psychosocial assessment should be part of both the pre-test and post-test genetic counselling process, beginning by identifying the patient's primary reason for seeking the consultation and enquiring about the patient's current understanding of cancer genetics risk assessment and testing process. The skills required by genetic counsellors are complex and far-reaching. The counsellor should address any misconceptions in a sensitive manner and help the patient with his/her cancer worry, intrusive thoughts, depression, anger, fear, guilt, family experiences with cancer, perception of risk for self and others, competence for giving informed consent, social stressors, supports and networks, family communications and readiness for testing.

IMMUNIZATION

Immunization is the procedure whereby those individuals who are most susceptible to contracting certain communicable diseases are administered a vaccine. This procedure is aimed at both the immediate protection of individuals and immunity across the whole community where the uptake rate is high. Over the years, various vaccines have been developed for specific diseases.

In the mid- to late nineteenth century several countries began to introduce vaccines to prevent specific diseases. In the UK, laws were passed making smallpox vaccination of children compulsory. However, this was not always met with approval and in some countries led to the development of anti-vaccination societies (Blume, 2006). This was perhaps not surprising in view of the organization of public health practice at that time, but gradually this opposition declined and a range of vaccines have been introduced over the past century. According to current public health agencies, immunization is now one of the most successful examples of the primary prevention of disease. However, as McKeown (1979) emphasized, the specific impact of vaccination programmes should not be confused with the health benefits of improvements in living and working conditions.

Despite the apparent success of mass immunization programmes (Figure 15.2), a substantial proportion of individuals are not immunized against certain diseases. Indeed, this has given rise to what has been described as a new anti-vaccination movement (Blume, 2006). An understanding of this participation of people in mass vaccination programmes requires an exploration of individuals' perceptions and the broader social context.

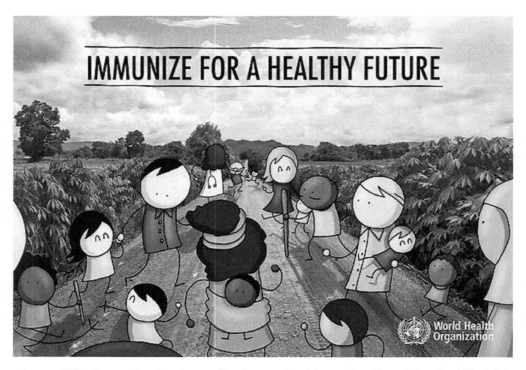

Figure 15.2   Immunization is an effective method for saving lives. Measles killed 2.6 million people before 1980 when the vaccine was introduced. That figure has dropped to around 100,000

Source: Poster produced by the World Health Organization: http://apps.who.int/immunization-week-posters

PSYCHOLOGICAL MODELS OF IMMUNIZATION

There is a large body of research using different social cognition models (SCMs) to predict uptake of vaccination. A common feature of these models is risk perception. In a meta-analysis of 48 such studies, Brewer et al. (2007) distinguished between three dimensions of risk that were termed perceived likelihood, perceived susceptibility and perceived severity. These dimensions are detailed in Table 15.1. A fourth dimension – perceived risk if you do not take the health-protection action – was also noted. However, since this dimension was seldom reported in research, it was not included in the meta-analysis.

The results of the meta-analysis showed that:

- Those perceiving a higher likelihood of getting an illness were more likely to be vaccinated.

- Those who perceived themselves to be more susceptible to a particular illness were more likely to be vaccinated.

- Those who perceived the severity of the particular illness to be higher were more likely to be vaccinated.

It could be argued that these relationships were simply *post-hoc* rationalizations for receiving the vaccinations, i.e., after being vaccinated the individuals justified their actions by emphasizing their perceived risk. However, the effect sizes for the prospective studies were larger than for the cross-sectional studies, suggesting that this was not the case.

Table 15.1   Dimensions of risk

Dimension	Description	Example
Perceived likelihood	Probability that one will be harmed by the hazard	'If I don't get immunized, there is a high chance I'll get the flu'
Perceived susceptibility	Constitutional vulnerability to a hazard	'I get sick more easily than others my age'
Perceived severity	Extent of harm that the hazard would cause	'The flu can kill you'

Source: Brewer et al. (2007)

It was also noted that the effect sizes were larger for influenza vaccination than for other forms of vaccination. This may have been due to a variety of factors, including:

- The non-flu studies included a wide range of vaccines, each with perceived characteristics.

- Flu vaccination is more familiar and contributes to a clearer perceived risk.

- The non-flu vaccines (e.g., hepatitis) require multiple vaccinations that may attenuate the risk perception.

Findings on the role of risk perception in explaining vaccination can be contradictory. For example, in an online experiment, Betsch and Sachse (2013) found that strong 'no risk' messages were followed by a higher perceived vaccination risk than weak 'no risk' messages.

Further, there is evidence that the role of risk depends upon who the risk is for – self or someone else. For example, in a survey of parents, Tang et al. (2014) found that they were more willing to vaccinate their child than themselves. It was suggested that parents were likely to take a risk of non-vaccination for themselves, but they were anxious about doing similar for their child. Some evidence of this was found in a Q-methodology study of parental understandings of child vaccination (Harvey et al., 2015a). In this study, parents completed a Q-sort task after their two-month-old infant had been immunized. Four factors were identified in the Q-sort as being important: A: 'Because the doctor told me to'; B: 'I know what's best for my baby'; C: 'Will they really be OK?'; and D: 'Why wouldn't you protect them?' While there were differences between parents in which factors they stressed, all agreed that vaccination provided unrivalled protection against disease. However, those parents with factor C also had feelings of uncertainty about vaccine safety and its side effects.

Recently there have been attempts to expand SCMs of health behaviour to include emotional components. In the case of immunization, this has included emotions such as worry and regret. In a study of university employees, Chapman and Coups (2006) found that anticipated regret and worry were stronger predictors of vaccination than perceived risk. This would confirm that humans are less concerned about statistical estimates of risk and more with how they feel about the likelihood of something happening.

SOCIO-CULTURAL CONTEXT OF IMMUNIZATION

As with our earlier discussion of screening, there is a need to locate the cognitive view of the risk associated with immunization within a broader understanding of the meaning of immunization and infectious diseases and the socio-cultural context.

The widespread introduction of immunization programmes over the past two centuries is a major example of the power of medical science. However, this power has not been accepted unquestionably. Blume (2006) has reviewed the growth of anti-vaccination movements over the past two centuries. When compulsory vaccination was introduced in the mid-nineteenth century it was opposed by a wide range of groups of people, including the middle class, who were concerned with threats to individual liberty, but especially by the organized working class, who opposed the growing power of the state in the disciplining of the body. In the 1970s the public concern about the safety of the pertussis vaccine led to a substantial fall in its uptake. More recently, moves to introduce a range of new vaccines have been met with varying degrees of support.

The swine flu vaccine was introduced into many countries in 2009. Although in some countries it was enthusiastically received, in others this was not the case. For example, in North America there were active campaigns for mass vaccination against swine flu, whereas in the UK, after some initial debate, support for it declined as evidence for the severity of the epidemic declined. This is probably a reflection of the greater medicalization of American society.

Dew (1999), in his review of changing media representations of measles, argues that the dominant approach of the media has been an acceptance of the medical viewpoint. However, in this age of risk (Beck, 1992) the media can become a forum for challenging the accepted medical approach. A review of British newspapers during the 1990s found a substantial increase in reportage of vaccine-related topics (Cookson, 2002). Of note was the finding that an increasing proportion of these articles dealt specifically with concerns about the safety of vaccines.

In addition, there are an increasing number of websites devoted to critical views of vaccination. This would suggest that the debates about the value of immunization that were current in the nineteenth century are again growing. It is within this context of confusion that individuals attempt to develop an approach that is personally and socially responsible.

IMMUNIZATION AMONG CHILDREN

Much of the debate and research on immunization has focused on children and their parents. The reason for this is that it is expected that from a very early age children receive immunization against a range of diseases, such as whooping cough, polio and measles. Despite substantial health care expenditure, immunization uptake among children is not comprehensive. For example, more than two-thirds of Primary Care Trusts (PCTs) in England (221 of 294) reported less than 85% coverage for MMR during 2003–2004. Indeed, the coverage fell below 70% in 19 PCTs (Henderson et al., 2008). As with adults, rates of immunization have been found to be lower among children from more disadvantaged communities and from certain minority ethnic communities.

New and Senior (1991) conducted detailed interviews with over 250 mothers from north-west England. They found that mothers with lower educational qualifications, mothers living alone, mothers with large families and mothers with a sick child were the best predictors of non-immunization. A study in the north of England (Reading et al., 1994) found that even after the establishment of an immunization programme, the relationship between immunization uptake and social deprivation remained. In this study, the immunization of four birth cohorts between 1981 and 1990 was examined. Although there was an overall increase in uptake, the rates remained lowest among the children from the most disadvantaged areas.

Several studies have identified a variety of reasons expressed by parents for not having their children immunized. These have been summarized by Meszaros et al. (1996) under five categories that focused on perceptions of risk and risk management (see Table 15.2).

Table 15.2 Parental reasons for non-immunization

Risk: benefit ratio	Perception that the risks of contracting the disease outweigh the benefits of being immunized
Individual risk	Belief that the societal statistics that public health planners use do not apply to their child. Further, the parents believe that they can protect the child from exposure
Ambiguity aversion	Aversity to options with ambiguous outcomes such that parents will prefer a straightforward Yes/No assessment of the likelihood of their child contracting a disease. When there is disagreement about potential risk they will err on the side of caution. Further, some parents may already be sceptical of medical information
Omission bias	Preference for acts of omission over acts of commission
'Free riding'	Assumption that since most of their children's peers have been vaccinated they are protected

Source: Meszaros et al. (1996: 698)

In their study, Meszaros et al. (1996) attempted to assess the relative importance of each of these explanations in a questionnaire survey of readers of *Mothering*, a popular magazine read by mothers in the USA. They found that the most important predictors of parents having their child immunized were the perceived dangers of the vaccine, doubts about medical claims that vaccines are effective, omission bias, belief that physicians overestimate the dangerousness of the disease, perceived ability to protect their child, and perceived assessment of the likelihood of their child contracting the disease.

Following a series of reports in the 1990s of a possible link between childhood vaccination and autism, vaccination rates dropped. Subsequent reports have been strongly challenged, and childhood MMR vaccination rates for England steadily increased from 85.2% in 2006–2007 to 92.7% in 2013–2014 but there was a slight decline in the following two years to 91.9% in 2015–2016 (NHS Digital, 2016). However, anti-vaccination organizations continue to report this link, promoting fear and anxiety among parents. According to a Swedish study by Dannetun et al. (2005), parents report obtaining information on vaccination from the media (82%) and the internet (36%). A study of websites on vaccination found that nearly half contained vaccine critical information (Davies et al., 2002). Further, these websites often use emotional appeals and personal stories coupled with photographs and pictures. In an experimental study, Betsch et al. (2010) found that accessing a vaccine critical website increased the perception of risk due to vaccination.

This fear of the adverse effect of immunization may be particularly high in certain communities. In a study in England (Loewenthal and Bradley, 1996) it was found that the uptake of childhood immunization was particularly low among orthodox Jews. It was suggested by the mothers who were interviewed that the main reason for their low uptake was their fear of a negative reaction, logistical difficulties and unsympathetic treatment by health staff. According to the health professionals, the mothers' fears were exaggerated because they lived in a close-knit community that perpetuated tales of bad reactions. A more recent study of a similar community by Henderson et al. (2008) emphasized the importance of the closed nature of the community, within which rumours about the harm done by immunization were combined with a general concern about the negative influence of the outside world on the Jewish community. Table 15.3 summarizes the main findings of the study.

Besides these factors, an additional element is the perceived relative risk. In a qualitative investigation of the views of a sample of inner-city parents in Baltimore, Keane et al. (1993) found that although some parents accepted that they or their children might be vulnerable to infectious diseases, other threats, such as drugs, street violence and 'the wrong crowd', were considered more severe. Further, vaccines were viewed as only partly successful. The continued occurrence of chickenpox was frequently cited as evidence of vaccine failure.

Table 15.3   Childhood immunization in an orthodox Jewish community

Social network	Advice circulated through local networks
Media	Stories from mass media coupled with negative feelings about outside world
Safety	Separation of community from outside influence led to feelings of safety
Danger	Immunization was perceived as 'putting the disease in the child'

Source: Henderson et al. (2008)

A frequent explanation given by mothers in several studies is the natural/unnatural distinction. This was alluded to in a large German study by Weitkunat et al. (1998). They found that the most significant predictors of measles immunization were parental natural health orientation, advice of paediatrician, birth-order position, dangerousness of measles, marital status, reliability of vaccination and smoking. They suggested that natural health orientation and advice of paediatricians may be interactive since individuals with a natural health orientation may select like-minded physicians. In a more detailed analysis of what they described as the subjective relevance of measles, they found that those who assessed the likelihood of contracting measles as high and the latency as low were more likely to have their children immunized. A more recent German study of Facebook groups (Betsch and Sachse, 2013) reported finding that those with a preference for conventional medicine also tended to have a positive attitude to vaccination.

Taken together these findings would suggest that while parents may be hesitant about having their child immunized because of their anxiety about the potential risk, this image is compounded by media speculation and by the contradictory advice they sometimes receive from health professionals. A study in the UK of parents who had had their child immunized found that most shared the view that vaccinations provided protection against disease (Harvey et al., 2015b). For these parents, the process was stress-free. A minority still held the view that there was some uncertainty about the vaccine and they worried about the possible side effects. However, most felt that it was the right thing to do – it was part of their job of being a parent. This would tally with Tickner et al.'s (2007) view that the uptake of immunization among children has become the social norm in the UK.

However, there remain cultural differences. For example, a study in Slovakia investigated the perceptions of mothers and university students of pro-vaccination messages (Massaryk and Hatokova, 2016). They found that the participants were generally concerned about vaccination and that the various pro-vaccination messages did not reduce these concerns and even increased them in some cases. They concluded that this reflected a critical attitude to health professions and to authority such that in the face of ambiguity about the supposed health benefits they adopt a critical and more negative attitude towards vaccination.

A last point needs to be made about a more recent form of childhood immunization. The recent introduction of HPV immunization for 11–12-year-old girls has attracted substantial media and increasing research interest. A survey of parents of adolescent girls resident in North Carolina (Reiter et al., 2009) found that the dimensions of the HBM were predictors of vaccine uptake by their daughters. Parents who reported their daughter had been vaccinated were more likely to perceive the HPV vaccine as effective, perceived fewer barriers and harms, and were also likely to be confident their insurance covered the cost. Although there has been media discussion about the sexual connotations of HPV immunization, they did not find that anticipated regret about greater sexual activity by their daughter was an independent predictor of HPV uptake. However, another study did find some evidence of such a relationship (Ziarnowski et al., 2000).

There remains considerable uncertainty about this new vaccine. A survey of mothers of teenage girls conducted in Texas (Baldwin et al., 2012) found that those parents who perceived their daughters as being vulnerable were more likely to talk with others and their physician about the vaccine. However, people from ethnic minorities were less likely to discuss this vaccine with others. This is a new form of immunization and the role of socio-cultural factors is of obvious importance.

Despite considerable efforts to promote this vaccine, several studies have confirmed that parents remain apprehensive. In a review of studies, Jacobson et al. (2013) identified that the three main perceptions discouraging mothers were the perception that the vaccine was not needed by their daughter, that it was potentially harmful, and that their child was too young because she was not sexually active. Related to the latter perception was the anxiety that having the vaccine might promote earlier sexual activity. There is no evidence for this concern.

Although the target population for HPV vaccination is 11–12-year-old girls, there have been programmes aimed at promoting its uptake among young women. The rates of uptake remain low, with an estimated 18–41% of 18–26-year-old women in the USA reporting uptake (Daley et al., 2010). A survey of college-age women in the USA (Schaefer Ziemer and Hoffman, 2013) found that although perceived benefits was the major predictor of vaccination intentions, many of the unvaccinated women expressed the view that it was not necessary for them since they did not perceive themselves as being at risk. Gerend et al. (2013), in a survey of young women, found that those not intending to be vaccinated cited global concerns about vaccine safety and low perceived need. A study in the UK found that although financial incentives increased uptake among young women, the overall uptake remained low (Mantzari et al., 2015).

ANTI-VACCINE CONSPIRACY THEORIES

One factor in people's resistance to vaccination stems from the belief that vaccinations are dangerous. This idea is promoted quite heavily on anti-vaccination websites and blogs on the internet. There are many prominent alleged conspiracies to be found there, such as the NASA moon landings of 1969 being televised from a film studio, President J.F. Kennedy murdering Marilyn Monroe, the CIA in turn murdering President Kennedy, the Duke of Edinburgh murdering Princess Diana, 9/11 being cleverly arranged by President Bush so companies he had an interest in could grab some oil wells in Iraq, and global warming being a total myth. Vaccination programmes have been the subject of some equally popular conspiracy theories, one of the main ones being that Big Pharma has created evidence supporting vaccinations purely to promote expensive but ineffective vaccines.

The potential impact of anti-vaccination conspiracy theories on vaccination intentions was investigated empirically by Jolley and Douglas (2014). The results suggest that conspiracy theories can be influential. In one study, British parents completed a questionnaire measuring beliefs in anti-vaccine conspiracy theories and the likelihood that they would have a fictitious child vaccinated. A significant negative relationship was found between anti-vaccine conspiracy beliefs and vaccination intentions mediated by the perceived dangers of vaccines, and feelings of powerlessness, disillusionment and mistrust in authorities. In a second study, participants read information that either supported or refuted anti-vaccine conspiracy theories, or a control condition. Participants who were exposed to material supporting anti-vaccine conspiracy theories showed less intention to vaccinate than those in the anti-conspiracy condition or controls. The effect was mediated by the same variables as in Study 1. Jolley and Douglas's findings point to the potentially detrimental impact of anti-vaccine conspiracy theories, and highlight their potential role in shaping health-related behaviours. Disinformation can be an effective influence on behavioural intentions, so it would seem.

In her review of the role of risk communication in vaccination decision-making, Reyna (2012) emphasized that people with limited knowledge of an issue are more likely to engage in superstitious thinking linking vaccination with adverse events that occur around that event. Downs et al. (2008) criticized official communication as being cryptic, while anti-vaccine communications were more coherent.

In the case of HPV vaccination, there remains substantial opposition to its promotion. Although there is evidence that HPV vaccination can reduce infections (Garland et al., 2016), opposition to its uptake is often from a moral standpoint because it is promoting greater sexual activity among young people. Here health psychology must balance the competing interests of medical/health and moral/cultural agendas, with the former enmeshed with the risk of the increasing medicalization of society (Hayes, 2016).

CONCLUSION ABOUT DISEASE PREVENTION

The development of screening and immunization programmes designed to prevent the onset of specific diseases is premised upon a scientific model of risk, with less attention being given to the social and psychological features. While psychological research has tended to focus on the role of individual perceptions of risk, these need to be studied within the broader socio-cultural context.

FUTURE RESEARCH

1. There is a need for further research on breast self-examination.

2. Modern health care is pervaded by notions of risk control. There is a need to critique the relative contribution of prevention programmes.

3. There are substantial social and ethnic variations in participation in screening and immunization programmes. Research needs to explain the varying meanings of these programmes to population sub-groups.

4. The media plays a significant role in shaping lay people's understanding of vaccination. There is a need for research to consider the influence of different forms of media, including conspiracy theories.

5. Genetic research has rapidly produced a host of social, psychological and ethical issues. There is a need for an expanded programme of research to investigate both professional and public perceptions of genetic screening and the impact on different populations.

SUMMARY

1. Many countries have implemented screening programmes for different forms of cancer. Participation in these programmes varies substantially.
2. Psychological factors associated with the use of these programmes connect with the socio-cultural context.

(Continued)

3. The health professional – especially the family doctor – is central to explaining participation in these programmes.
4. The so-called 'genetic' revolution has many implications for screening.
5. Both the public and people who are at risk of certain diseases have a variety of concerns about genetic screening.
6. A wide range of immunization programmes have been developed for adults and children.
7. A central feature in the uptake of immunization is perceived risk, but this needs to be considered within its socio-cultural context.
8. Parents have a range of fears and anxieties about childhood immunization.
9. Irrational fears and beliefs exert a powerful influence on intentions and decisions.

HEALTH PROMOTION

'Imagination lights the fuse of possibility.'

Emily Dickinson

OUTLINE

This chapter focuses on the psychological dimensions of health promotion. Two contrasting approaches to health promotion are described: the behaviour change approach and the community development approach. Health promotion interventions informed by each approach are described and critically examined. Criteria for the evaluation of the effectiveness of health promotion interventions are also presented. We conclude with discussions concerning healthist discourses in health promotion and the latter's wider implications on subject positioning and experience.

WHAT IS HEALTH PROMOTION?

Health promotion is any event, process or activity that facilitates the protection or improvement of the health status of individuals, groups, communities or populations. The objective is to prolong life and to improve quality of life, that is, to prevent or reduce the effects of impaired physical and/or mental health in those individuals who are directly (e.g., patients) or indirectly (e.g., carers) affected. Health promotion practice is often shaped by how health is conceptualized. While early models focused primarily on disease prevention (as influenced by the biomedical model), more recent models are influenced by the biopsychosocial model, which takes into account the psychological and social determinants of health.

In 1986, the Ottawa Charter for Health Promotion defined health promotion as 'the process of enabling people to increase control over, and to improve, their health' (World Health Organization, 1986: 1). The charter recognized that this process requires the strengthening of skills and capabilities of individuals, communities and social groups. This involves building healthy public policy, creating supportive environments, strengthening community actions, developing personal skills and reorienting health services. The Ottawa Charter also acknowledged that health is a *resource for everyday life*, not the object for living. It affirmed that the prerequisites for this state of well-being should include peace, shelter, education, food, income, a stable ecosystem, sustainable resources, social justice and equity. To achieve its goals, health promotion needs to: (1) advocate for health and create favourable social conditions; (2) enable individuals to achieve their fullest health potential by reducing inequalities and ensuring equal opportunities; and (3) mediate between all sectors of society and coordinate with people from all walks of life. A weighty agenda indeed!

Health psychologists can be involved in health promotion in different ways. There are specialists who have expertise on developing behaviour change techniques, while there are those who work within communities and provide support to other professionals in the health and social care arena (Lawrence and Barker, 2016). In this chapter, we present two commonly used approaches to health promotion: the **behaviour change approach** and the **community development approach**. While these approaches pursue different goals, utilize different means to achieve the goals and propose different criteria for **evaluation**, both aim to promote good health and to prevent or reduce the effects of ill health. Health promotion interventions informed by each approach are described and critically examined.

BEHAVIOUR CHANGE APPROACH

The goal of the behaviour change approach is to bring about changes in individual behaviour through changes in their cognitions. Based on the assumption that humans are rational decision-makers, this approach relies heavily upon the provision of information about risks and benefits of certain behaviours. As such, this approach to health promotion is synonymous with health education as it aims to increase individuals' knowledge about the causes of health and illness. Health information can be disseminated through leaflets, mass and social media campaigns, visual displays or one-to-one advice. Information is often presented as factual and attributed to an expert source. Health messages can be framed positively by highlighting the benefits of the behaviour, or negatively by emphasizing health risks (see Chapter 14). Through the provision of health information, this approach gives the illusion of patient empowerment by enabling individuals to make informed choices and to allow them to take more responsibility for their own health.

Social cognition models and behaviour change

As we saw in Chapter 8, theories about the relationship between knowledge, attitudes and behaviour are known as **social cognition models (SCMs)**. These have been researched in a wide range of preventive health behaviours, such as vaccination uptake, breast self-examination and contraceptive use. SCMs aim to predict the performance of behaviours and, by implication, to provide guidance as to how to facilitate their uptake by manipulating relevant variables (such as beliefs, attitudes and perceptions). A systematic review has shown that published interventions that aim to explain behaviour change and maintenance tend to focus mainly on motivation, self-regulation, resources, habits and social influences (Kwasnicka et al., 2016). It is suggested that there is a close relationship between people's beliefs, attitudes and their intentions to act in particular ways. Consequently, by bringing about changes in knowledge and beliefs, it is hoped to bring about behaviour change. Now that sounds as easy as falling off a log, but is it really?

To give an example, Cassidy et al. (2014) used the health belief model (HBM; Becker, 1974) to design an information-based intervention to promote HPV vaccine uptake. A brochure was given to parents of pre-teen girls, and electronic alerts promoted telephone reminders for dose completion. Using a quasi-experimental design to evaluate outcomes, results showed that parents who received the intervention were 9.4 times more likely to have HPV vaccine uptake and 22.5 times more likely to complete the dose. If these kind of outcomes could be obtained everywhere, that would be really exciting!

The theory of reasoned action (TRA; Fishbein and Ajzen, 1975) and its revised version, the theory of planned behaviour (TPB; Ajzen, 1985, 2002), have also been used extensively to predict health relevant behaviours and to use these as a framework to develop behaviour change interventions (see Chapter 8 for further details). For example, Giles et al. (2014) used the TPB to develop an intervention to improve young people's motivations to breastfeed. PowerPoint slides developed by the Health Promotion Agency (Northern Ireland) were initially used in the programme. This was further developed using information from focus groups and questionnaires with young people exploring their cognitions around breastfeeding. The findings were integrated into the final intervention. This was delivered as part of the Year 10 Home Economics curriculum in the school. To evaluate outcomes, questionnaires that included key components of the TPB were administered to control and intervention schools. Findings showed that female pupils from the intervention group had increased intentions to breastfeed, improved their knowledge, and had more positive attitudes and perceptions of subjective norms towards breastfeeding than those in the control group. The only trouble is we never know whether those good intentions will cash out in actual behaviour, as quite frequently they do not. This is known as the 'intention–behaviour' gap. In a systematic review, McDermott et al. (2016) found that although some behaviour change techniques had positive effects on intention, these did not have an impact on behaviour.

Theoretical developments in the use of SCMs to predict health-relevant behaviours have also seen extensions of existing models by incorporating additional variables (see Chapter 8). For example, Rogers' (1975) protection motivation theory expanded upon the HBM to include the role of fear in promoting behaviour intentions. This model had been influential in the use of fear tactics in persuading people to modify behaviours. One example is the use of graphic warnings in anti-smoking campaigns.

Ruiter et al. (2014) reviewed 60 years of fear appeal research and concluded that fear tactics may not be the most appropriate strategy to promote healthy behaviour. Presenting coping information that increases perceptions of response effectiveness may be more effective than presenting fear-arousing stimuli. Ethical issues also must be taken into consideration when using fear-arousing stimuli in health communication. Brown and Whiting (2014) argued that the use of fear tactics poses the potential risk of harming audiences who do not consent to being exposed to these campaigns and are unable to withdraw from them. Lupton's (1995) critique of the discourse of risk prevalent in contemporary health promotion proposed that 'risk, in contemporary societies, has come to replace the old-fashioned (and in modern secular societies now largely discredited) notion of sin' (Lupton, 1995: 89). This is achieved through the practice of health risk appraisals and screening programmes. Lupton likened these practices to religious confessions where sins are confessed, judgement is passed and penance is expected.

Lupton pointed out that risk discourse attributes ill health to personal characteristics such as lack of will power, laziness or moral weakness. In this way, those 'at risk' become 'risk takers' who are responsible for their own ill health as well as its effects upon others and society as a whole. Lupton argued that risk discourse can have detrimental consequences for those positioned within it: being labelled at risk can become a self-fulfilling prophecy since people may feel reluctant to seek medical advice for fear of being reprimanded. Also, it can give rise to fatalism, as well as anxiety, uncertainty and fear, as, for example, for women 'at risk' of breast cancer who can experience their 'at risk' status as a half-way house between health and illness (Gifford, 1986, cited in Lupton, 1995).

Despite the risks and criticisms associated with the use of fear tactics in health promotion, several campaigns still adopt this approach to influence behaviour change. To explore the reasons for the wide application of fear appeals in health risk communication, Peters et al. (2014) conducted semi-structured interviews with 33 stakeholders in behaviour change interventions in the Netherlands. The analysis suggested that the main reasons for using fear arousal were to attract attention and to encourage audiences to reflect about risks. Social dynamics and power structures in intervention development play a role. While those who were more closely involved in developing and implementing interventions were convinced that fear arousal should be avoided, often they were unable to convince funders, who preferred the use of fear appeals in health risk communication. Furthermore, non-researchers were unable to understand the research evidence about the use of fear tactics and the cognitive processes involved in behaviour change. The psychologist must learn the best ways to communicate evidence to programme investors in a convincing fashion, otherwise there can be conflicts.

Critique of behaviour change approaches to health promotion

The behaviour change approach has attracted many criticisms. First, it is unable to target the major causes of ill health. Individual behaviour change, even when successfully implemented, cannot address socio-economic factors such as poverty, unemployment or environmental pollution. Its objective is change within the individual rather than change in the individual's environment. Neglecting wider determinants of health poses the risk of generating further inequalities in health. As discussed in Chapter 4, there is an association between unhealthy behaviours and socio-economic status (SES). It can be argued that this can be explained by a wider intention–behaviour gap among lower SES groups. However, there is no evidence to support this.

Second, the choice of which behaviour to target lies with 'experts' whose task it is to communicate and justify this choice to the public. As a result, recommendations and advice provided 'from above' can be seen as incompatible with community norms.

Third, the behaviour change paradigm does not address the many variables other than cognitions that influence human actions. Despite the increasing range and complexity of SCMs, there are a number of shared characteristics on which to base a critique of the genre. For example, SCMs conceptualize the individual as a rational decision-maker and are only concerned with conscious, cognitively mediated health behaviours (e.g., the decision to buy a smoke alarm). However, many health habits occur routinely (e.g., brushing one's teeth in the morning) and do not involve conscious decision-making.

SCMs also assume that the same variables are universally relevant to diverse groups of people. The behaviour change paradigm tends to assume homogeneity among the receivers of its health messages. However, information is not received or processed uniformly by those to whom it is directed: mood, motivation, past experience, interest, perceived relevance, lay beliefs, group membership and many other factors mediate the way in which a message is 'heard' and interpreted. Translating and communicating information in a meaningful way is a complex undertaking affected by a multiplicity of factors, including health literacy, the media and the ubiquity of health information (see Chapter 14).

Considering all of these criticisms, it is not surprising that outcomes from interventions based on SCMs are unimpressive, so much so that they show no significant improvements beyond those obtained with interventions lacking any theoretical basis whatsoever. As the authors of one study concluded: 'interventions based on Social Cognitive Theory or the Transtheoretical Model were similarly effective and no more effective than interventions not reporting a theory base' (Prestwich et al., 2014). This is the disappointing legacy of half a century of research with SCMs. Alternative approaches need to be considered as the SCMs are quietly retired.

COMMUNITY DEVELOPMENT APPROACH

Health psychologists have explored different ways of understanding health and illness and engaged with different strategies for intervention with health and well-being. Throughout this book we emphasize the value of broadening the scope of health psychology by considering the social and cultural context within which health and illness are located and developing more socially collective strategies for promoting health. Recently, there has been increasing interest in the **community development approach** within health psychology.

The community development approach aims to improve and promote health by addressing socio-economic and environmental determinants of health within the community. These recognize the close relationship between individual health and its social and material contexts, which consequently become the target for change. Individuals act collectively in order to change their environment rather than themselves. Thus, it constitutes the interface between the environmental and behavioural approaches to health promotion in that it is concerned with the ways in which collectivities can actively intervene to change their physical and social environment. The psychologist serves as an agent of change.

Over the past 20 years there has emerged increasing interest in developing a community health psychology. This has been defined as 'the theory and method of working with communities to combat disease and to promote health' (Campbell and Murray, 2004: 187). As in community psychology itself, there are different orientations. The more accomodationist approach focuses on processes within the community, while the more critical approaches aim to connect intra-community processes with the broader socio-political context.

Theoretical influences in community health psychology

Community health psychology has deliberately attempted to connect with other developments in critical social and health psychology and with developments in community psychology. Paulo Freire's (1910–1990) critical pedagogy is one of the key theoretical influences of this approach. Freire was a Brazilian educator who argued that the campaign to increase literacy was a political struggle. He contrasted the traditional approach to literacy education with a more critical approach. In the former approach, the all-knowledgeable educator pours her/his wisdom into the empty vessels, who are the students. 'Education thus becomes an act of depositing, in which the students are the depositories and the teacher is the depositor' (Freire, 1970: 53). Freire described this as the 'banking' model of education. In the more critical approach, the educator engages with the student in an active dialogical manner to encourage them to consider the broader social and structural restraints on their lives and how they can begin to challenge these through collective action.

Freire used the term *conscientization* to describe this process of developing **critical consciousness**. He stressed that his work was 'rooted in concrete situations' and emphasized the collaborative nature of his work. He described the radical as someone who:

> does not become the prisoner of a 'circle of certainty' within which reality is also imprisoned. This person does not consider himself or herself the proprietor of history or of all people, or the liberator of the oppressed; but he or she does commit himself or herself, within history, to fight at their side. (Freire, 1970: 21)

These ideas were also developed further in the **liberation psychology** of Ignacio Martín-Baró (Box 16.1). While acknowledging Freire's ideas as a powerful starting point for advocacy and community development, Campbell (2014) also encouraged contemporary community health psychologists to develop approaches suitable for new century problems.

BOX 16.1

Liberation psychology

This approach draws its inspiration from the liberation theology developed by the worker-priest movement in different countries in Latin America during the 1950s and 1960s. This movement argued that it was the duty of Catholics to fight against social injustice and to adopt a *preferential option for the poor*. These ideas were given wider currency within psychology by Ignacio Martín-Baró (1942–1989), who was murdered by the Salvadoran army for his campaigning work in defence of the poor.

He developed a form of liberation psychology that set as its primary task the interests of the poor and oppressed. He criticized mainstream psychology for its scientistic mimicry and its lack of an adequate epistemology (including positivism, individualism and ahistoricism). This focus on individualism 'ends up reinforcing the existing structures, because it ignores the reality of social structures and reduces all structural problems to personal problems'. Instead he argued that psychologists need to 'redesign our tools from the standpoint of the lives of our own people: from their sufferings, their aspirations, and their struggles' (Martín-Baró, 1994: 25). He proposed three elements in this new liberation psychology:

1. *A new horizon*: psychology must stop focusing on itself and being concerned about its scientific and social status but rather focus on the needs of the masses.
2. *A new epistemology*: psychology needs to consider what psychosocial processes look like from the perspective of the dominated.
3. *A new praxis*: psychology needs to consider itself as 'an activity of transforming reality that will let us know not only about what is but also about what is not, by which we may try to orient ourselves toward what ought to be' (Martín-Baró, 1994: 29).

Eliot Mishler states in the preface to the collection of his writings that they 'challenge us to align ourselves, as he did in El Salvador, with those struggling for equality and justice in our own country' (Martín-Baró, 1994: xii). Cornish et al. (2014) proposed new ways of thinking about community mobilization by using the Occupy movement as an example (see Box 16.2). The authors argued that modernist conceptualizations of community mobilization tend to 'follow a linear logic, establishing a set of goals, objectives, indicators of success, and a clearly defined and hierarchical division of labour, with leaders on the top and frontline workers at the bottom' (Cornish et al., 2014: 62). However, as reflected in many community-based health interventions, processes tend to be messier and less straightforward than planned. Thus, the authors encouraged community health psychologists to explore alternatives to instrumental rationality. They suggested to 'trust the process' and to create mechanisms that enable people to decide on outcomes themselves. Creating a social space where people can come together for a common cause helped to develop a positive sense of community for Occupy participants (Permut, 2016).

BOX 16.2

Using the Occupy movement to reconceptualize community mobilization

The Occupy movement is a global protest against corporate greed and the unjust distribution of economic and political power in society. It was inspired by the Indignados' occupation of Madrid's Sol Square in mid-May 2011. The movement gained vast media attention when Occupy Wall Street began on 17 September 2011. United by the slogan 'We are the 99%', thousands of protesters camped in hundreds of cities around the world. On 15 October 2011, thousands gathered in London with the aim to occupy the London Stock Exchange (Figure 16.1). As the police blocked their access, the group settled and erected 250 tents in front of St Paul's Cathedral instead. The protesters were evicted four months later. However, during the course of their 'occupation', the group managed to establish a 'community', with common facilities, networks and processes in place to organize themselves.

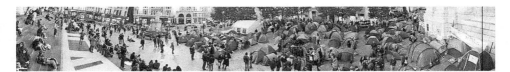

Figure 16.1   Protesters outside St Paul's Cathedral in London

Source: http://en.wikipedia.org/wiki/Occupy_London

This is a concrete example of a process-focused community mobilization wherein goals were developed as part of a process rather than being imposed from above. This movement also reconceptualizes the notion of community wherein shared practices define what it means to be part of a community rather than by similarities of identity, interest or geographical location.

Source: Cornish et al. (2014)

More recently, important developments in South Africa and other countries have served to revitalize community psychology in terms of its socio-political project. This includes projects concerned with the health challenges faced by indigenous people and also the issues of colonialism and post-colonialism (Duncan et al., 2007). These developments have introduced important ideas, such as those of Frantz Fanon (2008). Fanon developed a sophisticated understanding of the psychology of political oppression, in particular the processes by which oppressed people internalize ideas of inferiority and worthlessness.

Another concept relevant to this approach is that of social capital, referring to the community's ability to support empowerment through participation of local organizations and networks. Putnam (2000) discussed two kinds of social capital: *bonding social capital*, which refers to within-group social capital, and *bridging social capital*, which is concerned with linking with outside bodies with the power and resources to enable mutually interesting benefits to accrue. He argued that in modern society there has been a steady decline in social capital, which he characterized as the character of civic participation, trust in others and reciprocity within a community. Other work by Bourdieu has characterized social capital in terms of resources that can be drawn upon. In a systematic review, Samuel et al. (2014) explored social capital concepts related to health education and promotion. Trustworthiness, neighbourly reciprocity, reporting a good sense of community, neighbourhood collective efficacy and behavioural social norms were some of the concepts that were consistently associated with health-promoting behaviours.

Promoting healthy behaviour and well-being in communities

While the traditional focus of health psychology has been on promoting individual behaviour change, there have been various attempts to explore more community-based strategies. Previously, we have discussed how there have been various strategies designed to encourage behaviour change. However, these strategies have adopted the traditional individualist focus. Community health psychology attempts to work with groups or communities to identify how they see the issue and to explore opportunities for change.

Community participation in health promotion can involve various community members in the process – it is not just about community leaders and activists. For example, Dela Llagas and Portus (2016) described how enabling farmers to develop their knowledge and skills to think, communicate, decide and act upon their knowledge can help to successfully promote actions on malarial control among marginalized rural communities in the Philippines. Nakiwala (2016) also demonstrated how children can be actively involved as partners in malaria education in Uganda. In this context, children acted as health messengers, and offered peer support and environmental management. This helped to boost the children's knowledge about malaria, improved their self-esteem and developed their communication skills. Despite these positive outcomes, the programme also had its drawbacks due to hostility from some adults and time constraints due to tight school schedules.

Barbershops can also be used as a setting for health promotion. For example, in Phoenix, Arizona, Davis (2011) demonstrated how the barbershop can be used as a setting to improve health literacy and knowledge about the screening, treatment and control of high blood pressure among black barbershop owners and their clients. Barbers were trained by health care professionals to monitor and record customers' blood pressure scores. They were also trained to identify customers with untreated hypertension and to be able to advise those who might need to seek further medical attention. Barbers were given information about blood pressure disparities within African-American communities and the impact of tobacco use on cardiovascular health so that they could inform their customers about these issues as well.

Other contexts that can help to build social capital in the local community include playgroups (Strange et al., 2016), and 'Men's Sheds', which are community spaces that enable men to participate in a range of shared activities and interests in an inclusive and friendly environment (Wilson et al., 2016). It has been shown that social ties can be developed among Men's Sheds users and can improve members' physical, psychological and social health, as well as quality of life and willingness to accept health advice (Ford et al., 2015). Similarly, Camic et al. (2017) demonstrated how handling museum artefacts can be used to promote the well-being of people with dementia. The findings suggest that participants showed improvements in their well-being, particularly among those with early stage dementia.

Combatting structural determinants of health inequalities

A more critical community health psychology attempts at all times to connect local action with broader social change. The extent to which community health psychologists make connections with the broader social context depends upon opportunity as well as orientation. Indeed, while community action projects can enthuse the participants, they are often apprehensive about taking wider social action. The magnitude of the task is apparent in the various community projects that have sought to challenge social inequalities in health.

In previous chapters we have outlined the substantial social inequalities in wealth and health that exist both within and between societies. As we have argued, the traditional individualistic lifestyle approach to addressing these inequalities has met with limited success. There is a need to address the material and wider social factors within which these unhealthy lifestyles are located.

Critique of community development approaches to health promotion

It is clear that approaching health promotion using community health psychology as a framework is deeply political. It involves the collective organization of those who are traditionally excluded from decision-making processes and a direct and active challenge to power relations associated with health and illness. As a result, health promotion initiatives using this approach have the potential to come into conflict with interests that lie with the status quo, such as industry, employers, government departments and local councils that aim to make financial savings. Consequently, community action as a form of health promotion is vulnerable to lack of public funding and subject to resistance from dominant social groups (Stephens, 2014).

There is also a danger of '*professionalization creep*', whereby those involved in the initiative become removed from the grassroots concerns of those they set out to represent (Homans and Aggleton, 1988). Self-appointed community leaders or representatives can emerge who claim to speak for all members of the community, but in reality represent the dominant elites. Alternatively, because of the huge personal effort and sacrifice needed to make this type of project work, professionals tend to become emotionally involved, which may lead to *burn-out*. Community change also occurs as a consequence of a complex interplay of actors, circumstances and actions. Generally, community workers have a strong commitment to social justice and may experience tensions when attempting to overcome challenges on the ground (Murray and Ziegler, 2015). The aims and objectives may well be noble and virtuous, but the consequences are not predictable or certain. The outcome could possibly be to the benefit of some and to the detriment of others in unpredictable ways (Estacio and Marks, 2010). When facilitating equitable community partnerships, researchers need to tread carefully. They need to be cautious of project ownership and not make community members feel 'used or over-researched' (Matthew, 2017).

The ability of an intervention to improve the health of individuals suffering from an illness needs to be evaluated if we are to place any confidence in the community psychology approach in health care. Ideally, a similar, robust level of proof is required for all types of intervention, as assumed in the evidence hierarchy (Chapter 7). However, there is an 'uneven playing field' because the same high level of proof available for individual-level interventions is not feasible for community-level interventions. Individual-level interventions of the top-down variety can be studied in randomized controlled trials and the data can be synthesized in meta-analysis. This is because the parameters can be systematically varied in the design of any trial and the conditions controlled accordingly. Bottom-up community interventions are by definition unique to each particular community and circumstance, and the intervention(s) designed in light of the circumstances arising as the various stakeholders influence what actually happens.

A community intervention often feels very messy, fluid and difficult to control, and certainly not amenable to a randomized controlled trial. In fact, it is almost impossible to run trials using matched controlled conditions in bottom-up interventions of the kind reviewed here. When any intervention is truly bottom-up, there is hardly ever going to be the opportunity to provide a controlled evaluation. However, evaluation using other types of design is not precluded, and should ideally be carried out (e.g., processes and outcomes can be monitored and compared at different time points). Drawing upon Freire's later work, the *Pedagogy of Hope*, Nolas (2014) encouraged community health psychologists to engage with the messiness of practice and argued for a 'journey' approach to collective action. Since community health psychologists work with vulnerable groups and usually within multidisciplinary teams, it is important for the field to widen its research agenda and to be more open to interdisciplinary dialogue (Ferreira-Neto and Henriques, 2016). These have implications for the research choices we make, who we choose to work with and who remains neglected (Graham, 2017).

HEALTH PROMOTION EVALUATION

As discussed earlier, evaluation of the effectiveness of health promotion initiatives can be an extremely difficult undertaking. First, we need to differentiate between **outcome evaluation**, i.e., an assessment of changes brought about by the intervention, and **process evaluation**, i.e., an understanding of how and why the intervention worked. In addition, outcome evaluation can focus on a range of different criteria, such as behavioural (e.g., how many people have stopped smoking) or cognitive (e.g., the extent to which people's knowledge about the health risks of smoking has increased) or health status (mental or physical). Furthermore, there may be unintended consequences of an intervention, such as increases in anxiety that may be generated by provision of information about particular risks.

In recent years, increasing emphasis has been placed upon evaluation and the need for evidence-based health promotion. Within a climate of financial pressures and budget cuts, public service expenditure needs to be cost-effective. Governments and funding bodies are more likely to invest in health promotion projects that can be shown to work. In addition, there are ethical reasons for systematic evaluations: ineffective or counter-productive interventions should not be repeated, while effective interventions should be made available as widely as possible.

Evaluation of health promotion interventions can be complex, as some interventions may require multiple components, involving several partners, contexts, target groups or behaviours. Datta and Petticrew (2013) examined the challenges described by researchers when evaluating such interventions. Using extracts from published journal articles ($n = 207$) from January 2002 to December 2011, the analysis suggests that the content and standardization of interventions, development of outcomes measures, and methods used for evaluation were common issues in evaluation. Challenges associated with organizational factors such as the impact of the people involved (i.e., staff and patients) and the organizational context were also described.

In the UK, the Medical Research Council (MRC) (2000, 2008) developed a framework for funders, developers and evaluators of complex interventions (see Figure 16.2). It recognized the complexity of developing and evaluating interventions and acknowledged that this process will require several phases which may not necessarily follow a linear sequence. While experimental designs are preferred, particularly randomized controlled trials, the MRC framework also acknowledged that using experimental designs may not always be feasible. Thus, alternatives have been proposed such as quasi-experimental and observational designs (Craig et al., 2013).

RE-AIM is another framework that can be used to evaluate health promotion interventions. Originally developed by Glasgow et al. (1999), the acronym stands for:

> **R**each – The absolute number, proportion and representativeness of individuals who participate in a given initiative, intervention or programme.
>
> **E**ffectiveness/Efficacy – The impact of an intervention on important outcomes, including potential negative effects, quality of life and economic outcomes.
>
> **A**doption – The absolute number, proportion and representativeness of settings and staff who are willing to initiate a programme or approve a policy.
>
> **I**mplementation (at the setting level) – How closely staff members follow the programme that the developers provide, including consistency of delivery as intended and the time and cost of the programme.
>
> **M**aintenance (at the setting level) – The extent to which a programme or policy becomes part of the routine organizational practices and policies. At the individual level, this refers to the long-term effects of a programme on outcomes after six-month follow-up or more. (*Source*: www.re-aim.org)

The RE-AIM framework has been used for a wide range of health promotion interventions, including sugar-sweetened beverage interventions for children (Lane et al., 2016), older adult exercise programmes (Kohn et al., 2016), Type-2 diabetes primary care prevention (Sánchez et al., 2016), stroke research and education (Jenkins et al., 2016) and patient-centred fall prevention (Katsulis et al., 2016). More recently, it has been used to support the development of interventions and to translate research into practice. There are now over 100 publications that have used this framework.

As well as adopting a pluralistic approach to developing and evaluating interventions, evaluators need to be pragmatic by using data that can be realistically obtained yet remain meaningful and useful to the many key players in implementing the learning from evaluations. Often this is not an easy task. Failure to translate research evidence into practice and policy is not uncommon in clinical and health services (Grimshaw et al., 2012). Research evidence may not be accessible to practitioners and policy makers. It is also possible that practice is informed by other sources of knowledge apart from research (e.g., personal experience and interaction with others).

To bridge the evidence–practice gap, Klinner et al. (2014) recommended that conceptions of health promotion evidence need to be expanded. Furthermore, 'relationship-based' methods need to be harnessed to enable practitioners to document community interactions and to use these as research evidence. This requires developing organizational capacity to enhance practitioners' skills. Reforms in the research-to-practice pipeline are also needed to make research evidence more relevant and actionable in real-life contexts (Green, 2014).

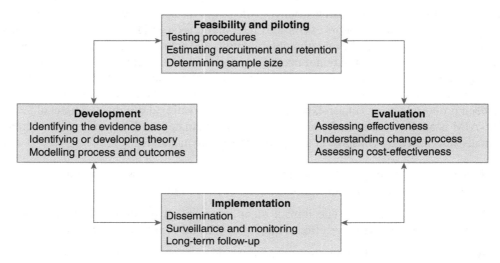

Figure 16.2   Key elements of the development and evaluation process

Source: Craig et al. (2013: 589)

CHALLENGING HEALTHISM IN HEALTH PROMOTION

Health promotion is concerned with strategies for promoting health. It is assumed that (1) good health is a universally shared objective, (2) there is agreement on what being healthy means, and (3) there is a scientific consensus about which behaviours facilitate good health. From this perspective, the real (and only) challenge for health experts and educators is to find effective ways of helping people to maximize their health.

However, there have been criticisms of this contemporary 'ideology of health promotion'. In 1980, Crawford coined the term '**healthism**', which refers to the ideology that situates health and disease within the context of the individual. He raised concerns regarding how healthist ideas could lead to the 'medicalization of everyday life' and reinforce neoliberal ideals by placing the emphasis on personal responsibility for health (see Chapter 4 for further critique of the ideology of the 'responsible consumer').

Evans (1988) argued that such an ideology can also begin to drive health promotion interventions that instead ought to be informed by scientific evidence (both biomedical and psychosocial). Evans drew attention to programmes directed at lifestyle changes that are not unequivocally justified by biomedical research evidence, such as the recommendation to reduce cholesterol levels in the blood to prevent heart disease. Evans worried that 'by increasingly promoting presumably non-risky behaviours, we may be contributing to a type of mass hypochondriasis resulting in an increasingly diminished freedom in human lifestyle and quality of life' (Evans, 1988: 207). This, he suggested, can result in an unhealthy obsession with exercise, an inability to enjoy a meal, as well as a reduction in spontaneity of lifestyle.

Recent critics of the healthist ideology draw upon critical theory to highlight how healthism is propagated in society and how this is used as a method of social control. For example, using critical discourse analysis and Bourdieu's theoretical framework, Lee and Macdonald (2010) explored how healthist discourses are maintained through young people's experiences in school physical education (PE). They interviewed rural young women and examined these alongside discourses from their school PE head of department (HOD). The analysis suggests that healthist discourses were evident in the way the participants discussed physical activity, health, fitness and their bodies. Health and fitness were constructed as important elements that enable them to control body shape and to conform to the 'ideal' feminine appearance. Furthermore, findings suggest that the school's PE curriculum is also being influenced by the HOD's own engagement with healthist discourses and that these too impact upon young people's understandings of health, wellness and their bodies.

The adoption of healthist ideas can also support and maintain social segregation. For example, Gurrieri et al. (2013) examined the impact of healthism-based campaigns on how women's bodies are portrayed, and its implications on subject positioning and experience. Drawing upon embodiment theory, the authors argued that some health promotion campaigns (e.g., breastfeeding, weight management and physical activity) may inadvertently construct women's bodies as sites of control. Using critical visual analysis, the authors showed that such campaigns can represent certain body types as less acceptable. Women who do not fit within the ideal body type or those who engage in activities that counter dominant health messages can become subject to stigmatization and exclusion. Thus the authors urged the emerging field of critical social marketing to develop a broader social justice agenda to address the societal impacts of health promotion campaigns.

Graham et al. (2015) explored the understanding of health among lesbian, gay, bisexual, pansexual, queer and transgender individuals in Aoteraroa/New Zealand. Twelve focus groups with 47 participants were held. Findings suggest that the participants also drew upon notions of healthism, such that health was perceived as holistic and that contextual factors created health risks. There is also a consistent view about the need to preserve health and how health promotion and education efforts are geared towards this purpose.

While healthist ideas can be used as a form of social control, Ayo (2012) argued that in the context of modern neoliberalism, healthism is shaping individuals into health-conscious citizens who willingly abide by society's prescribed norms. Healthy lifestyles are now 'being sold' by health promotion campaigners and other private companies wherein the responsible consumer is expected to buy into this lifestyle in the free market. Thus, social control is no longer constructed as something that is delivered forcefully. Rather, autonomous individuals wilfully obey the state and regulate their own behaviour as 'good and responsible citizens'.

Healthist ideas in health promotion have not gone unchallenged, however. Recent publications have explored the function and position of contemporary health promotion in an attempt to formulate alternatives to individualistic risk-based approaches (e.g., Stephens, 2008). Debates concerning the use of healthist ideas to promote neoliberal agendas have also sparked discussions and research into the politics of health promotion. For example,

Lovell et al. (2014) examined how political changes have impacted on health promotion in New Zealand. They conducted interviews and focus groups with health promotion practitioners between January 2008 and March 2009. While neoliberal reforms have been adopted to increase efficiency in the health care sector, participants from this study have responded critically to government restrictions. In the face of limited resources and budget constraints, health promotion practitioners often have become community advocates when neoliberal agendas have come into conflict with community priorities. In this respect, it is important for health promotion developers and practitioners to reflect upon their position and on how their work impacts upon the lived experiences of individuals and on society as a whole. Health promotion that is guided by evidence, ethics and values may be a good way forward (Carter et al., 2011). Otherwise, the healthist agenda could become yet one more mechanism for the creation of stigma, difference and discrimination.

FUTURE RESEARCH

1. Further development of critical social marketing is needed to encourage more discussion and consideration of wider social determinants of health in social marketing-based health promotion interventions.

2. Methodological developments in community-based research are needed to generate more robust evidence into the impact of community health promotion interventions.

3. Exploration of reforms is needed to encourage effective translation of research evidence into practice.

SUMMARY

1. Health promotion is any event, process or activity that facilitates the protection or improvement of the health status of individuals, groups, communities or populations.
2. Two commonly used approaches in health promotion are the behaviour change approach and the community development approach. Each pursues different goals, utilizes different means to achieve its goals and proposes different criteria for intervention evaluation.
3. The behaviour change approach aims to bring about changes in individual behaviour through changes in the individual's cognitions. Social cognition models are utilized in order to make the link between knowledge, attitudes and behaviour. However, attempts by SCMs to predict behaviour on the basis of cognitions has led to disappointing results.
4. Criticisms of the behaviour change approach include its inability to target socio-economic causes of ill health, its top-down approach to education, its exclusive focus upon cognitions, its assumption of homogeneity among receivers of health messages and its individualism.
5. The community development approach recognizes the close relationship between individual health and socio-economic factors. It aims to remove the socio-economic and environmental causes of ill health through the collective organization of members of the community.

6. Health promotion interventions that use the community development approach can encounter a number of difficulties. They can come into conflict with powerful bodies and they are vulnerable to lack of public funding and official opposition. Other problems include creeping professionalization and difficulties associated with defining and identifying communities.

7. Evaluation of the processes and outcomes of health promotion interventions can be a complex task as interventions may involve multiple components, involving several partners, contexts, target groups or behaviours.

8. Healthist discourses have sparked discussions concerning their role in social governance and control. It is important for health promotion developers and practitioners to reflect upon their values and the impact of their work on the lived experiences of individuals and on society as a whole.

STRESS AND DISEASE PREVENTION[1]

OUTLINE

Stress is a core topic within Health Psychology and deserves a chapter all on its own. Here we discuss theoretical approaches to the study of stress and resilience as determinants of physical illness. The stimulus, response and interactional perspectives and a critical analysis is followed by alternative approaches to stress management and assessments of their effectiveness. The methodological problems confronting research on stress and illness are considered in examining the evidence linking stress to cardiovascular disease, cancer and infectious diseases.

WHAT IS STRESS?

Stress is a word that pops up everywhere these days. In the authors' opinion, the word is overused. The current practice of classifying as a stressor any event that is accompanied by a change in behaviour is sustained by the desire for a simple term that might explain almost anything that feels bad; for example, 'the tension generated by the threat of terrorists, growing economic inequality, increased competiveness in the workplace or for admission to the best universities, rogue nuclear bombs, and media reports of threats to health in food and water. I believe that the concept stress should be limited to select events that pose a serious threat to an organism's well-being or discarded as too ambiguous to be theoretically useful' (Kagan, 2016; Appley and

---

[1]This chapter is an updated version of one contributed originally by Brian Evans to the 3rd and 4th editions. Feeling that the topic was no longer necessary, I fought to have the chapter removed and it was deleted from the 5th edition. However, by popular demand – students and lecturers said they must have it – and with one arm twisted behind my back, I updated it and put it back in (DFM). Will it survive into the 7th edition, I wonder?

Trumbull, 1967). One could say that the word 'stress' has been stressed too much in popular discourse about health and illness. For a spirited defence of the concept, see Cohen, Gianaros and Manuck (2016).

As this book goes to press, the word generates more than 1.5 billion documents on Google. People want to know the answers to questions such as the following:

What are the common signs of stress?

Can stress kill you?

What are the causes of stress?

How can we reduce stress?

Are some people more resilient to stress than others?

In spite of our questioning of the permissive use the term, we will do our best to answer these questions in this chapter. It is often assumed that **stress**[2] is caused by greed, selfishness, uncertainty, smoking, injustice, junk food, competition, family issues, deadlines/insufficient time, life–work balance, feeling stressed, other people stressed, negative thinking, negative emotions, lack of confidence, poor physical health, drinking too much, uncertainty, and a few other things as well. In Australia, many of these concepts were obtained in a qualitative study with students and experts by Kilby, Sherman and Wuthrich (2020).

Life today may be less obviously stressful than the life of our hunter-gatherer ancestors, but modern humans have created an environment that is far from optimal for mental and physical health, especially for people with a limited income. Stress is thought to be a principal cause of psychological distress and physical illness, and millions of working days every year are believed to be lost as a consequence of this. The ability to be resilient and cope successfully with stress is frequently held to be the key to a contented and happy life.

There are two sides to stress as a state or a process. On side one is the stress itself and the stressors that produce it. On side two is the ability to resist the stress or one's 'resilience' to it. Wu et al. (2013) describe resilience as follows:

> Stressful life events, trauma, and chronic adversity can have a substantial impact on brain function and structure, and can result in the development of posttraumatic stress disorder (PTSD), depression and other psychiatric disorders. However, most individuals do not develop such illnesses after experiencing stressful life events, and are thus thought to be resilient. Resilience as successful adaptation relies on effective responses to environmental challenges and ultimate resistance to the deleterious effects of stress, therefore a greater understanding of the factors that promote such effects is of great relevance.

The review by Wu et al. (2013) focuses on genetic, epigenetic, developmental, psychosocial and neurochemical factors that are considered essential contributors to the development

---

[2]The word 'stress' was borrowed from engineering – the ability to build bridges that don't collapse. The more accurate term to have borrowed would have been 'strain' (that which results from stress). Oh well, it's only a word, it is what it is. We will persevere using the term 'stress' even though, strictly speaking, it is incorrect.

of resilience. Increased understanding of resilience should lead to the development of new pharmacological and psychological interventions for enhancing resilience and mitigating the untoward consequences of stress (Wu et al., 2013). Today, researchers are as interested in resilience as much as stress itself.

But what exactly does the term 'stress' actually mean? Answers fall into three main categories (Table 17.1).

Table 17.1   Three perspectives on stress

Theoretical perspective	Popular conception	Major theories and techniques	Approaches to stress management
Stimulus-based	'When things are getting on top of you'	Life event stress scales; studies of workplace and environmental stress	Making jobs and physical environments less stressful
Response-based	'When you feel stressed-out'	Measuring physiological effects of stress; post-traumatic stress disorder	Biofeedback; relaxation and breathing exercises; yoga
Interactional	'When you think that you cannot cope'	Interactional theories; coping scales	Stress inoculation training; mindfulness-based stress reduction

The first answer is that stress occurs 'when you are under a lot of pressure', or 'when things are getting on top of you'. This is essentially the position taken by researchers who adopt a stimulus-based perspective. It is assumed that individuals have a certain tolerance for stress but will become ill when the stress is too great (Bartlett, 1998). Stimulus theorists have tried to devise measures of the relative stressful impact of different life events, ranging in severity from bereavement, divorce and job loss to problems in personal relationships, work pressures and environmental disturbances. These measures have in turn been used to investigate the role of stress as a cause of physical illness. Stimulus-based perspectives are associated with the work of occupational and environmental psychologists, seeking to reduce levels of stress by changing the structuring of jobs, and reducing stressful aspects of the physical environment.

The second answer concentrates on the physical and psychological feeling of 'being stressed' or 'completely stressed out', with symptoms such as anxiety, poor concentration, insomnia, bodily tension and fatigue. This position is taken by theorists who adopt response-based perspectives. They concentrate on the psychophysiology of stress and investigate possible mechanisms linking stress to physical illnesses such as coronary disease and viral infections, by way of the cardiovascular and immune systems respectively. Response-based perspectives have also provided the impetus for the introduction of stress-management programmes that focus on controlling the psychophysiology of stress using techniques such as relaxation and breathing exercises, yoga, aerobics and other forms of physical exercise.

The third answer is that stress is 'when you think you can't cope' or 'when you have too much strain put on you and you do not have the ability to deal with it'. This is the position developed in interactional perspectives by theorists who argue that stress occurs when there is an imbalance between the perceived demands placed on the individual and the ability to meet those demands, often described as *coping resources.* These theories are attractive because they overcome a problem inherent in stimulus and response perspectives; individuals differ as to what events or demands they find stressful and in the ways that they respond to them. Interactional perspectives have led to the study of coping and to the development of techniques such as **stress inoculation training** (Meichenbaum, 2014) aimed at helping individuals to overcome stress by increasing the effectiveness of their coping strategies.

The above three perspectives are not mutually exclusive and it is possible to contemplate the emergence of a very broad 'general theory of stress' which incorporates elements of all of them (e.g., see the General Theory of Behaviour below). However, the classification is useful because it enables us to focus on the three different styles of research and to discuss the criticisms that have been directed at them.

STIMULUS-BASED PERSPECTIVES AND LIFE EVENT SCALES

Holmes and Rahe (1967) conducted some influential research into the types of life events that people rate as being most stressful. They began by choosing 43 probably stressful life events, and then asked 400 US adults to rate the relative amount of readjustment that they judged would be required by each of the 43 events. They used their results to construct a social readjustment rating scale (SRRS) that assigns point values to different kinds of stress and which is still being used in research on the relationship between stress and physical illness.

Some researchers felt dissatisfied with the SRRS because many of the events listed in it occur relatively rarely in anyone's life. There was a need for a scale that reflected to a greater degree the day-to-day variation experienced by people in the levels of the stress to which they are exposed. This led Kanner et al. (1981), using similar techniques to those of Holmes and Rahe, to devise two further scales, a **hassles scale**, consisting of everyday events that cause annoyance or frustration, and an **uplifts scale**, consisting of events that make them feel good.

Much of the research linking physical illness to stressful life events has consisted of retrospective studies in which participants are asked about events occurring prior to the onset of physical illness. These studies have been criticized because people who have recently been ill may very well be predisposed to recollect and report recent stressful events to a greater extent than control group individuals who have remained well. Any such tendency will obviously lead to an overestimation of the association between stress and illness. The inclusion of vague and ambiguous items in the scales is clearly likely to maximize the differential reporting of stressful events.

The question as to whether the scales may be partially measuring neuroticism arises because they include a lot of items such as *too many things to do* or *troubling thoughts about the future*, which could equally find a place in scales designed to measure anxiety or depression. This leads to a problem in interpreting the results even of prospective studies that investigate the association between scores on life events and hassles scales and subsequently occurring physical illness over a period of time. In principle this can establish whether stress really does predict the development of illness. Most prospective studies have relied on self-reports of illness; but it is highly probable that neurotic individuals will not only give high scores on life events and hassles scales, but also be more likely to interpret minor symptoms as indicative of physical illness in comparison with individuals low on neuroticism. Here an empirical association between stress and illness may occur as a result of a reporting bias rather than a genuine causal link. A better approach is to rely on biologically verified assessments of illness.

An improvement on the traditional life events stress scales is the structured interview techniques developed by Brown and Harris. Their **life events and difficulties schedule (LEDS)** is used to assess, classify and rate the severity of each stressful event, making allowance for individual circumstances. Originally developed to study the social origins of depression in women, the LEDS has since been used to study links between life event stress and physical illness (Harris, 2007).

RESPONSE-BASED PERSPECTIVES AND THE PHYSIOLOGY OF STRESS

Since any catalogue of potentially stressful events is endless, and individuals differ greatly as to what they find stressful, an alternative is to seek to identify characteristic responses that occur for a range of stressful circumstances. This could theoretically include physiological, psychological and behavioural consequences of stress, although in practice researchers have tended to concentrate on physiological effects, especially those that may be associated with the development of physical illness. We will briefly consider the work of two historically significant contributors to this field, and then survey contemporary developments.

A pioneer in studying the physiology of stress was Hans Selye, whose work extended from the early 1930s until shortly before his death in 1982 (Selye, 1976). He argued for the existence of a generalized response, known as the **general adaptation syndrome (GAS)**, which is triggered by exposure to stress. The GAS occurs primarily in the pituitary-adrenocortical system and consists of three stages, an *alarm reaction* in which the body's defences are mobilized, a *resistance stage* in that the body adapts to the cause of stress, and an *exhaustion stage* in which the body's capacity to resist finally breaks down. Selye drew particular attention to the abnormal physiology that develops during the resistance stage, which if protracted, could lead to what he called the *diseases of adaptation*. These include ulcers, cardiovascular disease and asthma. Although Selye's views have been very influential in the history of stress research, they are no longer widely accepted following extensive criticism, particularly that of Mason (1971, 1975).

The tradition of psychosomatic medicine, described in more detail in Chapter 18, spans a similar historical period to the work of Selye. A key figure was Franz Alexander (1950), who drew a distinction between the temporary and biologically adaptive changes in the physiology of the animal facing an emergency necessitating flight or fight, and the protracted and maladaptive physiological changes taking place in the anxious or stressed human being. Of particular significance are the physiological changes that are activated by the sympathetic branch of the autonomic nervous system. The proponents of psychosomatic medicine emphasized the effects of stress and anxiety on the cardiovascular, gastro-enteritic and respiratory systems. Some of their theories have an attractive plausibility, but their broad theoretical sweep and the range of physiological mechanisms proposed were never matched by an appropriate level of careful empirical research (Holroyd and Coyne, 1987).

A brief summary of contemporary research findings on physiological pathways that may link stress to disease has been provided by Cohen et al. (2007). This research is based on physiological measures taken from stressed laboratory animals, and from human participants who have experienced a range of types of stress, both long term, such as caring for a relative with dementia, and brief but traumatic, such as experiencing a sexual assault. Cohen et al. note that the effects of stress have been demonstrated on two major endocrine systems which act in conjunction with the hypothalamus and autonomic nervous system. These are the *hypothalamic-pituitary-adrenocortical axis* (*HPA*) and the *sympathetic-adrenal-medullary* (*SAM*) *system*. Of specific relevance for links between stress and diseases to be considered in this chapter, both HPA and SAM influence the functioning of the immune and cardiovascular systems. Cohen et al. also point out that stress has demonstrable effects on *vagal tone*, a key component of para-sympathetic activity and strongly linked to cardiovascular processes.

One example of the causal relationship between stress and a chronic physical disorder is shown in Figure 17.1.

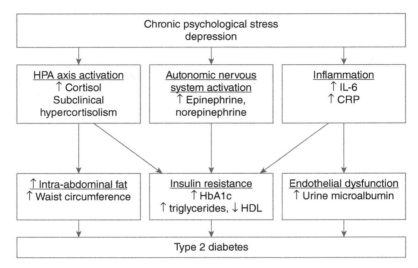

Figure 17.1   Hypothesized relationships among stress, depression, cortisol and diabetes (Reproduced from Joseph & Golden, 2017)

While contemporary research on the psychophysiology of stress is of a much higher quality than that of the early pioneers, there is at least agreement that the proposed mechanisms could lead to higher rates of cardiovascular disease (CVD) and Type 2 diabetes for individuals who experience stress, particularly long-term stress. Of course it is necessary not only to find evidence of plausible physiological mechanisms, but also to show that there actually is a demonstrable link between stress and CVD. In recent years there has also been a great deal of research into the effects of stress on the immune system, which indicates that stress may be responsible for a range of other diseases. This research is referred to as **psychoneuroimmunology (PNI)** (see Chapter 2).

INTERACTIONAL PERSPECTIVES AND COPING SCALES

A key problem for both stimulus- and response-based perspectives on stress is that of individual differences. Different people find different things stressful, and react to the same potentially stressful events and circumstances in different ways. A number of theorists have sought to overcome this problem by conceptualizing stress as a relationship between the individual and the environment and developing *interactional models*. The most influential of these was first put forward by Lazarus and developed by Lazarus and Folkman (1984). In this model psychological stress is defined as 'a particular relationship between the person and the environment that is appraised by the person as taxing or exceeding his or her resources and endangering his or her well-being' (p. 10). A distinction is made between *primary appraisal* whereby an event may be perceived as benign and non-threatening, potentially harmful, threatening to one's self-esteem, or challenging, and *secondary appraisal* in which an assessment is made of one's ability to cope with the threat or challenge. Stress occurs whenever the perceived threat exceeds the perceived ability to cope.

These ideas have been developed at considerable length in a number of books and articles, but they do raise the question as to whether they amount to much more than just another way of saying that stress occurs when you think you cannot cope, i.e., having low resilience. Although this may seem a modest enough assertion, it can in fact be criticized for its implication that stress results only from a purely subjective mismatch between demands and coping resources. One can ask, what about the person who thinks that they can cope when objectively the demands of the situation exceed their actual ability to cope? Are such optimists not stressed? This problem was partially solved by Trumbull and Appley (1986), who extended the model of Lazarus and Folkman by proposing that stress can occur whenever either the real or the perceived demands exceed either the real or the perceived capacity to cope. It might be felt that Trumbull and Appley's definition is so broad and all-encompassing that it amounts to no more than a statement of the obvious. A critical question might be, what is the relative importance of mismatches between real demands and coping resources and those between perceived demands and coping resources in determining whether an individual suffers the effects of stress?

A thoughtful and influential analysis of problems for interactional approaches has been given by Monroe and Simons (1991). While their analysis is primarily concerned with depressive disorders, it also has broader implications for stress theories. In particular, they devote their attention to the problems of separating the influence on stressed reactions of pre-existing individual characteristics, including personality, and of current stressors in all their variety. We have already touched on these issues in considering methods of measuring life events stress and on analysing the causes of post-traumatic stress disorder. The problems are further confounded if we bear in mind that pre-existing characteristics may very well determine not only whether people experience specific events as stressful, but also whether they actively seek stress, as is the case for some competitive personalities, or whether they seek to avoid it. We will consider these issues further later in this chapter, when examining the relationship between stress and physical illness, and also in Chapter 18, which is concerned with illness and personality.

In some ways it is probably better to think of interactional models of stress as *frameworks* for thinking about the subject rather than as specific and testable theories or models. Another way of representing an interactional framework is the flowchart of Cox (1978) shown in Figure 17.2. One of the useful features of this flowchart is that it incorporates feedback between responses, demands and appraisal. For example, behavioural responses, depending on whether they are appropriate or inappropriate, may result in a reduction or an increase in actual demand; psychological defence mechanisms may become activated, leading to changes in the cognitive appraisal of mismatches between perceived demand and perceived capability, and so on.

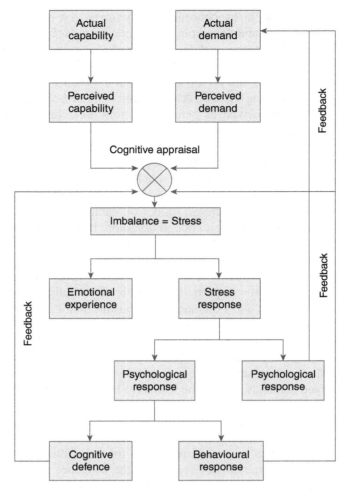

Figure 17.2   Flowchart for an interactional model of stress

Source: Cox (1978: 19). Reproduced with permission

One consequence of the emergence of interactional models of stress has been the development of checklists designed to assess the individual's predominant coping strategies. An example is the COPE questionnaire devised by Carver et al. (1989), which consists of 15 sub-scales each made up of a number of items for which the individual indicates agreement or disagreement on a four-point scale. The 15 sub-scales with an example of a checklist statement from each are shown in Box 17.1.

BOX 17.1

Assessing coping strategies: the COPE scale

In the COPE scale, you are asked how you respond when confronting difficult or stressful events in your life. To each item you use the following rating system:

I usually don't do this at all.

I usually do this a little bit.

I usually do this a medium amount.

I usually do this a lot.

The 15 COPE sub-scales with an example of a checklist from each (the complete version contained four items per sub-scale) are:

Active coping: I take additional action to get rid of the problem.

Planning: I try to come up with a strategy about what to do.

Suppression of competing activities: I put aside other activities in order to concentrate on this.

Restraint coping: I force myself to wait until the right time to do something.

Seeking social support for emotional reasons: I ask people who have had similar experience what they did.

Seeking social support for instrumental reasons: I talk to someone about how I feel.

Positive reinterpretation and growth: I look for something good in what is happening.

Acceptance: I learn to live with it.

Turning to religion: I seek God's help.

Focus on and venting of emotions: I get upset and let my emotions out.

Denial: I refuse to believe that it has happened.

Behavioural disengagement: I give up the attempt to get what I want.

Mental disengagement: I turn to work or other substitute activities to take my mind off things.

Alcohol-drug disengagement: I drink alcohol, or take drugs, in order to think about it less.

Humour: I make fun of the situation.

Source: Carver et al. (1989)

Problems and issues for coping research were discussed by Folkman and Moskovitz (2004). Coping scales have been criticized for adopting a 'blunderbuss' approach to the complex mechanisms involved in coping with different types of stress, and failing to take account of the fact that individuals may vary greatly in the way they cope with different stressful situations (Somerfield, 1997; Aldwin and Park, 2004). They may also be criticized for relying too much on introspective judgements unsupported by other types of evidence. If it is a feature of the psychology of stress that people tend to behave irrationally when exposed to high levels of stress, then the reports of individuals about their personal ways of coping may be particularly inaccurate. For example, *denial*, the refusal to acknowledge the existence of a real danger, may be observed when an individual ignores or denies the significance of symptoms of life-threatening disease, but it is unlikely to be a fully conscious process. How is such an individual likely to respond to the denial items on the COPE questionnaire when asked, for example, how often, when confronted with stressful life events, he or she 'refuses to believe that it has happened'? Surely the whole point about denial is that it only works as a defence if the person does not realize that she/he is doing it.

CONSERVATION OF RESOURCES THEORY

One of the most widely cited theories of stress is Conservation of Resources (COR) theory (Hobfoll, 1989). COR theory covers the entire stress spectrum from burnout to traumatic stress and led to the job demands-resources model. COR theory is a general theory in the sense that it makes hypotheses that are much broader than those offered by single focus theories. In this section, we present the principles and corollaries of COR theory that inform those more specific hypotheses, and review research in organizational behaviour that relies on the theory. First, here are the basic assumptions of the theory (Box 17.2; Hobfoll and Freedy, 2017).

BOX 17.2

Principles and corollaries of conservation of resources theory

Basic COR theory tenet: Individuals (and groups) strive to obtain, retain, foster and protect those things they centrally value.

Principles

Principle 1: Primacy of loss principle. Resource loss is disproportionately more salient than resource gain.

Principle 2: Resource investment principle. People must invest resources in order to protect against resource loss, recover from losses and gain resources.

Principle 3: Gain paradox principle. Resource gain increases in salience in the context of resource loss. That is, when resource loss circumstances are high, resource gains become more important – they gain in value.

Principle 4: Desperation principle. When people's resources are outstretched or exhausted, they enter a defensive mode to preserve the self which is often aggressive, and may become irrational.

Resource Caravans and Resource Caravan Passageways Principles

Resource caravans: Resources do not exist individually but travel in packs, or caravans, for both individuals and organizations.

Resource caravan passageways: People's resources exist in ecological conditions that either foster and nurture or limit and block resource creation and sustenance.

Corollaries

Corollary 1: Those with greater resources are less vulnerable to resource loss and more capable of resource gain. Conversely, individuals and organizations who lack resources are more vulnerable to resource loss and less capable of resource gain.

Corollary 2: Resource loss cycles. Because resource loss is more powerful than resource gain, and because stress occurs when resources are lost, at each iteration of the stress spiral individuals and organizations have fewer resources to offset resource loss, and these loss spirals gain in momentum as well as magnitude.

Corollary 3: Resource gain spirals. Because resource gain is both of less magnitude and slower than resource loss, resource gain spirals tend to be weak and develop slowly.

Source: Hobfoll and Freedy (2017)

COR theory is supported by multiple empirical studies. Freedy and Hobfoll (1994) evaluated two programmes designed to reduce stress among nurses by increasing their coping resources. The two interventions were based on principles of Stress Inoculation Training and Conservation of Resources stress theory. A dual resource intervention targeted the enhancement of both social support and mastery resource while a single resource intervention targeted the enhancement of only mastery resources. Both interventions were contrasted to a no intervention control condition. Participants receiving the dual resource intervention experienced significant enhancements in social support and mastery compared to the no intervention control. Those in the dual resource intervention with low initial levels of social support or mastery experienced significant reductions in psychological distress. Participants in the single resource intervention experienced a slight enhancement in mastery compared to the no intervention control.

The COR theory helps to explain the different people's suicide proneness after disasters, for example, the Deepwater Horizon oil rig explosion. In April 2010, the Deepwater Horizon oil rig exploded in the Gulf of Mexico, killing 11 people and excreting 4.9 million barrels of oil per day until the well was re-sealed several months later. A clean-up effort was launched and 1.84 million gallons of chemical dispersants were released into the water. Health effects were linked directly to the spill, as well as increased rates of mental health symptoms (e.g., depression, anxiety, post-traumatic stress symptoms) both immediately and over the following years in coastal communities. Bell, Langhinrichsen-Rohling and Selwyn (2020) invited 213 residents in affected areas to complete measures of resource stability, distress and coping 18 months after the disaster. Overall, 10% expressed clinically elevated suicide proneness and the COR model was found to have an excellent fit that accounted for 41% of inter-individual differences in suicide proneness. Consistent with the theory, residents lacking resources who experienced distress and coped by avoidance were more suicide prone. On the basis of this study, and in line with COR theory, the fostering of resource stability and constructive coping after catastrophe may help to prevent suicide in disaster-impacted citizens.

GENERAL THEORY OF BEHAVIOUR[3]

The General Theory of Behaviour (GTB) is a theory that applies to all behaviour in all situations in all conscious organisms and so it includes human stress and resilience. The GTB builds on a key point made by French philosopher, Jean-Paul Sartre, when he proclaimed that all of psychology can be explained with two simple words – *childhood decides* (Sartre, 1964). A large amount of research carried out over many decades finds this opinion to be correct. For example, Green et al. (2010) did a survey with a US representative sample of 9,282 adults to examine the joint associations of 12 retrospectively reported childhood adversities (CAs), aka 'early life stresses' (ELS), with the first onset of *Diagnostic and Statistical Manual of Mental Disorders,* fourth edition (DSM-IV) disorders (American Psychiatric Association, 1994). The CAs were highly prevalent and intercorrelated. The CAs in a maladaptive cluster (parental mental illness, substance abuse disorder and criminality; family violence; physical abuse; sexual abuse; and neglect) were the strongest correlates of disorder onset. Analysis suggested that CAs are associated with 44.6% of all childhood-onset disorders and with 25.9% to 32.0% of later-onset disorders. CAs have powerful associations with the onset of many types of largely primary mental disorders throughout the life course, for example mood 26.2%, anxiety 32.4%, substance use 21.0%, disruptive behaviour 41.2%.

Murgatroyd and Spengler (2011) argue that epigenetic mechanisms can mediate the gene–environment dialogue in early life and give rise to persistent epigenetic programming of adult physiology eventually resulting in disease. The most critical stages are the prenatal period continuing through the neonatal and early adolescent stages, during which the environment is able to fine-tune neural circuitry. The evidence suggests that ELS can induce persistent changes in the programming of neurobiological stress response systems, which could predispose a person to develop depression, especially when there is later additional exposure to stress.

A General Theory of Early Life Stress is presented in Figure 17.3.

Early life stress (ELS) has deleterious effects on the nervous, endocrine and immune systems, which can be permanently altered in structure and function by early life 'programming' (ELP). We describe a few findings emerging from recent studies of ELP in humans. One focus has been on the effect of ELS or glucocorticoids upon hypothalamus-pituitary-adrenal axis (HPA axis) activity. Targets suggested for ELP include glucocorticoid receptor gene expression and the corticotrophin-releasing hormone system. ELP of neuroendocrine systems and behaviour by stress and exogenous or endogenous glucocorticoids has been associated with the development of common disorders. It has been suggested that the glucocorticoid

---

[3]This section is reprinted from Chapter 10 of *A General Theory of Behaviour* (Marks, 2018).

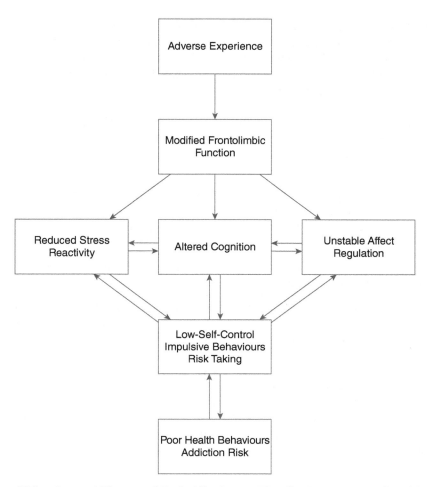

Figure 17.3   General Theory of Early Life Stress. The diagram summarizes how the experience of stressful events in childhood and adolescence may programme behaviour patterns towards addiction and other adverse health outcomes. Life experience is processed through the frontolimbic structures of the Central Homeostatic Network. Early life programming has three consequences: 1) stress reactivity is reduced; 2) cognitive processing is shifted toward a focus on short term goals and more impulsive response selection; 3) regulation of affect is less stable and prone to negative states. These three consequences result in an impulsive behavioural style of risk taking and reduced self-control. (From Marks, 2018. Adapted with minor amendments from the conceptual model published by William R. Lovallo, 2013.)

receptor- encoding gene, nuclear receptor subfamily 3 group C member 1 (NR3C1), is down-regulated in the hippocampus of individuals who have been exposed to ELS, which leads to an overactive HPA axis, the development of anxiety traits, and increased risk of suicidal behaviour (Turecki, 2014). Prenatal exposure to maternal depression may alter neonatal methylation of human glucocorticoid receptor gene (NR3C1) and thereby increase infant cortisol stress responses (Oberlander et al., 2008). Another study shows that altered stress reactivity following childhood trauma in humans is related to altered DNA methylation levels at the KITLG locus (Houtepen et al., 2016). The findings of many recent studies are converging on one simple principle: *All systems involving behavioural homeostasis are programmed by genetics, epigenetics and early life experience* (Marks, 2018). There are many implications of this principle, including these four:

1. Stable, secure and protective ELE produce high threshold REF reset values predictive of high resilience, stability and self-control that can impact on health throughout life due to a tendency to avoid use of alcohol, drugs and engaging in unhealthy behaviours such as smoking.

2. Unstable, insecure or adverse ELE produce low threshold REF reset values predictive of low resilience, impulsiveness and self-control that can impact on health throughout life due to a tendency to use alcohol, drugs and engaging in unhealthy behaviours such as smoking.

3. An overactive HPA axis and the development of anxiety traits predispose individuals to increased risk of depression and suicide.

4. ELP is expected to show the normally observed gradients across the population distribution of socioeconomic position, education and income, and to vary according to gender, ethnicity and other sociodemographic conditions.

Resilient ELP is a significant issue. It is also a policy matter about equity and social justice: the less fortunate sectors of the population do not have sufficient resources to provide a stable and secure foundation enabling infants, children and families to thrive. A minimum level of resources is required to provide shelter, water, food and sanitation as a foundation for human resilience at the bottom end of the needs pyramid. There is a long way to go before this foundation is universally available.

POST-TRAUMATIC STRESS DISORDER (PTSD)

PTSD is a special stress response in individuals who have been subjected to extreme levels of stress, such as soldiers, victims of rape, child abuse, other violent crimes, and survivors of disasters such as earthquakes, floods and nuclear accidents. The term 'PTSD' was introduced by researchers studying psychological symptoms reported by soldiers returning to the US from the Vietnam War and it was subsequently extended to studies of other types of traumatic stress. It was first accepted as a diagnostic label by the American Psychiatric Association in 1980. The symptoms that are most often used to characterize PTSD are insomnia, nightmares, flashbacks, problems of memory and concentration, acting or feeling as if the event is recurring and a greatly increased sensitivity to new stressful events (Posluszny et al., 2007).

Surveys of the general population have examined rates of exposure and PTSD in children and adolescents (Hamblen and Barnett, 2016). Results indicate that 15–43% of girls and 14–43% of boys have experienced at least one traumatic event in their lifetime. Of these, 3–15% of girls and 1–6% of boys could be diagnosed with PTSD. Rates of PTSD vary from 3–100%, e.g., 100% of children who witness a parental homicide or sexual assault develop PTSD. Similarly, 90% of sexually abused children, 77% of children exposed to a school shooting, and 35% of urban youth exposed to community violence develop PTSD (Hamblen and Barnett, 2016).

Our understanding of PTSD is always complicated by the existence of large individual differences. There are also large individual differences in the types of symptoms encountered and their severity. Some recent attempts have been made to review the voluminous literature on PTSD to establish whether differences in emotional reactions occurring at the time of and immediately after traumatic stress can predict the subsequent development of PTSD, although so far with little agreement (Harvey and Bryant, 2002; Ozer et al., 2003). Neither is it clear whether reactions to different kinds of traumatic stress are basically the same or whether they depend on the particular type of stress involved.

The psychophysiological differences found between those who suffer from PTSD and those who do not are real enough, but it has not been established whether they have occurred purely as a result of exposure to traumatic stress, or whether they are at least partly determined by pre-existing characteristics of the individuals who develop PTSD. It is quite often found that these individuals have a history of psychological problems, including childhood trauma, abnormal adolescent development, and depression and anxiety disorders (Posluszny et al., 2007). This in turn raises the question, in any particular case, as to whether the traumatic stress is the primary cause of subsequent psychological reactions or the final trigger at the end of a series of causal influences.

To what extent is PTSD associated with the development of physical illness in addition to psychological problems? A number of studies have sought to answer this question but with mixed results. The main focus has been on cardiovascular disease (CVD). Qureshi et al. (2009) analysed a selection of studies published between 1981 and 2008 and found a conflicting mixture of positive and negative findings. Dedert et al. (2010) conducted a detailed review of research published between 2002 and 2009, concluding that there was evidence of an association but that it could not be relied on because the research had a range of methodological shortcomings. Other studies of PTSD and physical illness have usually found positive associations where the measures of illness are patients' subjective reports, but few or no associations where objective physicians' reports have provided the data. Rytwinski et al. (2014) utilized both subjective and objective measures for a sample of 200 PTSD sufferers. They found that PTSD severity is associated with subjectively assessed but not objectively assessed health, a finding which suggests that the effects of traumatic stress are primarily psychological. At the same it should be noted that long-term psychological problems, especially anxiety and depression, have themselves been found to be associated with CVD (see Chapter 18).

Numerous guidelines have been developed regarding treatments for PTSD. Extensive reviews have been conducted on treatments for people with PTSD, for example, Cusack et al. (2016). This review included 64 trials with patients who generally had severe PTSD. The review evidence supported efficacy of exposure therapy, cognitive therapies, eye movement desensitization and reprocessing, and narrative exposure therapy. Thus, several psychological treatments are effective for adults with PTSD.

POST-TRAUMATIC GROWTH (PTG)

Just as resilience is on the other side of the stress coin, PTG is on the other side of the PTSD coin. In fact, one response to trauma and stress is post-traumatic growth (PTG) and it can modify the intensity of PTSD over time. Xu et al. (2020) evaluated PTG in Chinese adolescent earthquake survivors (n = 5,195) and relationships among self-esteem, post-traumatic stress disorder (PTSD) and PTG. The prevalence of PTG among adolescent survivors was

14.8%. PTG was independently associated with self-esteem, severity of exposures and avoidance facets of PTSD. PTSD was found to be partially mediated by self-esteem on PTG, and PTSD was also a mediator between earthquake exposure and PTG. Future longitudinal research and clinical practice should explore whether promoting self-esteem can enhance PTSD treatment.

STRESS MANAGEMENT

The most obvious approach to stress management is to deal with the causes of stress – prevention rather than treatment. For example, an occupational psychologist can analyse stress in the workplace to advise on how restructuring could reduce the amount of stress experienced by employees. This would be of benefit both to employees and employers because employees will likely be more productive when less stressed. However, everything depends on the specific nature of the job, the work environment and the workers themselves. Environmental planning is also highly task specific, considering the design of housing, thoroughfares and public spaces to reduce levels of stress that may be related to noise, pollution, overcrowding, and exposure to crime and other physical dangers. At the other end of the spectrum, where stress is unavoidable, stress management needs to be based on efforts to modify the psychophysiology of stress, including the use of physical exercise, breathing and relaxation techniques. In practice these methods have normally been incorporated into the main interactional approaches to stress management.

Stress management often makes use of techniques based on of **cognitive behavioural therapy (CBT)**. One version of CBT is **stress inoculation training (SIT)** (Meichenbaum, 1996). Using an interactional perspective, the aim of SIT is to help people to cope after exposure to stressful events and to improve already existing coping skills so that they become more readily available for dealing with continuing and future stressors. In the first or *conceptualization* phase, the therapist/trainer aims to educate the client to treat threats as soluble problems and to clarify those stressors and responses which are potentially changeable and those which are not. The second phase then concentrates on *skills acquisition* and *rehearsal*, in which effective skills are practised, first in training sessions and subsequently in real situations. Skills may include methods for relaxation and anxiety reduction, cognitive restructuring and interpersonal skills using social support networks. In the third and final phase of *application* and *follow-through*, clients are taught to apply their expanded coping skills to increasingly high levels of stress, using imagery, rehearsal, modelling and role playing. They are also taught how to identify high-risk situations to prevent relapse to previous and inadequate methods of coping, and to deal with relapse if and when it does occur. At this stage they may be encouraged to help others with similar problems. SIT has been used for individuals and in groups of various sizes, and for a range of time scales, from single 20-minute sessions when preparing patients for stressful surgery to regular weekly and bi-weekly 1-hour sessions, up to 40 sessions in some cases.

Mindfulness

An increasingly widely used technique in recent years is based on the concept of *mindfulness*. An influential pioneer of this approach is Jon Kabat-Zinn, a molecular biologist and Buddhist, who introduced **mindfulness-based stress reduction (MBSR)** in 1979. Kabat-Zinn has written a series of popular accounts (e.g., Kabat-Zinn, 1990). Mindfulness is a central feature of

Buddhist meditation, especially in Theravada Buddhism, but Kabat-Zinn and practitioners of similar programmes, now collectively referred to as *mindfulness-based therapies*, emphasize that they can be practised with equally good effect without any commitment to Buddhist beliefs. Keng et al. (2011) describe the practice as follows:

> The elements of mindfulness, namely awareness and nonjudgmental acceptance of one's moment-to-moment experience, are regarded as potentially effective antidotes against common forms of psychological distress – rumination, anxiety, worry, fear, anger, and so on – many of which involve the maladaptive tendencies to avoid, suppress, or over-engage with one's distressing thoughts and emotions. (2011: 1042)

Mindfulness-based therapists, like Buddhist teachers, may recommend the initial practice of hatha yoga and concentration on breathing as a preliminary step in developing attention, but the practice of observing the mind is regarded as the central therapeutic procedure. It is instructive to contrast this with traditional forms of cognitive behavioural therapy, stress management and self-help manuals, in which the emphasis is on the cultivation of positive thinking and desirable habits, and the elimination of negative ones. For the mindfulness-based therapist the practice of self-observation will inevitably lead to beneficial outcomes as the practitioner becomes increasingly aware of the maladaptive nature of his or her problematic states of mind. They may simply be dropped with no further effort required. For Buddhist monks the cultivation of mindfulness is often regarded as a preliminary to deeper spiritual practices, perhaps leading to the ultimate goal of enlightenment/salvation, while for the mindfulness-based therapist, as indeed for many Buddhists, mindfulness may be regarded as sufficient in itself. The non-directional character of mindfulness training is in some ways comparable with the psycho-analytic procedure of free association, although without the additional requirement for analysis and interpretation. Perhaps the results of observing the mind are self-evident.

There have been a number of recent reviews of studies into the efficacy of mindfulness-based therapies, including MBSR. Keng et al. (2011) examined 18 randomized controlled studies of MBSR and 14 of mindfulness-based cognitive therapy (MBCR) and found evidence of increased subjective well-being and reduced levels of anxiety, depression, anger and perceived stress. Khoury et al. (2013) examined 209 studies, of which 109 were randomized controlled studies. They concluded that mindfulness therapies are moderately or largely effective for treating anxiety, depression and stress, but no more effective than traditional cognitive behavioural therapies (CBT). Goyal et al. (2014) examined 47 studies, concluding that mindfulness is moderately effective for anxiety, depression and pain control, but less effective for stress and mental-health-related quality of life. They found no evidence that meditation is more effective than drugs, exercise and other behavioural therapies.

One recent study carried out in Sussex, UK, systematically reviewed mindfulness-based interventions (MBIs) (Gu et al., 2015). The reviewers concluded as follows:

> This review identified strong, consistent evidence for cognitive and emotional reactivity, moderate and consistent evidence for mindfulness, rumination, and worry, and preliminary but insufficient evidence for self-compassion and psychological flexibility as mechanisms underlying MBIs.

A positive result.

DOES STRESS INCREASE SUSCEPTIBILITY TO PHYSICAL ILLNESS?

To put the question more bluntly, can stress actually kill us? This topic has generated a great deal of research and it is easy to see why. If stress can be shown to be an important influence on our susceptibility to disease, then the possibility exists that interventions designed to reduce stress, or to help individuals to cope better with unavoidable stress, may lower the incidence of disease and assist the recovery of those who are already ill. The popular belief that stress is a major cause of physical illness is not convincingly supported by existing research findings, but neither is the opposite belief that stress plays only an insignificant role. The problem is that it is extremely difficult to carry out well-controlled research in this area and most of what has been done is open to a range of possible interpretations. We have already noted two shortcomings that apply to the majority of studies. First, retrospective studies may have a substantial response bias because people are more likely to recall experiencing stress in periods preceding illness than at other times. Second, all studies that rely on self-reports of illness may have a response bias because people who consider themselves to be suffering from stress are more likely than non-stressed individuals to interpret minor ailments as symptoms of illness.

The better designed studies that investigate the association between exposure to stress and subsequent and biologically verified illness may still present problems of interpretation. For example, it has been shown that people who are experiencing stress are more likely than others to indulge in health hazardous behaviour such as heavy smoking, a high-fat diet and lack of exercise (Ng and Jeffery, 2003). Thus it could be that stress acts only indirectly as a cause of illness insofar as it influences health behaviour, rather than through direct physiological pathways.

Methodological problems are all likely to lead to inflated estimates of the strength of the association between stress and illness. Further issues have been raised that point in the opposite direction, to the possibility that current research may produce underestimates. These issues derive partly from work on the relationship between personality and illness considered in Chapter 18. One argument is that some individuals possess personal characteristics that make them resistant to the effects of stress. Among the personal characteristics that have been suggested as having this function are **conscientiousness, self-efficacy, hardiness**, resilience and **sense of coherence**. If stress only causes illness in people with vulnerable personalities, then it may be misleading to calculate the size of the effect of stress on illness by using general population samples that include many who are relatively insensitive to these effects. A further issue is the potential mediating effect of *social support* on the relationship between stress and illness. There is extensive evidence that people with strong networks of social support live longer and enjoy better health than relatively isolated individuals (Cohen, 2004). In seeking to explain this relationship, Cohen argues that social support has a *buffering effect* against the effects of stress, so that stress is only likely to cause illness among individuals with relatively low levels of support.

If the above considerations are valid, then stress is only likely to have a strong effect on susceptibility to illness among individuals who score low on conscientiousness, self-efficacy, hardiness and sense of coherence, and who have a low level of perceived social support. Therefore, studies of stress–illness links that are based on representative population samples may greatly underestimate the potential effects of stress because they include many individuals for whom the effect is likely to be small. Would-be researchers, who consider these issues alongside our previous observations on factors that may lead to overestimates, could be excused if they were to throw up their hands in despair. As a research topic it is not an easy one and certainly no study published to date has succeeded in overcoming all or even most of the potential problems. Nevertheless, recent and relatively well-designed studies have thrown up a number of interesting findings, particularly in the areas of **coronary heart disease (CHD)**, cancer and infectious diseases, and to these we now turn. For further discussion of chronic conditions, see Chapters 20 to 24.

Coronary Heart Disease (CHD)

Studies of the relationship between stress and subsequent CHD have produced a mixture of positive and negative findings. In a 12-year follow-up study of 6,935 healthy men, Rosengren et al. (1991) found that those who had initially reported substantial stress were more likely to experience coronary artery disease subsequently, after controlling for the effects of smoking, alcohol consumption and lack of physical exercise. In contrast, in a six-year follow-up of 12,866 men who were at high risk, Hollis et al. (1990) found no relationship between stress and subsequent mortality. Macleod et al. (2002) described a 21-year follow-up study of 2,623 Scottish men in which self-reported stress was strongly associated with subsequent angina but not with objective measures of CHD, including mortality. However, the diagnosis of angina is usually based on self-reported chest pain and Macleod et al. conclude that the stress–angina relationship probably results from a tendency of participants reporting higher stress to also report more symptoms.

There has also been extensive research into the possible relationship between occupational stress and CHD (Byrne and Espnes, 2008). Studies of workers in European countries, with follow-up periods ranging from five to ten years, all found an association between assessments of job strain and subsequent risk of CHD (e.g., Kivimäki et al., 2002; Kuper and Marmot, 2003), but Reed et al. (1989) found no association in an 18-year follow-up of 8,006 Hawaiian men of Japanese ancestry and Eaker et al. (2004) found no association in a 10-year follow-up of 1,711 men and 1,328 women in the USA.

In view of the conflicting nature of these findings it is obviously not possible to draw any definite conclusions as to whether stress increases susceptibility to CHD. However, two recent meta-analyses concur in finding a modest prospective relationship between perceived stress and objective measures of CHD, including mortality. Richardson et al. (2012) analysed studies with a combined total of 118,696 participants and found that individuals with high perceived stress were 27% more likely than those with low perceived stress to be diagnosed with or die as a result of CHD at least six months later. Kivimäki et al. (2012) pooled results from 13 European studies comparing risk of heart attack for people in high stress versus low stress jobs. Out of a total of 197,473 participants there were 2,358 heart attacks in an average follow-up period of 7.5 years, with those reporting high job strain at a 23% increased level of risk compared with those reporting no job strain, an increased risk which is quite similar to that estimated by Richardson et al. Kivimäki et al. conclude that prevention of workplace stress might decrease disease incidence but to a much smaller extent than tackling standard risk factors, such as smoking.

Cancer

Studies that have considered that the subsequent occurrence of all forms of cancer following periods of stress have generally failed to find evidence of an association. The few positive findings have come from small and poorly designed studies, whereas large prospective studies have produced negative findings. There is, for example, no indication of a higher cancer rate among the bereaved (Jones et al., 1984; Fox, 1988), and Keehn (1980) found no increased rate of cancer among former prisoners of war, men who had suffered extreme forms of mental and physical hardship. Joffress et al. (1985) found no relationship between stressful life events and subsequent cancer in a study of Japanese men living in Hawaii. More recently Heikkilä et al. (2013) conducted a meta-analysis of 12 European cohort studies including 116,056 participants who were initially free from cancer when assessed for self-reported job strain. The follow-up period was for a median time of 12 years, during which 5,765 cases of cancer were recorded from hospital admission and death registers. Heikkilä et al. found no clear evidence for an association between job strain and risk of cancer.

With regard to the prognosis for individuals already suffering from cancer, the most impressive study involved over 14,000 women in Norway and found no increased risk of recurrence or death for those who had lost a spouse or had been divorced (Kvikstad et al., 1995) or who had lost a child (Kvikstad and Vatten, 1996). Reviewing the evidence from 26 studies on coping styles and survival and recurrence in people with cancer, Petticrew et al. (2002) conclude that there are few indications of significant associations.

Particular attention has been given to the possible relationship between stress and breast cancer. McGee, Hevery and Horgan (1999) note that speculation about stress as a cause of breast cancer may be found in medical opinion at least as far back as 1893. He gives examples of relatively recent poorly designed studies which sometimes produce dramatic positive findings, while large prospective studies have not found an association. Duijts et al. (2003) confirmed this conclusion in a detailed meta-analysis, with the single exception that there was a significant, albeit modest, association with death of a spouse. Fallah et al. (2016) also studied the associations between incidence and survival in breast cancer patients and stressful life events. They used a structured telephone interview with 355 women with breast cancer and 516 women with benign breast diseases who were matched on demographic characteristics to collect information about the experience of major stressful events in the years before the diagnosis. Only 'severe interpersonal problems with spouse' was significant. A definite answer to the question 'Can stress kill you via cancer?' seems a long way off. Cancer certainly kills, but we simply do not know whether any cancers are definitely caused by stress. The provisional answer is maybe yes, but we need a lot more well-designed prospective studies.

Infectious Diseases

If stress causes changes in the immune system, then this could obviously lead to altered susceptibility to infectious diseases. We have already seen that there is extensive evidence that stress does have statistically significant effects on a variety of measures of immune functioning, but that these effects are generally well within the range of normal variation for healthy people. This leaves the question open as to whether they are sufficiently large to lead to altered susceptibility to disease. The obvious way to find out is to examine the evidence for a direct relationship between stress and the incidence of infectious disease. Over the last 30 years Sheldon Cohen and his associates have been conducting a thorough and detailed analysis of this issue.

Cohen and Williamson (1991) dismissed evidence drawn from retrospective studies and all studies that rely on self-reported illness for reasons that we have already explained. Much of the research in this area is concerned with minor viral infections, such as the common cold, and these are likely to be particularly susceptible to reporting bias. For example, a mild sore throat and headache may be self-diagnosed as a viral infection by the more hypochondriacal individual, while others will attribute the same symptoms to staying up too late at a party or pollution from traffic fumes. It is easy to see how correlations may occur between such self-reported illness and perceived levels of stress, even if there is no true causal relationship between stress and susceptibility to viral infections.

A large prospective study was carried out by an international group of researchers called the 'TEDDY Study Group' (Roth et al., 2019). The group conducted a prospective analysis of the association between Negative Life Events (NLEs) and respiratory infections in 5,618 children genetically at risk for islet autoimmunity (IA) and Type 1 diabetes (T1D) for at least one to four years. All models were adjusted for demographics, day care, season of infection and psychosocial factors associated with the rate of child RIEs between study visits. This large-scale prospective study confirmed that stress may increase the susceptibility for infections in paediatric populations and suggested at least one mechanism by which stress could increase risk for IA and T1D in genetically at-risk children.

In light of the above study, can stress kill via infections? The answer to the question must be positive.

FUTURE RESEARCH

1. Studies focusing on the psychological and physiological effects of different types of stress (e.g., bereavement, excessive work load, physical assault).

2. Prospective stress-disease studies that combine measures of a wide variety of physiological characteristics (e.g., of the immune system) with biologically verified assessments of disease status.

3. Research into the effects of stress on the gastro-enteric and respiratory systems (like the TEDDY group study) in addition to its effects on the cardiovascular and immune systems.

4. Assessment of the effectiveness of stress-management programmes for those already suffering from stress-related diseases. This research should examine the psychological benefits of the programmes as well as their effect on disease prognosis.

SUMMARY

1. The 'glass half empty' approach focuses on stress and PTSD. The 'glass half full' approach focuses on resilience and post-traumatic growth. Health psychology contributes to both halves of the glass.

2. Stress is sometimes conceptualized as environmental stimuli or life events that impinge on the individual, sometimes as a particular type of response or reaction to stressful events, and sometimes as a mismatch between demands placed on the individual and the perceived ability to cope with these demands.

(Continued)

3. Various methods have been proposed for assessing life events stress. The main problem is that individuals differ greatly as to what they find stressful. For this reason structured interviews are to be preferred to standardized questionnaires.

4. Significant effects of stress on the immune system have been demonstrated, although it is not yet clear whether these effects are large enough to alter susceptibility to disease.

5. A variety of physiological and psychological effects associated with exposure to traumatic stress have been shown to exist, although it is arguable whether they can be used to establish post-traumatic stress disorder as a clinical syndrome.

6. Interactional models of stress are intrinsically attractive because they take account of individual differences in reactions to stress and methods of coping. They have the disadvantage that they depend very much on the reliability of subjective assessments and, for this reason, may not be scientifically testable.

7. Empirical studies of the relationship between stress and disease have frequently been unsatisfactory because they are retrospective and rely on self-reported stress and illness. They also frequently fail to distinguish between physiological effects of stress and influences on health behaviour.

8. Theoretical models of the relationship between stress and disease are difficult to test because they involve complex interactions between stress, social support and personality variables.

9. There is conflicting evidence as to whether stress does or does not contribute to risk of coronary heart disease. Recent meta-analyses concur in finding a moderate increase in risk, although much less than major risks such as smoking.

10. There is no convincing evidence for a significant role of stress in the aetiology and prognosis for cancer, but for infections the evidence is much stronger.

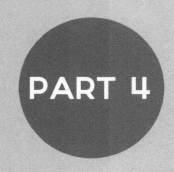

PART 4

ILLNESS EXPERIENCE AND HEALTH CARE

In Part 4 we turn to some of the major issues and syndromes, acute and chronic, that are a significant part of the work of clinical health psychologists.

In Chapter 18 we examine the claimed associations between individual differences in personality and other psychological characteristics on susceptibility to illness.

In Chapter 19 we discuss the complexities of pain. Some of the main psychological and social processes that mediate and moderate pain behaviour and experience are considered along with the pros and cons of different pain assessment methods.

In Chapter 20 we consider the nature of that most dreaded of disorders, cancer, and the relevant risk factors. We continue by discussing what it is like to live with cancer and to care for someone with cancer, and we introduce the design and testing of a specific psychological intervention.

In Chapter 21 we consider one of the major diseases of the cardiovascular system, coronary heart disease (CHD), the nature and causes of the illness and its major risk factors. We discuss the psychosocial issues of living with CHD, caring for someone with CHD, and the design and testing of interventions.

In Chapter 22, we consider one of the most highly stigmatized conditions of modern times, HIV-seropositivity and AIDS. We describe the nature and causes of the illness, the main risk factors and at-risk groups, the psychosocial issues of people living with HIV infection/AIDS and of people caring for someone with the condition, and also interventions.

In Chapter 23, we review two long-term conditions that are increasingly diagnosed: diabetes and myalgic encephalomyelitis/chronic fatigue syndrome (ME/CFS). The former has causes that are understood while the latter is not at all well understood. Lack of understanding is one aspect of ME/CFS that patients can find highly stressful in their interactions with medics. Neither condition can be cured using current treatments and both require a health care approach based on the biopsychosocial model.

Finally, in Chapter 24 we review research on the psychological aspects of end-of-life care, dying and death. We consider the concept and meaning of a 'good death' and the 'quality of death and dying'.

ILLNESS AND PERSONALITY

'The virtues of science are skepticism and independence of thought.'

Walter Gilbert, 1986

OUTLINE

In this chapter, we examine claimed associations between individual differences in personality and other psychological characteristics on susceptibility to illness. This is a field of high expectations and false hopes. For this reason, we adopt a sceptical attitude towards some of the worst examples of hyped science, wishful thinking and blatant exaggeration. We discuss the scientific problems involved in investigating and explaining links between personality and physical illness. We assess contemporary research on personality and illness with particular reference to coronary heart disease and cancer.

This chapter critically reviews the literature on personality, health and illness. As we have seen in other chapters, the 'biopsychosocial model' (BPSM) has been proposed as an alternative to biomedicine. The banner status of the BPSM has opened the floodgates to the idea that psychological processes can directly or indirectly influence well-being and the course of illness. However, there have been many difficulties establishing any solid findings. 'Exciting' new findings on the 'power of the mind' to cure cancer, to prevent heart disease and to live a long and happy life are frequently reported in the media but rarely are these substantiated in dispassionate reviews. What we can learn from this field is a valuable object-lesson in sceptical science. An evidence-based and critical appreciation of current knowledge serves as a shield against the bad science and flawed studies put out by journals and media that put hype before truth. A recent example of distorted reviewing by a well-known health psychology journal is described in Box 18.1.

BOX 18.1

Misleading review on slowing cancer progression and increasing survival time using psychological intervention

Some researchers have extravagantly claimed that their interventions extended their patients' survival but, apart from this one highly publicized report, the evidence is *non-existent*. Spiegel et al. (1989) reported a positive effect of psychosocial treatment on the survival of patients with metastatic breast cancer, claiming an increased survival time of about 18 months. Although the findings have never been replicated, it raised many false hopes among cancer sufferers, a false hope that became reinforced by practitioners offering hyped-up and glamorous-sounding but totally ineffective therapies. Edwards et al. (2004) and Chow et al. (2004) both reported systematic reviews of psychosocial interventions in which effects on survival proved statistically non-significant.

This review by Spiegel (2014) in the *British Journal of Health Psychology* repeats the misleading claim of Spiegel et al. (1989) that cancer progression can be slowed by psychological intervention. The review provides an instructive example of how the national psychological society representing the science and practice of psychology in the UK, the British Psychological Society, lends credence to a distorted view of scientific evidence. The journal has allowed privileged access to the author by inviting his paper. The publication repeats a misleading claim originally made by the same author 25 years earlier concerning alleged survival benefits of psychotherapy in a manner that could be detrimental to patients and their families. The review is biased in numerous ways: only supportive studies are cited; no reference is made to their statistical and methodological flaws; and finally, important studies that produced negative findings are not cited but are ignored, even when they are of high quality. The truth is that there is no evidence from properly controlled trials that psychological intervention prolongs survival in cancer.

BIOPSYCHOSOCIAL MODEL AS A 'BLUEPRINT'

Biomedicine is based on the belief that physical illness has physical causes and requires physical treatment. While there is increasing acceptance of the importance of health behaviours, emotions and social issues among the causes of illness, the assumption remains that the actual mechanisms are physical, including such things as viruses, bacteria, carcinogens and physiological abnormalities. Partly as a result of DNA research and the influence of the pharmaceutical industry, this *physicalist* approach is increasingly being applied to psychological disorders, and conditions ranging from schizophrenia to mild cases of depression are commonly attributed to biochemical imbalances, often thought to be genetic.

Engel (1977: 132) famously proposed a biopsychosocial model (BPSM) that purported to provide 'a blueprint for research, a framework for teaching, and a design for action in the real world of health care'. Engel claimed that BPSM is a scientific model. However, Engel's so-called BPSM is really a *framework* (see Chapter 1) within which true models and theories can be created. Engel's BPSM does not meet the necessary criteria for a scientific model, which would be the capability to explain and predict observed phenomena. The BPSM offers no such capability because it is only a 'framework for teaching', an idea about how to approach the business of health care. BPSM offers an open invitation to health care practitioners to consider psychological and social experience as complementary to the biological condition of the physical body. Although the BPSM does not enable prediction or explanation, it has provided a rationale, a banner for the role of emotion, thought and behaviour in the study of health and illness.

A popular belief is that people with certain dispositions may be particularly susceptible to heart disease or cancer and that psychological disturbances may be a cause of much physical illness. People talk of 'mental toughness', being 'strong willed', 'centred', 'resilient' or 'positive'. Alternative treatments and complementary therapies for physical diseases often have psychological components, including stress-management programmes, relaxation, breathing exercises and meditation. It is claimed by some proponents of such treatments that they are capable of correcting 'psychic' or 'energy' imbalances that have triggered the symptoms in the first place. Others claim to be able to train people to become more 'positive' and to improve resilience to the impact of serious illnesses such as cancer. These claims rest on a bedrock of folklore, myth and 'old wives' tales' that persist to the present day.

Before jumping to judgement on these fanciful claims, we must take stock of some of the far-fetched claims put out today under the umbrella of 'Positive Psychology'. Many beliefs that psychologists study are entrenched in popular narratives about mind, body and spirit. These cultural heirlooms do not simply lie down and die when a few negative findings are published. False beliefs and fanciful tales are highly resilient. The inkblot that is the biopsychosocial model facilitates their survival.

EXPLAINING LINKS BETWEEN PERSONALITY AND PHYSICAL ILLNESS

It is generally agreed that the psychosomatic approach in psychoanalysis and the proponents of **psychosomatic medicine** failed to produce convincing evidence of any causal connections between psychological characteristics and physical illness, or to demonstrate that their therapeutic interventions were effective (Holroyd and Coyne, 1987). The period since the 1960s has seen the growth of a large empirical literature on the statistical relationship between personality, as assessed by a wide variety of standardized tests, and physical illness. These studies often derive their hypotheses from the earlier speculations of the psychosomatic approach but seek to rectify its defects by carefully analysing statistical evidence. There is, however, one major defect that cannot be overcome because it is intrinsic to this type of research. The evidence is obtained from correlational investigations rather than true experiments and, as a consequence, findings are open to a wide range of interpretations. Obviously, no ethical investigator can assign people with different personalities at random to experimental participants and then study their subsequent proneness to illness. All that the investigator can normally do is to administer personality tests to the participants and obtain measures of their illness status. If the personality and illness scores are obtained at the same time, then this is a **cross-sectional** or **correlational study**. In a **prospective study**, personality scores are taken at time 1 (T1) and health outcomes are measured at time 2 (T2). The prospective study is a statistically more powerful methodology because it allows for the possibility of analysing causal relationships between antecedent (T1) measures and outcome measures at T2. Owing to the more complex and resource-intensive nature of prospective studies, cross-sectional studies are far more common.

There are several possible mechanisms that could mediate associations between personality and illness, including accumulated stress, disruption of the immune and endocrine systems, and increased chronic inflammation. Personality may influence cancer risk indirectly via poor health behaviours, such as smoking and not participating in screenings.

It is not possible to infer causation from such correlation and, in the case of personality–illness correlations, it is possible to illustrate this by considering a range of important problems of interpretation. The issues are perennial problems in the literature and are essentially logical in nature. We summarize these in Table 18.1 along with safeguards that readers of research papers need to apply when interpreting study findings.

Direction of causality

Psychological characteristics may be a cause of physical illness, but they can also be a consequence of it. This is a particular problem for cross-sectional studies that simultaneously assess personality traits and illness. For example, if patients with a history of coronary illness have higher scores on anxiety and depression than healthy controls, should we conclude that anxiety and depression are risk factors for coronary illness or that a history of coronary problems can cause people to become more anxious and depressed? Obviously, the existence of any causal relationship cannot be inferred from this type of study. The flaw may seem trivially obvious, but it is surprising how many cross-sectional studies are to be found in the research literature on associations between personality and illness.

The problem cannot always be resolved by conducting prospective studies to investigate the extent to which the current personalities of healthy participants are predictive of future illness. The reason for this is that many major illnesses take a long time to develop and it is frequently the case that patients have experienced unusual and disturbing symptoms for some time before a diagnosis is given. It is therefore possible that psychological characteristics that appear to be a cause of subsequent illness are in fact a consequence of symptoms of developing illness occurring prior to diagnosis. Prospective studies are clearly far superior to cross-sectional studies, but they do not necessarily eliminate the problem of how to determine the direction of causality.

Self-reporting of illness

Stone and Costa (1990) and Cohen and Williamson (1991) pointed out that much health psychology research relies on self-reported illness rather than biologically verified disease. This does not only apply to minor ailments such as colds and flu. The diagnosis of angina pectoris, for example, is frequently based solely on patients' reports of chest pain. Stone and Costa argue that this reliance on self-reported illness is particularly unsatisfactory when considering research into links between personality and illness. They point out that there is extensive evidence that psychological distress is associated with somatic complaints but not with organic disease. Since many personality test scores may be interpreted, at least to some extent, as measures of distress, it follows that correlations between test scores and self-reported illness may provide a false indication of a link between personality and disease when all that they really show is that neurotic

Table 18.1 Problems of interpretation in research on personality and illness and safeguards for readers of research reports

Type of problem	Statement of the problem	Reader's safeguard
Direction of causality	Cross-sectional studies are correlational and so there can be no certainty as to the direction of causality, as to what may be a cause and what may be an effect. There may be no causal relationship between the two variables whatsoever	Substitute all usage of terms such as 'causes', 'leads to', 'influences', 'produces' or 'creates' with 'associated with', 'correlated with' or 'related with'
Background variables	Two variables (A and B) that are associated together may both be related to a third, background variable (C) that has not been measured and may not even be known to be relevant	Always seek the possible existence of confounding or background variables and, whenever possible, expect to see them controlled in a second analysis
Self-reporting of illness	Health psychology research often relies upon self-reported illness that has not been verified by objective medical tests	Whenever possible seek objective measurement of outcomes
Dimensions of personality	The number and nature of different personality variables to evaluate remains controversial	Recognize the limitation of a study that is based on a particular theory of personality if measures from other theoretical approaches are not available
Physiological mechanisms versus health behaviour	It is difficult to determine whether associations between personality and illness are mediated by physiological differences or health behaviour or something else altogether	Always seek the possible existence of confounding or background variables such as health behaviours, and, whenever possible, control for them in a second analysis
Data mining, HARKing (hypothesizing after the results are known) and *p*-hacking (collecting or selecting data or statistical analyses until non-significant results become significant)	The investigator selects only positive, confirming evidence for publication from a larger array of findings and fails to reveal the existence of negative, disconfirming evidence	Almost impossible to safeguard. Expect the investigator to state in advance the hypotheses and the operational definitions of the dependent and independent variables. Replication is necessary
Minimally significant effect (*p* < .05)	The minimum level of statistical significance may be a Type I error (a 'false positive')	Replication is necessary
Fabrication/ fraud	The investigator may conspire, with or without others, to fabricate data in support of a theory or hypothesis	If the results look too good to be true, they probably are too good to be true. Replication is necessary

individuals are the ones most likely to complain of being ill. Friedman and Kern (2014) consider these issues in some detail, and recommend that personality–illness research should focus primarily on mortality and longevity as outcome measures. However, it should not be assumed that any discrepancy between self-reported illness and biologically verified illness is necessarily an indication of neuroticism. Adler and Matthews (1994) noted that there is evidence that perceived health predicts mortality independently of biological risk factors, leading them to conclude that self-reported health provides useful information over and above direct biological indications. The association between perceived health and mortality has now been confirmed by many studies, and Jylhä (2009) provides a detailed analysis of possible reasons for it.

Dimensions of personality

Personality testing is an inexact science with little agreement as to what the basic dimensions of personality really are, or even whether the question is worth asking. Three influential theories have been those of Eysenck, who argued initially that there were only two dimensions, extraversion and neuroticism, and subsequently added a third, psychoticism; Cattell, who believed he had identified 18; and McCrae and Costa (2003), who settled for five. These so-called 'Big Five' personality traits have generated a considerable amount of recent research. They consist of extraversion/introversion, agreeableness/antagonism, conscientiousness, neuroticism/emotional stability, and openness to experience.

A problem that arises in research using personality tests is that similar items can often be found in tests that are supposed to be measuring different traits so that, not surprisingly, scores for the same group of individuals given both tests may be highly intercorrelated. Consider some of the measures that are frequently used in research into the links between personality and illness. The individual who scores high on anxiety is also likely to score high on depression, neuroticism and **pessimistic explanatory style**, and correspondingly low on **self-esteem**, **self-efficacy, hardiness** and **sense of coherence**. The common element that may run through all of these measures is probably best labelled, following Stone and Costa (1990), as *distress proneness or negative affectivity.* Suls and Bunde (2005) discuss this issue in a detailed review of research linking anger/hostility, anxiety and depression with cardiovascular disease. They note that strong correlations exist between all three traits that make it difficult to establish which of the associations with cardiovascular disease is of primary importance, or whether a more general trait of negative affectivity is the key variable.

Physiological mechanisms versus health behaviour

Psychological characteristics may be linked to illness, either by way of physiological variables with which they are associated or, more indirectly, by way of their relationship to health behaviour. Health psychologists who conduct research into the relationship between personality and illness are also primarily interested in physiological pathways. However, it is generally acknowledged that more prosaic explanations for correlations between personality and illness may be derived from the fact that personality differences are often associated with differences in health behaviour (Suls and Rittenhouse, 1990; Miller et al., 1996; Stone and McCrae, 2007). Characteristics such as anxiety, depression, neuroticism and hostility have been variously shown to be associated with levels of smoking and alcohol consumption, diet and exercise, sleep disturbance, likelihood of seeking medical advice in the early stages of a disease and the likelihood of adhering to recommendations subsequently. Any of these variables, or some combination of them, could be invoked to account for an empirical correlation between personality and illness.

Data mining, *p*-hacking and data selection

Questionable research practices including data mining (also known as data dredging, fishing or snooping, and *p*-hacking) is the seeking of patterns in data that can be presented as statistically significant without first devising a specific hypothesis as to the underlying causality. It is a process of falsification that can be completely hidden from external observers and that is guaranteed to produce publishable results. Results obtained using these methods will almost always be unrepeatable.

Minimally significant effect

Any study with a finding based on a single *p* level of .05 must be interpreted cautiously. There are many different reasons why a single $p < .05$ finding may find its way into print. The only way to support a single $p < .05$ finding is replication. Without that, it is prudent to ignore the finding.

Fraud

Fraud involves the fabrication of data to present a positive confirmation of a hypothesis or desired outcome. Fortunately, known cases of fraud are relatively rare, but they do exist. Retractions of 'unsafe' papers by the late Hans J. Eysenck and R. Grossarth-Maticek followed an enquiry by King's College London (Marks, 2019) after exposure by Pelosi (2019) of a huge array of 'impossible' findings concerning personality and fatal illnesses.

THE IMPORTANCE OF INTERVENTION STUDIES

The following brief survey of statistical studies of the associations between personality and physical illness indicates a number of promising findings. However, for the reasons that have been presented, all of these findings are subject to a range of interpretations so that true causal links have not yet been definitively established.

Friedman and Kern (2014) concluded that, in order to make a convincing case for causality, it is necessary not only to demonstrate the existence of an association, but also to show that interventions designed to reduce a 'toxic' aspect of personality, or enhance a beneficial one, have the effect of reducing disease risk and increasing longevity. Interventions may obviously be of value in reducing distress in individuals suffering from serious illness, but the question that also needs to be addressed is: Can they produce an improved prognosis for the disease in question? Sadly, this has not yet been convincingly shown in any study. We now review the evidence in order to indicate the areas that look most promising for future research using interventions.

THE TYPE A PERSONALITY, HOSTILITY AND CORONARY HEART DISEASE

Type A and B personalities

Speculation about an association between the Type A and Type B personalities and coronary heart disease (CHD) has a history that dates back more than 50 years (Riska, 2000). The distinction between the two personalities was introduced in the mid-1950s by cardiologists

Meyer Friedman and Ray Rosenman, although, as already noted, their ideas can be traced back further to the work of Alexander in psychosomatic medicine. The Type A personality, thought to be at greater risk of CHD, is described as highly competitive and achievement oriented, not prepared to suffer fools gladly, always in a hurry and unable to bear delays and queues, hostile and aggressive, inclined to read, eat and drive very fast, and constantly thinking what to do next, even when supposedly listening to someone else. In contrast to this, the Type B personality is relaxed, laid back, lethargic, even-tempered, amiable and philosophical about life, relatively slow in speech and action, and generally has enough time for everyone and everything. The Type A personality has much in common with Galen's choleric temperament, the Type B with the phlegmatic (see Table 1.1). It is well known that men are at greater risk of CHD than women, and Riska (2000) made an interesting argument for the view that the concept of the Type A personality was an attempt to 'medicalize' and 'pathologize' traditional concepts of masculinity.

The key pioneering study of Type A personality and CHD was the Western Collaborative Group Study (WCGS), in which over 3,000 Californian men, aged from 39 to 59 at entry, were followed up initially over a period of 8.5 years, later extending over 22 years. When results were reported at the 8.5-year follow-up, it appeared that Type As were twice as likely compared with Type Bs to suffer from subsequent CHD. Of the sample, 7% developed some signs of CHD and two-thirds of these were Type As. This increased risk was apparent even when other risk factors assessed at entry, such as blood pressure and cigarette smoking, were statistically controlled for. Similar results were subsequently published from another large-scale study conducted in Framingham, Massachusetts, this time with both men and women in the sample, and by the early 1980s it was confidently asserted that Type A characteristics were as much a risk factor for heart disease as high blood pressure, high cholesterol levels and smoking.

However, later research failed to support these early findings. When Ragland and Brand (1988) conducted a 22-year follow-up of the WCGS, using CHD mortality as the crucially important measure, they failed to find any consistent evidence of an association. Much further research continued to be published up to the late 1980s, yielding few positive findings. Reviewing this evidence, Myrtek (2001) suggests that the modest number of positive findings that did exist were the result of over-reliance on angina as the measure of CHD. As we have already pointed out, this is an unreliable measure because it is frequently based solely on self-reported chest pain. Considering studies that adopted hard criteria, including mortality, Myrtek concludes that we can be confident that the Type A personality is not a risk factor for CHD.

Hostility

It can take a long time for a popular belief to fade away when there is a lack of evidence to support it. The extensive coverage still given to the Type A–CHD hypothesis by textbook writers is a good illustration of this. Researchers may be a little quicker to react, as is indicated by the decline in publications in this field from the early 1990s. In fact, it was largely replaced by an alternative hypothesis that was itself generated by the analysis of Type A–CHD research. This hypothesis is that hostility is the key dimension of personality that is associated with CHD.

The Type A personality, as described briefly in the last section, contains a number of components that are not necessarily closely correlated. Measures of Type A and B personalities often included sub-components that could be separately analysed for their association with subsequent CHD. When this was done it emerged that there was only one component that did seem to have some predictive power, and this component was anger or hostility. Research into links between anger/hostility and CHD became as popular in the 1990s as Type A research had been in previous years, but unfortunately with a very similar conclusion. By the end of the decade a number of reviews, including that of Myrtek (2001), found the studies to be of very mixed quality, with inconsistent results. There was some evidence of a statistically significant but very weak relationship for prospective studies of initially healthy individuals, but not for studies that have followed up patients already diagnosed with CHD.

In a curious mirroring of the breakdown of the Type A personality into sub-components, which led to the hostility–CHD research, the hostility researchers themselves reacted to disappointing findings by breaking hostility down into separate components. These included cynicism, mistrust, verbal and physical aggressiveness, and overt and experienced aggressiveness. It was proposed that more attention should be given to these sub-components in order to discover which are the most hazardous for health. However, when reviewing this area of research, Suls and Bunde (2005) noted that there is considerable overlap between measures of these sub-components of anger/hostility, with similar items being included in ostensibly different measures. Suls and Bunde also confirm Myrtek's earlier conclusion that evidence of an association between hostility, however measured, and subsequent CHD suggests a weak relationship, possibly no more than a side effect of the correlation of hostility measures with anxiety and depression, characteristics that will be considered later in this chapter because they appear to have a more substantial association with CHD.

SUPPORT OF THE TOBACCO INDUSTRY FOR PERSONALITY–ILLNESS RESEARCH

In view of the disappointing results achieved by research into the Type A personality, hostility and CHD, it may well be asked why it obtained so much publicity over more than 40 years. The reason may be connected with the high level of support this research has received from the US tobacco industry. Petticrew et al. (2012) have established this by analysing material lodged at the Legacy Tobacco Documents Library, a vast collection of documents that the companies were obliged to make public following litigation in 1998. These documents show that, for over 40 years from the 1950s, the industry heavily funded research into links between personality and both CHD and cancer, hoping to demonstrate that these personality variables were associated with cigarette smoking, thereby undermining claims about causal links between smoking and disease. Thus, for example, if it could be shown that Type A personalities were both more likely to smoke than Type Bs, and more likely to develop CHD, then it could be argued that smoking might be just an innocent background variable. Further to this, the Philip Morris company funded Meyer Friedman, the originator of Type A research, for the Meyer Friedman Institute, conducting research aiming to show that Type A personalities could be changed by interventions, thereby presumably reducing proneness to CHD even if they continued to smoke. Petticrew et al. also show that, while most Type A–CHD studies were not funded by the tobacco industry, most of the ones that found positive results were tobacco-funded. As has been pointed out in many areas of science, positive findings invariably get a great deal more publicity than negative findings and rebuttals.

DEPRESSION, STRESS AND CORONARY HEART DISEASE

There have been a number of reviews that have concluded, on the basis of prospective studies, that there are substantial associations between both anxiety and depression and subsequent CHD (Hemingway and Marmot, 1999; Krantz and McCeney, 2002; Wulsin and Singal, 2003; Lett et al., 2004; Suls and Bunde, 2005). These associations have been found in studies of patients with clinically diagnosed distress and in general population studies. Anxiety seems to predict sudden cardiac death rather more than other types of CHD, and phobic, panic-like anxiety is a particularly strong predictor: Haines et al. (1987) found that sufferers were three times more at risk of sudden cardiac death over the next seven years compared with non-sufferers. Very similar results were subsequently found by Kawachi et al. (1994) in a two-year follow-up of 33,999 initially healthy US male health professionals.

Depression is predictive of a wider range of CHD than anxiety. In a UK study with 19,649 participants who were initially free of clinical manifestations of heart disease, Surtees et al. (2003) found, with an average follow-up period of 8.5 years, that those assessed as suffering from a major depressive disorder were 2.7 times more likely to die from ischaemic heart disease over the follow-up period than those who did not, independently of age, sex, smoking, systolic blood pressure, cholesterol, physical activity, body mass index, diabetes, social class, heavy alcohol use and antidepressant medication use. In a very large prospective study of 96,376 post-menopausal women, Wassertheil-Smoller et al. (2004) report that depressive symptoms were substantially associated with death from cardiovascular disease after adjusting for age, race, education, income, diabetes, hypertension, smoking, cholesterol level, body mass index and physical activity.

These findings for anxiety and depression are impressive, but they should be considered alongside our earlier discussion of problems in interpreting personality–illness correlations. Hemingway and Marmot (1999) point out that these problems are particularly acute in this area. Anxiety and depression are certainly consequences of CHD as well as possible causes of it. Furthermore, symptoms of incipient CHD, such as breathlessness and chest pains, may occur for years prior to diagnosis, and lead in turn to experienced anxiety and depression. In this way, prospective studies could give the impression that anxiety and depression are causes of CHD, when in fact the direction of causality is the other way around.

Stress is often cited as a causal factor in coronary heart disease. Possible neurobiological pathways are illustrated in Figure 18.1. The neurobiological model of stress, unlike the BPSM, is a genuine scientific model. It enables predictions to be tested, shows relationships between processes that can be observed, and combines biological and psychosocial processes in a single system.

> According to the neurobiological model: the stress response involves the central activation of brain systems responsible for the analysis of the environment. This response is important and appears not to be deleterious, as it promotes a physiological balance in response to classic and normal environmental stressors. However, in the case of chronic and mainly psychosocial stressors, the allostatic system may be overwhelmed with hyperactivation of the hypothalamic–pituitary–adrenal axis and the autonomic nervous system with dysregulation of blood pressure and cortisol levels. In addition, an immuno-inflammatory response occurs with the production of inflammatory cytokines. If this phenomenon lasts for a long time because of chronic adversity (work or social stress, for instance), the pathophysiological effects

can lead to metabolic disturbances (glucose and lipid dysregulation), metabolic syndrome and cardiovascular disease. Then, psychological factors like perceived stress, coping style, personality traits, or social support might modulate the stress response. (Chauvet-Gelinier and Bonin, 2017)

As Miller et al. (2009) pointed out, one practically useful way of resolving some of the methodological problems in interpreting findings in this area would be a robust demonstration that interventions designed to reduce stress in patients suffering from CHD could produce an improved prognosis. Unfortunately, the two most substantial trials that have been conducted so far, each targeting depression and with more than 2,000 participants, showed no effect of interventions. Berkman et al. (2003) evaluated a programme that included cognitive behavioural therapy supplemented with antidepressants for the more severely depressed patients. Van Melle et al. (2007) evaluated an intervention consisting simply of treatment with antidepressants.

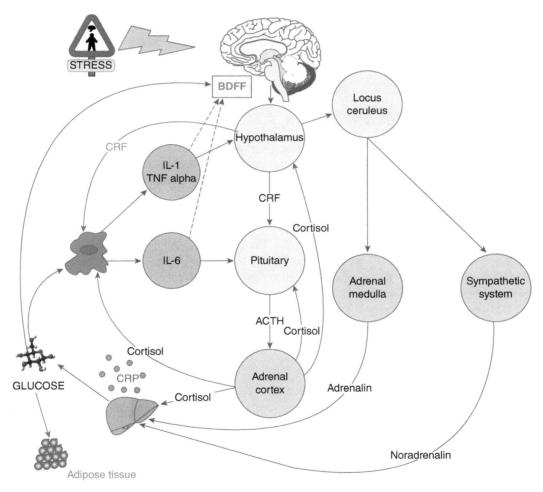

Figure 18.1   Neurobiological action of stress

Source: Reproduced from Chauvet-Gelinier and Bonin (2017)

Sin et al. (2016) prospectively examined relationships of depressive symptoms with behavioral and lifestyle factors among 667 patients with stable coronary heart disease. The lifestyle behaviours consisted of physical activity, medication adherence, body mass index, waist to hip ratio, sleep quality and smoking status. These were assessed at baseline and five years later. Sin et al. found that greater depressive symptoms at baseline predicted poorer lifestyle behaviours five years later (less physical activity, lower medication adherence, higher body mass index, higher waist to hip ratio, worse sleep quality and smoking). Baseline lifestyle behaviours predicted five-year change in depressive symptoms.

Some studies have indicated that the relationship between emotional distress and illness is not restricted to heart disease. Mykletun et al. (2007) examined data from a population-based health study of 61,349 participants. With a mean follow-up of 4.4 years, they found that depression was equally associated with all disease-related causes of death, not just CHD. They did not find any evidence of an association with anxiety. On the other hand, Grossardt et al. (2009), in a follow-up of 7,080 participants originally tested between 1962 and 1965, found that pessimistic, anxious and depressive personality traits were each predictive of all-cause mortality. Further research is obviously needed to clarify reasons for the differences between the findings of the two studies. However, they both suggested that the association between psychological distress and disease-related death extends beyond CHD.

DEPRESSION, HOPE AND CANCER

The widely held belief that depression is also an important factor in the onset and subsequent development of cancer has received little support from research. Adler and Matthews (1994) reviewed three large-scale prospective studies of the relationship between depression and both the incidence of and mortality from cancer. In these studies, initially healthy samples of up to 9,000 were followed up over periods ranging from 10 to 20 years and no associations were found between depression and either cancer onset or mortality. Since then two large-scale studies have produced conflicting results. Penninx et al. (1998) carried out a prospective study of 1,708 men and 3,117 women aged 71 and over. They found a significantly increased incidence of cancer for those who were diagnosed as suffering from chronic depression, indicated by repeated assessments of symptoms over six years. On the other hand, Whooley and Browner (1998) undertook a prospective study over six years of 7,519 women aged 67 or over and analysed the relationship between depression and subsequent mortality from (a) cancer, (b) cardiovascular disease and (c) all other diseases. They found no relationship between depression and cancer, but a strong relationship with both cardiovascular disease and all other diseases.

Negative findings have also been reported from follow-up studies of patients who have been treated for cancer. For example, Barraclough et al. (1992) followed up 204 patients who had received surgery for breast cancer over 42 months after surgery. They used a very detailed interview schedule, which included the assessment of prolonged major depression before surgery and during the follow-up period. They found no relationship at all between depression and relapse. Relapse was also unrelated to stress, including bereavement, long-term social difficulties and lack of a confiding relationship.

Coyne et al. (2007) noted the persistence of the belief that psychotherapy promotes survival in people with cancer in the face of contradictory findings. They provide a systematic critical review of the relevant literature and conclude:

> No randomized clinical trial designed with survival as a primary endpoint and in which psychotherapy was not confounded with medical care has yielded a positive effect. Among the implications of the review is that an adequately powered study examining effects of psychotherapy on survival after a diagnosis of cancer would require resources that are not justified by the strength of the available evidence. (Coyne et al., 2007: 367)

Psychological resources such as hope, mindfulness and spirituality, have been identified as potential resources for patients to cope with the course of cancer and its treatment by alleviating emotional distress and improving quality of life (Aspinwall and MacNamara, 2005; Coughlin, 2008; Hou et al., 2010; Lim et al., 2016). These resources are said to be amenable to individual control and have been suggested as targets for psychosocial interventions (Pitceathly et al., 2013). Mahendran et al. (2017) followed a sample of newly diagnosed Asian cancer patients over a one-year period to identify early opportunities to improve patient outcomes. They aimed to investigate the relative predictive value of hope, mindfulness, spirituality and life satisfaction on cancer mortality. They hypothesized that metastatic and advanced stage cancer predict higher cancer mortality, and greater availability of psychological resources predict lower cancer mortality. Mindfulness, spirituality and life satisfaction were all non-significant as predictors of cancer mortality. They found that metastatic cancer, advanced stage cancer and hope predicted cancer mortality after adjusting for socio-demographic and medical variables. However, this result must be interpreted with caution as it was significant at only the .05 level, and could have been a Type I error. Also, cancer mortality was evaluated over a single year of follow-up with newly diagnosed patients, and the association between psychological resources and mortality over five or ten-year follow-up remains unknown. Finally, Mahendran et al.'s (2017) study did not include potential moderating variables such as health behaviours or social support.

Schofield et al. (2016) investigated associations between resources of hope, optimism, anxiety, depression, health utility and survival in patients starting first-line chemotherapy for metastatic colorectal cancer. This cross-sectional study included 429 patients with metastatic colorectal cancer in a randomized controlled trial of chemotherapy with a median follow-up of 31 months. They completed questionnaires assessing hopefulness, optimism, anxiety and depression, and health utility. Univariable analyses showed that overall survival was associated negatively with depression and positively with health utility and hopefulness. Schofield et al. (2016) concluded that depression and health utility, but not optimism, hope or anxiety, were associated with survival after controlling for known prognostic factors in patients with advanced colorectal cancer. This was not a randomized clinical trial designed with survival as a primary endpoint.

It would be a sensible strategy to switch the effort and research funds expended on cross-sectional studies of cancer survival and psychological resources to high-powered prospective studies using randomized controlled trials.

CONSCIENTIOUSNESS AND LONGEVITY

Conscientiousness is one of the five factors of personality proposed by McCrae and Costa in their influential theory that was originally developed in 1985. A considerable amount of research has shown that this characteristic is associated with longevity. Many studies, including some long-term prospective ones, have found positive evidence for an association between conscientiousness and longevity.

In a meta-analysis that pooled the results of 20 independent samples, Kern and Friedman (2008) found a modest but significant correlation of 0.11 between conscientiousness and longevity. In a subsequent review, Friedman and Kern (2014) drew attention to more research that confirms the existence of this relationship, which also extends from childhood through adult life. They suggest a number of pathways mediating the association. An important one is health behaviour. For example, Bogg and Roberts (2004) pooled the results from 194 studies that incorporated measures of conscientiousness-related traits and assessments of any of the leading behavioural contributors to mortality (tobacco use, diet and activity patterns, excessive alcohol use, violence, risky sexual behaviour, risky driving, suicide and drug use). They found that conscientiousness-related traits were negatively related to all risky health-related behaviours and positively related to all beneficial health-related behaviours.

A major 40-year prospective study in Hawaii investigated a lifespan health behaviour mechanism relating childhood conscientiousness to adult clinical health (Hampson et al., 2015). Children in entire elementary school classrooms on two Hawaiian islands were assessed between 1959 and 1967 on their personality traits by their teachers towards the end of one school year. Then in 1998, efforts were made to find these same people, who by then were middle-aged adults. There were 2,418 in the original child cohort, 79 of whom were already deceased and 19 only had first names recorded, leaving 2,320 to locate. Of these, an amazing 1,938 (84%) were found. From those successfully identified, 36 refused further contact and one was illiterate, reducing the sample to 1,901. Of these, 1,387 (73%) were recruited and completed at least one questionnaire. To be included in the study, participants had to have participated in the medical and psychological examination at 51 years, and to have completed the first questionnaire. These requirements limited the sample to 372 men and 387 women ($n = 759$).

The investigators studied the associations between the Big Five personality traits at mean age 10, adult Big Five personality traits, and adult clinically assessed 'dysregulation' at mean age 51. Dysregulation was defined as a summary of dysregulated blood glucose, blood pressure and lipids. A retrospective, cumulative measure of lifespan health-damaging behaviour (lifetime smoking, physical inactivity, and body mass index from age 20) was assessed in the Hawaii Personality and Health Cohort ($n = 759$). Structural equation modelling was used to test the conceptual model with direct and indirect paths from childhood Conscientiousness to adult Conscientiousness, lifespan health-damaging behaviours, educational attainment, adult cognitive ability and adult clinical health.

For both men and women, childhood Conscientiousness influenced health-damaging behaviours through educational attainment, and lifespan health-damaging behaviours predicted dysregulation. Although childhood Conscientiousness predicted adult Conscientiousness, the latter did not predict any other variables in the model. The pathways of influence differed between the two genders. For men, childhood Conscientiousness predicted dysregulation through educational attainment and health-damaging behaviours. For women, childhood Conscientiousness predicted dysregulation through educational attainment and adult cognitive ability.

According to Hampson et al. (2015), childhood Conscientiousness appears to influence health assessed more than 40 years later through complex processes including educational attainment, cognitive ability and the cumulative effects of health behaviours, but not adult Conscientiousness. However, it must be noted that the effects are relatively small. The models account for only 7.4% of the variance in dysregulation for women and 16.5% of the variance in dysregulation for men.

A question that naturally arises at this point is: Can interventions be developed to increase conscientiousness, thereby potentially leading to improved health? Here there are grounds for scepticism. Given that health behaviours play an important role in mediating the association, it is likely to be more productive to focus on health promotion campaigns and interventions aimed directly at specific behaviours, such as dysregualtion, smoking, drinking, diet and exercise, rather than programmes aimed at conscientiousness as a general characteristic.

POSITIVE PSYCHOLOGY: A CAUTIONARY TALE

In contrast to the focus on the health consequences of negative characteristics, such as anxiety and depression, a considerable amount of recent research within 'Positive Psychology' has been concerned with the potential health benefits of positive characteristics, such as optimism, life satisfaction and self-esteem. There has been a massive amount of hype about positive psychology, but is there any solid evidence to support these conjectures?

One example is the work of Surtees et al. (2003) on sense of coherence and health. Originally proposed as a measurable characteristic by Antonovsky (1979), sense of coherence is described as the ability to perceive one's world as meaningful and manageable. Surtees et al. carried out a prospective study over six years of the relationship between sense of coherence and mortality from all causes for a very large UK sample of 20,579 participants aged 41–80 years. They found that a strong sense of coherence was associated with a 30% reduction in mortality from all causes and also, more specifically, for cardiovascular disease. The explanation for this probably lies in the fact that sense of coherence is inversely correlated with anxiety and depression. In a study conducted in Finland of 4,642 men and women aged from 25 to 74, Konttinen et al. (2008) found inverse correlations of 0.62 between sense of coherence and depression for both men and women; the inverse correlations between sense of coherence and anxiety were 0.57 for men and 0.54 for women. It follows that the findings of Surtees et al. could be basically the corollary of the positive correlations already discussed between anxiety and depression and both cardiovascular disease and all-cause mortality.

Boehm and Kubzansky (2012) provide a broad critical review of research on the association between psychological well-being and cardiovascular health. They note the existence of many findings that confirm this association, while pointing out the potential significance of the correlations between psychological well-being and the health behaviours that are already known to be associated with cardiovascular health. It has not been demonstrated that changes to an individual's psychological well-being, whether the result of interventions or for other reasons, have a direct effect on cardiovascular health, independently of known risk factors such as smoking, diet and exercise.

Coyne and Tennen (2010) examined four widely accepted claims in the positive psychology literature regarding beneficial adaptational outcomes among individuals living with cancer:

1. The alleged role of positive factors such as a 'fighting spirit' in extending the life of persons with cancer.

2. The alleged effects of interventions cultivating positive psychological states on immune functioning and cancer progression and mortality.

3. The alleged value benefit finding.

4. The alleged post-traumatic growth following serious illness such as cancer and other highly threatening experiences.

Coyne and Tennen's analysis suggested that these four types of claim are routinely made in the positive psychology literature but none is supported by the available evidence. In particular, they found that claims about the adaptational value of benefit-finding and post-traumatic growth among cancer patients and the implausibility of claims that interventions that enhance benefit-finding improve the prognosis of cancer patients by strengthening the immune system lacked coherence. Coyne and Tennen (2010: 16) concluded by urging positive psychologists to 'rededicate themselves to a positive psychology based on scientific evidence rather than wishful thinking'.

MORE NULL RESULTS

The role of personality in cancer risk has been controversial, and, as we have seen, the evidence remains inconclusive. Jokela et al. (2014) pooled data from six prospective cohort studies (British Household Panel Survey; Health and Retirement Study; Household, Income and Labour Dynamics in Australia; Midlife in the United Survey; Wisconsin Longitudinal Study Graduate; and Sibling samples) in a meta-analysis to examine whether personality traits of the Five Factor Model (extraversion, neuroticism, agreeableness, conscientiousness and openness to experience) were associated with the incidence of cancer and cancer mortality in 42,843 cancer-free men and women at baseline (mean age 52.2 years, 55.6% women). For an average follow-up of 5.4 years, there were 2,156 incident cancer cases. In a meta-analysis adjusted for age, sex and race/ethnicity, none of the Big Five personality traits were associated with the incidence of all cancers or any of the six site-specific cancers included in the analysis (lung, colon, breast, prostate, skin and leukaemia/lymphoma). In the three cohorts with cause-specific mortality data (421 cancer deaths among 21,835 participants), none of the personality traits were associated with cancer mortality. These data suggest that personality is *not* associated with increased risk of incidents of cancer or cancer-related mortality. It is fanciful, irresponsible and actually unethical to suggest that interventions based on the belief that cancer can be beaten by 'mind power' have any effect on cancer mortality. Positive psychologists please take note! If only this null effect were more widely appreciated, sufferers would be spared from wasting their money on expensive private treatments based on unsubstantiated claims and also, perhaps more seriously, be spared from blaming themselves for having become ill in the first place, and for failing to get better. As a service to patients, national professional psychological societies such as the British Psychological Society and the American Psychological Association should promote a balanced view of the evidence rather than promote 'quack' psychological interventions for physical illnesses such as cancer.

FUTURE RESEARCH

1. Investigations are needed to distinguish between personality variables that are associated with biologically verified illness and those that are associated only with self-reported illness.

2. There is a need for studies to establish which dimensions of personality are directly associated with health-relevant physiological variables, and to distinguish them from those that are primarily associated with health behaviours.

3. Outcome studies are needed to assess the effectiveness of interventions designed to modify psychological characteristics that are suspected of being hazardous to health.

4. In the case of anxiety and depression, interventions would obviously be worthwhile if they relieve these conditions, whether or not they influence health outcomes.

SUMMARY

1. From the ancient Greeks to modern times, medical practitioners have usually believed that there is a physical basis to all illness, including psychological disorders. In contrast to this, there has also been a holistic tradition that has placed an emphasis on the role of psychological factors.

2. Health psychologists have found it very difficult to determine whether personality is associated with susceptibility to physical disease directly through physiological mechanisms or indirectly by way of health behaviour, or whether the data are best explained by statistical artefacts and flaws in the design of the studies from which they are obtained.

3. Early indications that the Type A personality is a risk factor for CHD were not confirmed by later studies. Attention then shifted to hostility, but this variable now seems only to be a weak predictor, if a predictor at all.

4. Anxiety, especially phobic, panic-like anxiety, and depression are both associated with an increased risk of CHD, although a number of different interpretations of these associations are possible.

5. There is no clear-cut evidence to support the view that personality variables are associated with risk of cancer or of relapse following treatment. Interventions based on treatment for depression have not been shown to improve the survival chances of cancer sufferers.

6. There is substantial evidence that 'positive' psychological characteristics, including sense of coherence, are associated with reduced risk of CHD and all-cause mortality. This may be the inverse of the parallel findings for anxiety and depression, which have strong negative correlations with positive characteristics.

7. Conscientiousness has been shown in many studies to be predictive of longevity. A major reason seems to be that this characteristic is negatively related to many risky health-related behaviours and positively related to beneficial health-related behaviours.

8. The study by Jokela et al. (2014), which pooled data from six prospective studies, suggests that personality is *not* associated with increased risk of incidents of cancer or cancer-related mortality. Interventions based on the belief that cancer can be beaten by 'mind power' have no effect whatsoever on cancer mortality.

9. As a service to patients, national professional psychological societies such as the British Psychological Society and the American Psychological Association need to promote a balanced view of the scientific evidence and avoid occasionally giving the impression of promoting 'quack' psychological interventions for physical illnesses such as cancer.

PAIN AND PAIN CONTROL

'[M]edicine has overlooked the fact that the activity of this (pain) apparatus is subject to a constantly changing influence of the mind.'

Bonica (1990: 12)

OUTLINE

In this chapter, we discuss the complex and multifactorial nature of pain, starting with the direct line of transmission, pattern and multi-dimensional gate control theories. Psychological and social processes that mediate and moderate pain behaviour and experience are considered. We summarize the pros and cons of different pain assessment methods. The fear-avoidance model and relevant empirical evidence are reviewed. Finally, we explore psychological techniques used in pain management and the evidence for their effectiveness. The postscript discusses recent uses of torture and interrogation.

WHAT IS PAIN?

According to the Institute of Medicine (2011), chronic pain affects approximately 100 million Americans. This is higher than the number of diabetes, heart disease and cancer sufferers combined. The cost to the US economy of chronic pain, including health care and lost productivity costs, was estimated to be between US$560 billion and $635 billion annually. In Europe, one study found that 19% of adults suffered from chronic pain of moderate-to-severe intensity and nearly half received inadequate pain management (Breivik et al., 2006). One in five Australians will expect to suffer chronic pain in their lifetime, and it is estimated to cost the economy AU$34 billion per annum (Pain Australia, 2010). One scientific problem is that pain is subjective.

> We know that pain is a highly adaptive but complex and multifaceted phenomenon that is poorly understood by many health care practitioners, especially physicians. As a consequence, many of those afflicted by pain suffer prolonged periods without understanding, care and support. This can cause conflict, irritability and even anger. It has been wisely asserted by two leading experts that:pain is not a monolithic entity. Pain is, rather, a concept used to focus and label a group of behaviours, thoughts and emotions. Pain has many dimensions, including sensory and affective components, location, intensity, time course, and the memories, meaning, and anticipated consequences that it elicits … no isomorphic relationship exists among tissue damage, nociception, and pain report. (Turk and Wilson, 2013: 314)

The pain experience is also difficult to disentangle from the language we use to describe it. The socio-cultural context, consisting of beliefs and explanations, may be implicit in the description. A physician is unlikely to be able to allocate the time necessary to analyse all of the variables that influence the waxing and waning of chronic pain reported by an individual sufferer. The physician may simply ask 'Is it painful? and/or 'Where is the pain?'.

An account of the initiation, exacerbation and maintenance of pain is a compelling and engaging task for the patient and her/his carers. If they are lucky, they will have access to a health professional with training in chronic pain management. However, such expertise is rare, and millions of patients globally receive inadequate care and are left to their own devices. Bring out the paracetamol!

It is frequently asserted that pain is a biological safety alarm to warn us when something is physically wrong, allowing us to act to alleviate the problem. Pain serves an essentially homeostatic function. Its importance can be seen when cases of congenital universal insensitivity to pain (CUIP) are considered. Most cases of CUIP involve premature death. A different concept, 'psychological pain', is used to refer to mental anguish or suffering. Pain expression is a performance of affliction of a person in a social situation, suggesting that pain can influence any aspect of existence, not only the physical body. In this chapter we discuss only physical pain, not mental anguish, although the first may lead to the other.

Pain experience is uniquely personal. It can be described in many ways, including:

- An aversive, personal, subjective experience, influenced by cultural learning, the meaning of the situation, attention and other psychological variables, which disrupts ongoing behaviour and motivates the individual to attempt to stop the pain (Melzack and Wall, 1982/1988).

- Whatever the person experiencing it says it is, existing whenever the experiencing person says it does (McCaffery and Thorpe, 1988).

- An unpleasant sensory and emotional experience associated with actual or potential tissue damage, or described in terms of such damage (Merskey, 1996).

Such definitions highlight the subjective, emotional and multi-dimensional nature of pain experience. Pain is further classified as either acute or chronic, differentiated only by a duration of six months (acute being under six months and chronic over six months). The six-month cut-off is highly arbitrary; other suggested cut-off points are 30 days, 3 months or 12 months.

Acute pain is a useful biological response provoked by injury or disease (e.g., broken leg, appendicitis), which is of limited duration (International Association for the Study of Pain, 2010). It tends to be amenable to pharmacological treatment. **Chronic pain** is described as pain persisting for six months or more and tends not to respond to pharmacological treatment. The time continuum is imperfect because there are many cases of acute recurrent pain, e.g., migraine headaches, and also pain from progressive illnesses such as metastatic cancer.

Further useful distinctions include:

- malignant (associated with progressive illness, e.g., cancer);

- benign (not associated with progressive illness, e.g., lower back pain, LBP);

- progressive (becomes worse over time, e.g., arthritis);

- intractable (resistant to treatment, e.g., LBP);

- intermittent (pain that fluctuates over time and in intensity, e.g., fibromyalgia);

- recurrent (acute pain occurring periodically, e.g., migraine);

- organic (involving observable tissue damage, e.g., arthritis);

- psychogenic (absence of demonstrable pathology, e.g., fibromyalgia);

- referred (pain originating in one body area which is perceived as originating from another, e.g., perceiving an 'earache' that originates from a bad tooth).

Pain can affect anyone at any time and can be highly disabling, often involving all aspects of a person's life, including physical, psychological and emotional states, disrupting daily activities, work, finances, social, marital and family life and relationships (e.g., Marcus, 2000). In addition to its association with many chronic illnesses (e.g., cancer, HIV/AIDS, sickle-cell anaemia), particular groups appear more likely to experience chronic pain, especially the elderly and many disabled people, even in the absence of illness (e.g., pain from braces or harnesses).

Pain is simply suffering for the person with it, but it is an extremely interesting phenomenon for physicians, physiologists and psychologists alike: *pain is perceived in the body, produced by the central nervous system, and processed by the mind.* To the pain sufferer, however, pain can be the primary determining influence on quality of life and well-being. Talking about pain is always a tricky problem. Discussing it with the sufferer in simple terms or using tired clichés should always be avoided. It is lamentable to 'psychologize' pain; little else can be more infuriating to a pain sufferer.

One response to pain is to misinterpret it as a catastrophe, a sign of serious injury or pathology over which one has little or no control. This can lead to an excessive fear of pain that gradually extends to a fear of physical movements such that people will avoid physical activities that they presume will worsen their problem, and as their inactivity is reinforced, their disablement worsens as a consequence. We review in a later section the fear-avoidance model (FAM) (Asmundson et al., 1999; Vlaeyen and Linton, 2000; Crombez et al., 2012).

PAIN ASSESSMENT

Pain **assessment** is not a simple process. The inherent difficulty is trying to interpret a uniquely individual experience related by another person. Assessment is crucial to the understanding and treatment of pain, including its underlying mechanisms and mediating factors, as well as the development of effective treatment programmes.

Assessments are mostly undertaken for medical, research or compensation claim purposes and the purpose will influence the type of assessment used. Assessment measures may include intensity, psychological and functional effects and pain behaviours. Assessment methods can generally be grouped under one of four categories: physiological measures, pain questionnaires, mood assessment questionnaires and observations (direct observations or self-observations).

Table 19.1 summarizes some of the common measures that have been described in the literature. Medical examinations form the backbone of clinical pain assessments and include joint mobility and heart rate. Physiological measures attempt to objectively measure responses to pain. Psychological measures assess pain using psychometric instruments of different kinds.

Pain questionnaires present commonly used descriptive words that the individual uses to communicate their current experience. The words may be presented in rating scales or descriptive lists. The McGill Pain Questionnaire (MPQ; Melzack, 1975; Melzack and Katz, 2013) is the most frequently used questionnaire. In this, descriptive terms are clustered in groups of two to five. Participants circle the words that describe their pain, one word from each group. Then they must go back and circle the three words in groups 1–10 that most convey their pain response, two words in groups 11–15 that do the same thing, and one word in group 16. Finally, they are asked to pick one word in groups 17–20. At the end, they should have seven words that they can take to their doctor that will help describe the nature and intensity of the pain. Examples are as follows: Group 1 – Flickering, Pulsing, Quivering, Throbbing, Beating, Pounding; Group 2 – Jumping, Flashing, Shooting; Group 3 – Pricking, Boring, Drilling, Stabbing; Group 19 – Cool, Cold, Freezing; Group 20 – Nagging, Nauseating, Agonizing, Dreadful, Torturing (Melzack, 1975).

Table 19.1 Summary of common pain-assessment measures

Physiological measures	Questionnaires assessing pain	Questionnaires assessing mood and pain-related attitudes	Observations – direct or self
Medical examination, including pain sites, joint mobility, history, etc.	McGill Pain Questionnaire (MPQ) (Melzack, 1975)	Beck's Depression Inventory (Beck, 1977)	Activity levels
Muscle tension – electromyography (EMG)	Multidimensional Pain Inventory (MPI) (Kearns et al., 1985)	Hospital Anxiety and Depression Scale (Zigmond and Snaith, 1983)	Standing and sitting time (uptime and downtime)
Heart rate	Sickness Impact Profile (SIP) (Follick et al., 1985)	Pain Anxiety Symptoms Scale (McCracken et al., 1992)	Sleep patterns
Hyperventilation	Survey of Pain Attitudes (Jensen et al., 1987)	Well-being Questionnaire (Pincus et al., 1997)	Sexual activity

Physiological measures	Questionnaires assessing pain	Questionnaires assessing mood and pain-related attitudes	Observations – direct or self
Galvanic skin response (GSR)	Pain Information and Beliefs Questionnaire (Shutty et al., 1990)	Chronic Pain Acceptance Questionnaire (McCracken et al., 2004a)	Medication requests and usage
Electroencephalograph (EEG)	Pain diagram (Chan et al., 1993)		Normal household activities Appetite and eating
Pedometer	Bio-behavioural Pain Profile (Dalton et al., 1994)		Leisure activities

Fear of pain has been implicated in chronic pain behaviour. McCracken et al. (1992) developed an instrument to measure fear of pain across cognitive, behavioural and physiological domains – the Pain Anxiety Symptoms Scale (PASS). Related to fear of pain is acceptance of chronic pain, which occurs when an individual reduces avoidance or control and tries to focus on carrying out activities in the pursuit of personal goals. McCracken et al. (2004b) investigated the psychometric properties of the Chronic Pain Acceptance Questionnaire (CPAQ). They found that factors assessing (a) the degree to which one engaged in life activities regardless of the pain and (b) the willingness to experience pain were both positively related to patient functioning.

Other methods include verbal rating scales, visual analogue scales and a pain diagram that shows front and back outlines of a body on which patients can mark areas where pain is felt. Visual analogue scales may be most appropriate with diverse cultural groups, children, the elderly and people with communication difficulties. They are easy to use and therefore frequent ratings can be made then averaged, or peak times and triggers identified. Most pain questionnaires attempt to assess sensory, affective and evaluative dimensions of pain. They can be completed by the individual or as part of an interview. Specific types of pain seem to be described using similar words, and questionnaires have been found to discriminate between different pain populations.

Observations of individual pain behaviours and functional levels are also used in assessments, either direct observations by another person (e.g., a nurse on a hospital ward), or self-observations (e.g., in diaries or logs). However, direct and self-observations have drawbacks. Direct observations can never elicit unbiased data, being influenced by the setting in which they occur (e.g., clinical setting, home), the purpose of the assessment (e.g., benefit claim versus treatment assessment) and assessor characteristics (e.g., gender, ethnicity). Similarly, self-observations (e.g., pain diaries) may be inaccurate or overly subjective. Scales exist for patients and carers to rate their ability, on a 0–10 scale, to carry out everyday tasks such as sitting, car riding, dressing, sleeping, having sex, walking, housework, getting up from a chair or bed, shopping and carrying out light work, e.g., the Activities of Daily Living Scale (Linton, 1990).

An alternative approach is to use interviews to assess all aspects of the pain experience, including a full pain history, emotional adjustment and pre- and post-pain lifestyle. However, interviews need to be structured or they tend to tail off in different directions as sufferers need to talk about their pain and disrupted life experience at length, often because they don't feel listened to by doctors. In the vast majority of cases, physicians and surgeons care only about one thing: reducing pain using medication. They don't get paid for, or care too much about, discussing the finer distinctions about where pain is, what it feels like, or even what is causing it; they just want it gone. Hence, there is a niche for the more empathic health psychologist.

Issues in pain assessment

Many assessment instruments are insensitive to age, disability and culture. For groups who have communication difficulties, due to age, language problems, or sensory or cognitive deficits, assessment may require extended assessment time to enable rapport building. Herr et al. (2006) found that there is no standardized tool based on non-verbal/behavioural pain indicators in English that can be recommended for clinical practice. It is necessary to rely on the reports of significant others (e.g., a carer or interpreter), which has additional challenges of perception, interpretation and motivation. More work is required to address issues around the impact of the situational context and assessor characteristics on the assessment process. Further investigation is needed of the influence of assessment, including the impact of compensation claim assessments, and of the need to prove the existence of pain and how it restricts the sufferer's daily activities.

MECHANISMS, MEDIATORS AND MODERATORS OF PAIN

A useful framework for conceptualizing pain includes attention, expectations, beliefs, knowledge, emotions, coping strategies, along with cultural and family influences, which can all play a role in mediating and moderating pain experience (Linton and Shaw, 2011). The diagram in Figure 19.1 is self-explanatory. All of the processes are familiar ones. However, moving from a framework to a scientific model and then to a theory are massive steps that have yet to be convincingly taken. A few faltering steps have been made, but there is thin ice afoot for the unwary. We are not even going to begin to discuss here the philosophical complexities, but they are substantial.

The **biopsychosocial model** (see Chapter 1) encapsulates the contemporary view that chronic pain and disability have multiple causes: biological, psychological and social. Psychosocial factors are important predictors of chronic pain and disability early in acute and sub-acute stages of pain (Boersma et al., 2014). The transition from acute to chronic pain and to disability is moderated by depression, anxiety, pain beliefs, catastrophizing and coping behaviours. All of the factors shown in Figure 19.1 are embodied in a single nervous system to produce the pain experience. An external observer can only guess at the resulting experience from the subject's verbal and non-verbal behaviour.

Theories about pain production are few in number, and none to date are able to explain all of the known facts. The specific mechanisms for the transmission and perception of pain are not well understood, although knowledge in the form of empirical data is expanding. Three main theories have been proposed: specificity theory, pattern theory and gate control theory.

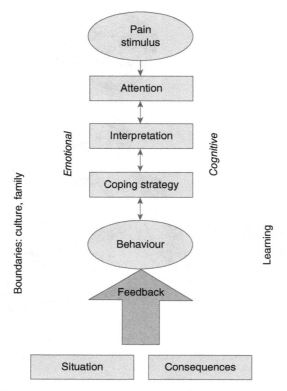

Figure 19.1   Psychosocial mechanisms involved in the perception and performance of pain

Source: Linton and Shaw (2011)

Specificity theory

Specificity theory was suggested by René Descartes in 1664 (Figure 19.2) and taken up by von Frey in 1894. This theory describes a direct causal relationship between pain stimulus and pain experience. Stimulation of specific pain receptors (nociceptors) throughout the body sends impulses along specific pain pathways (A delta fibres and C fibres) through the spinal cord to specific areas of the sensory cortex of the brain. Stimulus intensity correlates with pain intensity, with higher stimulus intensity and pain pathway activation resulting in a more intense pain experience. Failure to identify a specific cortical location for pain, realization that pain fibres do not respond exclusively to pain but also to pressure and temperature, and the disproportional relationship between stimulus intensity and reported pain intensity (e.g., injured soldiers reporting little pain while similarly injured civilians require substantial medication) led to specificity theory losing favour. To put it bluntly, the theory is simply wrong.

Pattern theory

Pattern theorists proposed that stimulation of nociceptors produces a pattern of impulses that are summated in the dorsal horn of the spinal cord. Only if the level of the summated output

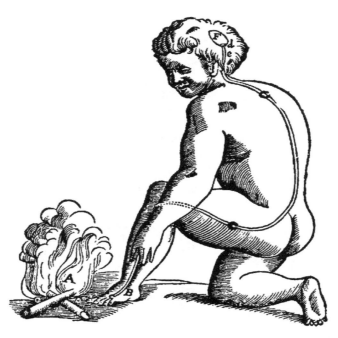

Figure 19.2   The pain pathway in René Descartes' *Traité de l'homme* (1664). The specificity view of pain has been replaced with more complex theories

exceeds a certain threshold is pain information transmitted onwards to the cortex, resulting in pain perception. Evidence of deferred pain perception (e.g., soldiers not perceiving pain until the battle is over), intact pain transmission systems where pain is perceived without injury (e.g., phantom limb) and injury without pain perception (e.g., CUIP) raised questions about pattern theories. In addition, there was growing evidence for a mediating role for psychosocial factors in the experience of pain, including cross-cultural differences in pain perception and expression. The theory was inadequate.

Gate control theory

Conscious experience, whether pain or otherwise, is derived from a multiplexed array of afferent information arriving via sensory transducers allied with cognitive and emotional information about the context, history and future implications of the stimulus environment. The growing body of evidence contradicting the direct line of transmission and pattern theories culminated in the development of the **gate control theory** by Melzack and Wall (1982/1988). In the gate control theory, pain is viewed as a multi-dimensional, subjective experience in which ascending physiological inputs and descending psychological inputs are equally involved. The gate control theory posits that there is a gating mechanism in the dorsal horn of the spinal cord that permits or inhibits the transmission of pain impulses (see Figure 19.3).

The dorsal horn receives inputs from nociceptors that it projects to the brain via a neural gate. The dorsal horn also receives information from the brain about the psychological and emotional state of the individual. This information can act as an inhibitory control that closes the neural gate, preventing the transmission of the nociceptive impulses and thus modifying the perception of pain. The mechanism operates based on the relative activity of the peripheral nociceptor fibres and the descending cortical fibres. Pain impulses must reach conscious awareness before pain is experienced. If awareness can be prevented, the experience of pain is decreased, eliminated or deferred.

The gate control theory has been an influential theory that continues to inform theoretical and empirical work. Gate control theory offers substantial explanatory power by acknowledging a role for descending control and psychological, social and behavioural factors. However, the absence of any direct evidence of a 'gate' in the spinal cord is a problem. Also, gate control theory is unable to explain several chronic pain problems, such as phantom limb pain.

Melzack (1999; see also Melzack and Katz, 2014) updated gate control theory by describing a 'body-self neuromatrix', in place of the gate. The body-self neuromatrix is a proposal that pain is a multi-dimensional experience produced by characteristic 'neurosignature' patterns of nerve impulses generated by a widely distributed neural network in the brain. These neurosignatures may be triggered by sensory inputs or generated independently of them. Pain is produced by a 'widely distributed neural network in the brain rather than directly by sensory input evoked by injury, inflammation or other pathology' (Melzack, 1999: 880).

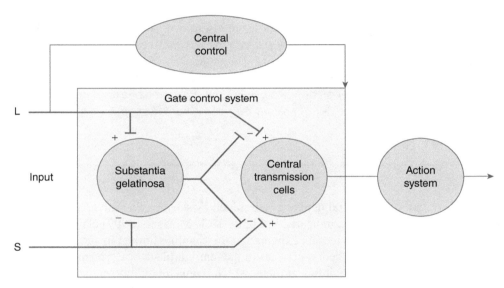

Figure 19.3   The Melzack–Wall gate control theory of pain

Source: Melzack and Wall (1967: 975, Figure 4)

BOX 19.1

KEY STUDY: How can we know when another person really experiences pain?

First-person introspection is necessary for communicating the pain experience to a third-person observer. Therefore, can we ever be sure they are not fabricating? This study by

(Continued)

Coghill et al. (2003) identified the neural correlates of an individual's subjective experience of pain. Seventeen healthy volunteers (eight women and nine men of mean age 26) participated in a psychophysical and functional magnetic resonance imaging (fMRI) study of individual differences in pain sensitivity. Thermal stimuli were delivered and assessed with a ten-unit mechanical VAS for pain intensity. Thirty-two stimuli (35°C, 43–49°C, 5-second duration) were applied to their non-dominant ventral forearm. Each participant underwent functional imaging during thermal stimulation of the skin of the right lower leg. For painful stimulation, five 30-second duration epochs of 49°C stimulation were interleaved with six 30-second duration epochs of 35°C stimulation. At the end of each 330-second series, participants provided a rating of pain intensity. Participants were assigned to a high- (mean VAS rating = 7.43), moderate- (mean VAS rating = 4.44) or low-sensitivity (mean VAS rating = 2.43) sub-group. To identify brain regions that were activated more frequently in the high-sensitivity individuals, the frequency map of the low-sensitivity group was subtracted from that of the high-sensitivity group.

Cortical regions involved in sensation, attention and affect were activated more frequently in pain-sensitive individuals than in those who were insensitive. The most robust difference between high-sensitivity and low-sensitivity sub-groups was located within a portion of the anterior cingulate cortex, where six out of six of the highly sensitive volunteers, but none of the insensitive volunteers, displayed statistically significant activation. This study shows that individuals with similar subjective reports of pain evoke similar patterns of activation magnitude, suggesting that people can accurately represent their conscious experience via introspection.

Source: Coghill et al. (2003)

Pain is the output of this neural network determined by sensory, cognitive, affective, experiential and genetic influences, as indicated in Figure 19.1. Melzack (1999) claims that the new 'theory' of a 'neuromatrix' provides an explanation for phantom limb pain and pain experience more generally. However, the 'theory' consists of the familiar black box type model of overlapping circles with some arrows pointing at them, which seems incredibly vague, and, one might ask, what exactly is the 'theory' saying and which predictions does it make? It is a truism that pain experience must be coded in the nervous system. Using the definitions and terminology of Chapter 1, the 'neuromatrix' is not a theory but a framework summarizing one knowledgeable scientist's ideas about pain. A 'work in progress' is a phrase that springs to mind. There appear to be no definite predictions that can be based upon it, which means that the search for the neural networks of pain will go on, but without any specific guidance from this particular approach.

NEURAL CORRELATES OF PAIN

What kind of neural networks exist in the brain that may help to explain how pain is coded? Are differences in self-reported pain associated with measurable neural differences? Coghill et al. (2003) used psychophysical ratings to define pain sensitivity, and functional magnetic resonance imaging (fMRI) to assess brain activity. They found positive evidence that individuals who were more sensitive to pain stimuli exhibited more frequent and more robust pain-induced activation of the primary somatosensory cortex, anterior cingulate cortex and prefrontal cortex than did insensitive individuals. Coghill et al. identified objective neural correlates of subjective differences, validating the use of self-reported pain from introspection as a method of communicating a first-person experience.

On the other hand, Mouraux et al. (2011) found that the largest part of the fMRI responses elicited by phasic nociceptive stimuli reflected non-nociceptive-specific cognitive processes, i.e., nociceptive and non-nociceptive stimuli triggered overlapping sets of brain activity. The search for nociceptive-specific brain activities continues. Meanwhile, millions of chronic pain patients deserve better health care and support. Enter the health psychologists.

PSYCHOLOGICAL FACTORS IN CLINICAL PRACTICE

Many psychosocial factors have been investigated in relation to pain and these appear to exert independent effects on the experience of pain. The most significant determinant of pain chronicity appears to be the level of impact on activities of daily living, the functional disability associated with the pain. While the role of psychological factors in the experience of pain is now generally accepted, discussion of psychological inputs to pain is likely to provoke passionate responses and/ or denials from sufferers, who fear invalidation of their very real experiences as 'all in the mind'. Health professionals need to be sensitive to this fear and present psychological issues skilfully, in ways that cannot be interpreted as invalidating the experience of the individual. Eccleston (2001) provided a helpful set of guidelines for the clinical care of patients with pain (Table 19.2).

COGNITION AND EMOTION

Cognition influences emotion to produce pain-related behaviour. An individual's cognitions influence the experience of pain, particularly the appraisal of situations for their significance and meaning (e.g., association of pain and sexual pleasure for masochists). Three aspects of cognition that have received attention in relation to pain are attention, interpretation, with or without dysfunctional thinking, and coping style.

Table 19.2   Using psychological factors in clinical practice

Vigilance to pain	Patients are distracted by the pain and are urged to react. Pain patients will have impaired concentration as they are being interrupted constantly by an aversive stimulus. Keep all communications clear and brief. Repeat key points often. Expect patients to talk about the pain often, as it is being brought repeatedly into attentional focus for them. This is not a sign of a somatization disorder or hypochondria.
Avoidance	Patients will naturally avoid pain and painful procedures. Be aware that this will occur and plan for it. Painful treatments will be avoided and patients will compensate for any disability caused by avoidance (e.g., shifted body weight distribution). If a habitual pattern of avoidance develops, this may lead to chronic pain. Patients must be given an understanding that pain does not necessarily equal damage. A credible medical authority must deliver this message.

(Continued)

Table 19.2   (Continued)

Anger	Patients with pain may shout at you, abuse you and generally be hostile to you. If they are hostile to you, they have probably been hostile to everyone. Most often this will have nothing to do with you, and you will need to understand that anger normally means extreme frustration, distress and possibly depression. Anger functions to push people away and isolate a person. The angry pain patient is therefore less likely to have received or heard any information about their problems and be more confused than the non-angry patient.
Involve the patient	First, assess the patient's normal way of coping with pain by simply asking how he or she has coped with predictable pain, such as a visit to the dentist. Second, match your strategy to the patient's preference. If the patient needs information, inform them how much pain they may expect to feel, what it may feel like and, critically, for how long (if this information is known). Always slightly overestimate the time rather than underestimate it. Finally, if possible, involve the patient in the delivery of any pain management strategy.
Make sense of the pain	Always ask the patient what they know and fear about the cause of the pain, the meaning of the pain and the time course of the pain. Expect the unexpected. What makes sense to one person is nonsense to another. What matters is that it is their understanding, not yours, that will inform their behaviour. Uncertain diagnoses or unknown diagnoses will lead to increased vigilance to pain and increased symptom reporting.
Consistency	Develop a consistent approach to clinical information, patient instruction and patient involvement within pain management. Practice should be consistent over time for each patient and from each member of the pain team.

Source: Eccleston (2001). Reproduced by permission

Increased attention to pain has been associated with increased pain perception. Pain demands or draws attention to itself, reducing the ability to focus on other competing activities, and therefore increasing pain perception. This may explain why distraction techniques are useful in combating pain. However, the role of attention may differ for acute and chronic pain. In acute pain, taking attention away from pain (e.g., via distraction) appears to be associated with reduced anxiety and depression, whereas it has an opposite effect for chronic pain patients, for whom attending to rather than avoiding the pain may be more adaptive.

Dysfunctional thoughts, attitudes and beliefs about pain are automatic patterns of thinking that block the attainment of an individual's goals (e.g., participating in work or social activity). A major form of dysfunctional thinking that influences the pain experience is **catastrophizing** (e.g., 'It's hopeless, pain has ruined my life, I can't cope, it will never get better'). Catastrophic thinking has been found to increase the likelihood of chronicity and the level of perceived intensity and disability, and even to have a small association with pain onset (e.g., Crombez et al., 2003). Other dysfunctional thoughts include negative mental bias, discounting the positive, fortune telling and magnification.

Cognitive coping styles are strategies that an individual uses in an attempt to deal with their pain. They can be divided into active and passive coping. Both can be functional or dysfunctional. Active coping might include keeping oneself busy or taking recreational drugs, which could easily become dysfunctional. Passive coping might include resting, which would be useful in the early stages of pain but could become dysfunctional if continued for too long. In general, active coping styles have been found to be associated with improved coping, reduced pain intensity and improved recovery rates. However, McCracken and Eccleston (2003) suggest that acceptance of pain and its incorporation into one's sense of self appears to be an adaptive cognitive technique for chronic pain. Specific coping techniques are detailed below under pain management.

LEARNING: PREVIOUS EXPERIENCE AND CONDITIONING

Previous experience of pain is a significant factor in current pain experience. Both **classical** and **operant conditioning** have been implicated in the aetiology of chronic pain via the association of behaviour and pain. In classical conditioning theory, a particular situation or environment may become associated with pain (e.g., the dentist) and therefore provoke increased anxiety and pain perception. Jamner and Tursky (1987) reported that even the words used by migraine sufferers to describe their pain appear to reinforce the experience by provoking stronger physiological responses than non-pain words. In operant conditioning theory, pain stimuli are perceived as sensations and unpleasant effects that generally evoke responses like grimacing or limping, demonstrating that the person is in pain. Pain behaviours become conditioned responses through positive (e.g., attention, medication, time off work) and negative (e.g., disapproval of others, loss of earnings) reinforcements. Pain behaviours may be functional and appropriate (e.g., removing a hand from a burning source of heat), or they may be less functional and therefore pain maintaining (e.g., avoidance, alcohol).

SECONDARY GAINS

The role of secondary gains in the development and maintenance of pain and illness behaviours has been described. Secondary gain relates to social rewards accruing from the demonstration of pain behaviours (e.g., receiving attention, financial benefits, time off work). These secondary gains are thought to reinforce pain behaviours and thus maintain the condition. For example, receipt of financial disability compensations has been associated with slower return to work and increased pain. However, this may actually reflect that those in receipt of compensation can allow themselves appropriate time to recover and says nothing about the quality of life of those who returned to work earlier. For many individuals, pain results in the loss of jobs, social contact, leisure activities, valued identities, reduced incomes and concomitant reduced standard of living. Such losses are very real and distressing and are often associated with substantial hardships, lowered mood and loss of self-esteem, which are unlikely to be outweighed by incidental benefits.

MOOD

The most common moods that have been associated with pain are anxiety and depression. Where these moods are present, pain appears to be increased. It has been reported that acute pain increases anxiety but once pain is decreased through treatment the anxiety also decreases, which can cause further decreases in the pain – a cycle of pain reduction. Alternatively, chronic pain remains unalleviated by treatment and therefore anxiety increases, which can further increase the pain, creating a cycle of pain increase. Research has shown that anxiety increases pain perception in children with migraine and people with back pain and pelvic pain (McGowan et al., 1998).

Anxiety is normally a result of fear. Pain-related fear can be specific or general (e.g., 'The pain is going to get worse' or 'What will the future be like?'). The fear-avoidance model of pain suggests that fear of pain amplifies perception and leads to pain avoidance behaviours in some people, especially those with a propensity to catastrophic thinking (Vlaeyen and Linton, 2000). This cycle results in pain experience and behaviours becoming separated from pain sensation through exaggerated pain perception. A prospective study by Klenerman et al. (1995) found fear-avoidance variables correctly predicted future outcome in 66% of patients. A more recent prospective study (Linton et al., 2000) also found that higher baseline scores for fear-avoidance in a non-pain population were associated with double the likelihood of reporting back pain in the following year and a significantly increased risk of reduced physical functioning.

While correlations between mood states and pain have been found, the causal direction and the nature of the relationships remain unclear. Most recent work appears to indicate that negative mood states are an outcome of chronic pain rather than a cause.

FEAR-AVOIDANCE MODEL

The fear-avoidance model (FAM) explains how individuals develop chronic musculo-skeletal pain as a result of avoidance of activities based on their fear of pain (Lethem et al., 1983). This model helps to explain how individuals experience pain *despite the absence of pathology*. If an individual experiences acute pain and manages the situation by using avoidant behaviour, a lack of pain increase reinforces this behaviour. However, this avoidant behaviour causes the individual to decrease exercise, which may in turn lead to increased disability (Figure 19.4).

Vlaeyen and Linton (2000) explained how and why some individuals with musculo-skeletal pain develop a chronic pain syndrome using the FAM of exaggerated pain perceptions. 'Confrontation' and 'avoidance' are postulated as the two extreme responses to the fear of pain. While the former leads to the reduction of fear over time, avoidance leads to the maintenance or even exacerbation of fear. Possible precursors of pain-related fear include negative appraisal of internal and external stimuli, negative affectivity and anxiety sensitivity. Subsequently, a number of fear-related processes ensue, including escape and avoidance behaviours resulting in poor behavioural performance, hypervigilance to internal and external illness information, muscular reactivity, and physical disuse in terms of deconditioning and guarded movement. Vlaeyen and Linton (2000: 317) concluded that 'Pain-related fear and avoidance appear to be an essential feature of the development of a chronic problem for a substantial number of patients with musculo-skeletal pain'. A substantial body of evidence to date supports the FAM of chronic pain. Waddell et al. (1993) developed the 'Fear-Avoidance Beliefs Questionnaire' (FABQ) to investigate the role of fear-avoidance beliefs in chronic LBP and disability.

Wertli et al. (2014) carried out a systematic review of RCTs that suggested that fear-avoidance beliefs are associated with poor treatment outcome in patients with LBP of less than six months. Patients with strong fear-avoidance beliefs are more likely to improve when fear-avoidance beliefs are addressed in treatments than when these beliefs are ignored, and treatment strategies should be modified if fear-avoidance beliefs are present. The findings of Wertli et al. (2014) support the FAM in suggesting that early treatment, including interventions to reduce fear-avoidance beliefs, may avoid delayed recovery and chronicity.

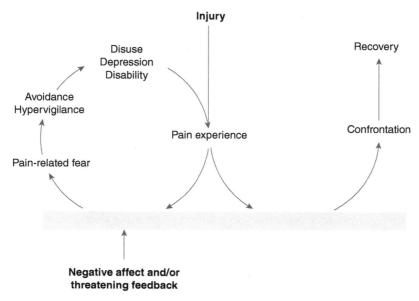

Figure 19.4   The fear-avoidance model

If pain, from an injury or other cause, is interpreted as threatening (pain catastrophizing), fear evolves – which leads to avoidance behaviours and hypervigilance to bodily sensations. This may lead to disability, disuse and depression. The latter will maintain the pain experience, fuelling a vicious circle of increasing fear and avoidance. In non-catastrophizing patients, no pain-related fear and rapid confrontation with daily activities is likely to occur, leading to fast recovery. Pain catastrophizing is assumed also to be influenced by negative affectivity and threatening illness information

Source: Vlaeyen and Linton (2000)

BOX 19.2

CLINICAL CASE STUDY: Chronic pain response and reduced quality of life following an accidental injury

A woman, Miss D, aged 75, was a spectator at a yacht race where she was struck at close quarters with a piece of fast-moving shrapnel from a starting cannon. Fortunately, the physical injury itself was slight, leaving a small red mark in close proximity to a scar from a cancer operation on her right breast. However, the trauma would bring profound changes to Miss D's quality of life.

A health psychologist at a multidisciplinary pain clinic diagnosed Miss D as suffering from **chronic pain** syndrome as a direct consequence of the accident. This syndrome was

(Continued)

triggered initially by an intense fear that she would suffer a recurrence of breast cancer. While this fear may seem irrational, for Miss D it was a very palpable consequence of being struck with some force.

The mechanism for the development of the chronic pain syndrome can be explained by the FAM. Since the accident, Miss D progressively decreased her activity levels to avoid the pain that was mysteriously appearing in different parts of her body. This complex of unexplained pain led to a vicious circle of pain–fear–avoidance of activity–more pain.

Miss D gave up many of her normal daily physical activities, which included walking, cycling, yoga and dancing. Starting with the trauma, triggering her fear of cancer recurrence, her consequent avoidance of activity to prevent pain, hyper-vigilance to internal and external illness information, sleeplessness, disuse of her body, depression and finally progressive disability. The quality of life for Miss D had been significantly lowered by the incident and her suffering seemed likely to continue until a suitable treatment could be identified. Cognitive behavioural therapy and graded exercise were offered and these led to a partial recovery. However, following legal compensation and treatment, Miss D believes that she will never make a full recovery from what was an unlucky 'wrong place at the wrong time' chance event.

Social interaction has a critical influence on experience and expression of pain, particularly during early development. Children's and adolescents' cognitions and beliefs about pain, including fear-avoidance beliefs, develop within the family context. Asmundson et al. (2011) amended the FAM for paediatric populations. The paediatric model recognizes distinct fear/escape and anxiety/avoidance pathways and increases the possible influences of predispositional and current psychological factors. The paediatric FAM emphasizes the two-way relationship between parental pain management behaviour (e.g., protectiveness, solicitousness), parent psychological responses (e.g., parent catastrophizing, anxiety sensitivity, general distress) and child/adolescent psychological responses (e.g., catastrophizing, acceptance, anxiety sensitivity) in influencing child/adolescent escape and avoidance behaviours. In this paediatric model, both child/adolescent and parent psychological responses encompass the individual's overt expression of pain and/or fear. The child/adolescent escape and avoidance behaviours can directly impact parent psychological responses and, indirectly, through parent psychological responses, impact parent pain management behaviours. Furthermore, the model includes the likely effect that parent pain management behaviours (e.g., removing children and adolescents from pain-inducing activities) would have on child/adolescent escape and avoidance behaviours.

Crombez et al. (2012) argue that the FAM needs to be extended by adopting a motivational perspective on chronic pain and disability. They propose that the next generation of the FAM needs to adopt an explicit motivational perspective built around goals and self-regulatory processes. This might yield a better understanding of how the disruptiveness of pain to an individual's life goals can be overcome by successful problem solving, moving away from efforts to remove pain to fostering acceptance and palliation.

INTERVENTIONS

Before the complex and multi-dimensional nature of pain had been accepted, pain was treated through the administration of analgesic drugs, surgery and rest. Today pain management programmes seek to address the pain experience utilizing psychological and physical interventions, with considerable emphasis on psychology and weaning patients off opiates. The historical aim of pain management was to eliminate pain. More recently, the aims have shifted towards acceptance of pain, reducing pain perception, improving coping ability, increasing functional ability, and decreasing drug reliance and distress. Many commonly used pain management strategies are listed in Table 19.3.

Table 19.3   Common pain management strategies

Behavioural	Cognitive	Pharmacological	Physical	Other
Operant conditioning	Cognitive restructuring	Non-opioid analgesics	Surgical	Hypnosis
Contingency management	Cognitive coping skills training, e.g., distraction	Paracetamol, NSAIDs, e.g., ibuprofen, aspirin	Transcutaneous electrical nerve stimulation (TENS)	Other alternative therapies, e.g., Reiki, Chinese medicine, music therapy
Graded exercise	Acceptance	Opioid analgesics: morphine and derivatives, e.g., codeine	Acupuncture, physiotherapy, heat and cold	Support groups
Biofeedback	Imagery	Local anaesthetics	Vibration, massage, aromatherapy	Internet advice
Autogenic training	Meditation and prayer	Indirect action drugs, e.g., sedatives, antidepressants, tranquillizers	Spinal cord stimulation	Self-help books
Relaxation	Information	Placebos	Reflexology	Spiritual, including prayer
Progressive muscle relaxation	Stress management	Self-medications, e.g., cannabis, alcohol, heroin	Mobility-enhancing exercise	
Acceptance and Commitment Therapy	Increase engagement in activities that bring meaning, vitality and value			

Whether prescribed by health professionals or independently adopted by the individual, any pain management strategy has the potential to improve the situation (e.g., numbing pain sensations with drugs or improving mood with aromatherapy). Equally, any strategy can worsen the situation, as with medication side effects or lowered mood induced by substance abuse. It is important that an individual's own attempts at self-management are respected and that health professionals work in partnership with the individual to identify the optimum programme for that person.

Behavioural strategies

Most behavioural strategies are based upon operant learning processes, like using operant conditioning in which pain behaviours are ignored (negative reinforcement) and improved activity is praised (positive reinforcement). Conditioning is integral to contingency management. Typically, this is a two- to six-week inpatient programme, during which nursing staff would ignore medication requests, reinforce targeted 'well' behaviours, introduce increasing exercise quotas and employ a fixed-schedule 'pain cocktail'. The pain cocktail delivers medication within a strong-tasting masking fluid that allows medication dosages to be reduced without the patient noticing. While such programmes have had good (even dramatic) short-term results, they have been less successful in maintaining such gains, possibly due to non-generalization outside the hospital environment. It is rare for programmes today to focus solely on conditioning methods.

Graded exercise strategies involve setting a starting level of activity that the person can manage and then developing a schedule to gradually increase the length of time and intensity of the exercise. The schedule allows the person to gain the confidence to handle each new level before the next increment.

Cognitive strategies, cognitive behavioural therapy and mindfulness

Cognitive strategies work on the principle that cognitions (thoughts and beliefs) are responsible for the consequences of events, not the event itself, and if these cognitions can be changed, the consequence(s) will also change. In relation to pain management, cognitive strategies aim to help the individual identify and understand their cognitions and their connection with their experience of pain and then change negative cognitions to improve it. This includes teaching individuals to identify and challenge distorted thinking (e.g., catastrophizing) – a process known as cognitive restructuring, an active coping technique that promotes the internal attribution of positive changes.

While coping strategies can be helpful, there is growing evidence that pain control efforts directed at uncontrollable pain can come to dominate an individual's life and distance them from important and valued aspects of their lives, such as family, friends and work.

Cognitive behavioural therapy (CBT) utilizes the full range of cognitive and behavioural techniques already described in individualized programmes that emphasize relapse prevention strategies. The literature on CBT and pain suggests considerable promise as an effective treatment for pain in adults (Eccleston et al., 2002). It forms the major component of most current pain management programmes. Improved mood, affect, function and coping have been associated with CBT in up to 85% of pain patients. While there is some support for the efficacy of CBT for the control of headache pain in children, there is a paucity of research relating to other pain conditions in children, as well as CBT for pain in the elderly and people with intellectual or communication difficulties, probably as it may be assumed not to be an appropriate treatment option for these groups. Acceptance and Commitment Therapy (ACT) and mindfulness-based approaches, which can be seen as sub-types of CBT, may hold more potential for future progress (McCracken and Vowles, 2014).

Another approach is based on **mindfulness** meditation. The concept follows the Buddhist tradition of living in the present. Mindfulness is the practice of 'observing' physical symptoms, emotions or thoughts. The goal is to change how pain is experienced and the influences it exerts on behaviour. Brown and Ryan (2003) developed a Mindful Attention Awareness Scale (MAAS) containing items such as: 'I find it difficult to stay focused on what is happening in the present', 'I rush through activities without being really attentive to them', 'I find myself preoccupied with the future or the past.' In a study of chronic pain, McCracken et al. (2007) found that mindfulness was associated with measures of depression, pain-related anxiety, as well as physical, psychosocial and 'other' disability. In each instance greater mindfulness was associated with better functioning. However, the results from systematic reviews are mixed. For example, Rajguru et al. (2014) found that mindfulness meditation has minimal effects on chronic pain. Hilton et al. (2016) reviewed 38 randomized controlled trials and found low-quality evidence that a small decrease in pain is associated with mindfulness meditation compared with controls. Small but statistically significant effects were also found for depression symptoms and quality of life.

Imagery

Imagery involves forming and maintaining a pleasant, calming or coping image in the mind. In guided imagery attention is guided away from an undesirable sensation or mood (e.g., pain) by another person, who verbally describes the image while the patient relaxes. Most imagery involves relaxation and employs images of a peaceful, safe, pain-free place, which the individual focuses upon while relaxing. The person may also be guided to visualize energy flowing into their body and pain flowing out. The benefits derived from this type of imagery are probably due to relaxation and distraction effects. Alternatively, confrontational imagery may be employed, for example visualizing white blood cells as an army attacking the source of pain (e.g., a tumour). Imagery has been found to be effective for the treatment of pain. The benefits of imagery may relate to relaxation, distraction effects and an active stance, increasing feelings of self-efficacy. As imagery generally involves elements of relaxation, it is unclear what unique and independent effects it has. Syrjala et al. (1995) compared relaxation and imagery with cognitive behavioural training to reduce pain during cancer treatment in a controlled clinical trial. Results confirmed that patients who received either relaxation and imagery alone or patients who received the package of cognitive behavioural coping skills reported less pain than control patients. Adding cognitive behavioural skills to the relaxation with imagery did not further improve pain relief.

Meditation also frequently forms part of relaxation training and involves the individuals focusing their attention on a simple stimulus, such as a meaningless monosyllable or disyllabic sound repeated slowly and continuously (aloud or in their head) to the exclusion of all other stimuli. Prayer is another common coping strategy that patients have reported to be helpful in response to pain, including headaches, neck pain and back pain (McCaffery et al., 2004). Both meditation and prayer inherently involve some distraction and possibly aspects of relaxation, although this is far from consistent.

Information provision has been shown to reduce pain reports and intensity, possibly by alleviating the fear and anxiety of not knowing what to expect for acute and postoperative pain (Williams et al., 2004). The widespread interest in self-help literature, internet information and support groups may be indicative of the desire of people in pain to understand their experience, what to expect and potential treatment options.

Pharmacological strategies

Various analgesics and anaesthetics are prescribed for the treatment of pain. Anaesthetics (local or central) are used to numb the sensation of pain. The identification of endogenous opioid mechanisms has confirmed the status of opioid analgesics as an effective pain treatment.

However, the associated perceived high risk of addiction has resulted in their use being restricted to severe pain cases, such as cancer, a perception challenged by the findings from studies of patient-controlled analgesia and low-dose opioid treatment that suggest the risk of addiction may not be very high (e.g., Urban et al., 1986). Non-opioid analgesics, NSAIDs (non-steroidal anti-inflammatory drugs) and drugs that control pain indirectly (e.g., antidepressants, sedatives) are commonly used. Drugs with indirect effects may be beneficial due to their action on higher brain regions, modulating the downward transmission of pain, or due to their modulating effects on negative mood states.

Another aspect relating to drugs is the placebo effect. It has been shown that substantial pain relief occurs in about 50% of patients when they are treated with an inert compound rather than the drug they are expecting, often equalling the relief felt by those receiving the actual medication (Melzack and Wall, 1982/1988). The effect is strongest with high doses, when it is injected, and depends upon the individual believing they are receiving a pain-relieving substance. Unsurprisingly, the effect rapidly declines with repeated use: you cannot fool all of the people all of the time!

In addition to prescribed drug treatments, many individuals self-medicate with recreational drugs like alcohol and cannabis to alleviate their pain. However, there is considerable anecdotal evidence for cannabis as an effective pain control treatment, and an endogenous cannabinoid pain control system has now been identified. This system functions as a parallel but distinct mechanism from the opioid system in modulating pain (Notcutt, 2004). Cannabinoids have been authorized for the treatment of pain and other conditions in a number of countries and states, including the Netherlands, many states in the USA, and the UK. While current research may result in new cannabinoid-based NSAID-like treatments in the future, problems with the restricted range of dosages that allow pain control before producing psychotropic effects, and concerns about the incidental condoning of recreational cannabis use, mean this is far from being certain. The informal use of cannabis for pain control and its interaction with other pain control strategies warrants further investigation (Eisenberg et al., 2014).

Physical strategies

Surgical control of pain mainly involved cutting the pain fibres to stop pain signal transmission. However, it provided only short-term results and the risks associated with surgery mean it is no longer viewed as a viable treatment option (Melzack and Wall, 1982/1988).

Physiotherapy may be used to increase mobility and correct maladjusted posture, encourage exercise and movement (often despite pain), and education. In addition, individuals may be taught safe ways to function (e.g., stand up, sit down, lift objects). Physiotherapy is about maintaining mobility, increasing function and helping the individual manage their life (e.g., Eccleston and Eccleston, 2004).

An additional strategy is the promotion of mobility-enhancing exercise to help retain and improve physical function and prevent lack of mobility from exacerbating pain problems. General practitioners can refer pain patients to specialist rehabilitation classes at local fitness centres, which has shown some success for older people with musculo-skeletal disorders (Avlund et al., 2000).

Interdisciplinary pain rehabilitation programme

Originally run as inpatient programmes, pain management programmes tend to be run in specialist pain management or rehabilitation centres. Interdisciplinary teams may include doctors, nurses, physiotherapists, psychologists, psychiatrists, occupational therapists and counsellors, and provide a range of management techniques usually underpinned by CBT. An interdisciplinary chronic pain rehabilitation programme (IPRP) is a partial-hospitalization programme in which patients with chronic non-cancer pain who are resistant to opiate management, steroid injections and surgery receive a tailored combination of interventions. Programmes aim to improve quality of life by reducing pain as far as possible, increasing activity and coping, restoring function, and promoting self-efficacy and self-management. The patient receives a full history-taking assessment, education, skills training, exercise schedules, relapse prevention and family work. Multidisciplinary rehabilitation programmes represent the most comprehensive approach to date, by targeting the individual's specific pain experience and tailoring appropriate treatment combinations.

Pain treatment facilities are both scarce and in high demand according to a review by Fashler et al. (2016). Access varies by country, with 1 per 310,000 people in Australia, 1 per 258,000 people in Canada, and 1 per 200,000–370,370 people in the UK. With an estimated 37% of the world population suffering from chronic pain, this indicates poor availability of services for pain sufferers. The high demand for multidisciplinary pain treatment facilities is reflected in the wait times, which have a median of 100–150 days in several countries (Fashler et al., 2016)

Bosy et al. (2010) described a private, intensive eight-week IPRP with a CBT emphasis and the results obtained with a cohort of 338 consecutive patients who completed the programme over a three-year period. Improvements in vocational status occurred in 75% of patients with chronic pain; pain levels were reduced by 16%; levels of anxiety and depression were reduced by 13% and 17%, respectively; and 61% of patients were able to reduce or eliminate their pain medications.

Vowles et al. (2014) studied Acceptance and Commitment Therapy in 117 completers of an interdisciplinary programme. A significant change in at least one measure of functioning (depression, pain anxiety and disability) was achieved by 46.2% of patients. Changes in psychological flexibility were found to mediate changes in disability, depression, pain-related anxiety, number of medical visits and the number of classes of prescribed analgesics.

Such programmes are economically unaffordable on a mass scale. A health economist noted that 'there is still a long way to go to understand the economic implications of interdisciplinary rehabilitation from the perspectives of society, the health insurers, and the patients' (Becker, 2012: 127). Demand far outstrips supply.

Treatment issues

Pain management can be a particularly controversial issue. Evidence suggests that in many circumstances pain is under-treated. Some of the reasons for this include inadequate services, lack of assessment, focus on underlying pathologies, negative stereotypes and erroneous assumptions about certain population groups, addiction fears, the inappropriateness of non-pharmacological treatments and patients' inability to verbalize pain information or requests for medication (e.g., Greenwald et al., 1999). Many medical professionals have their own benchmarks concerning acceptable pain behaviour and medication levels for different conditions. It has also been shown that many prejudices and misconceptions operate in the treatment of pain patients, with various populations (e.g., children, people with communication difficulties and the elderly) being under-treated for pain (Todd et al., 2000). For example, sickle-cell patients are often assumed to be drug addicts and their pain outcries to be drug-seeking behaviour, resulting in inadequate medication being administered. Similarly, pain has only recently been recognized as part of the symptom repertoire of people with HIV infection or AIDS, and therefore up to 85% of people with HIV infection or AIDS receive inadequate pain management (Marcus et al., 2000).

Pain is sometimes deemed to be psychogenic, resulting from emotional, motivational or personality problems. The distinction between 'organic' and 'psychogenic' pain has little practical value and can be highly stigmatizing and alienate patients. A number of diseases where pain was not thought historically to be a valid symptom have subsequently had a physiological basis for pain identified, including multiple sclerosis and HIV/AIDS (e.g., Marcus et al., 2000). Pain designated as 'psychogenic' may relate to as-yet-undetected or unidentified organic pathology. Health psychologists must endeavour to promote the sensitive and respectful treatment of individuals reporting pain in terms of research, intervention development and treatment.

FUTURE RESEARCH

1. A testable theory of the neural coding of pain needs to be developed.

2. Long-term, prospective studies are required to understand the relationships between psychosocial factors and pain, particularly in diverse sub-groups within the chronic pain population.

3. Additional research is needed regarding the pain experience of under-represented groups, especially those who are verbally challenged (e.g., babies, older people, people with disabilities, people with a diagnosis of dementia), including the development of improved measurement instruments and assessing the efficacy of CBT in these groups.

4. The FAM requires refinement and extension to provide a better understanding of unexplained sources of pain.

SUMMARY

1. Pain is a complex and multi-dimensional phenomenon that includes biological, psychological and social components.
2. Early pain theories proposed that pain was a sensation that involved a direct line of transmission from the pain stimulus to the brain. This theory is unsupported by evidence of psychological elements to pain.
3. The growing evidence on the psychological mediation of pain has seen the development of the gate control theory. However, the absence of any direct evidence of a 'gate' in the spinal cord is a problem. Also, gate control theory is unable to explain several chronic pain problems, such as phantom limb pain.
4. Many psychological variables that influence the pain experience have been examined, including cognitions, prior experience, conditioning, secondary gains, personality and mood.
5. Particular groups appear to be under-represented in the pain literature, including ethnic minorities, children, the elderly, some disabled people and people with certain medical conditions (e.g., dementia, HIV and chronic fatigue syndrome (CFS)).

6. Assessment of pain is difficult and various techniques are used singly or in combination, such as medical examinations, observations, questionnaires, diaries and logs, and interviews.

7. A wide variety of pain management strategies exist. Currently, the most successful approach appears to be tailored programmes that use cognitive behavioural therapies fostering acceptance and the reduction of fear. There is no panacea, including medications.

8. Demand for services far outstrips supply. More resources need to be put into health care provisions internationally for patients suffering from unexplained pain.

9. Health psychologists can make a genuine, significant contribution in promoting sensitive and respectful research and treatment for people experiencing long-standing painful conditions.

CANCER

20

'I asked the doctor – I looked him straight in the face and I asked "Is it cancer?" and he said, "Yes." Well, I'd rather know the truth – it's better than imagining all the time. I asked my own doctor in the first place, "Was it ... ?" and I didn't get to say the word, and he said "We don't know," so naturally I thought it must be. If I'm ill I'd rather know what I'm suffering from, because you don't die any sooner for knowing about it.'

Aitken-Swan and Easson (1959: 779)

OUTLINE

In this chapter, we consider the nature of cancer, risk factors, living with cancer, caring for someone with cancer, and the design and testing of a psychological intervention. Cancer refers to a collection of 100–200 dread diseases caused by the uncontrolled division of cells. There are multiple risk factors, including genetic, environmental and behavioural toxins. The disease can have profound physical, psychosocial and existential impacts. The evidence suggests that psychosocial interventions have not yet demonstrated their full potential. The quality of evaluation research with psychosocial interventions has generally been rather poor and the findings inconclusive. We analyse a case study of a randomized controlled trial with an intervention designed to alleviate stress in breast and colon cancer patients. This RCT illustrates methodological issues with small samples and a lack of appropriate controls, problems that are impeding progress in the field of interventions.

WHAT IS CANCER?

Cancer is the name given to a collection of related diseases.[1] In all types of cancer, some of the body's cells begin to divide without stopping and spread into surrounding tissues. Cancer can start almost anywhere in the human body, which is made up of trillions of cells. Normally, human cells grow and divide to form new cells as the body needs them. When cells grow old or become damaged, they die, and new cells take their place. There are more than 100 types of cancer. Types of cancer are usually named for the organs or tissues where the cancers form. For example, lung cancer starts in cells of the lung and brain cancer starts in cells of the brain. Cancers also may be described by the type of cell that formed them, such as an epithelial cell or a squamous cell.

Carcinoma

Carcinomas are the most common type of cancer. They are formed by epithelial cells, which are the cells that cover the inside and outside surfaces of the body. There are many types of epithelial cells, which often have a column-like shape when viewed under a microscope.

Carcinomas that begin in different epithelial cell types have specific names:

Adenocarcinoma is a cancer that forms in epithelial cells that produce fluids or mucus. Tissues with this type of epithelial cell are sometimes called glandular tissues. Most cancers of the breast, colon and prostate are adenocarcinomas.

Basal cell carcinoma is a cancer that begins in the lower or basal (base) layer of the epidermis, which is a person's outer layer of skin.

Squamous cell carcinoma is a cancer that forms in squamous cells, which are epithelial cells that lie just beneath the outer surface of the skin. Squamous cells also line many other organs, including the stomach, intestines, lungs, bladder and kidneys. Squamous cells look flat, like fish scales, when viewed under a microscope. Squamous cell carcinomas are sometimes called epidermoid carcinomas.

Transitional cell carcinoma is a cancer that forms in a type of epithelial tissue called transitional epithelium, or urothelium. This tissue, which is made up of many layers of epithelial cells that can get bigger and smaller, is found in the linings of the bladder, ureters and part of the kidneys (renal pelvis), and a few other organs. Some cancers of the bladder, ureters and kidneys are transitional cell carcinomas.

Sarcoma

Sarcomas are cancers that form in bone and soft tissues, including muscle, fat, blood vessels, lymph vessels and fibrous tissue (such as tendons and ligaments).

Osteosarcoma is the most common cancer of bone. The most common types of soft tissue sarcoma are leiomyosarcoma, Kaposi sarcoma, malignant fibrous histiocytoma, liposarcoma and dermatofibrosarcoma protuberans.

---

[1]This chapter covers a vast subject with 100–200 types of cancer. At the time of writing, Google Scholar listed 4.77 million publications on 'cancer', while 'psychosocial issues of cancer' yielded 603,000 results (accessed on 19 February 2017). The section on 'What is cancer?' is courtesy of the National Institute of Health National Cancer Institute: https://www.cancer.gov [Public domain].

Leukemia

Cancers that begin in the blood-forming tissue of the bone marrow are called leukemias. These cancers do not form solid tumours. Instead, large numbers of abnormal white blood cells (leukemia cells and leukemic blast cells) build up in the blood and bone marrow, crowding out normal blood cells. The low level of normal blood cells can make it harder for the body to get oxygen to its tissues, control bleeding or fight infections.

There are four common types of leukemia, which are grouped according to how quickly the disease gets worse (acute or chronic) and on the type of blood cell the cancer starts in (lymphoblastic or myeloid).

Lymphoma

Lymphoma is cancer that begins in lymphocytes (T cells or B cells). These are disease-fighting white blood cells that are part of the immune system. In lymphoma, abnormal lymphocytes build up in lymph nodes and lymph vessels, as well as in other organs of the body.

There are two main types of lymphoma:

Hodgkin lymphoma – People with this disease have abnormal lymphocytes that are called Reed-Sternberg cells. These cells usually form from B cells.

Non-Hodgkin lymphoma – This is a large group of cancers that start in lymphocytes. The cancers can grow quickly or slowly and can form from B cells or T cells.

Multiple myeloma

Multiple myeloma is cancer that begins in plasma cells, another type of immune cell. The abnormal plasma cells, called myeloma cells, build up in the bone marrow and form tumours in bones all through the body. Multiple myeloma is also called plasma cell myeloma and Kahler disease.

Melanoma

Melanoma is cancer that begins in cells that become melanocytes, which are specialized cells that make melanin (the pigment that gives skin its colour). Most melanomas form on the skin, but melanomas can also form in other pigmented tissues, such as the eye.

Brain and spinal cord tumours

There are different types of brain and spinal cord tumour. These tumours are named according to the type of cell in which they formed and where the tumour first formed in the central nervous system. For example, an astrocytic tumour begins in star-shaped brain cells called astrocytes, which help keep nerve cells healthy. Brain tumours can be benign (not cancerous) or malignant (cancerous).

Germ cell tumours

Germ cell tumours are a type of tumour that begins in the cells that give rise to sperm or eggs. These tumours can occur almost anywhere in the body and can be either benign or malignant.

Neuroendocrine tumours

Neuroendocrine tumours form from cells that release hormones into the blood in response to a signal from the nervous system. These tumours, which may make higher-than-normal amounts of hormones, can cause many different symptoms.

Carcinoid tumours

Carcinoid tumours are a type of neuroendocrine tumour. They are slow-growing tumours that are usually found in the gastrointestinal system (most often in the rectum and small intestine).

RISK FACTORS FOR CANCER

The following are risk factors for cancer:

- growing older;
- tobacco use;
- sunlight, sunlamps and tanning machines, i.e., ultraviolet (UV) radiation;
- ionizing radiation, e.g., radioactive fallout, radon gas, X-rays;
- certain chemicals and other substances, e.g., asbestos, benzene, benzidine, cadmium, nickel or vinyl chloride;
- some bacteria (e.g., *helicobacter pylori*);
- some viruses (e.g., hepatitis B virus, human papillomavirus, human immunodeficiency virus, *helicobacter pylori*, and others);
- certain hormones;
- family history of cancer;
- alcohol;
- poor diet, lack of physical activity, or being overweight.

The study of the psychosocial aspects of cancer care and treatment is referred to as '**psycho-oncology**'. Psycho-oncology is concerned with (1) the psychological responses of patients, families and caregivers to cancer at all stages of the disease, and (2) the psychosocial factors that may influence the disease process. A key concept is **quality of life (QoL)**.

Table 20.1   Incidence of new cases and estimated cancer deaths in the US in 2016

	Common types of cancer	Estimated new cases 2016	Estimated deaths 2016
1.	Breast cancer (female)	246,660	40,450
2.	Lung and bronchus cancer	224,390	158,080
3.	Prostate cancer	180,890	26,120
4.	Colon and rectum cancer	134,490	49,190
5.	Bladder cancer	76,960	16,390
6.	Melanoma of the skin	76,380	10,130
7.	Non-Hodgkin lymphoma	72,580	20,150
8.	Thyroid cancer	64,300	1,980
9.	Kidney and renal pelvis cancer	62,700	14,240
10.	Leukemia	60,140	24,400
	–	–	–
	Cancer of any site	**1,685,210**	**595,690**

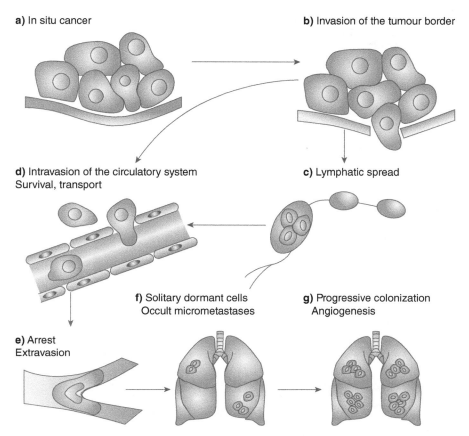

a) In situ cancer

b) Invasion of the tumour border

d) Intravasion of the circulatory system
Survival, transport

c) Lymphatic spread

f) Solitary dormant cells
Occult micrometastases

g) Progressive colonization
Angiogenesis

e) Arrest
Extravasion

Figure 20.1   A schematic of cancer and the metastatic process

Metastasis is a complex, multistep process. (a) An in situ cancer surrounded by an intact basement membrane. (b) Invasion requires reversible changes in cell–cell and cell–extracellular-matrix adherence. Metastasizing cells can (c) enter via the lymphatics, or (d) directly enter the circulation. (e) Survival and arrest of tumour cells, and extravasion of the circulatory system. (f) Metastatic colonization of the distant site progresses through single cells and (g) progressively growing angiogenic metastases

Source: Steeg (2003). Reproduced with permission

Unfortunately, many cancer patients remain untreated owing to stigmatization and lack of resources to diagnose, treat and support. Cancer causes anxiety and depression in more than one-third of patients and often affects the sufferer's family emotionally, socially and economically. Inequalities in cancer treatment and care occur across different regions and social groups. In spite of increased publicity and reduced incidence of breast cancer, breast self-examination has not been proven to prevent cancer (Gøtzsche, 2013).

There are several aspects of the cancer experience that psychological expertise can help to understand, especially pain, fatigue, depression and anxiety. Treatments with chemotherapy (CT) and radiotherapy (RT) tend to be aggressive, and a decline of psychosocial function before, during and after treatment is quite common.

The research literature is limited by methodological issues: most studies are cross-sectional, meaning that problems reported may not be caused by cancer and its treatment; many studies

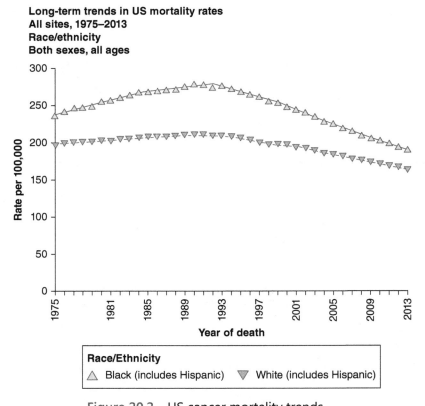

Figure 20.2 US cancer mortality trends

Source: US Mortality Files, National Centre for Health Statistics, CDC

involve women only; most studies are conducted in the USA or Canada; and the majority of studies include mainly white people, with few participants from ethnic minority groups.

We turn to some of the main issues that arise in living with cancer: diagnosis, treatment and survivorship. End-of-life care is reviewed in Chapter 24.

LIVING WITH CANCER

Diagnosis

The diagnosis of cancer is a significant and emotionally charged event in anybody's life. The 'C-word' on the lips of a doctor is the thing that most patients absolutely dread. Every two minutes someone in the UK is diagnosed with cancer. About half of people born after 1960 will develop some form of cancer during their lifetime (NHS Choices, 2017). Two million people are living with or beyond cancer in the UK (Macmillan Cancer Support, 2015). Higher incidence, an ageing population and improved survival rates mean that this figure will double to 4 million over the next 20 years. In the USA, the number of people living with a history of cancer was estimated to be 13.7 million in 2012 which will rise to 18 million by 2022.

A cancer diagnosis affects everyone differently, but it is common to experience shock, sadness, fear about the future, anger, guilt, denial, confusion, stress, anxiety and depression, or many of these rolled into one. Cancer diagnosis has been recognized as a stressor that can potentially precipitate post-traumatic stress disorder (PTSD; Kangas et al., 2002).

Early diagnosis gives people the best possible chance of survival. However, cancer is still a relatively unusual condition for an individual GP to encounter. An Electronic Cancer Decision Support tool is being used by GPs across England and currently is focused on five cancer types, including lung cancer. Diagnosis by computer may also become more possible in the future. For example, skin cancers can already be detected using image analysis alone and machines can already identify certain cancers as successfully as skin-cancer doctors (Leachman and Merlino, 2017).

Treatment

The main treatments are surgery, chemotherapy, radiation therapy, immunotherapy or targeted therapy. Most people have a combination of treatments, such as surgery with chemotherapy and/or radiation therapy. Some patients also choose complementary therapies to support the physical therapies obtained in hospital. The treatments all bring significant uncertainties, side effects and stress.

Surgery

If the cancer is completely contained in a specific area and has not spread, surgery treats the part of the body where the tumour is located. Usually, the earlier a cancer is found the easier it is to remove it. The surgeon removes the tumour and some normal tissue from around the cancer (a 'clear margin') and may also remove the **lymph nodes** nearest to the cancer, in case they contain cancer cells.

The surgeon sends the tissue that they remove to a laboratory for examination under a microscope. The findings help the surgeon to decide whether any further treatment is required to reduce the risk of the cancer coming back. Some people have treatment before surgery to help shrink a cancer and make it easier to remove, which is called **neoadjuvant treatment**.

During an operation, surgeons may find that a cancer has spread further than expected, in which case the operation might take longer than planned or may have to be terminated. If cancer has spread to another part of the body, surgery cannot usually cure it. With some types of cancer, surgery can help people to live for a long time and may sometimes lead to a cure. When a cancer has spread, a treatment that works throughout the body, such as chemotherapy, biological therapy or hormone therapy, is likely to lead to a better outcome. Radiotherapy can control symptoms caused by areas of cancer elsewhere in the body.

Radiotherapy

Radiotherapy (RT) is used in a variety of ways depending on the specific features of the case. Curative or radical radiotherapy treatment aims to cure a patient of their cancer by destroying a cancerous tumour. The length of the course of treatment depends on the size and type of the cancer and its location. Curative radiotherapy may be combined with other treatments, such as surgery, chemotherapy, hormonal therapy or biological therapy. Radiotherapy can also be used to relieve symptoms, for example to reduce pain, a form of **palliative treatment**.

Radiotherapy is sometimes given before or after surgery. Preoperative radiotherapy is given to shrink a tumour and make it safer and easier to remove or to reduce the risk of the cancer spreading during surgery. Postoperative or adjuvant radiotherapy is given to kill off any remaining cancer cells after the operation with the aim of lowering the risk of the cancer coming back. It will often be used in breast cancer, rectal cancer and cancers of the head and neck area.

Chemotherapy

Chemotherapy (CT) can be given before, during or after a course of radiotherapy. Chemotherapy and radiotherapy given together is called chemoradiotherapy or chemoradiation. In cancer treatment, chemotherapy means treatment with cell-killing (cytotoxic) drugs. A single chemotherapy drug may be administered or a combination of drugs. There are more than 100 different drugs currently available. Whether chemotherapy is suitable, and which drugs might be offered, depends on many factors, such as the type of cancer, the origin of the cancer, the grade of cancer, whether it has spread and the patient's general health.

Biological therapy

Biological therapy (BT) can be administered singly or in combination with radiotherapy to treat some types of cancer. These therapies act directly on processes in cells in an attempt to stop cancer cells from dividing and growing, to seek out cancer cells and kill them or to encourage the immune system to attack cancer cells. Whether a patient is offered biological therapy depends on the type of cancer, the stage of cancer and the other cancer treatments the patient has had.

Total body irradiation

Total body irradiation (TBI) may be given to patients having a bone marrow transplant or stem cell transplant, for example for some types of leukaemia or lymphoma. The treatment destroys the bone marrow cells. New bone marrow or stem cells must then be supplied into the bloodstream. The bone marrow or stem cells are obtained from the patient's own body or from a donor.

Shared decision-making

With such a broad and complex array of treatments, it is easy to understand if the cancer patient feels a degree of trepidation about the outcome. The significant uncertainties can best be dealt with in an open and transparent relationship with the responsible health professionals. An important concept in cancer care is shared decision-making. Shared decision-making (SDM) involves mutual engagement and participation, in which information is shared in a context that acknowledges the different values and preferences of both parties (Mahmoodi and Sargeant, 2017). A description of what SDM meant to one patient, 'Jane', follows:

> I wanted to take part in decision-making, have discussions and ask questions about the different treatments so I could better understand my options. But when it actually came down to deciding which treatment was best for me, I decided to share that task with my oncologist. I think it's a difficult one to make on your own and I am happy I decided to make it with my doctor. I felt much supported that way. Choosing to share the responsibility of decision-making made the task so much easier. (Mahmoodi and Sargeant, 2017: 4)

However, not all patients want to share in decision-making. For example, here are the views of 'Charlotte':

When I got diagnosed, I was given a big information booklet which I didn't look at. I had so many opportunities to have a say, to discuss the options with my oncologist and be a part of decision-making process, but I didn't want to. I didn't want to absorb any knowledge that could worry me more. … I chose not to be involved in decision-making full stop, let alone share decision- making. I totally avoided having those conversations together, and just let him decide. (Mahmoodi and Sargeant, 2017: 5)

In some cases, an oncologist may decide on the treatment and then simply inform and explain to the patient, which the patient accepts as sharing.

The later reduced version of SDM may often be the only pragmatic way of proceeding in many cases and is quite well accepted by patients.

Side effects

Cancer treatments can cause many different side effects – problems that occur when treatment affects healthy tissues or organs. When one considers all of these possible unpleasant side effects that treatment can often bring, the case for SDM is a strong one. Ultimately, it is the patient's choice whether to accept a treatment that is offered. Side effects vary from person to person, even among those receiving the same treatment. Some people have very few side effects while others have many. The type(s) of treatment received, as well as the amount or frequency of the treatment, age and general health of the patient, may also influence the type and severity of the side effects.

Often, treatment is feared as much as the illness itself. Common side effects caused by cancer treatment include:

- Anaemia;
- Appetite loss;
- Bleeding and bruising (thrombocytopenia);
- Constipation;
- Delirium;
- Diarrhoea;
- Fatigue;
- Hair loss (alopecia);
- Infection and neutropenia;
- Lymphoedema;
- Memory or noncentration problems;
- Mouth and throat problems;
- Nausea and vomiting;
- Nerve problems (peripheral neuropathy);
- Oedema;
- Pain;

- Psychosocial issues;
- Sexual and fertility problems (men);
- Sexual and fertility problems (women);
- Skin and nail changes;
- Sleep problems;
- Urinary and bladder problems.

Psychosocial issues in cancer treatment

Psychosocial issues are commonly encountered in cancer treatment. They include depression, anxiety, PTSD, insomnia, fatigue, pain, hopelessness, sexual concerns, identity problems, body image disturbances and social isolation. In a review of 97 studies, Hess and Chen (2014) reported that approximately one-third of radiotherapy patients experienced some form of psychosocial function decline. Their review indicated that anxiety may dissipate after initiation of RT, whereas depression tends to persist throughout and after RT. They reported that severe physical symptoms and time-related factors predicted psychosocial function decline, which can be improved by psychotherapy and interventions aimed at improving patient education. It has been suggested that differences in coping with cancer occur between people with different **attachment styles** (Jimenez, 2016; Nissen, 2016).

Lack of consistency across studies, however, suggests that measurement, conceptual and methodological issues remain unsolved. Hess and Chen (2014) reported that no less than 86 different assessment tools were being used to monitor RT-related psychosocial function decline, with the Hospital Anxiety and Depression Scale (HADS; Zigmond and Snaith, 1983) (25.8%) and the psychiatric interview (22.6%) being most utilized.

Qualitative studies of patient experience provide an essential perspective, complementing the more statistical approach of quantitative research. In a qualitative analysis of patients' psychosocial experiences with cancer during the course of oncology treatment with curative intent, Aldaz et al. (2016) identified six themes.

Theme I: diminished sense of well-being caused by physiological and psychological changes, including fatigue, gastrointestinal symptoms (e.g., nausea, reflux and constipation), changed perception of taste, anxiety, insomnia and perceived slower cognitive functioning. Patients described their well-being and enjoyment of day-to-day life as hindered by the uncontrollability of treatment-associated symptoms and subsequent reduced sense of agency and autonomy.

Theme II: perceived role changes in intimate relationships with their partners, who felt the need to provide constant care to them. Both participants and partners reported that caregiving affected partners' ability to carry on with their own interests and work commitments. Participants perceived their partners as suffering from emotional distress and having fearful thoughts about losing them to cancer.

Theme III: heightened awareness of limited time and future uncertainty in which the nature of cancer treatment has an 'embedded element of uncertainty about the probabilities of remission and recovery'. Such uncertainty appears to act as a catalyst to an expansion of participants' present time 'here and now' awareness.

Theme IV: a new order of priorities is required. Participants not only worry a lot, they also have to consider the possibility of a shortened life expectancy and take action according to their new order of priorities. They reprioritized what was most important to them in life by reordering priorities from reluctantly giving up work in favour of recovery, making effort to spend time with family and/or going on an overseas holiday sooner than planned.

Theme V: 'taking things as they come':

> I don't treat anything in life as, I just take things as they come and I don't sit and wonder oh what would've happened if I hadn't had it. I'm not that type of person. I'm very much if there's an issue, you deal with it, you move on and that's what I've always done throughout my whole life. So this is just a small chapter in my life and so I'll move on from here. (Aldaz et al., 2016: 8)

Theme VI: development of trust in health professionals. This last theme concerned the trust they felt with their oncologists, acknowledging their high regard for their expert advice and guidance. They valued having the possibility to openly discuss treatment issues and the wider impact on their lives with a professional who showed knowledge and expertise and also a friendly manner of approachability.

Patients' perspectives of qualitative issues in their care can be very informative and helpful in making improvements to services by plugging unmet needs.

Psychiatric issues

Derogatis et al. (1983) examined 215 randomly accessed US cancer patients, who were new admissions to three collaborating cancer centres, for the presence of psychiatric disorder. Each patient was assessed in a psychiatric interview using standardized psychological tests. The *Diagnostic and Statistical Manual of Mental Disorders,* third edition (*DSM-III*) (American Psychiatric Association, 1980) was used in making the diagnoses. A total of 47% of the patients received a *DSM-III* diagnosis, with 44% being diagnosed as manifesting a clinical syndrome and 3% with personality disorders. Approximately 68% of the psychiatric diagnoses consisted of adjustment disorders and 13% major affective disorders (depression). The remaining diagnoses were divided between organic mental disorders (8%), personality disorders (7%), and anxiety disorders (4%). Of those patients with a positive psychiatric condition, 85% were experiencing a disorder with depression or anxiety as the central symptom.

Kissane et al. (2004) assessed psychiatric disorder in women with early stage and advanced breast cancer. Similar figures were obtained for psychiatric illness to those found by Deragotis et al. (1983). A total of 303 women with early stage breast cancer were psychiatrically assessed at baseline and compared with 200 women with advanced breast cancer. The early stage patients (mean age 46 years) were an average of three months post-surgery and had an overall prevalence of *DSM-IV* (American Psychiatric Association, 1994) psychiatric diagnosis of 45%. The metastatic patients (mean age 51 years) were on average 63 months post-primary diagnosis and had an overall prevalence of *DSM-IV* diagnosis of 42%. The difference was not statistically significant. In women with early stage breast cancer, 36.7% had mood disorders, 9.6% with major depression and 27.1% with minor depression. In the metastatic sample, 31% had mood disorders, 6.5% with major depression and 24.5% with minor depression. Anxiety disorders were present in 8.6% of the early stage group and 6% of women with advanced disease. Fatigue, a history of depression and helplessness, hopelessness or resignation were associated with depression in both groups. The rates of psychosocial distress were high and similar across patients with both early and advanced stage breast cancer.

Miovic and Block (2007) reviewed evidence that around 50% of adult patients with advanced cancer met the criteria for a psychiatric disorder, the most common being adjustment disorders (11–35%) and major depression (5–26%). The large majority of the conditions suffered by cancer patients is highly treatable.

All three of the above studies found similarly high rates of psychiatric illness among adult cancer patients of 45–50%, wherein affective disorders are the most prevalent. Vigilance is needed to detect the signs and symptoms of affective disorders among cancer patients as early as possible so that appropriate treatment can be given. Few instruments exist for evaluating psychiatric illness in children and adolescents, older adults, individuals with cognitive impairments, and individuals from different ethnic and cultural groups. These gaps need to be filled.

Survivorship

As a consequence of improvements in treatment, an increasing number of patients complete their treatment and spend many years living as cancer survivors. The number of people living with cancer in the UK will double from today's 2 million to 4 million in the next 20 years (Macmillan, 2015). The number of individuals living with a history of cancer was estimated to be 13.7 million in the USA in 2012 and to rise to 18 million by 2022. The good news is that adults diagnosed with cancer generally show satisfactory psychosocial adjustment over time. However, as a consequence of long-term or late effects of cancer and its treatment, a group of patients are at risk for compromised psychological and physical health. The fear of recurrence is common among cancer survivors. They may also experience survivor guilt.

Stanton et al. (2015) describe survivorship after medical treatment in three phases that they call 're-entry', 'early survivorship' and 'long-term survivorship'. They describe the psychosocial and physical experiences facing adults during these three periods (Figure 20.3).

The re-entry period can be a mixed blessing. Re-entry is the transition from 'cancer patient' to 'person with a history of cancer'. It covers the point from completion of major cancer treatments, which can take from a few weeks to more than one year, and the next several months. The transition is often a difficult one. The patient is 'handed over' from the strict and structured protocols of hospital treatment to the more loose 'trial and error' world of recuperation at home. Patients may be ill-prepared for the re-entry period, where cancer survivors and loved ones may have unrealistic expectations of a rapid recovery and be surprised by their feelings as treatment ends. McKinley (2000: 479) wrote: 'I thought I would feel happy about finally reaching the end of treatment, but instead, I was sobbing. … Instead of joyous, I felt lonely, abandoned, and terrified. This was the rocky beginning of cancer survivorship for me.'

As shown in Figure 20.3, the early survivorship period extends from several months after diagnosis to approximately five years after diagnosis. Treatment-related acute physical illnesses have diminished for most survivors, who will have consolidated and come to terms with the cancer experience psychologically. The whole experience will have 'gelled' as a profound life event and the survivor will be feeling new hope and expectations for the future, having passed through the zone of greatest existential uncertainty. However, not all is peace and tranquility, because psychosocial and physical consequences can persist or arise periodically. For example, routine cancer surveillance appointments may prompt fear of recurrence. Cancer survivors may often experience 'islands' of psychosocial disruption after they have recovered from primary treatments (Andersen et al., 1989).

Long-term survivorship is defined by Stanton et al. (2015) as the experience beyond five years after diagnosis, by which time many survivors can expect to attain near-normative values on measures of health-related QoL. However, the five-year marker for long-term survivorship does not imply that psychological or physical recovery is complete. Long-term treatment effects can be evident even many years after cancer diagnosis.

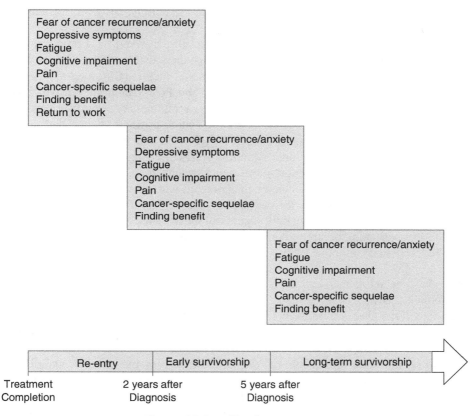

Hypothesized periods of cancer survivorship and associated sequelae: an evolving heuristic model

Figure 20.3   Life after treatment

Source: Stanton et al. (2015). Reproduced by permission

ALLEGED 'BENEFIT FINDING' AND 'POST-TRAUMATIC GROWTH'

Experiences associated with significant life disruption, threat, distress or adversity can lead to positively evaluated 'growth' outcomes (Tedeschi and Calhoun, 2004). It has been observed for centuries that benefit finding and **post-traumatic growth (PTG)** can follow the occurrence of traumatic events, including accidents, warfare, death of a loved one, and cancer diagnosis and treatment). The alleged benefit finding and growth represent a fundamental restorative principle of homeostasis that is continually active towards the achievement of stability, equilibrium and well-being. Adaptation to any life-threatening illness, such as cancer, is facilitated by homeostasis systems that include the drive to find meaning, exert mastery or control over the experience and bolster self-esteem. Growth and benefit finding are frequently reported by cancer survivors as they gain awareness of their illness, its treatment and prognosis. The theoretical model of PTG proposed by Tedeschi and Calhoun suggests that growth can occur in different ways through developing new relationships with others, finding a new appreciation for life, new meanings in life, discovering personal strength, experiencing spiritual change and realizing new opportunities. The experiences of benefit finding and growth are undeniable. The methods currently used for their study, however, raise more questions than answers.

Among cancer populations, reported prevalence rates of perceived PTG range from 53% to 90% and vary according to the type of cancer, time since diagnosis, heterogeneity and ethnicity of the sample, choice of measurement, and many personal factors (Coroiu et al., 2016). Post-traumatic growth is measured using scales such as 'The Post-Traumatic Growth Inventory' (PTGI), a 21-item measure of positive change following a traumatic or stressful event (Tedeschi and Calhoun, 1996). Respondents rate the degree to which positive change had occurred in their life 'as a result of having cancer'. A total PTGI score and five sub-scale scores (New possibilities, Relating to others, Personal strength, Spiritual change and Appreciation of life) are calculated. Women generally report more benefits than men, and persons experiencing traumatic events report more positive change than persons who have not experienced extraordinary events. It has been suggested by the developers that the Post-Traumatic Growth Inventory 'appears to have utility in determining how successful individuals, coping with the aftermath of trauma, are in reconstructing or strengthening their perceptions of self, others, and the meaning of events' (Tedeschi and Calhoun, 1996: 455).

> Critics have been less than enthusiastic about measuring PTG in this manner. Coyne and Tennen (2010: 23) argue that: Every PTG scale asks participants to rate how much they have changed on each scale item as the result of the crisis they faced. Thus, a respondent must: (a) evaluate her/his current standing on the dimension described in the item, e.g., a sense of closeness to others; (b) recall her/his previous standing on the same dimension; (c) compare the current and previous standings; (d) assess the degree of change; and (e) determine how much of that change can be attributed to the stressful encounter. Psychological science, which purportedly guides positive psychology, tells us that people cannot accurately generate or manipulate the information required to faithfully report trauma- or stress-related growth (or to report benefits) that results from threatening encounters. … The psychological literature demonstrates consistently that people are unable to recollect personal change accurately.

The five steps (a)–(e) certainly are a tall order, and it seems highly doubtful that anybody could achieve them with any accuracy of judgement. It seems naïve to analyse the numbers that research participants place on scales from the PTGI as though they are valid and authentic representations of 'post-traumatic growth' when there is no attempt being made to validate these measures in the manner of Frazier et al. (2009). In spite of criticisms of the methodology, which suggest that the PTGI and other retrospective measures of PTG do not appear to measure actual pre- to post-trauma change, many studies have been conducted using the PTGI scale.

CARING FOR SOMEONE WITH CANCER

The stress experienced by family members of cancer sufferers is often high. The condition fosters emotional turmoil, with fear, anxiety, stigma, depression, isolation, hopelessness, fatigue, burn-out and insomnia all entering the arena at various stages. The social support provided by immediate family and friends can be a key factor in promoting the patient's adaptation and QoL. However, 'caregiver burden' can be high, and interventions are needed on a wider scale to support the informal caregiver.

Soylu et al. (2015) explored the psychological distress and loneliness in 100 caregivers of advanced oncological inpatients in Turkey. The study examined the relationships among levels of loneliness, anxiety, depression and other variables on primary caregivers and cancer inpatients. Loneliness and anxiety scores were significantly higher for the primary caregivers of inpatients with terminal stage cancer than primary caregivers of inpatients with advanced stage cancer.

A qualitative study examined the nature and consequences of cancer on the relationship between informal carers and the person with cancer in Australia (Ussher et al., 2011). There were 62 carers (42 women and 20 men) from a range of cancer types, stages and relationship dyads who took part in semi-structured interviews. Not surprisingly, participants indicated that cancer had led to a change in roles and in dynamics of the relationship, including the taking of quasi-medical tasks and decisions, neglect of the self and other relationships, changes to emotions or even personality of the person with cancer, changed communication patterns, and changes to sexuality and intimacy. The impacts of these changed relationships included sadness, anger and frustration, as well as feelings of love and being closer together, resulting in relationship enhancement. Women more frequently reported changes in the person with cancer and were more likely to mourn the previous relationship, while more men reported relationship enhancement.

The US Institute of Medicine (IOM) (2007a) report, *Cancer Care for the Whole Patient: Meeting Psychosocial Health Needs*, concluded that despite the evidence for the effectiveness of services, cancer care often fails to meet patients' psychosocial needs. One possible reason for this failure is the tendency of cancer care providers to underestimate patients' distress (Falomir-Pichastor et al., 2015) and to not link patients to appropriate services when their needs are identified (Institute of Medicine, 2007b).

The IOM report recommends a model for the elective delivery of psychosocial services with a five-step sequence of processes:

1. Identify each patient's psychosocial needs.

2. Link patients and families to needed psychosocial services.

3. Support patients and families in managing the illness.

4. Coordinate psychosocial and biomedical care.

5. Follow up on care delivery to monitor the effectiveness of services and make modifications if needed.

Northouse et al. (2012) reviewed research that suggested that caregiver stress leads to psychological and sleep disturbances, changes in caregivers' physical health and immune function, and reduced financial well-being. Interventions for caregivers of patients with cancer or other chronic illnesses can reduce many of the negative effects and improve caregivers' coping skills, knowledge and quality of life. However, the authors concluded that these interventions are seldom implemented in practice. To help solve this problem, they recommended: the publication of standardized guidelines that address caregiver assessment, education and resources; the identification of 'caregiver champions' in practice settings; the provision of referrals to established support organizations for caregivers (e.g., Cancer Support Community, Cancer Care); and collaboration among caregiving, professional and cancer-related organizations to advocate policy and practice changes for family caregivers.

CASE STUDY OF INTERVENTION

It has been estimated that more than half the variance in psychosocial adjustment to breast cancer may be attributed to coping styles (Glanz and Lerman, 1992). Cancer patients who use coping strategies characterized as hopelessness/helplessness, fatalistic, pessimistic and anxious preoccupation report greater levels of stress than patients who use coping strategies characterized as active, problem-focused and confrontational (Greer et al., 1992; Schnoll et al., 1998). Patients using passive coping styles are more distressed than patients who confront their problems directly and seek solutions (Dunkel-Schetter et al., 1992). Active problem-solving coping has a positive effect on well-being, whereas passive, avoidant strategies had a relatively large negative effect in another study (De Ridder and Schreurs, 1996). The use of avoidant coping is predictive of poorer adjustment to breast cancer (Carver et al., 1993; Stanton and Snider, 1993; McCaul et al., 1999).

Meyer and Mark (1995) synthesized the findings of RCTs of psychosocial interventions with adult cancer patients using meta-analysis. A total of 45 studies reporting 62 treatment–control comparisons were included. Samples were predominantly white, female, and from the USA. Beneficial effect size ds^2 were 0.24 for emotional adjustment measures, 0.19 for functional adjustment measures, 0.26 for measures of treatment- and disease-related symptoms, and 0.28 for compound and global measures.

Carrying out research to evaluate interventions for cancer patients can be a highly complex and difficult project even for an experienced investigator. It is not something to be undertaken lightly. We illustrate here the design and testing of an intervention for cancer patients carried out at McGill University in Canada where 'NUCARE' (a neologism formed from '**NU**rsing, **CA**ncer and **RE**search') has been proposed as a psycho-educational intervention based on cognitive behavioural principles (Box 20.1). The study provides an instructive lesson on the difficulties that can occur in running trials of this type. We discuss this trial in some detail to enable the key issues and complexities to be critically appraised.

BOX 20.1

The Nucare intervention

The Nucare intervention incorporates two areas: the enhancement of a sense of personal control and the learning of emotional and instrumental coping responses. The intervention was based on the McGill Model of Nursing, which stresses a partnership with the patient and family where situation responsive learning about healthy behaviours and coping can occur.

---

[2]Cohen's d is a measure of an effect size determined by calculating the mean difference between two groups, and then dividing the result by the *pooled* standard deviation.

The intervention may be effective for reducing patient distress, enhancing a sense of control and managing distressing side effects of treatment.

The model emphasizes individual strengths, the labelling of positive behaviours by providing feedback, working with the agenda of the patient, providing learning experiences at appropriate, teachable times, considering the individual as a member of a family or larger social system, and a focus on good coping. The Lazarus and Folkman conceptual model of coping guided the development of Nucare (1984).

The NUCARE intervention emphasizes training in seven skills:

> *Problem-solving techniques*: Each patient was taught a specific series of steps in problem solving. *Goal setting*: Setting graduated and attainable goals provides a means of accomplishing tasks that provide a sense of perceived personal control. *Cognitive reappraisal*: Patients were taught to be more cognizant of and identify those thought patterns that contribute to negative mood. The awareness that patients could have control over their thoughts was often sufficient to provide positive change and improved mood. Patients practised identifying facts, thoughts and feelings. *Mindfulness. Relaxation training* was a second step in problem solving (i.e., taking time out to develop a different perspective). Progressive muscle relaxation with guided imagery was used with an audiotape for home use. *The effective use of social support*: Learning how to use 'I' statements, develop assertive behaviours and determine the adequacy of one's own social support network. *The use of resources*: A comprehensive booklet outlining all the resources available to patients with cancer and their families within the hospital setting and in the wider community was presented.

A published version of the workbook is entitled *Mastering the Art of Coping in Good Times and Bad* (Edgar, 2010).

Source: Edgar et al. (2001)

Edgar et al. (1992) tested the effects of the Nucare intervention in an individual and group format.

The Nucare intervention focuses on enhancement of a sense of personal control and emotional and instrumental coping responses (Edgar et al., 2001; Rosberger et al., 2002). There is evidence suggesting that the intervention enhances QoL and reduces distress in patients with cancer (Edgar et al., 1992; Allison et al., 2004; Vilela et al., 2006). The intervention is based on the coping model and Ways of Coping Questionnaire of Folkman and Lazarus (1988).

Edgar et al. (2001) designed an RCT to compare the relative effectiveness of both an individual and a group presentation of the Nucare intervention, along with an unstructured peer support group (which attempted to control for the non-specific effects of group process) and a no treatment arm, which serves as a no-treatment 'control'.

The latter basically informs the investigators of the outcome of not giving any intervention. This feature can be ethically controversial because, if the interventions are effective, then the control participants have been deliberately denied beneficial health care.

Edgar et al. stated that they wanted to investigate the outcomes of functional well-being and emotional distress on patients over the course of one year. Participants with breast or colon cancer were assessed four months after diagnosis, and every four months for a total of four evaluation points. Edgar et al. (2001) hypothesized that the effectiveness of Nucare presented in group format on psychosocial outcomes would be equal to or better than Nucare presented in a one-to-one format, and better than both the unstructured support group and the no treatment arm for breast and colon cancer patients. They investigators also hypothesized that patients who received the Nucare intervention would achieve greater improvements in emotional distress and functional well-being than patients in the control arm.

The patient sample was recruited from the Department of Oncology of the Sir Mortimer B. Davis Jewish General Hospital, Montreal, Quebec, Canada. Edgar et al. were granted access to the Tumour Registry of the hospital, where all cancer patients were registered; consequently, they could report on the entire population from which the sample was drawn. (A definite advantage compared to many similar studies.) All patients meeting the following criteria were invited to participate: (1) at least 18 years of age; (2) able to speak and read English or French; (3) accepting medical treatment and follow-up at the study site; (4) diagnosed with breast or colon cancer within the previous four months and about to begin treatment on or off a clinical trial protocol. They limited their focus to breast and colon cancer patients to increase the homogeneity of the sample and hence the power of the analysis, while studying two different cancer sites.

The RCT design contained four arms (i.e., treatments or procedures). All patients from the Tumour Registry were contacted if they met criteria (1) and (4). Research assistants then determined whether criteria (2) and (3) were satisfied before continuing the recruitment process. The physicians of the potential participants were notified of the study. They respected the wishes of a few physicians who stated that there was no need for the study for their patients. All other patients were contacted by a research assistant, oncology nurse or physician to begin the process of recruitment. [*Note in the following that the Edgar et al. referred to 'subjects' instead of 'participants', indicating a somewhat diminished status for the patients.*] After the 'subjects' received a complete description of the study, they obtained written informed consent. The authors go on to state that the 'procedures followed were in accordance with the ethical standards of the Research Committee of the Hospital' [*This statement suggests the possibility that no formal application may have been made to an Institutional Review Board for ethical approval. Concerning, if true.*] Following the baseline interview:

> patients were randomized into one of four arms using a block randomization procedure. The four arms consisted of (1) individual Nucare; (2) Nucare presented in a group format; (3) a supportive, unstructured group; (4) a no intervention control arm. When the randomization envelope specified either the group Nucare or unstructured support group arm, the subsequent eight subjects would be allocated to that arm to facilitate the formation of a group of sufficient size within our estimation of a reasonable time frame (a mean of six months following the baseline interview). (Edgar et al., 2001: 292)

All patients were interviewed and completed questionnaires to measure well-being and psychological distress four times: at baseline four months from diagnosis prior to the intervention; and subsequently every four months up to one year. The five-session interventions were completed within a six-month period following the first data-collection point.

The research assistants for the study were two nurses and a social worker. They conducted the four interviews at the study centre or occasionally in the patient's home. The questionnaires were completed by the patient in the interviewers' presence and demographic data were collected in an open-ended fashion. The 'subjects' met with the same interviewer over the four data collection points. The intervention educators were a nurse, two social workers and a psychologist, who were all experienced in individual and group work with cancer patients. Two educators led the individual and group Nucare sessions and two others led the unstructured support groups.

In these last two sentences, we learn of a potentially fatal flaw in the study design. Different treatments were administered by different personnel. Therefore, there is no way of knowing whether any differences between the treatments administered by the different personnel are due to the characteristics of the treatment *per se* or to the characteristics of the personnel delivering those treatments.

The Nucare intervention was as described in Box 20.1 except it left out the Mindfulness component.

We turn now to the measures taken. Interviewers blind to what intervention arm the 'subjects' belonged to conducted the following measures: (1) Demographic and Disease Data: age, gender, education, marital status, religion, hours of paid work per week, disease, staging, treatment information, and disease severity according to the three-stage nuclear grade system (good, medium or poor); (2) Profile of Mood States (POMS) – emotional distress was measured by the POMS; a five-point response ranging from 1 (not at all) to 5 (extremely) was used for items on six sub-scales: depression, anxiety, confusion, anger, fatigue and vigour; (3) the Functional Assessment of Cancer Therapy (FACT) scale, measuring actual and perceived impact in five domains – functional, physical, social and emotional well-being, the physician–patient relationship and a global assessment of adjustment with items rated on a five-point scale. The first of the reported findings related to the sample characteristics:

> During the two-year accrual period there were just over 1200 breast and colon patients registered with the Tumour Registry of the hospital. We are able to report on the entire cohort of patients diagnosed with breast and colon cancer during the accrual phase, in marked contrast to most published studies which rely on referrals from the health care team or a public relations approach. Five hundred and thirty-three of the 1200 patients were ineligible due primarily to the severity of their illness or difficulty comprehending the project, leaving a possible total of 667 eligible subjects. We were able to recruit 225 of the remaining 667 for a response rate of 33 percent. Four hundred and forty-two patients declined to participate including a small number to whom we were denied access by their physicians. Of those who declined, 40% were not interested in the study, 20% were not comfortable communicating in English or French, 20% felt they were too ill to participate, 10% felt they were too old, and 10% lived too far away to travel to the study site. There were no significant ANOVA differences between the participants and those who declined to join according to age or gender (for colon cancer patients). The known participation and accrual rates in oncology clinical trials range between 3 and 14 percent. (Edgar et al., 2001: 295)

Aspects of this description are concerning. Only 225 patients from a total of more than 1,200 patients were recruited. That is <18.75% of patients on the Tumour Registry. If we accept that only 667 patients were eligible, that is still only 33.7%, almost exactly one-third. We are given, in round numbers, reasons for non-participation, but these numbers are high, and one is left wondering how well the study findings would generalize to the entirety of the patient population. Unfortunately, there is no way of knowing because these participants were self-selected.

An alternative method of evaluating interventions is to carry out an observational study in which patients are offered a range of treatments and are free to choose which one they prefer. The results that are obtained may be closer to what happens in the 'real world'.

Another concern regarding the details of the sample is the low number of male patients. Only 41 males were recruited to the study along with 184 female patients. This gender split is destined for serious problems, as we shall see below. It would have been better to have dropped all of the males out of the study or gone the 'extra mile' to recruit males in much larger numbers. We are informed also that:

> Thirty-six ($n = 19$ breast; $n = 17$ colon) patients withdrew over the course of the year: Nine patients were too ill or died, 5 moved away from the area, and 22 were not interested in following the study to its year completion. There were no significant differences in numbers of subjects, reasons for withdrawal, or in demographics between dropouts and participants among the four arms. The dropouts were distributed across the treatment groups from Nucare individual, Nucare group, unstructured group and control arm as follows: 9, 9, 10, and 8. (Edgar et al., 2001: 296)

Thirty-six withdrawals is 16% of the total sample, quite a high proportion. We are not informed about the gender of the colon patient drop-outs, but if the majority of the 17 was male, then the sample size of male colon patients will have been too small to analyse, which transpired to be the case.

The reported results were outcome differences over one year for the POMS and FACT scales. The results suggested that breast cancer patients who received individual Nucare had made the most improvements in their well-being and adjustment as measured by the FACT scale. These positive effects were maintained over the one year of the study. Contrary to the investigators' expectations, individual, face-to-face Nucare was found to be more effective at every time point than group Nucare, unstructured group or no-treatment arm in improving functional, physical and general well-being, and in the domain of depression at 8 months, vigour at 12 months, and emotional well-being at 8 and 12 months. The authors state:

> Before the analyses began, we became aware that we had failed to create and sustain functioning groups of patients with colon cancer within the constraints of the research design; therefore we had a situation where there was no clear treatment to evaluate in the group arms. We were distressed to find that patients with colon cancer did better in the no treatment arm than in either of the two group arms. The attendance of those patients with colon cancer for the two group conditions was significantly lower ($M = 2.5$) than for individual Nucare ($M = 4$), and clinically, the educators informed us of the reluctance expressed by the subjects who had been randomized to the group conditions to participate. (Edgar et al., 2001: 300)

Alarm bells are ringing loudly at this point. The drop-out rates for the colon groups were very high: 6/16, 10/21 and 4/21 for the group Nucare, support group and control interventions, respectively. These rates provide interesting information. The support group in particular was not greatly supported by the colon patients with nearly half leaving before the end of the trial. Were these mainly males? The many empty cells in the results table that presented the outcomes for colon patients suggests that there were no male colon patients left to analyse in these cells. This was a disastrous feature of the trial, as was the finding that a no-treatment control condition did better than the two group intervention arms for the colon patients.

The study results were egregious for the Nucare intervention as the patients with colon cancer did not benefit from either the individual or group arms. They 'voted with their feet' in withdrawing in high numbers from the study. In the debriefing sessions with the educators, the investigators learned that the men with colon cancer in the individual sessions seemed to 'build a protective barrier around them to prevent having to engage in learning coping skills. There was a consensus that the men gave "lip service" to the concepts under discussion but did not practice the skills away from the sessions' (Edgar et al., 2001: 300). Colon cancer patients of both sexes were dealing with a variety of physical problems, such as dietary issues and diarrhoea, that interfered with any interest they might otherwise have had about their psychosocial concerns. The educators reported that the mixing of males and females in the colon cancer groups inhibited the 'subjects' from sharing their thoughts. There were 20 groups during the study but these were all mixed sex groups due to the small numbers available. The lack of choice in receiving group or individual sessions may also have been a deterrent to participation, especially in the colon patients.

The authors were fully cognizant of many of the problems with this study. They acknowledged that they were attempting two contradictory goals for the groups within an unrealistic time frame: to foster group processes and social support, and to present the Nucare intervention in a didactic way. They acknowledged that they were unable to create a naturalistic setting for the groups and were aware of the gap between the constraints of a randomized clinical trial and the real world where patients decide for themselves whether or not to participate and when. A 'real-world' evaluation of the intervention may well have obtained very different results and, quite possibly, results that were more in line with the investigators' predictions. Real-world and RCT studies often do produce different findings.

The authors point to problems caused by the large variances in the baseline scores and the mean changes. When combined with the small samples, the high variances at baseline became a fatal flaw. Had Edgar et al. limited recruitment to patients who were clinically distressed at baseline, there would have been scope for more statistically significant changes attributable to the interventions. The possibility of an unknown systematic bias from the participation of 33% of the invited sample may also have existed as patients self-selected themselves into the clinical trial.

Edgar et al. (2001) are to be applauded for publishing their study in all humility under the title 'Lessons Learned'. In so doing, other investigators can learn from their mistakes and the quality of future trials can be raised.

Methodological issues

Jacobsen (2009) discussed reasons why evidence-based psychosocial care for cancer patients is not more widely promoted and adopted by clinicians. First, there are inconsistent findings, attributable, at least in part, to differences in demographic, disease and treatment characteristics of the samples, and the type of outcome assessments employed. Considerable variation also exists across studies in the number and content of sessions for interventions that share the same name, e.g., relaxation training. Inadequate reporting of study methodology and lack of transparency in reports of trials are problems for anybody wishing to replicate an intervention (Marks, 2009). Newell et al. (2002) found that only 3% of trials provided sufficient information to permit an evaluation of ten indicators of study quality.

Methodological issues are common. For example, the majority of studies fail to account for patients lost to follow-up in the outcome analyses. This means that it is impossible to calculate with accuracy the odds ratio for a treatment compared to the control condition. Seitz et al. (2009) systematically reviewed psychosocial interventions for adolescent cancer patients. The authors concluded that:

> Taken together, the findings point out that there is a lack of intervention research in psycho-oncology with adolescents. So far, there is only limited evidence for the effectiveness of psychosocial interventions to improve coping with cancer-associated problems in adolescent patients. ... In order to establish more conclusive results, larger samples and interventions particularly designed for adolescent patients ought to be studied. (Seitz et al., 2009: 683)

As we have seen, much of the evidence concerning the alleged benefits of psychological interventions (reviewed in Chapter 19) remains unconvincing. Coyne and Tennen (2010) examined four widely accepted claims in the positive psychology literature regarding adaptational outcomes among individuals living with cancer. These claims from positive psychology were found to be wanting. Coyne and Tennen (2010: 16) noted:

> incoherence of claims about the adaptational value of benefit finding and post-traumatic growth among cancer patients, and the implausibility of claims that interventions that enhance benefit finding improve the prognosis of cancer patients by strengthening the immune system. ... We urge positive psychologists to rededicate themselves to a positive psychology based on scientific evidence rather than wishful thinking.

The current prominence of concepts such as 'being positive', 'fighting spirit', 'post-traumatic growth' and 'benefit finding' in the popular literature about cancer has little or no basis in science. A more sceptical, evidence-based approach is necessary if we are to avoid the dissemination of inaccurate information and the raising of false hopes.

Influence of the internet

As internet access increases throughout the world, the internet is a major source of health information for patients and their families, particularly for serious life-threatening conditions such as cancer. Eysenbach (2003) explored the impact of the internet on cancer outcomes. He distinguished four areas of internet use: communication (electronic mail), community (virtual support groups), content (health information on the World Wide Web) and e-commerce. Eysenbach estimated that, in the developed world, 39% of cancer patients were using the internet, and approximately 2.3 million persons living with cancer worldwide were online. These figures will be vastly higher today, with perhaps 50% of the global population online. Recent systematic reviews of online support have yielded mixed outcomes (Hong et al., 2012; Kuijpers et al., 2013). A trial by Bantum et al. (2014) reported significantly greater reductions in insomnia and greater increases in vigorous exercise and stretching compared to controls (based on self-reports).

Beekers et al. (2015) hypothesized that dissatisfaction with health care information provided by professional providers may be one driver for cancer survivors seeking health information on the internet. All individuals diagnosed with endometrial or colorectal cancer between 1998 and 2007 or lymphoma or multiple myeloma between 1999 and 2008 in Eindhoven were invited to participate; 4,446 cancer survivors received questionnaires, including the 25-item European Organization for Research and Treatment of Cancer Quality of Life Group Information questionnaire and the Hospital Anxiety and Depression Scale (HADS; Zigmond and Snaith, 1983).

Beekers et al. found that patients having anxious or depressive symptoms or both were less likely to have experienced helpfulness in the received information. Having depressive symptoms or having both depressive and anxious symptoms were negatively associated with satisfaction with information, and having depressive symptoms was negatively associated with disease-related internet use.

Alsaiari et al. (2017) evaluated the content and quality of health information on adult kidney cancer websites found on Google, Yahoo and Bing using two terms: 'kidney cancer' and 'renal cell carcinoma'. They reviewed the top 30 hits consisting of 35 websites. Content was assessed using a 22-item checklist adapted from the American Cancer Society. The average website had 16 of 22 content items, while 6 websites fulfilled all 22 items. The average website readability was at the ninth-grade reading level. However, some websites were difficult to read without a high school education.

As internet access increases throughout the world, the internet will play an increasing role as an information source for people with illness. There are many excellent websites provided by governmental and third-sector organizations offering information based on the best scientific evidence. Regulation is needed to remove quack websites that exploit people with offers of 'snake oil' placebos, phoney services and fake cures.

FUTURE RESEARCH

1. Research that uses sensitive and robust designs, both quantitative and qualitative in nature, is required to understand illness experience at different stages of diagnosis, treatment and survival.

2. Research on interventions for patients and caregivers is also needed to improve services at different stages of the illness, especially the re-entry phase, which has been somewhat neglected.

3. Few instruments exist for evaluating psychiatric illness in children and adolescents, older adults, individuals with cognitive impairments, and individuals from different ethnic and cultural groups, and these gaps need to be filled.

4. More research is needed on methods to enhance critical thinking and scepticism about 'quack science' in medicine and psychology.

SUMMARY

1. Cancer occurs when cells keep dividing and forming more cells without internal control or order. This cell growth is known as a 'tumour' or 'neoplasm' and can be benign or malignant.
2. Approximately one out of every two men and one out of every three women have cancer during their lifetime.
3. Risk factors for cancer are many and various, and include genetic, environmental, viral and behavioural toxins, such as smoking and sunbeds.
4. Diagnosis may trigger psychological and existential threat, leading to an outpouring of emotions.
5. Treatments aim to cure cancer, control it, or treat its symptoms. The type of treatment depends on the type of cancer, the stage of the cancer, and individual factors such as age, health status, and the personal preferences of the patient and his/her family.
6. Most patients prefer shared decision-making, wherein the professionals engage the patient in making treatment choices.
7. The four major treatments for cancer are surgery, radiation, chemotherapy, and biological therapies such as hormone therapies (e.g., tamoxifen) and transplant options (e.g., with bone marrow or stem cell therapy).
8. The prominence of concepts such as 'being positive', 'fighting spirit', 'post-traumatic growth' and 'benefit finding' has little or no basis in science. A sceptical, evidence-based approach is required if we are to avoid dissemination of inaccurate information and false hope.
9. The internet is playing an increasing role as an information source for people with illness. Regulation is needed to remove fake services and information.

CORONARY HEART DISEASE

21

'The heart has reasons that reason cannot know. ... We know the truth not only by the reason, but by the heart.'

Blaise Pascal

OUTLINE

In this chapter, we consider one of the major diseases of the cardiovascular system, coronary heart disease (CHD). We describe the nature and causes of the illness and its major risk factors. Then we discuss the psychosocial issues of living with CHD, caring for someone with CHD, and the design and testing of interventions. We describe research on cardiac rehabilitation for myocardial infarction and angina patients and the results of recent meta-analyses. The ability to offer interventions that are effective and cost-efficient is a challenge that potentially can be solved using a combination of professional, lay and web-based provision.

WHAT IS CORONARY HEART DISEASE?[1]

Cardiovascular disease is a broad category that involves diseases affecting the heart or blood vessels. CHD, also known as 'coronary artery disease', includes angina and myocardial infarction (heart attack). Other major cardiovascular diseases are stroke, heart failure, hypertension,

---

[1]Figure 21.1 and descriptive material on CHD are courtesy of the National Heart, Blood and Lung Institute: www.nhlbi.nih.gov/health/health-topics/topics/cad [Public domain].

rheumatic heart disease, cardiomyopathy, heart arrhythmia, congenital heart disease, valvular heart disease, caritis, aortic aneurisms, peripheral artery disease and venous thrombosis.

CHD occurs when the walls of the coronary arteries become narrowed by a gradual build-up of fatty material called atheroma. **Myocardial infarction (MI)** occurs when one of the coronary arteries becomes blocked by a blood clot and part of the heart is starved of oxygen. It usually causes severe chest pain. A person having a heart attack may also experience sweating, light-headedness, nausea or shortness of breath. A heart attack may be the first sign of CHD in many people. Over time, CHD can weaken the heart muscle and cause heart failure and arrhythmias.

When plaque builds up in the arteries, the condition is called **atherosclerosis**. The build-up of plaque occurs over many years. Over time, plaque can harden or rupture. Hardened plaque narrows the coronary arteries and reduces the flow of oxygen-rich blood to the heart. If the plaque ruptures, a blood clot can form on its surface. A large blood clot can mostly or completely block blood flow through a coronary artery. Over time, ruptured plaque also hardens and narrows the coronary arteries.

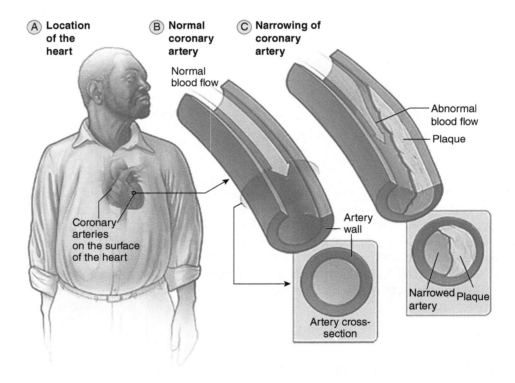

Figure 21.1   Coronary heart disease

(A) shows the location of the heart in the body. (B) shows a normal coronary artery with normal blood flow. The inset image shows a cross-section of a normal coronary artery. (C) shows a coronary artery narrowed by plaque. The build-up of plaque limits the flow of oxygen-rich blood through the artery. The inset image shows a cross-section of the plaque-narrowed artery

Source: National Heart, Blood and Lung Institute (2017). Public domain

If the flow of oxygen-rich blood to your heart muscle is reduced or blocked, **angina pectoris** or a **heart attack** can occur.

A heart attack occurs if the flow of oxygen-rich blood to a section of heart muscle is cut off. If blood flow is not restored quickly, the section of heart muscle begins to die. Without quick treatment, a heart attack can lead to serious health problems or death. Over time, CHD can weaken the heart muscle and lead to heart failure and arrhythmias. **Heart failure** is a condition in which the heart cannot pump enough blood to meet the body's needs. **Arrhythmias** are problems with the rate or rhythm of the heartbeat.

Angina pectoris is characterized by a heavy or tight pain in the centre of the chest that may spread to the arms, neck, jaw, face, back or stomach. Angina symptoms occur when the arteries become so narrow from the atheroma that insufficient oxygen-containing blood can be supplied to the heart muscle when its demands are high, such as during exercise. There are two categories of angina: stable or unstable angina. Stable angina is characterized by chest pain relieved by rest, resulting from the partial obstruction of a coronary artery by atheroma. Unstable angina occurs with lesser degrees of exertion or while at rest. This type increases in frequency and duration and worsens in severity. Unstable angina is an acute coronary syndrome requiring immediate medical attention. This is usually caused by the formation of a blood clot at the site of a ruptured plaque in a coronary artery. If left untreated, it can result in heart attack and irreversible damage to the heart.

Treatments for CHD include lowering blood pressure, preventing blood clots which can lead to heart attack or stroke, preventing or delaying the need for a stent or percutaneous coronary intervention (PCI), or surgery, such as coronary artery bypass grafting (CABG). Invasive treatment may be necessary when medication alone does not relieve angina. Referral to a cardiologist or a heart surgeon may be required for further treatment to gain effective control of angina symptoms and for some people to prolong life. Invasive revascularization treatment may include either a PCI or CABG surgery.

Globally, CHD is recognized as the leading cause of death and is predicted to remain so for the next ten years. Each year, approximately 3.8 million men and 3.4 million women die from CHD. In 2020, it is estimated that CHD will be responsible for a total of 11.1 million deaths globally. Someone suffers a coronary event every 26 seconds, and someone dies from one every minute in the USA. In Europe, between one in five and one in seven European women die from CHD, and the disease accounts for between 16% and 25% of all deaths in European men (Mathers and Loncar, 2006). Angina is the most common form of CHD, with 10 million people in the USA and 2 million in the UK suffering from it. Angina is common among older adults. In England, 1 in every 12 men and 1 in every 30 women between 55 and 64 years of age have angina. This figure rises to 1 in every 7 men and 1 in every 12 women who are over 65 years of age. Angina is more common in men than women. Figure 21.2 shows observed age-adjusted death rates for cancer and heart disease since 1969 and projected to 2020.

The 'bad news' in Figure 21.2 is the increasing deaths from cancer (see Chapter 20). The 'good news' is that the incidence of heart disease, including CHD, is declining. Another piece of good news is that CHD, along with most cardiovascular diseases, can be prevented by addressing behavioural risk factors such as tobacco use, unhealthy diet, obesity, inactivity and abuse of alcohol. There is a major role for health psychology in the design and dissemination of high-quality, evidence-based interventions. Another role for health psychology is that people with cardiovascular disease and people at high cardiovascular risk require early detection and management using counselling and medicines.

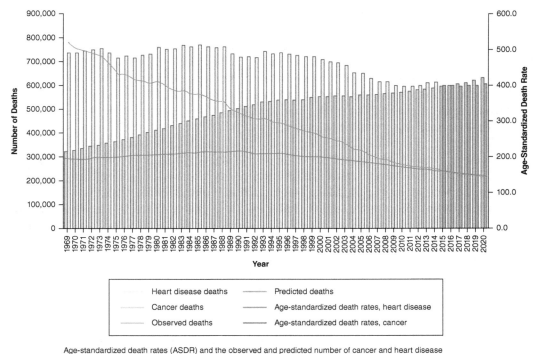

Age-standardized death rates (ASDR) and the observed and predicted number of cancer and heart disease deaths from 1969 through 2020 for men and women combined.

Figure 21.2   The changing incidence of cancer and heart disease rates in the USA

Source: Weir et al. (2016). Public domain

Risk factors for CHD include:

- increasing age;
- male sex;
- heredity;
- tobacco smoking;
- high blood cholesterol;
- high blood pressure;
- physical inactivity;
- obesity and overweight;
- diabetes mellitus;
- high alcohol consumption;
- insomnia;
- sleep disordered breathing;

- low social support/isolation;

- oxidative stress;

- C-reactive protein concentration;

- hostility;

- work stress/burnout/vital exhaustion;

- caregiving for a disabled or ill spouse for more than nine hours per week;

- depression.

Many of these risk factors are well established. However, others on the list overlap with each other so are difficult to completely disentangle as independent risk factors. Recent studies have focused on psychosocial and behavioural risk factors. Enter the health psychologist.

Kivimäki and Siegrist (2016) reviewed evidence on work stress as a risk factor for CHD and stroke, with a particular emphasis on 'effort–reward imbalance' (ERI). Their findings from meta-analyses of cohort studies suggested that individuals with ERI or job insecurity have an increased risk of CHD, while those working long hours appear to be at an increased risk of stroke. They concluded that excess risk associated with ERI was not attributable to other well-established work stressors, such as job strain.

Another alleged risk factor is Type D or 'distressed' personality (Denollet et al., 1996; see below). The size of the effect of Type D on prognosis appears to have been overestimated and claims have decreased as more studies have been conducted (Grande et al., 2012).

Similarly, depression has been controversial as a risk factor for CHD. Nicholson et al. (2006) carried out a meta-analysis of depression among 146,538 participants in 54 observational studies of CHD. Results needed to be adjusted for left ventricular function, a risk factor for CHD, but such results were available in only eight studies. It was concluded that depression had yet to be established as an independent risk factor for CHD. However, more recent studies with large samples appear to be more conclusive.

Daskalopoulou et al. (2016) examined the risk of 12 cardiovascular diseases according to depression status, whether historical or new onset. They carried out a cohort study of a large sample of nearly 2 million adult men and women, free from cardiovascular disease at baseline, using linked UK electronic health records between 1997 and 2010. The exposures were new-onset depression based on a new GP diagnosis of depression and/or prescription for antidepressants during a one-year baseline, and history of GP-diagnosed depression before baseline. The primary endpoint was initial presentation of 12 cardiovascular diseases after baseline. Over a median of 6.9 years of follow-up, 18.9% had a history of depression and 94,432 cardiovascular events occurred. After adjustment for cardiovascular risk factors, history of depression was associated with stable angina, unstable angina, myocardial infarction, unheralded coronary death, heart failure, cardiac arrest, transient ischemic attack, ischemic stroke, subarachnoid haemorrhage, intracerebral haemorrhage, peripheral arterial disease, and abdominal aortic aneurysm. New-onset depression developed in 2.9% of people, among whom 63,761 cardiovascular events occurred. New-onset depression was similarly associated with each of the 12 diseases, with no evidence of stronger associations compared to a history of depression. The strength of association between depression and these cardiovascular diseases was not found to differ between women and men. The results of this large, well-controlled study seem fairly conclusive and depression can be accepted as a risk factor for a range of cardiovascular diseases. The precise mechanism remains uncertain.

LIVING WITH CHD

The way a person adjusts to CHD is dependent on many different factors, including their personality, support mechanisms, habits and work–life balance. Some research has focused on 'cognitive adaptation', which can be scored and used as a predictor of psychological adjustment. Helgeson and Fritz (1999) tested whether people with high cognitive adaptation scores would be less vulnerable to a new coronary event due to restenosis within six months of initial PCI. Three components of cognitive adaptation were measured: self-esteem, optimism and control. Patients with a low cognitive adaptation score were more likely to have a new cardiac event even when demographic variables and medical variables thought to predict restenosis were statistically controlled.

Depression

Waiting for invasive treatment to improve or prolong life can be very stressful and have deleterious effects on the quality of daily life. The association between CHD and depression has been a major topic for research.

Pre-surgical depression predicts cardiac hospitalization, continued surgical pain, failure to return to previous activity and depression at six months (Burg et al., 2003). Arthur et al. (2000) conducted a trial of a multi-dimensional pre-operative intervention on pre-surgery and post-surgery outcomes in low-risk patients awaiting elective CABG. The intervention consisted of individualized, prescribed exercise training twice per week in a supervised environment, education and reinforcement, and monthly nurse-initiated telephone calls to answer questions and provide reassurance. Patients who received the intervention spent one day less in the hospital and less time in the intensive care unit. Patients in the intervention group reported a better QoL during the waiting period than the control group. The improved QoL continued up to six months after surgery. Using outcome measures such as length of hospital stay as well as QoL measures provides evidence of cost-effectiveness, which is helpful for budget holders wondering whether to invest in such interventions.

Rutledge et al. (2006) carried out a meta-analytic review of prevalence, intervention effects and associations with clinical outcomes of depression in heart failure. Clinically significant depression was present in at least one in five patients with heart failure, but rates can be higher among patients screened with questionnaires. The authors concluded that the relationship between depression and poorer heart failure outcomes is consistent and strong across multiple end points. Unsurprisingly, then, depression is a common response to heart disease.

A special committee of the American Heart Association (AHA) published recommendations for the screening, referral and treatment of depression in heart patients (Lichtman et al., 2008). The committee recommended the following:

1. Routine screening for depression in patients with CHD in settings including the hospital, physician's office, clinic and cardiac rehabilitation centre.

2. Patients with positive screening results should be evaluated by a qualified mental health professional.

3. Patients with cardiac disease who are under treatment for depression should be carefully monitored for adherence to their medical care, drug efficacy and safety with respect to their cardiovascular as well as mental health.

4. Monitoring mental health may include, but is not limited to, the assessment of patients receiving antidepressants for possible worsening of depression or suicidality, especially during initial treatment when doses may be adjusted, changed or discontinued.

5. Coordination of care between health care providers is necessary in patients with combined medical and mental health diagnoses.

In 2013 the National Heart Foundation of Australia proposed similar guidelines to screen CHD patients for depression. It led to more referrals to hospital-based, community and private psychologists.

The AHA recommendations were evaluated using more recent evidence The review of the evidence four years later by Thombs et al. (2013) suggested that the evidence base for this advisory has not, after all, been sufficiently established. Thombs et al. (2013) systematically reviewed evidence on depression screening in CHD by assessing (1) the accuracy of screening tools, (2) the effectiveness of treatment, and (3) the effect of screening on depression outcomes. The authors found few examples of screening tools with good sensitivity and specificity using a priori-defined cut-offs in more than one patient sample. Treatment with antidepressants or psychotherapy generated only modest symptom reductions among post-MI and stable CHD patients, but antidepressants were not reported to improve symptoms more than placebo in two heart failure (HF) trials. Thombs et al. reported that depression treatment did not improve cardiac outcomes. There was evidence that treatment of depression results in modest improvement in depressive symptoms in post-MI and stable CHD patients, although not in HF patients. The authors concluded that 'there is still no evidence that routine screening for depression improves depression or cardiac outcomes. The AHA Science Advisory on depression screening should be revised to reflect this lack of evidence' (Thombs et al., 2013: 1).

Anger and hostility

Almost 60 years ago Friedman and Rosenman (1959) showed that patients who exhibited the 'Type A behaviour pattern' – characterized by competitiveness, excessive drive and an enhanced sense of time urgency – had more risk factors for CHD and were more likely to suffer from major adverse cardiovascular events than patients without the Type A behaviour pattern. Many studies since have found that anger and hostility, as components of the Type A pattern, are associated with the incidence of CHD in both older and younger people.

Kawachi et al. (1996) examined prospectively the relationship of anger to CHD incidence in the Veterans Administration Normative Aging Study with an ongoing cohort of older (mean age, 61 years), community-dwelling men: 1,305 men who were free of diagnosed CHD completed the revised Minnesota Multiphasic Personality Inventory (MMPI-2) in 1986. The participants were categorized according to their responses to the MMPI-2 Anger Content Scale, purporting to measure problems with anger control. During an average of seven years of follow-up, 110 cases of incident CHD occurred, with 30 cases of non-fatal myocardial infarction (MI), 20 cases of fatal CHD, and 60 cases of angina pectoris. Compared with men reporting the lowest levels of anger, the relative risks for men reporting the highest levels of anger were 3.15 for total CHD (non-fatal MI plus fatal CHD) and 2.66 for combined incident coronary events, including angina pectoris. A dose–response relation was found between level of anger and overall CHD risk, suggesting that the higher the level of expressed anger, the higher the risk for CHD among older men.

Pollock et al. (2016) used longitudinal measures to examine the prospective influence of anger in young adults. From 1985 to 1986, 768 young adults from the Bogalusa Heart Study completed the State Trait Anger Expression Inventory (STAXI) and were followed for cardio-vascular risk factors. The STAXI score is summed from a ten-item test with four response options (1 = 'never angry'; 2 = 'sometimes angry'; 3 = 'often angry'; 4 = 'almost always angry'). The study population was 63.3% female and 23.2% black. At baseline, age ranged from 17 to 27 years with a mean of 22.7, and the mean STAXI score was 18.6. After a median follow-up of 18 years, anger as a young adult was found to be strongly associated with risk of CHD, with 'always angry' people having a greater Framingham risk score at follow-up compared to those who were 'never angry'. This result corresponded to a four-fold increase in a ten-year risk of incident CHD (4% versus 1%, respectively). Pollack et al.'s analysis showed that the relationship between anger and CHD risk may be detectable in young adulthood.

Hostility is another significant predictor of mortality and cardiovascular events in patients with CHD, as indicated by many studies, but the exact mechanisms are uncertain. Wong et al. (2013) evaluated potential mechanisms of association between hostility and adverse cardiovascular outcomes. They prospectively examined the association between self-reported hostility and secondary events (myocardial infarction, heart failure, stroke, transient ischemic attack and death) in 1,022 outpatients with stable CHD. Baseline hostility was assessed using the eight-item Cynical Distrust scale. During a follow-up time of 7.4 ± 2.7 years, the age-adjusted annual rate of secondary events was 9.5% among people in the highest quartile of hostility and 5.7% among people in the lowest quartile. After adjustment for cardiovascular risk factors, participants with hostility scores in the highest quartile had a 58% greater risk of secondary events than those in the lowest quartile. Wong et al. found that the association was mainly moderated by poor health behaviours, specifically physical inactivity and smoking.

Social support

Living with CHD is often associated with fear, anxiety, depression and stress. The sufferer may worry about heart problems or making lifestyle changes that are necessary for his/her health. Social support from family and friends can be a great help in relieving stress and anxiety. Talking and sharing are both excellent ways of reducing the burden of an illness such as CHD.

Social support is of key importance in moderating the influence of negative affect on the person's well-being. Mookadam and Arthur (2004) systematically reviewed social support and its relationship to morbidity and mortality after acute myocardial infarction. Having low social support networks was a predictor of one-year mortality following acute myocardial infarction. Low social support is equivalent to many 'classic' risk factors, such as elevated cholesterol level, tobacco use and hypertension. Another review found that low functional social support is associated with prevalence of CHD and all-cause mortality, but concluded that it remained uncertain whether low structural social support causally increases mortality in patients with CHD (Barth et al., 2010).

Lack of social support predicts mortality in population studies. Orth-Gomér et al. (1993) measured emotional support from very close persons ('attachment') and the support provided by the extended network ('social integration'). They studied a random sample of 50-year-old men born in Gothenburg, Sweden, in 1933. All men ($n = 736$) were followed for six years and the incidence of myocardial infarction and death from CHD was determined. Men who contracted CHD had both lower 'attachment' and 'social integration' scores. When controlling for other risk factors, both factors remained significant predictors of new CHD events. Smoking and lack of social support were the two leading risk factors for CHD in these middle-aged men.

Fear of dying

Experiencing an acute coronary syndrome (ACS) can provoke a range of negative emotional responses, including acute distress and fear of dying. The heart is accurately viewed as the organ most essential for the preservation of life. Any perceived disturbances to the heart, especially pain, can easily trigger a fear of dying. Whitehead et al. (2005) examined the presence and severity of the fear of dying and acute distress in 184 patients with ACS. Intense distress and fear of dying was reported by 40 patients (21.7%) and moderate fear and distress by 95 patients (51.6%). Intense distress and fear were associated with female gender, lower levels of education, greater chest pain and emotional upset in the two hours before onset of ACS. Having no acute distress or fear was more common in patients who exercised regularly and who did not initially attribute the chest pain to cardiac causes. Acute distress and fear of dying predicted greater depression and anxiety one week after ACS and elevated levels of depression at three months, after adjustment for age, gender and negative affect. The authors concluded that distress and fear during the initial stages of an ACS may trigger subsequent depression and anxiety, promoting poorer prognosis and greater morbidity with time.

Malinauskaite et al. (2017) investigated whether the fear of dying after ACS can be used to predict later post-traumatic stress symptoms. They enrolled 90 patients hospitalized with a main diagnosis of ACS and assessed baseline characteristics. One month after discharge, they collected data using the Posttraumatic Stress Scale. A total of 24 patients (26.7%) were found to have developed post-traumatic stress symptoms one month after the ACS event. These patients reported significantly greater fear of dying, helplessness, avoidance-focused coping and severe anxiety.

Type D personality

Personality test scores correlate with the mental and physical health of coronary patients. Interest has been focused on 'Type D' (distressed) personality, a joint tendency towards negative affectivity and social inhibition. The DS14 scale is used to measure Type D personality. The scales for Negative Affectivity include items 2, 4, 5, 7, 9, 12 and 13. The content of some of these overlaps with the symptoms of depression, i.e., 'I often feel unhappy' (4), 'I take a gloomy view of things' (7), 'I am often in a bad mood' (9), 'I am often down in the dumps' (13). The fact that Type D and depression scores are positively associated is not very surprising. However, Type D personality scores can 'predict' illness responses independently of depression scores. That said, lest there be any doubt, we do not interpret these correlations as anything other than associations, and certainly not as causes.

Personality and depression have been empirically associated in patients treated with PCI. AL-Qezweny et al. (2016) investigated the association between Type D personality at six months post-PCI (baseline) and depression at ten-year follow-up. A secondary aim tested the association between Type D personality at baseline and anxiety at ten-year follow-up. The study was done with a cohort of surviving consecutive patients ($N = 534$) who had undergone PCI between October 2001 and October 2002. Patients completed the Type D personality scale (DS14), measuring Type D personality at baseline, and the Hospital Anxiety and Depression Scale (HADS; Zigmond and Snaith, 1983), measuring anxiety and depression at baseline and at ten years post-PCI. At baseline, the prevalence of Type D was 25%. Type D patients were more often depressed (42%) than non-Type D patients (9%). Response rate of anxiety and depression questionnaires at ten years was 75%. At ten-year follow-up, 31% of Type D personality patients were depressed versus 13% of non-Type D personality patients. After adjustments, baseline Type D personality remained independently associated with depression at ten years. Type D showed a similar association with anxiety at ten years, albeit somewhat lower. The authors concluded that PCI patients with Type D personality had a 3.69-fold increased risk for depression and a 2.72-fold increased risk for anxiety at ten-year follow-up. There are several possible reasons for these associations other than causation, one being that Type D and depression scores are both related to a third, backgound variable yet to be determined.

CARING FOR SOMEONE WITH CHD

Caring for a person with CHD at home can often be a stressful and distressing experience. Caregivers of CHD and stroke patients report a high level of emotional stress. And they have many unmet needs.

Anderson et al. (1995) studied factors associated with emotional distress in caregivers one year after stroke in patients with residual handicap. Their main caregivers were interviewed as part of the follow-up activities for patients ($n = 492$). They assessed emotional distress in caregivers using the HADS and the 28-item General Health Questionnaire. Of 241 patients who survived one year after stroke and were living outside an institution, 103 patients (43%) were handicapped, of whom 84 patient/caregiver units were assessed. Anderson et al. reported that almost all caregivers reported adverse effects on their emotional health, social activities and leisure time, and more than half reported adverse effects on family relationships. Altogether, 46 caregivers (55%) showed evidence of emotional distress, particularly if they were caregiving for patients with dementia and/or abnormal behaviour.

Moser and Dracup (2004) compared the emotional responses and perception of control of MI and revascularization patients and their spouses, and examined the relationship between spouses' emotional distress and patients' emotional distress and psychosocial adjustment to their cardiac event. They found that spouses had higher levels of anxiety and depression than the patients. There were no differences in level of hostility. The patients also had a higher level of perceived control than did the spouses. Spouse anxiety, depression and perceived control were correlated with patient psychosocial adjustment to illness even when patient anxiety and depression were kept constant. The patients' psychosocial adjustment to illness was worse when spouses were more anxious or depressed than patients. Attention should be given to the psychological needs of spouses of patients who have suffered a cardiac event. Moser and Dracup also found that patients' psychosocial adjustment was best when patients were more anxious or depressed than spouses. This finding suggests that interventions that address the psychological distress of spouses may well improve patient outcomes.

One problem for evaluation of cardiac patients' experience of QoL is identifying an instrument that is not only reliable and valid, but also responsive to change. Instruments that are not very responsive will tend to under-represent the benefits of programme attendance. Research indicates that the most responsive instruments are the Beck Depression Inventory, Global Mood Scale, Health Complaints Checklist, Heart Patients' Psychological Questionnaire and Speilberger State–Trait Anxiety Inventory.

Rees et al. (2004) reviewed psychological interventions for CHD, typically stress-management interventions. They included randomized controlled trials, either single modality interventions or a part of cardiac rehabilitation with a minimum follow-up of six months. Stress management (SM) trials were identified and reported both in combination with other psychological interventions and separately. The quality of many trials was poor, making the findings unreliable. The authors concluded that psychological interventions showed no evidence of effect on total or cardiac mortality, but small reductions in anxiety and depression in patients with CHD. Similar results were seen for SM interventions when considered separately.

INTERVENTIONS FOR CHD

People with suspected CHD usually undergo several different tests for absolute diagnosis and to determine the best treatment to relieve symptoms. These include stress **exercise tolerance test (ETT), electrocardiogram (ECG)** and **coronary angiogram.** Seeking a diagnosis can be a stressful time for people with suspected CHD and their family and friends. Patients commonly feel apprehension about the procedure and find some parts of the procedure are unexpected, with doctors' technical language being an obstacle to understanding.

Many people with CHD are recommended to make lifestyle changes and take a regime of medication such as **ACE (angiotensin converting enzyme) inhibitors,** statins, anticoagulant drugs and beta-blockers. Clinical guidelines are not always implemented because of a lack of time for physicians, who only have a few minutes to discuss risk factors, lifestyle changes or treatment. This may not be an appropriate time to discuss such issues with a patient, who may well feel shocked by the diagnosis of being at risk of CHD and they may also show low levels of compliance with physician advice.

Riesen et al. (2004) acknowledged that, although high rates of compliance with lifestyle changes and lipid-lowering agents are reported in clinical trials, rarely are the findings reproduced in regular practice. They recommended the use of educational materials as well as regular telephone contact to improve compliance. However, further research is needed into the causes of poor compliance and methods of improving adherence with lipid-lowering agents. We now turn to discuss interventions for the two main categories of CHD patients: those with MI and those with angina.

Myocardial infarction

Guidelines for the management of CHD recommend cardiac rehabilitation, or 'cardiac rehab' (CR). This is a structured programme of rehabilitation for people who have had a heart attack, heart failure, heart valve surgery, coronary artery bypass grafting or PCI. It involves making changes towards a more 'heart-healthy' lifestyle to reduce established risk factors for cardiovascular disease. CR will typically include exercise training, education on heart-healthy living and counselling to reduce stress. CR aims to improve the participants' health and quality of life, reduce the need for medication, decrease heart or chest pain and the chance of recurrence. CR is usually provided in an outpatient clinic or hospital rehab centre. The CR team includes doctors, nurses, exercise specialists, physical and occupational therapists, dietitians or nutritionists, and mental health specialists. A standard CR programme includes 36 supervised sessions over 12 weeks.

A large number of MI patients do not return to work or regain normal functioning, despite being physically well. There is evidence that CR programmes can reduce distress and disability, increase confidence and improve modifiable risk factors. However, many patients do not attend rehab programmes after their MI. Patients' beliefs about their illness are alleged to be determinants of recovery after an MI. Petrie et al. (2002) evaluated a brief hospital intervention designed to alter patients' perceptions of their MI. The content of the intervention was individualized according to the patients' responses on the Illness Perception Questionnaire (Weinman et al., 1996). The intervention caused significant positive changes in patients' views of their MI. The intervention group reported being better prepared for leaving hospital and subsequently returned to work at a significantly faster rate than the control group. At the three-month follow-up, the intervention group reported a significantly lower rate of angina symptoms.

Stewart et al. (2004) found a difference in the health information needs between men and women recovering from an acute coronary event. Men who had received significantly more information reported greater satisfaction with health care professionals meeting their information needs. Women reported wanting more information than men concerning angina and hypertension. Men wanted more information about sexual function. Patients who reported receiving more information reported less depressive symptomatology. Most patients of both sexes preferred a shared decision-making role with their doctor. The majority felt their doctor had made the main decisions. CR that is individualized to patients' needs may be more attractive and effective than thinking of CR as a place to do exercise and be informed about lifestyle changes. However, individually tailored CR is costly and demand far outstrips supply.

Evaluations of CR have used a variety of methods, including RCTs, observational studies and qualitative studies. RCTs of cardiac rehabilitation following MI typically demonstrate a lower mortality in treated patients, but a statistically significant reduction is generally lacking. In an early review, Oldridge et al. (1988) carried out a meta-analysis on the results of ten RCTs that included 4,347 patients (control: 2,145 patients; CR: 2,202 patients). The pooled odds ratios of 0.76 for all-cause death and of 0.75 for cardiovascular death were significantly lower in the rehab group than in the control group, with no significant difference for non-fatal recurrent MI. The results suggested that comprehensive CR has a beneficial effect on mortality but not on non-fatal recurrent MI.

However, findings concerning CR have been modest and not always consistent, and doubts about the applicability of evidence from existing meta-analyses of exercise-based CR have been raised. In addition, the current model of CR delivery (e.g., 36 exercise and educational sessions delivered 3 weekly for 12 weeks) no longer appears to be financially viable or sustainable due to multiple factors, as recently reviewed in detail (Arena, 2015; Sandesara et al., 2015). Also, only a fraction of eligible patients are able to participate in and complete CR.

One of the primary sources for state-of-the-art reviews of therapies is Cochrane, previously known as the Cochrane Collaboration. Cochrane is an independent, non-profit, non-governmental organization consisting of a group of around 40,000 volunteers in more than 130 countries. Cochrane was founded in 1993 and conducts systematic reviews of RCTs of health care interventions and diagnostic tests.

Anderson et al. (2016) updated the Cochrane systematic review and meta-analysis of exercise-based CR for CHD. They included RCTs with at least six months of follow-up, comparing CR to no-exercise controls following myocardial infarction or revascularization, or with a diagnosis of angina pectoris or CHD defined by angiography. A total of 63 studies with 14,486 participants with median follow-up of 12 months were included. CR was associated with a reduction in cardiovascular mortality (relative risk: 0.74) and the risk of hospital admissions (relative risk: 0.82). However, no significant effect occurred on total mortality, myocardial infarction or revascularization. The majority of studies (14 of 20) also showed higher levels of health-related QoL following exercise-based CR compared with control conditions. This study confirmed in a fairly conclusive manner that exercise-based CR reduces cardiovascular mortality, hospital admissions and improvements in quality of life. According to the reviewers, these benefits were consistent across patients and intervention types and were independent of study quality, setting and publication date.

The Cochrane review by Anderson et al. led to a call in the *Journal of the American College of Cardiology* to 'rebrand and reinvigorate' CR. Lavie et al. (2016: 14) have suggested that:

> Alternative secondary prevention models do not need to replace conventional CR, but they should be used to reach a much larger patient population over an extended duration, that is, well beyond the traditional 12-week window. With such efforts, not only will CR be increasingly employed, but also an enhanced and invigorated CR brand may transform its effect from the individual to the population level and re-establish, or even improve upon, the previously reported overall mortality benefits of this intervention.

Angina

Angina affects more than 50 million people worldwide. Some of the major concerns for people living with angina are the regular occurrence of chest pain, anxiety, fear of dying and depression. Providers of interventions have needed to consider efficient ways of reaching the maximum audience in the most cost-effective manner.

One intervention in the UK has combined professional and lay practitioners. Lewin et al. (2002) evaluated the efficacy of a cognitive behavioural therapy (CBT) disease management programme, the **Angina Plan** (AP; Box 21.1), to aid the psychological adjustment of patients with newly diagnosed angina. At six-month follow-up, AP patients showed a significantly greater reduction in anxiety, depression, frequency of angina, use of glyceryl trinitrate and physical limitations. They were also more likely to report a change in diet and they increased their daily walking.

BOX 21.1

The Angina Plan: A psychological disease management programme for people with angina

The Angina Plan (AP) consists of a patient-held booklet and audio-taped relaxation programme. Before commencing the 30–40-minute AP session, the patient is sent a questionnaire designed to establish whether she/he holds any of the common misconceptions about angina (e.g., each episode is a mini-heart attack or angina is caused because the heart is worn out). The patient's partner or a friend is invited to the session.

After blood pressure has been taken and body mass index has been recorded, the AP facilitator discusses any misconceptions that were revealed in the questionnaire with the patient and, if possible, his or her partner in an effort to correct their understanding. Personal risk factors are identified and personal goals to reduce the risk factors are then set. They are provided with a relaxation tape and encouraged to use it. The Plan also contains written information, such as the role of frightening thoughts and misconceptions in triggering adrenaline (epinephrine) release and anxiety, and how this can result in poor coping strategies.

(Continued)

The patient is contacted by the facilitator at the end of weeks 1, 4, 8 and 12. During these phone calls, the patient is praised for any success. They are also asked whether they want to extend successful goals. Unsuccessful goals can be revisited. Adding procedures that encourage specific implementation intentions to this programme could well improve the success of the AP.

Zetta et al. (2011) carried out a trial to evaluate the AP against standard care (SC) with 218 hospitalized angina patients assessed pre-discharge and six months later. A structured interview, self-report and physiological measurement were used to assess between-group changes in mood, knowledge and misconceptions, cardiovascular risk, symptoms, QoL and health service utilization. The intention-to-treat analysis found no reliable effects on anxiety and depression at six months. However, Zetta et al. found that AP participants reported increased knowledge, less misconceptions, reduced body mass index, increased self-reported exercise, less functional limitation, as well as improvements in general health perceptions and social and leisure activities compared to those receiving SC.

Source: Lewin et al. (2002)

Nelson et al. (2013) conducted a qualitative study as part of an RCT comparing a lay-facilitated Angina Plan with usual care. The aim was to explore participants' beliefs, experiences and attitudes to the care they had received during the trial, particularly those who had received the angina management intervention. They ran four participant focus groups during 2008; three were with people randomized to the intervention ($n = 10$) and one with those randomized to control ($n = 4$). The authors state that both similarities and differences were observed between control and intervention groups. Similarities included low levels of prior knowledge about angina, whereas differences included a perception among intervention participants that lifestyle changes were more easily facilitated with the help and support of a lay worker. Nelson et al. concluded that lay facilitation with the Angina Plan is perceived by the participants to be beneficial in supporting self-management. However, clinical expertise is required to meet the more complex information and care needs of people with stable angina.

Another method has been to provide an internet-based intervention. Devi et al. (2014) evaluated the effectiveness of a web-based CR programme for people with angina. They conducted an RCT recruiting angina patients from GPs in primary care to an intervention or control group. The intervention group were offered a six-week web-based rehabilitation programme ('ActivateYourHeart'). The programme was introduced face-to-face and then delivered via the internet without further face-to-face contact. The programme contained information about CHD and set goals around physical activity, diet, managing emotions and smoking. Performance against goals was reviewed during the programme and goals were reset as they went along. Participants completed an exercise diary and communicated with rehab specialists through an email link/chat room. The control group continued with GP treatment as usual, which consisted of an annual review. Outcomes were measured at six-week and six-month follow-ups during face-to-face assessments. A total of 94 participants were recruited and randomized to the intervention ($n = 48$) or the usual care ($n = 46$) group; 84 and 73 participants completed the six-week and six-month follow-ups, respectively.

The average number of log-ins to the programme was 18.68, an average of three per week per participant. Change in daily steps walked at the six-week follow-up was +497 in the intervention group and –861 in the control group. Significant effects were observed at the six-week follow-up in energy expenditure, duration of sedentary activity, duration of moderate activity, weight, self-efficacy, emotional QoL score and angina frequency. Significant benefits in angina frequency and social QoL scores were also observed at the six-month follow-up. The results of this trial suggest that an internet-based secondary prevention intervention is both feasible and acceptable to people with angina, although it is necessary to run a trial with a larger sample. The use of the internet for CHD interventions has good potential.

FUTURE RESEARCH

1. We need to know more about the potential role of lay practitioners in the delivery of angina and MI interventions on a wider scale than is possible at present.

2. The association and role of depression in recurrence of CHD episodes needs further study in large-scale trials with robust designs.

3. The delivery of web-based systems of intervention and support using social media and apps warrants in-depth examination.

4. More qualitative research is necessary to enable interventions to be fine-tuned to meet the unmet needs of patients.

SUMMARY

1. CHD is a leading cause of death which can bring many medical and psychosocial issues into the lives of patients and their caregivers.
2. The two main forms of CHD are myocardial infarction and angina, which are both related to a narrowing of coronary arteries caused by plaque.
3. Decreases in CHD death rates are mainly due to reduction of a few major risk factors, principally smoking.
4. Seeking treatment for CHD can be stressful for both people with CHD and their family members.
5. Psychological disease management can help angina patients to adjust, but psychological services are currently patchy and inadequate.
6. The positive role of social and emotional support from family and friends has been repeatedly demonstrated in relief of stress and anxiety.
7. Cardiac rehabilitation has been shown to be effective in reducing cardiovascular mortality, hospital admissions and improvements in quality of life, but it is accessible to only a minority of cardiac patients.
8. An angina self-management plan has been shown to enable significant gains, including increased knowledge, reduced body mass index, less functional limitation and improvements in general health perceptions.
9. The challenge of delivering interventions that are effective and cost-efficient can be met using a combination of professional, lay and web-based provision.

HIV INFECTION AND AIDS: THE PINNACLE OF STIGMA AND VICTIM BLAMING

'Although stigma is considered a major barrier to effective responses to the HIV/AIDS epidemic, stigma reduction efforts are relegated to the bottom of AIDS programme priorities.'

Mahajan et al. (2008: S67)

OUTLINE

In this chapter, we consider the most highly stigmatized conditions of modern times, HIV-seropositivity and AIDS. We describe the nature and causes of the illness, the main risk factors and at-risk groups. We discuss the psychosocial issues of people living with HIV infection/AIDS and of people caring for someone with the condition, and interventions. We also discuss stigmatization from the viewpoint of the socio-cognitive and structural approaches. Research on different types of intervention for different population groups and the results of recent meta-analyses of interventions for stigma reduction indicate limited impact, leaving major challenges for the care of people living with HIV and AIDS.

WHAT ARE HIV INFECTION AND AIDS?

HIV infection and AIDS constitute a worldwide pandemic that has infected around 60 million people and has become the fourth largest killer in the world. There are estimated to be around 2 million new cases each year and about 1 million deaths annually from **AIDS (acquired immune deficiency syndrome)**. **HIV (human immunodeficiency virus)** is a retrovirus that infects and colonizes cells in the immune system and the central nervous system (T-helper and monocyte macrophage cells). Initial flu-like symptoms are followed by a quiescent, asymptomatic period (lasting years) during which the immune system battles the virus. Eventually, the virus compromises the immune system and the individual becomes symptomatic. The immune system is overwhelmed and the individual becomes vulnerable to opportunistic diseases, signifying the development of AIDS and, eventually, likely resulting in death.

An HIV particle is around 100–150 billionths of a metre in diameter, one-seventieth the size of a human CD4+ white blood cell. HIV particles are coated with fatty material known as the viral envelope or membrane; 72 spikes, formed from the proteins gp120 and gp41, project out of the membrane. Below the viral envelope is the matrix layer, made from protein p17. The core is usually bullet-shaped and made from the protein p24. Inside the core there are three enzymes, called reverse transcriptase, integrase and protease, together with HIV's genetic material, consisting of two identical strands of ribonucleic acid (RNA).

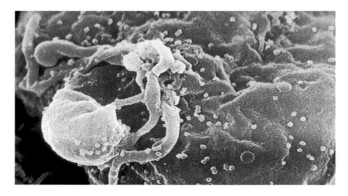

Figure 22.1   The human immunodeficiency virus

Scanning electron micrograph of HIV-1 (in light grey) budding from cultured lymphocyte. Multiple round bumps on cell surface represent sites of assembly and budding of virions

Source: Centers for Disease Control and Prevention (2010)

INCIDENCE AND PREVALENCE

HIV infection rates vary across different regions. By the end of 2014, an estimated 36.9 million people were living with HIV worldwide, an increase of 24% since 2001. The number of deaths peaked in 2004 and since then have declined slightly. This was the result of the continued large number of new HIV infections and significant expansion of access to combination antiretroviral therapy (cART), which has helped to reduce AIDS-related deaths. Part of the large number of new infections can be attributed to increased access to testing. An estimated 34 million people worldwide have died of AIDS-related illnesses since the beginning of the epidemic, with tuberculosis (TB) being the most common cause of death among people living with HIV.

The number of people with HIV has risen in every region of the world in the past decade. In 2015, the global prevalence of HIV infection was 0.8%. The vast majority of this number live in low- and middle-income countries. In the same year, 1.1 million people died of AIDS-related illnesses (UNAIDS (Joint United Nations Programme on HIV/AIDS), 2016). Since the start of the epidemic, an estimated 78 million people have become infected with HIV and 35 million people have died of AIDS-related illnesses. An estimated 25.5 million people living with HIV live in sub-Saharan Africa. The vast majority (an estimated 19 million) live in East and Southern Africa, which saw 46% of new HIV infections globally in 2015. Around 40% of all people living with HIV do not know that they have the virus (Figure 22.2).

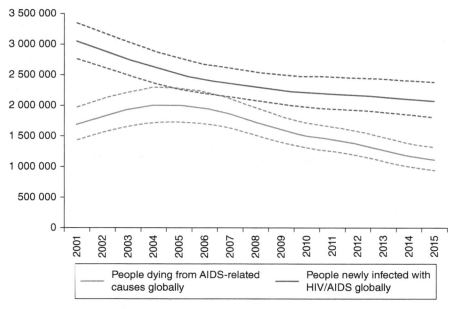

Figure 22.2 Numbers of people newly infected with HIV and numbers dying from AIDS-related causes globally

Source: UNAIDS, 2016. Public domain

Unprotected sexual intercourse is commonplace in many regions, which creates a health burden from people with HIV infection. The figures for developing countries are high, and the high cost of medicines is prohibiting the most effective forms of treatment. For example, in South Africa, where most HIV care is provided on an outpatient basis, hospitals continue to treat serious HIV-related admissions. This inpatient treatment is relatively resource-intensive and expensive. The three most common reasons for admission are tuberculosis and other mycobacterial infections (18%), cardiovascular disorders (12%) and bacterial infections (12%) (Long et al., 2016). African herbal medicines are often used to treat people living with HIV infection and their efficacy is non-existent (Mills et al., 2005).

cART

In 1996, the introduction of combination antiretroviral therapy (cART), also referred to as 'ART' or 'HAART', redefined the illness and improved the outlook for infected individuals. cART refers to the use of combinations of antiretroviral drugs with different mechanisms of action to treat HIV. cART is the treatment of choice for HIV or AIDS, and has to be taken every day for the rest of a person's life. The aim of antiretroviral treatment is to keep the amount of HIV in the body at a low level. This stops the weakening of the immune system and allows it to recover from any damage that HIV may have caused. However, antiretrovirals do not eliminate the virus, they only suppress it, and currently only four in ten who need the treatment actually receive it. HIV persistence eventually causes disease in all infected persons (Sleasman and Goodenow, 2003).

cART was given to 13.5 million people from low- and middle-income countries in 2015. The number of people becoming infected with HIV continues to fall, but more rapidly in some countries than others. HIV rates have fallen by 50% or more in 26 countries since 2001. There has been a significant reduction in areas such as the Caribbean and among newborn babies. However, there has also been a substantial increase in regions such as the Middle East and North Africa, and in Eastern Europe and Central Asia. Denial has been a factor in reducing access to cART in South Africa, and access to cART in African countries, India and China is still far below optimum levels (Figure 22.3).

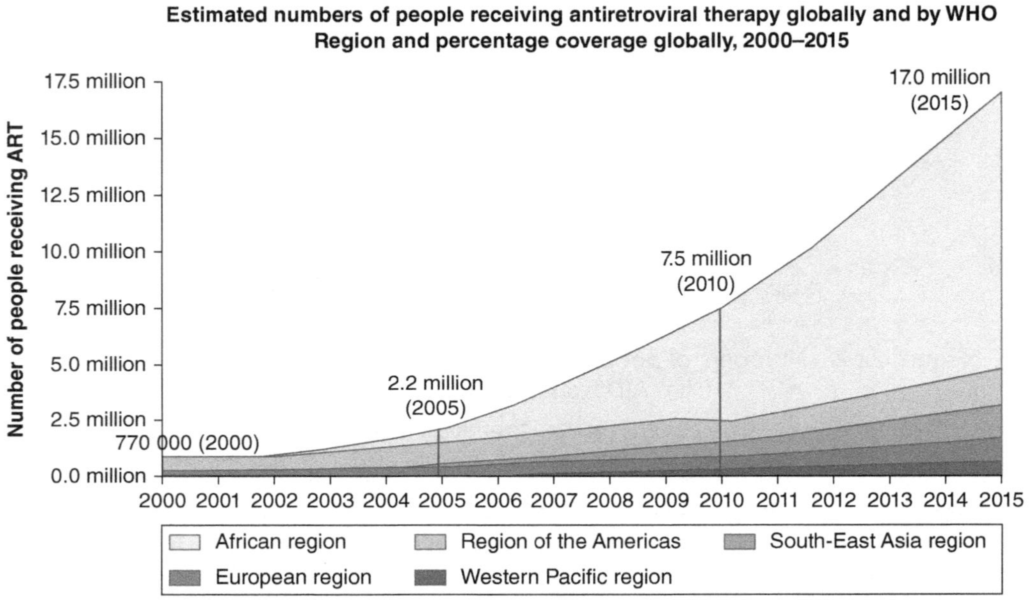

Estimated numbers of people receiving antiretroviral therapy globally and by WHO Region and percentage coverage globally, 2000–2015

Figure 22.3   Estimated numbers of people receiving cART and percentage coverage globally

Source: UNAIDS (2016). Public domain

One concern has been that, following the arrival of cART, people at risk might increase the already high rate of unprotected sex. This phenomenon of '**risk compensation**' has been observed in a variety of situations where new protective measures are introduced, such as the wearing of safety helmets by cyclists (Gamble and Walker, 2016).

Crepaz et al. (2004) conducted meta-analyses to determine whether (1) being treated with cART, (2) having an undetectable viral load, or (3) holding specific beliefs about cART and viral load were associated with increased likelihood of engaging in unprotected sex. Twenty-five English-language studies were screened and information from eligible studies was abstracted independently by pairs of reviewers using a standardized spreadsheet. The findings suggested that the prevalence of unprotected sex was not higher among persons with the human immunodeficiency virus (HIV) receiving cART than among those not receiving cART, or among HIV-positive persons with an undetectable viral load versus those with a detectable viral load. However, the prevalence of unprotected sex was elevated by 82% in HIV-positive, HIV-negative and unknown serostatus persons who believed that receiving cART or having an undetectable viral load protects against transmitting HIV, or who had reduced concerns about engaging in unsafe sex given the availability of cART. The authors concluded that 'people's beliefs about cART and viral load may promote unprotected sex and may be amenable to change through prevention messages' (Crepaz et al., 2004: 224).

Adherence to cART is necessary for the prevention of AIDS and adherence rates are strongly related to the degree of protection afforded (Bangsberg et al., 2001). Medication side effects are the most significant deterrent to adherent use of any medicine, including cART. Ammassari et al. (2001) examined the expected association between non-adherence and self-reported side effects of the medication: 358 persons were enrolled, of whom 22% reported non-adherence and were 51% less likely to have HIV RNA <500 copies/ml.[1] Frequency of moderate/severe symptoms or medication side effects in non-adherent participants ranged from 3.6% to 30%. On univariate analysis, nausea, anxiety, confusion, vision problems, anorexia, insomnia, taste perversion and abnormal fat distribution were significantly associated with non-adherence. Non-adherent persons had a higher mean overall symptom score and mean medication side effect score when compared with adherent participants. In the multivariate analysis, nausea, anxiety, younger age, unemployment, not recalling the name, colour and timing of drugs, running out of pills between visits and being 'too busy' were independently associated with non-adherence over the previous three days.

Vian et al. (2016) explored the role of motivation in predicting cART adherence in China. They tested whether self-determination theory could predict adherence behaviour among 115 HIV-positive patients. The study formed part of the 'China Adherence through Technology Study', a randomized controlled trial of an intervention using text reminders and supportive counselling to increase adherence. The treatment had a significant effect on improving adherence, although self-determination theory failed to predict adherence in HIV-positive patients.

Houston et al. (2016) examined the role of depressive symptoms and treatment self-efficacy in cART adherence. Depression is often associated with poor HIV treatment adherence. Using a sample of 84 cART patients with depressive symptoms, they examined whether patients with optimal adherence differed from those with suboptimal adherence in terms of type of depressive symptoms and treatment self-efficacy. There were no significant differences between participants with regard to types of depressive symptom. Patients with high treatment self-efficacy were more likely to report optimal levels of adherence than patients with low self-efficacy.

One strategy in research on HIV prevention is to focus on risk factors and at-risk groups.

RISK FACTORS AND AT-RISK GROUPS

Risk factors for HIV infection are: unprotected intercourse, injection drug use, sexually transmitted infections (STIs), blood exposure, mother–foetus transmission, mother–infant childbirth transmission and breastfeeding transmission. For nearly all of these risks, stigmatization and

---

[1] A viral load of 500 or fewer HIV RNA copies per mL is considered to be low, while a viral load of 40,000 or more HIV RNA copies per mL is considered high.

victim-blaming have been as damaging to those affected as the disease process itself. The reasons are not difficult to comprehend, as contemporary society becomes ever more divisive with privileged elites controlling ever more power and wealth while the '99 percent' at the bottom of the pyramid are feeling increasingly alienated and dispossessed.

The classic formulation of stigma is that of Erving Goffman (1963: 3), wherein stigma is 'an attribute that is deeply discrediting' and that reduces the bearer 'from a whole and usual person to a tainted, discounted one'. Society stigmatizes on the basis of what is considered as 'difference' or 'deviance', and results in a 'spoiled identity'. The label of 'deviance' requires stigmatized individuals to view themselves as discredited or undesirable. Goffman's theorization of stigma was extended by theorizing the origins of stigma in human cognition. This socio-cognitive, individualistic framework constrained the concept of H/A stigma (the stigmatization of people living with HIV and AIDS) to an examination of how people living with HIV infection or AIDS (PLHA) are labelled and stereotyped by the public, based on their incorrect beliefs and attitudes, and/or a focus on the specific emotions and cognition of PLHA (Majahan et al., 2008). This approach limited H/A stigma reduction interventions to strategies aiming to increase empathy and altruism towards as well as reduce the anxiety and fear of PLHA among the general population, or individual-based interventions to assist PLHA to cope with perceived or experienced stigma. In their review, Mahajan et al. (2008) observed that the great majority of articles on H/A stigma measurement and reduction interventions either implicitly or explicitly utilized a socio-cognitive conception of stigma. These approaches exclude consideration of structural aspects of stigma – the dynamic social/economic/political processes that simultaneously produce and intensify stigma and discrimination.

Adopting a structural approach, Parker and Aggleton (2003) conceptualized stigmatization as intimately linked to the *reproduction of social difference*. They suggested that 'stigma feeds upon, strengthens and reproduces existing inequalities of class, race, gender and sexuality' (Parker and Aggleton, 2003: 13). They highlighted the limitations of individualistic modes of stigma alleviation and called for a new approach wherein the resistance of stigmatized individuals and communities can be a resource for social change. Stigmatization, they argued, is linked with the workings of social inequality by its capacity *to cause some groups to be devalued and other groups to feel that they are superior*. In viewing stigma at the intersection of culture, power and difference, Parker and Aggleton argued that stigmatization reinforces the constitution of the prevailing social order. Stigma, in this formulation, is a scaffolding of power and preserves the status quo. For this reason, one can understand why the main approach to reducing stigma is akin to tinkering rather than to target root-and-branch change of the causal processes.

Following Parker and Aggleton, a review by Mahajan et al. (2008) supported the idea that stigma is a structural issue wherein power differentials are reproduced between different societal groups. The framework for the production of stigmatization proposed by Mahajan et al. is shown in Figure 22.4. The Mahajan et al. framework shows the production of stigma across a number of domains at both individual and structural levels. We have a stepped pyramid from the bottom to the pinnacle of stigmatization.

Starting from the foundations of power at the foot of the pyramid, there is the structural violence of racism, sexism and poverty along with pre-existing stigma against groups that are seen as deviant, such as commercial sex workers, injecting drug users and men who have sex with men (MSM). Going up a level, people are labelled on the basis of HIV status or their risk of infection and insulted with terms like 'scum' or 'dirty' or 'queer'. Up another level and there is an 'othering' of 'them' versus 'us', a crucial step towards full-blown stigmatization.

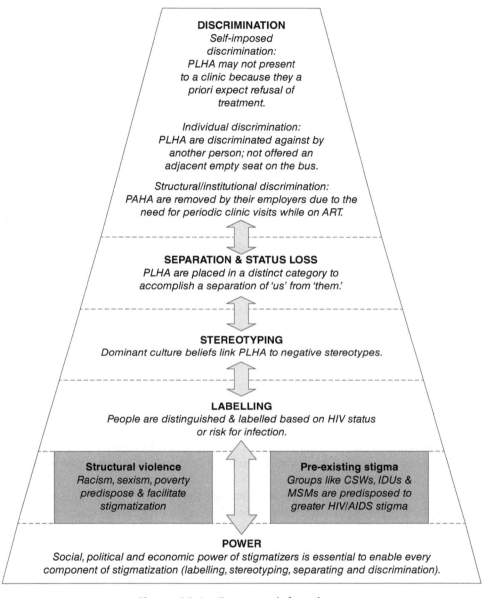

Figure 22.4   Framework for stigma

Up to the pinnacle, and we observe discriminating and devaluing behaviours which make the covert processes of the lower levels completely overt, along with self-imposed discrimination (e.g., non-presentation at clinics), individual discrimination (e.g., not being offered a seat on a bus), and structural or institutional discrimination (e.g., being fired by employer for absenteeism).

In spite of decades of health education, there is still widespread ignorance about STIs and HIV. The National AIDS Trust (2011) reported that one in five people still did not realize that HIV infection can be passed on through sex without a condom between a man and a woman, and worryingly, knowledge of this fact had fallen by 11% in the previous decade. One in ten people incorrectly believed HIV infection can be transmitted through impossible routes, such as kissing (9%) and spitting (10%), and these figures had doubled since 2007 (from 4% and 5%, respectively). In the field of HIV/AIDS, health education has been an expensive but disastrous failure. We turn to consider reasons why this might be the case by considering different population groups who are at risk of HIV infection.

Mother–foetus transmission

Routinely offering HIV testing to pregnant women during their first antenatal visit and retesting them in the third trimester and during breastfeeding is the gold standard in high-incidence settings (World Health Organization, 2015a). Some countries have inadequate health care infrastructure, poor linkages between HIV and maternal and child health services, and lack of awareness of the importance of routinely offering HIV testing, which prevents many women living with HIV from being reached. Traditional beliefs, cultural practices, stigma and discrimination, lack of confidentiality within health care settings, and transportation challenges also hinder access and contribute to the under-utilization of services (Njau et al., 2014).

Pregnant women may avoid medical help due to fear of stigma, discrimination and violence when disclosing their HIV status. Going against community norms of feeding leads to questions about a mother's HIV status, unwanted disclosure, and fear of stigma from partner, family and the community (Mahajan et al., 2008). Community-level education targeting pregnant women, community leaders and people of childbearing age is critical to improving acceptability of services and diminishing the effects of stigma.

Mother–infant transmission

Antiretroviral medicines need to be provided during pregnancy and delivery to minimize the risk of transmission to infants. HIV-negative new mothers at high risk of HIV are also insufficiently tested while they are breastfeeding. As a result, infants are exposed unknowingly to HIV during breastfeeding, with half of all mother-to-child HIV transmissions occurring during this period (World Health Organization, 2015a).

Many women living with HIV are not aware that they need to remain in treatment while breastfeeding, and opportunities to reinforce the adherence messages and resupply women with medication are fewer once the baby is born, as women reduce their contact with the health system. Even when the baby is immunized, it may not be the mother who makes the visit to the clinic, relying instead on an older sibling or a grandparent while the mother works. Side effects from cART and personal perception of wellness can also lead mothers to stop taking their medication (Kim et al., 2016). Insufficient adherence support of breastfeeding women living with HIV has seen postnatal HIV transmissions from mother to child remain higher than 5% in 8 of 21 high-priority countries (UNAIDS, 2016).

Although AIDS-related deaths among children have reduced dramatically in recent years, the vast majority of deaths still occur during the first five years of life. Early HIV diagnosis and early antiretroviral therapy greatly reduce infant mortality and HIV progression. Without antiretroviral therapy, 50% of children living with HIV die before their second birthday. Tuberculosis (TB) is a common killer. In 2015, about 40,000 children living with HIV died from TB. Coverage of early infant diagnosis remains low, however: only 4 of 21 priority countries – Lesotho, South Africa, Swaziland and Zimbabwe – provided HIV testing to more than half the infants exposed to HIV within their first eight weeks (UNAIDS, 2016).

TB is common among PLHA. Among pregnant women living with HIV, TB is associated with higher maternal and infant mortality. Maternal TB is also independently associated with a 2.5-times increased risk of HIV transmission to exposed infants. All pregnant women and new mothers living with HIV should be screened for TB symptoms, and children living with HIV should be fully investigated if they have signs or symptoms suggestive of TB (UNAIDS, 2016).

Men who have sex with men

Men who have sex with men (MSM) have been a focus for much research. AIDS prevention among MSM has overwhelmingly focused on sexual risk alone. Stall et al. (2003) measured the extent to which psychosocial health problems have an additive effect on increasing HIV risk among MSM. They conducted a cross-sectional household probability telephone sample of MSM in Chicago, Los Angeles, New York and San Francisco. Stall et al. measured poly-drug use as use of three or more recreational drugs (e.g., marijuana, cocaine, crack cocaine, heroin, hallucinogens, inhalants, amphetamines, methamphetamine, MDMA ['ecstasy'], barbiturates or tranquilizers and painkillers) in the past six months. They also used the Center for Epidemiological Studies–Depression scale to score levels of depression, with scores greater than 22 indicating depression. In addition, they measured partner violence as the experience of any form of violence, whether symbolic, physical or sexual, in the past five years with a primary partner, and also childhood sexual abuse as the experience of being 'forced or frightened by someone into doing something sexually' with a partner more than 10 years older than the respondent when the respondent was aged 16 years or younger. Psychosocial health problems were found to be highly intercorrelated among urban MSM. Greater numbers of health problems were positively associated with high-risk sexual behaviour and HIV infection.

Other studies have focused upon how MSM may attempt to reduce HIV risk by adapting condom use, partner selection or sexual position to the partner's HIV serostatus. This practice is known as 'serosorting'. Vallabhaneni et al. (2012) assessed the association of serosorting practices with HIV acquisition in 12,277 US participants, with 663 HIV-positive conversions. No unprotected anal intercourse (UAI) was reported in 47.4% of intervals; UAI with some seroadaptive practices in 31.8%; and UAI with no seroadaptive practices in 20.4%. Vallabhaneni et al. found that serosorting appeared to be protective when compared with UAI without serosorting, but serosorting appeared to be twice as risky as no UAI. Condom use and limiting the number of partners should remain the first-line prevention strategy, but serosorting reduces risk of harm for men at greatest risk.

Low Literacy

An important barrier to risk reduction is low literacy. Kalichman et al. (1999) tested the significance of health literacy relative to other predictors of adherence to treatment for HIV infection and AIDS. Kalichman et al. studied a community sample of HIV-seropositive men and women taking a triple-drug combination of antiretroviral therapies for HIV infection; 60% were from ethnic minorities and 73% had been diagnosed with AIDS. The findings showed that education and health literacy were significant predictors of treatment adherence after controlling for age, ethnicity, income, symptoms of HIV infection, substance abuse, social support, emotional distress and attitudes towards primary care providers. They found that people who were low in literacy were more likely to miss treatment doses because of confusion, depression and the desire to cleanse their body than were participants with higher health literacy. The authors concluded:

> People of lower literacy may benefit from pictorial displays of their medications, accurate in color and size, with graphic illustration of the instructions including the number of pills to be taken, and at what times. In addition, videotapes tailored to different levels of comprehension may provide a more effective medium than pamphlets and brochures for educating patients about their treatments. Intensive case management and assertive assistance programs may be required for those persons with the greatest difficulty understanding their treatment regimen and the importance of adherence. (Kalichman et al., 1999: 271)

Hittner and Kryzanowski (2010) investigated academic performance, residential status, class rank and gender as predictors of risky sexual behaviour under two different substance use contexts: being 'drunk or high' and 'not drunk or high'. Results indicated that gender moderated the association between residential status and risky sex, such that males living on-campus engaged in more frequent casual sex than males living off-campus. All studies on sexual behaviour using self-reports tend to find disparities between the males' and females' reports in line with gender stereotypes in which it has traditionally been 'macho' to report plenty of encounters and 'feminine' to report few, a well-known 'double standard'.

Denialism

A more insidious barrier to risk behaviour reduction is pseudoscience and the associated 'denialism', the organized, widespread form of denial such as occurred in South Africa and to a lesser extent in other regions, including the USA. Deniers promote the idea that HIV infection is a myth or that HIV treatments are poison. Their position is fuelled by pseudoscience, faulty logic, conspiracy theories, homophobia and racism (Kalichman, 2009). Individuals may refuse to be tested, ignore their diagnoses or reject the treatments that could save their lives based on pseudoscientific misinformation propogated by powerful figures such as President Mbeki in South Africa. Against the consensus of scientific opinion, Mbeki argued that HIV infection was not the cause of AIDS and that antiretroviral (ART) drugs were not useful for patients, and so he declined to accept freely donated nevirapine and grants from the Global Fund. It has been estimated that more than 330,000 lives or approximately 2.2 million person-years were lost because a feasible and timely ART treatment programme was not implemented in South Africa between 2000 and 2005 (Chigwedere et al., 2008).

Inconsistent condom usage and other risk behaviours are not caused only by lack of awareness or knowledge, or optimistic bias (e.g., Chapin, 2001). They can be influenced by misinformation and phony science. Motivational and emotional factors play a very significant role, as do cultural and sub-cultural norms. Explaining and reducing sexual risk taking is a significant challenge. The simplest 'take-home message' is to use protection at all times.

LIVING WITH HIV INFECTION OR AIDS

People living with HIV infection or AIDS (PLHA) face the general stressors of the chronically ill and may face additional stresses unique to HIV infection and AIDS, e.g., additional uncertainty and decision-making due to rapidly changing treatment developments/outlook, infectivity persistence, the imperative for major behaviour change (e.g., sexual behaviour), anticipatory grief and the excessive stigma associated with the condition. The quality of life of PLHA is severely compromised, particularly in the later stages of the disease, due to pain (experienced by 30–90% of PLHA), discomfort and mobility difficulties (e.g., Hughes et al., 2004).

The major stressors encountered by PLHA are summarized in Box 22.1. Different stressors may be experienced at different stages of the illness, with stress peaks at initial diagnosis, onset of symptomology, sudden immune system cell (CD4) count decline, onset of opportunistic infections and diagnosis of AIDS.

BOX 22.1

Stressors related to HIV infection and AIDS

Disease-related stressors

Being tested and receiving test results

Diagnoses – seropositivity, symptomatic phase and AIDS

Treatment commencement

Intermittent symptoms and opportunistic disease

Emergence of new symptoms

For children, neurocognitive and emotional developmental problems

Developing drug resistance and treatment failures

Co-infections (e.g., hepatitis)

Further exposure to the virus

Medication side effects

Pain, discomfort, sexual difficulties, mobility restrictions and progressive physical deterioration

Complications from ongoing substance use

Drug trials and drug holidays

External life-stressors

Enacted H/A stigma (e.g., ostracism and discrimination)

Disclosure reactions

Bereavement

Substance use

Employment changes

(Continued)

Reduced income

Loss/lack of health insurance

Access to treatment

Rejection and loss of social support

Uncertainty

Emotional/psychological stressors

Felt H/A stigma (internalization, fear, shame, guilt)

Disclosure decisions

Reproductive decision-making

Grief

Risk behaviour and decision-making

Anger

Rejection and isolation

Changing expectations

Preparing for death

Guilt

Few conditions have provoked such unprecedented levels of stigma, fear and uncertainty as HIV infection and AIDS, even in the well-informed. These fears are layered on top of pre-existing stigmas and moral judgements associated with particular groups, including gay men, sex workers, drug users and people with mental illnesses, reinforcing existing social inequalities.

Disclosure

The decision to disclose HIV-positive status can be a daunting and multifaceted issue that recurs throughout the course of the disease. Non-disclosure increases the likelihood of infecting others and denies knowledge to previous sexual partners, so represents a major barrier to controlling the pandemic. Non-disclosure also decreases social support and access to services. Disclosure decisions are often conflated with simultaneous disclosure of lifestyle choices (e.g., sexuality, drug use) to family and friends. Disclosure decisions may revert to someone other than the PLHA, particularly regarding children, when family members make decisions, including whether to tell the child of their own serostatus (DeMatteo et al., 2002).

Disclosing an HIV-positive status to intimate partners is of crucial importance in addressing the HIV epidemic, H/A stigma, and the psychological and physical well-being of people living with the condition.

Smith et al. (2017) carried out a qualitative cross-sectional study that aimed to provide a nuanced account of the disclosure process within an intimate partner (IP) relationship. A total of 95 people living with HIV answered a series of open-ended questions enquiring into their last experience of disclosing to an IP. Using thematic analysis, the investigators found that disclosure became a salient issue when the discloser acknowledged their relationship as being meaningful. The decision to tell was

> mostly made to build a foundation for the evolving relationship. Once the decision was made, it was enacted via one of two mechanisms (self-initiated or opportunistic) and partners' reported reactions fell within one of four main reaction types. In the long-term for couples who remained together, disclosure was understood to have brought them closer. However, for both those whose relationships remained intact, and for those whose relationship had since broken down, sexual difficulties associated with being in a sero-discordant partnership pervaded. At a personal level, the experience resulted in increased confidence in living with the diagnosis, and an increased sense of disclosure mastery. (Smith et al., 2017a: 110)

The authors concluded that disclosure is a highly nuanced process. In particular, it was found to be largely characterized by the IP relational context in which it was occurring. The process was found to be largely influenced by the discloser's subjective experience of the intimate partnership. The findings suggest a need for an intervention that supports couples longitudinally.

Adaptation to HIV infection and AIDS

Post-cART, AIDS has been defined as an incurable, chronic and life-threatening illness. Coping with HIV infection and AIDS is a complex, multi-dimensional phenomenon that is influenced by personality as well as contextual and cultural factors. It involves a process of continual adjustment in response to stress, challenging life events, and personal and interpersonal issues. Multiple stressors and negative psychological outcomes are deterrents to successful adjustment. Adaptation is also influenced by health behaviours, which have a bidirectional influence on mood states (e.g., depressed people drink more, which increases depression, resulting in increased alcohol consumption as well as increased risky sex behaviours). An increased number of symptoms and onset of the symptomatic stage are key predictors of adjustment. Factors associated with good psychosocial adjustment to HIV infection and AIDS include healthy self-care behaviours (medical care, healthy lifestyle, awareness and ability to take action to meet personal needs), a sense of connectedness (one close confidante, openness, disclosure), a sense of meaning and purpose (cognitive appraisal that there is something to live for, optimistic attitude) and maintaining perspective (realistic acceptance, e.g., not viewing the condition as imminently fatal). Adaptive coping skills have consistently been associated with increased self-esteem, increased self-efficacy and perceived control. They include active behavioural strategies (planning, help and information seeking, relaxation exercises) and cognitive strategies (cognitive reframing, finding meaning, emotion work, problem solving). Problem-focused coping appears more appropriate for situations that cannot be changed, whereas emotion-focused coping is more suitable where change is not possible (Park et al., 2001).

Adaptive coping strategies along with good social support can mediate the negative effects of stress. These strategies have also been associated with health-related benefits. Finding meaning in the experience of HIV infection and AIDS has been associated with maintaining immune system cell (CD4) levels, optimism with higher CD4 counts, medication adherence and lower distress, and perceived control, problem-focused coping and social support associated with longer survival. Adaptive and maladaptive coping strategies are not mutually exclusive, co-occuring or changing depending on context. Maladaptive coping strategies have been associated with poor adjustment, including lower fighting spirit, higher hopelessness, anxious preoccupation and a fatalistic attitude. Passive and avoidant coping, psychological inhibition and withdrawal have been associated with increased risk behaviours, distress and more rapid disease progression (Stein and Rotheram-Borus, 2004).

Another factor associated with successful adaptation is social support. Zuckerman and Antoni (1995) reported that seven social support criteria were especially related to optimal adjustment to HIV infection and AIDS: feeling supported, satisfaction with support received, perceived helpfulness of peers, total perceived availability and individual dimensions of support, absence of social conflict, greater involvement of AIDS-related community activities and greater number of close friends. These criteria were related to adaptive coping strategies, increased self-esteem and sense of well-being, as well as decreased depression, hopelessness, anxiety, mood disturbances, dysphoria and risk behaviour. Parental adaptation and support may be the most important influences on the adaptation of children and adolescent PLHA.

The internet has had a massive influence on public perception and awareness of HIV infection and AIDS, not all entirely positive. Kalichman et al. (2003) surveyed 147 HIV-positive persons to examine factors associated with internet use. The authors found that internet use was associated with HIV disease knowledge, active coping, information-seeking coping and social support among persons who were using the internet. These preliminary findings suggest an association between using the internet for health-related information and health benefits among people living with HIV infection and AIDS, supporting the development of interventions to close the digital divide in the care of PLHA.

Testing for HIV infection

HIV testing has been available from the beginning of the epidemic, but a significant proportion of people at risk have not presented themselves for testing. HIV testing is a necessary step for receiving HIV treatment and care among those who are HIV-positive. Early diagnosis and access to treatment reduce the likelihood of onward transmission, improve the response to cART, and reduce mortality and morbidity (Evangeli et al., 2016). However, many people living with HIV are unaware of their status. The World Health Organization estimates that less than half of those infected with HIV have been diagnosed (World Health Organization, 2014c).

It is important to learn why this might be the case. Bond et al. (2005) determined the overall prevalence of HIV testing within heterosexual men and women at high risk for HIV infection, and analysed the gender-specific individual- and structural-level barriers and facilitators to testing. Data consisted of 1,643 interviews in Philadelphia between 1999 and 2000. Of the participants, 79.4% had ever taken an HIV test, with women being significantly more likely to have been tested than men. Among the individual-level factors they examined, very few, including sexual and drug-using risk behaviours, were significantly associated with an increased likelihood of ever being tested for HIV. Structural factors, such as access to health care, were important correlates of HIV testing for both women and men.

Lorenc et al. (2011) systematically reviewed qualitative evidence concerning the views and attitudes of MSM concerning HIV testing in high-income countries since 1996. The authors' findings correlate with many other studies discussed in this chapter:

> The uncertainty of unknown HIV status is an important motive for testing; however, denial is also a common response to uncertainty. Fear of the consequences of a positive HIV test is widespread and may take several forms. A sense of responsibility towards oneself or one's partner may be a motive for testing. The perception of stigma, from other gay men or from the wider culture, is a barrier to testing. Gay and other MSM have clear preferences regarding testing services, particularly for those that are community based, include non-judgemental and gay-positive service providers, and offer a high degree of confidentiality. (Lorenc et al., 2011: 834)

Evangeli et al. (2016) systematically reviewed quantitative studies on psychological (cognitive and affective) correlates of HIV testing. A total of 62 studies were included, of which 56 were cross-sectional. Most studies measured lifetime testing. The most commonly measured psychological variables were HIV knowledge, risk perception and H/A stigma. The relationships between HIV knowledge and testing and between HIV risk perception and testing were both positive and significant but with small effects. Other variables, with a majority of studies showing a relationship with HIV testing, included perceived testing benefits, testing fear, perceived behavioural control/self-efficacy, knowledge of testing sites, prejudiced attitudes towards people living with HIV, and knowing someone with HIV.

Pellowski and Kalichman (2016) explored health behaviour predictors of medication adherence among low health literacy people living with HIV/AIDS. For these individuals, medication taking needs to be simplified as much as possible by integrating medication adherence into routine health behaviours. Adults living with HIV completed intake measures and three months of unannounced pill counts. Reported diet and exercise behaviours at intake predicted higher medication adherence, over and above other known predictors of medication adherence such as HIV symptoms, depression, social support and stress. The results support the idea of integrating medication management into routine health practices to improve adherence.

Stigma of living with HIV infection

From a psychological perspective, HIV stigma is composed of three distinct conceptual dimensions: 'internalized', 'anticipated' and 'enacted' stigma (Earnshaw et al., 2013). 'Internalized' stigma is the adoption of negative beliefs associated with having HIV about oneself and is the most common reaction to being diagnosed with HIV. 'Anticipated' HIV stigma is the expectancy of discrimination due to having HIV. 'Enacted' HIV stigma is the experience of being stereotyped or discriminated against for having HIV. Enacted stigma most closely corresponds to poorer mental health, especially depression (Bogart et al., 2011). Enacted stigma may influence health care utilization, treatment adherence, and the overall health and well-being of PLHA (Chambers, Rueda et al., 2015).

Stigma is a major factor in depression of PLHA. It is established as one of the most common psychiatric comorbidities among persons living with HIV (Nanni et al., 2015). Meta-analysis suggested that the frequency of major depression disorder is almost two times higher among persons living with HIV than their uninfected counterparts (Ciesla and Roberts, 2001). Depression risks increase in parallel to the progression of HIV infection and can lead to poorer HIV-related health outcomes. Hernandez and Kalichman (2017) explored the associations between depression among PLWH, HIV stigma, alcohol use, poorer social support and food insecurity. The study demonstrated a mediation effect of HIV stigma on depression through social support, which is additionally moderated by food insecurity. Hernandez and Kalichman's (2017) study observed that people who experience HIV stigma have less support than those who report not experiencing HIV stigma, and the less social support reported, the more depression increases. The effect of HIV stigma on depression through social support was also shown to be dependent on and moderated by level of food insecurity wherein poorer food insecurity resulted in decreases in social support and increases in depression. Their model demonstrates the complexity of depression and how recourses, such as social support and food insecurity, can impact and exacerbate depression in PLWH.

Studies suggest that fear of stigmatization is especially strong among migrants. This is 'stigma amplification', which occurs when there is more than one type of difference. For example, Arrey et al. (2015) found very high levels of non-disclosure among sub-Saharan African migrant women living with HIV/AIDS in Belgium. Non-disclosure to their friends and family averaged at a high level of 75–80%.

Owuor et al. (2016) investigated concealment, communication and H/A stigma from the perspectives of HIV-positive immigrant black African men, originally from East Africa, and their partners living in the UK. The data consisted of in-depth interviews involving 23 participants. They found widespread selective concealment of HIV-positive status. A few respondents had come out publicly about their condition. The authors concluded that: 'HIV prevention initiatives should recognise concealment as a vital strategy in managing communication about ones HIV-positive status' (Owuor et al., 2016: 3079).

Multiplied stigma is evident also among the LBGTQ community. Prevalence of anxiety and mood disorders (AMDs) in HIV-infected individuals in gay and bisexual men (GBM) was studied by Moore et al. (2016) in 557 HIV-infected and 1,325 HIV-uninfected GBM in Sydney, Australia. They observed 300 hospitalizations for AMDs in 15.3% of HIV-infected and 181 in 5.4% of HIV-uninfected participants. Being infected with HIV was associated with a 2.5-fold increase in risk of hospitalization for AMDs.

HIV PREVENTION USING PRE-EXPOSURE PROPHYLAXIS (PREP)

Pre-exposure prophylaxis (or PrEP) is when people at very high risk for HIV take HIV medicines daily to lower their chances of getting infected. PrEP can stop HIV from spreading throughout the body. A combination of two HIV medicines (tenofovir and emtricitabine) is approved for daily use as PrEP to help prevent an HIV-negative person from getting HIV from a sexual or injection-drug-using partner who is positive. Studies have shown that PrEP is highly effective for preventing HIV if it is used as prescribed. PrEP is much less effective when it is not taken consistently (CDC, 2016b).

In the USA over 30,000 people are taking PrEP. PrEP is available in the UK, especially for gay men. PrEP is necessary in the UK because while condoms testing and treating HIV-positive people are containing the HIV epidemic, infections in gay men are not decreasing. A recent study showed that compared to other HIV prevention measures, PrEP is most effective (Punyacharoensin et al., 2016). For each individual who acquires HIV, the personal impact is considerable. However, the cost to the NHS is high – one person's treatment costs around £360,000 over their lifetime (Nakagawa et al., 2015).

A concern is that PrEP could lead gay men to abandon condoms in a form of risk compensation. However, PrEP will most likely be used by people who already have difficulty in consistently using condoms. Another concern is that PrEP could lead to people catching more STIs such as chlamydia and gonorrhoea. Golub et al. (2010) surveyed 180 HIV-negative high-risk MSM in New York City between September 2007 and July 2009. Around 70% of participants reported that they would be likely to use PrEP if it were at least 80% effective in preventing HIV. Of those, over 35% reported that they would be likely to decrease condom use while on PrEP. Behavioural interventions are needed to accompany wide-scale provision of PrEP in high-risk populations.

INTERVENTIONS FOR PLHA

MSM are the fastest growing population group receiving a diagnosis of HIV-seropositivity. In 2015 there were 25,000 new cases in the USA, 17,000 of whom were black or Hispanic/Latino. While accounting for just 14% of the US population, blacks represent close to half of all new HIV infections and AIDS deaths every year. By risk group, gay and bisexual men continue to be at greatest risk for HIV – accounting for the majority of all new HIV infections. Black heterosexual women are also a growing group of people diagnosed with HIV seropositivity, with 4,142 new cases in 2015 (CDC, 2017a). HIV rates are becoming higher among both MSM and heterosexual women in many regions of the world (Figure 22.5).

Interventions have been designed for PLHA at different societal levels, including communities, groups and individuals. To the best of our knowledge, there are no documented examples of PLHA interventions at a structural level. Community interventions have been relatively rare. The majority of efforts have been directed at an individual level.

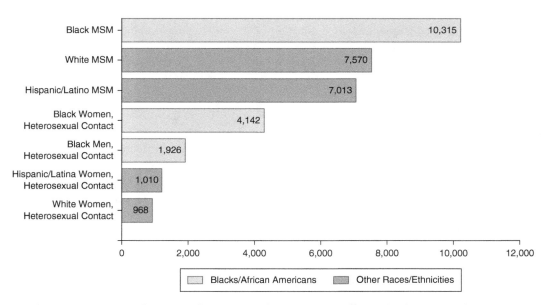

Figure 22.5   HIV diagnoses in the USA for the most-affected sub-populations, 2015

Source: CDC (2017a). Public domain

Community-level intervention

One example of a health promotion intervention that deals with the wider social determinants of health inequalities is Lubek et al.'s (2003, 2014) multi-sectoral participatory action research (PAR) in Cambodia (see Box 22.2). The intervention aims to empower local women who have been placed increasingly at risk using a culturally and gender-sensitive programme, which eventually can be made self-sustaining. This approach succeeds best by facilitating collaboration between grassroots organizations and local and international corporate industries.

BOX 22.2

CASE STUDY: Confronting HIV infection and alcohol in Cambodia

In rural Cambodia, where non-literacy rates are as high as 75%, female workers face risks selling beer brands in restaurants. These 'beer girls' or 'beer promotion women' are underpaid by about 50%, and are sometimes forced to trade sex for money. Of these women, 20% are HIV-seropositive, quickly die and are replaced by younger girls from the countryside. 'Beer girls' must wear the uniforms of the international beer brands that they sell in restaurants and beer gardens.

In 2002, 'beer girls' were set a sales quota of 24 33cl. cans/small bottles per night – each selling at US$1.50 on average, totalling daily beer sales worth $36 or $13,000 annually. In 2004–2005, Heineken and Tiger Beer promotion women were put on fixed salaries of around US$55 per month. This amount is about half the income they need to support their families. One-third of the women support children as single mothers and 90% support rural families. About half became indirect sex workers, exchanging money for sex to supplement their income.

'Beer girls' also consume unsafe quantities of alcohol when working, drinking over 1.2 litres of beer (about five standard drinks) nightly 27 days a month (Schuster et al., 2006). Condom use following beer drinking is lowered, increasing risk of HIV infections, AIDS and STIs. Averaged over seven years, 20% of the 'beer promotion women', in Cambodia are seropositive for HIV/AIDS (Lubeck, 2005). It was estimated that in 2005 there were approximately 200,000 people living with HIV infections and AIDS in Cambodia, with 10,000 in Siem Reap.

A clone of the life-prolonging cART costs approximately US$360 per year. The annual wage of US$600–$800 means that cART is not an option for 'beer girls'. Death can follow three months to two years after diagnosis. Médicins Sans Frontières and other NGOs provide free clone cART for a small number of Cambodians with HIV infections and AIDS.

The spread of HIV infections and AIDS is accelerated by sex tourism, poverty and lack of condom use. HIV sero-positivity rates averaged 32.7% (1995–May 2005) for brothel-based (direct) sex workers. Siem Reap is the largest tourist site in Cambodia and hosted 354,000 people in 2001 and over 1 million in 2004. Many male tourists are 'sex tourists'. In 2001, 23 brothels were registered in the 100% condom-use programme, employing 250 direct sex workers. An additional 350 indirect sex workers were 'beer promotion women' or worked as massage workers and karaoke singers (Lubek, 2005). Infection patterns reflect a 'bridging' pattern involving sex tourists, indirect and direct sex workers, local men, their wives and

---

newborns. Married women, men and young persons are increasingly at risk, with fewer than 10% of the estimated 10,000 persons living with HIV infection or AIDS in Siem Reap in 2006 being given antiretrovirals.

Using participatory action research to promote health interventions

In 2006–2008, the Siem Reap Citizens for Health, Educational and Social Issues (SiRCHESI) organization partnered with three Siem Reap hotels in a hotel apprenticeship programme. This removed women from risky beer-selling jobs, sending them every morning to SiRCHESI's school to learn English, Khmer reading, health education, and social and life skills. New advocacy, political and policy-formation skills and activism include trade union activities for beer sellers, meetings with government legislators, supplying data to ethical shareholder groups, and debating international beer executives in the press and scientific journals. Multiple actions were organized to tackle the issue on a number of different levels:

workshops training women at risk for HIV infection and AIDS to be peer educators about health and alcohol overuse;

workshops to prevent the sexual exploitation and trafficking of children;

company sponsorship of HIV infection-prevention health education;

fair salaries to enable the women to adequately support their dependents;

monitoring voluntary HIV testing (serology);

free antiretroviral therapy (ARVT) for 'promotion girls' who are HIV positive;

breathalyser testing in bars;

changes in community health behaviours and attitudes;

fundraising through the sale of fair trade souvenirs.

Evaluation of project outcomes showed changes in health-related knowledge, behaviour, self-image and empowerment (Lee et al., 2010). As reflected in this case study, Lubek et al. (2014) demonstrated how community health psychology can help to address critical community health issues by adjusting its research and practices to approaches that are guided by grassroots and locally defined interventions.

Source: Lubek et al. (2014)

Mize et al. (2002) carried out a meta-analysis of the effectiveness of HIV prevention interventions for women. The authors evaluated five ethnic groupings (all ethnicities combined, African-American, white, Hispanic and a mixed ethnicity group) over four time periods (post-test, less than 2 months after the intervention, 2–3 months after the intervention and 6–24 months after the intervention) on three HIV-related sexuality outcome variables (HIV infection and AIDS knowledge, self-efficacy and sexual risk-reduction behaviour). The HIV interventions appeared effective at improving knowledge about HIV infection and AIDS and increasing sexual risk-reduction behaviours for all ethnicities, except that the findings for self-efficacy were less consistent. The interventions were less consistently effective for African-American women, for whom significant improvements in feelings of self-efficacy were only seen six months or longer after the intervention.

Interventions for increased adherence

Adherence rates for cART tend to be suboptimal. Fogarty et al.'s (2002) review yielded 200 variables associated with adherence to HIV medication regimens falling into four broad categories: regimen characteristics, psychosocial factors, institutional resources and personal attributes. Of the psychosocial factors reported, positive disease and treatment attitudes, good mental health and adjustment to HIV were positively associated with adherence, while perceived negative social climate was negatively associated. Lack of access to institutional resources (financial, institutional, medical) was negatively associated with adherence. Finally, non-adherence was linked to personal attributes of younger age, minority status and history of substance use. Patients' active involvement in their medical care and treatment decision-making also promotes adherence, while low health literacy is associated with poor adherence.

Many studies have reported that stress accelerates disease processes in a variety of diseases, including HIV. The chronic status of HIV infection and AIDS and the limited accessibility to cART for many people living with HIV infection or AIDS means that psychosocial support interventions are increasingly important. Programmes of pain management, stress management, coping effectiveness training, sleep disorders and exercise promotion have been found to enhance immune system function, medication adherence and adaptive coping, and to decrease anxiety, stress and depression (Chesney et al., 2003). Supportive interventions, especially those that improve function and self-management and maximize independence, represent an essential part of treatment for people living with HIV infection or AIDS.

In cART for the management of HIV infection, stress may increase viral replication, suppress immune response and impede adherence to cART (Riley and Kalichman, 2014). Stressful living conditions caused by poverty and dealing with a chronic life-threatening illness and H/A stigma all can exacerbate chronic stress in HIV-affected populations. Interventions to reduce stress among PLHA have been explored as an adjunct to pharmacotherapy. Scott-Sheldon et al. (2008) reviewed stress-management interventions for HIV-positive adults as evaluated in trials from 1989 to 2006. The authors were interested in measuring the impact of stress-management interventions designed to enhance the psychological, immunological and hormonal outcomes among HIV-positive adults. The findings indicated that, in comparison to controls, stress-management interventions reduced anxiety, depression, distress and fatigue, and improved quality of life. However, stress-management interventions did not appear to affect immunological or hormonal processes compared with controls.

Men who have sex with men are increasingly using smartphone apps, such as Grindr, to meet sex partners (Holloway et al., 2014). Casual sex with 'hook-ups' is often associated with alcohol and drug use. Scott-Sheldon et al. (2013) observed that perceived stress in PLHA was associated with an increase in the frequency of alcohol use (drinking days, intoxication and drinking in shebeens/taverns). They found that stress mediated the association between HIV status and alcohol use.

In a systematic review, Riley and Kalichman (2014) identified 11 studies that have examined mindfulness-based stress reduction (MBSR) as an intervention for HIV-positive populations. The preliminary outcomes supported MBSR to decrease emotional distress, with mixed evidence for impact on disease progression. However, effect sizes were generally small to moderate in magnitude. The number of PLHA who are likely to access such interventions, even if shown to be effective, is likely to be only a tiny proportion of the total number who are at risk.

Interventions for caregivers

The burden of care for people with HIV infection or AIDS, both formal and informal, is being borne primarily by lay caregivers within the family or community, the majority of whom are women and girls (UNAIDS, 2016). There is some evidence, especially in Africa and Asia, that the least acknowledged caregivers are children (caring for a lone or surviving parent) and that older women, already vulnerable through higher levels of chronic poverty, lack of resources and their own substantial health problems, are disproportionately affected.

Caring involves a broad spectrum of psychological, spiritual, emotional and practical work throughout the course of the illness. It can be a rewarding undertaking from which caregivers derive a sense of purpose and self-esteem, and close bonds can become even stronger. However, the caring literature consistently reports the inherently stressful nature of caring for someone with a chronic illness (e.g., Chesler and Parry, 2001). Many of the stressors and negative psychological outcomes experienced by PLHA equally affect their caregivers. Caring is associated with anxiety, depression, overwork, fatigue, fear of death, decreased libido, helplessness, frustration and grief. While other care domains may be similar (e.g., cancer), the greater dependence of PLHA, and involvement and identification with them, result in increased patient contact and a higher intensity of emotional work, increasing the negative consequences. Neurological and/or cognitive symptoms associated with AIDS (from direct effects, opportunistic diseases or other causes) can make the burden of care especially arduous. The effects of multiple bereavements and the caregivers' own health problems (including their own HIV-positive status) also increase mental health problems. The circumscribing effects of H/A stigma create barriers to accessing social support and resources for caregivers.

The needs of caregivers are rarely prioritized and 'burnout' is common. Burnout is defined as emotional exhaustion, depersonalization and a damaged sense of personal accomplishment (e.g., Maslach and Jackson, 1981). Emotional support and stress management can prevent stress, depression and burnout in caregivers if they are lucky enough to access it.

Interventions to reduce stigmatization

Throughout history certain diseases have carried significant levels of stigma: leprosy, tuberculosis, cancer, mental illness and many STIs. Stigmatization of people living with HIV and AIDS (H/A stigma) has been a barrier to effective governmental and medical responses to the HIV epidemic. A relatively small number of studies have been published on interventions designed to reduce H/A stigma. Few such interventions and programmes described in the literature have been rigorously evaluated, in part due to the intrinsic difficulties of measuring stigma (Mahajan et al., 2008). Brown et al. (2003) could identify no studies testing national-level interventions to combat H/A stigma. They had expected to find studies on the effect of mass media campaigns on H/A stigma, but if the programmes do exist, they have not been evaluated or documented in the published literature. Mass media programmes could have potential for helping to reduce H/A stigma but they are not being funded. Mahajan et al. (2008) found that the majority of H/A stigma reduction interventions use cognitive behavioural and socio-cognitive models, employing activities such as information dissemination, empathy induction, counselling and cognitive behavioural therapy focused on individuals. They argued that new models for advocacy and social change in response to HIV/AIDS-related stigma should be encouraged.

The Greater Involvement of People Living with HIV (GIPA) has been advocated as a principle for effective social programmes to reduce H/A stigma (UNAIDS, 2007). The GIPA programme aims to reinforce the rights and responsibilities of PLHA, including the right to self-determination and participation in decision-making processes that affect their lives (UNAIDS, 2007). The GIPA principle called for a greater involvement of PLHA at all levels and the creation of supportive political, legal and social environments (UNAIDS, 2007). Public participation of PLHA at community and social levels would not only promote individual-level responses to internalized stigma on the part of PLHA, but could also prove a powerful deterrent to stigmatizing impulses of the general population.

Anti-discrimination legislation

One of the most powerful tools against stigma and discrimination is anti-discrimination legislation. The Equality Act 2010 made certain types of discrimination unlawful in the UK, including discrimination on the basis of HIV status. The Americans with Disabilities Act (ADA) guarantees equal opportunity for individuals with disabilities in public accommodations, employment, transportation, state and local government services and telecommunications (US Department of Justice, 2016). People with HIV, both symptomatic and asymptomatic, are protected by the ADA. The ADA also protects persons who are discriminated against because they have a record of or are regarded as having HIV, or they have a known association or relationship with an individual who has HIV. Similar legislation was passed in Nigeria in 2015.

FUTURE RESEARCH

1. The long-term impact of interventions to reduce stigma training is unknown and should be evaluated.

2. Innovative approaches of stigma reduction are required at a structural level.

3. The impact of recent anti-stigma legislation requires evaluation.

SUMMARY

1. HIV infection and AIDS constitute a worldwide pandemic that has infected around 80 million people and has become the fourth largest killer in the world. There are around 2 million new cases each year.
2. HIV (human immunodeficiency virus) is a retrovirus that infects and colonizes cells in the immune system and the central nervous system (T-helper and monocyte macrophage cells). Initial flu-like symptoms are followed by a quiescent, asymptomatic period (lasting years) during which the immune system battles the virus.

3. Gay and bisexual men, particularly young African-American gay and bisexual men, are most affected. Heterosexual women of colour are also a high-risk group.
4. HIV-seropositivity and AIDS are two of the most stigmatized conditions in health care. The majority of interventions to reduce H/A stigma have been at an individual level. Outcomes have generally been modest and short-lasting.
5. The most effective treatment consists of combination antiretroviral therapies (cART) that decrease an individual's HIV viral load to undetectable levels, reducing associated morbidity and mortality.
6. Pre-exposure prophylaxis (PrEP) provides high-risk individuals with HIV medicines daily to lower their chances of becoming infected.
7. The burden of care for people living with HIV-seropositivity or AIDS, both formal and informal, is being borne primarily by lay caregivers within the family or the community, the majority of whom are women and girls.
8. Caring is associated with anxiety, depression, overwork, fatigue, fear of death, decreased libido, helplessness, frustration and grief. While other care domains may be similar (e.g., cancer), the greater dependence of PLHA results in increased contact and higher intensity emotional work, increasing the negative consequences.
9. A major element of research has been concerned with medication adherence. Of the psychosocial factors reported, positive disease and treatment attitudes, good mental health and adjustment to HIV were positively associated with adherence, while perceived negative social climate was negatively associated.
10. One of the most powerful tools against stigma and discrimination is anti-discrimination legislation. The Equality Act 2010 (UK) and the Americans with Disabilities Act (US) make certain types of discrimination unlawful, including discrimination on the basis of HIV status.

LONG-TERM CONDITIONS: DIABETES AND ME/CFS

'I have high blood sugars, and Type 2 diabetes is not going to kill me. But I just have to eat right, and exercise, and lose weight, and watch what I eat, and I will be fine for the rest of my life.'

Tom Hanks

'No one chooses to have ME – everything changed when I became ill.'

Tom Kindlon (2015)

OUTLINE

In this chapter, we review two long-term conditions that are diagnosed in increasing numbers of patients: diabetes and ME/CFS. Neither can be cured using currently available treatments and both require an approach that utilizes the biopsychosocial model. The two conditions can often cause distress, with major reductions in quality of life, and involve significant care commitments from informal, family caregivers. We review each condition in turn, including the causes, the risk factors, the experience of living with the condition, interventions to ameliorate the symptoms and informal carers' experiences.

INTRODUCTION

Long-term or chronic illnesses have replaced acute illnesses as the predominant disease pattern. Greatly improved longevity and higher cancer survival rates have meant an increased prevalence of cancer, coronary heart disease, AIDS, diabetes and myalgic encephalomyelitis/chronic fatigue syndrome (ME/CFS). We reviewed the first three of these conditions in Chapters 20–22. In this chapter, we review the remaining two.

As life expectancy of the human population increases, so does the prevalence of diseases of older age. Long-term illness typically involves restrictions on activities of daily living, and increases in pain, fatigue, depression and anxiety. Patients need to cope daily with a changing array of ongoing symptoms, the life threat involved and the requirements of treatment. Maintaining effective relationships with health-service personnel, family and friends requires many adaptations and there is a need to continuously make adjustments. One of the greatest sources of worry is uncertainty around prognosis.

If one needs a litmus test of the current level of acceptance of the biopsychosocial model (BSM), then the manner in which long-term conditions without medical cures are perceived and managed provides a good indication. Neither diabetes mellitus nor ME/CFS can be cured using available treatments within biomedicine and both require an approach based on the biopsychosocial model. Diabetes has known causes but no known cure. ME/CFS has no known causes and no known cure. Unsurprisingly, ME/CFS receives little attention in the medical curriculum. A study by Stenhoff et al. (2015) found that medical students acquired their knowledge and attitudes from mainly informal sources and expressed difficulty understanding ME/CFS within the biomedical framework. ME/CFS patients were even perceived by some medical students as 'time-wasters'. Teaching about unexplained medical symptoms needs to be integrated into the medical curriculum, but to date this has not been happening. Unfortunately, lack of knowledge among physicians about ME/CFS and other long-term conditions increases the already high levels of distress and uncertainty for these patients and their families.

In the USA in 2012, about half of all adults – 117 million people – had one or more chronic health conditions. One in four adults had two or more chronic health conditions (Ward et al., 2014). Seven of the top ten causes of death in 2010 were chronic diseases. Two of these chronic diseases – cancer and heart disease – together accounted for nearly 48% of all deaths (CDC, 2013a) (see Chapters 20 and 21).

Obesity is a serious health concern, as we have seen earlier in this book. During 2009–2010 more than one-third of adults, or about 78 million people, were obese (defined as body mass index [BMI] ≥ 30 kg/m2). Nearly one in five youths aged 2–19 years was obese (BMI $\geq$ 95th percentile) (CDC, 2013b) (see Chapter 10).

Arthritis is the most common cause of disability (Hootman et al., 2009). Of the 53 million adults with a diagnosis of arthritis, more than 22 million say they have trouble with their usual activities because of it (Barbour et al., 2013).

Diabetes is the leading cause of kidney failure, lower-limb amputations other than those caused by injury, and new cases of blindness among adults (CDC, 2013c).

Chronic illnesses often strike in middle and older age and, while they can prove fatal, most people with a chronic illness live for many years with the condition. Genetic factors and diet-related behaviours are two primary determinants of diabetes, but the causes of ME/CFS remain a complete mystery. The focus of this chapter will be on the psychological aspects of disease management and treatments based on the BPSM. Management of fatal or chronic diseases is a principal feature in the lives of 10–15% of the population. The primary health care system is of great importance in long-term conditions. Patient-centredness has been strongly emphasized in offering care to patients with chronic conditions. Further research is needed on developing applications of the BPSM that are acceptable to patients.

The Chronic Care Model (CCM) was proposed as a possible solution to the rising prevalence of chronic diseases and has been widely advocated in order to improve quality of care for the chronically ill (Wagner et al., 2001). In the CCM, the health care system is viewed as one part of a larger community and health care practice or 'health organization':

> Effective self-management support and links to patient-oriented community resources help to activate and inform patients and families to better cope with the challenges of living with and treating chronic illness. Traditional patient education emphasized knowledge acquisition and didactic counselling. Mounting evidence indicates that while such interventions increased knowledge, they were unsuccessful in changing behaviour or improving disease control and other outcomes. More recent theoretical and empirical research has shifted the focus from patients' knowledge of the disease and its treatment to their confidence and skills in managing their condition. The interventions that have emanated from this research reinforce the patient's (and family's) crucial role in managing the condition, help patients to set limited goals for improving their management of their illness, identify barriers to reaching their goals, and develop a plan to overcome the barriers. (Wagner et al., 2001: 64)

CCM includes formal health care combined with informal self-care and care by family members or friends. The latter occurs almost invisibly with little recognition or financial support from society at large. In all life-threatening conditions, family members can experience significant emotional, economic and social challenges, as can the person with the illness. Caregiving is often seen as 'women's work'. Research indicates that around 3.1% of females provide informal care compared to around 1.6% of males (Mathiowetz and Oliker, 2005). More than 25 million family members provide informal care to disabled or ill family members in the USA (Levine, 2000). More than half of American women will care for a sick or disabled family member at some point during their adult lives (Moen et al., 1994). The economic value of informal care is estimated at $196 billion (in 1997 dollars), which is equivalent to 18% of the total national health care expenditure (Arno et al., 1999). One survey reported that women are twice as likely to care for someone for more than 20 hours a week and are 1.5 times more likely than men to perform more labour-intensive or intimate care tasks (Levine et al., 2000).

We discuss the psychological aspects of informal caregiving in more depth in the following sections.

DIABETES MELLITUS

The role of homeostasis in the maintenance of health and well-being has been a significant theme in our review of health psychology. Diabetes mellitus is a condition caused by a breakdown of homeostasis, in this case, at a physiological level. In Type 1 diabetes mellitus blood glucose homeostasis ceases to function because the beta cells of the pancreatic islets are destroyed. In Type 2 diabetes mellitus the pancreas loses its ability to secrete enough insulin in response to meals or to control the body's glucose level. The condition is fatal if left untreated.

What is diabetes?[1]

Diabetes mellitus is a chronic disease in which blood glucose (sugar) levels are above normal (hyperglycaemia). People with diabetes have problems converting food to energy. After a meal, food is broken down into a sugar called glucose, which is carried by the blood to cells throughout the body. Insulin, a hormone made in the pancreas, allows glucose to enter the cells of the body where it is used for energy. People develop diabetes because the pancreas produces little or no insulin or because the cells in the muscles, liver and fat do not use insulin properly. As a result, the glucose builds up in the blood, is transported into the urine and passes out of the body. Thus, the body loses its main source of fuel even though the blood contains large amounts of glucose. When insulin is no longer made, it must be obtained from another source – insulin injections or an insulin pump. When the body does not use insulin properly, people with diabetes may take insulin or other glucose-lowering medications. Neither insulin nor other medications, however, are cures for diabetes; they only help to control the disease.

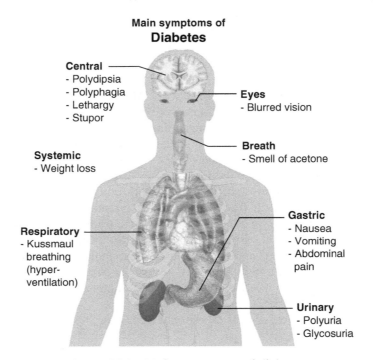

Figure 23.1   Main symptoms of diabetes

Source: Mikael Häggström (2009). Public domain

Taking care of diabetes is important. Over the years, ongoing high blood glucose, also called hyperglycaemia, can lead to serious health problems. If not managed effectively, diabetes can affect the blood vessels, eyes, kidneys, nerves, gums and teeth, making it the

---

[1]This primer text on diabetes is extracted from the US National Diabetes Education Program 'Diabetes Primer for School Personnel' (2017), which is in the public domain.

leading cause of adult blindness, kidney failure and non-traumatic lower limb amputations. Diabetes also increases a person's risk for heart disease and stroke. Some of these problems can occur in teens and young adults who develop diabetes during childhood. The good news is that research shows these problems can be greatly reduced, delayed or possibly prevented through intensive treatment that keeps blood glucose levels near normal. There are three main types of diabetes.

Type 1 diabetes mellitus (T1DM), formerly called juvenile diabetes, is a disease of the immune system, the body's system for fighting infection. In people with Type 1 diabetes, the immune system attacks the beta cells (the insulin-producing cells of the pancreas) and destroys them. Because the pancreas can no longer produce insulin, people with Type 1 diabetes must take insulin daily to live. Type 1 diabetes can occur at any age, but onset of the disease occurs most often in children and young adults. Most cases of diabetes in children under age 10 are Type 1. In adults, Type 1 diabetes accounts for 5–10% of all cases of diagnosed diabetes.

The symptoms of Type 1 diabetes are due to an increase in the level of glucose in the blood and include increased thirst and urination, weight loss, blurred vision and feeling tired all the time. These symptoms may be mistaken for severe flu or another rapid-onset illness. If not diagnosed and treated with insulin, the child with Type 1 diabetes can lapse into a life-threatening condition known as diabetic ketoacidosis or DKA. Signs of DKA include vomiting, sleepiness, fruity breath, difficulty breathing and, if untreated, coma and death.

Although scientists have made much progress in predicting who is at risk for Type 1 diabetes, they do not yet know what triggers the immune system's attack on the pancreas's beta cells. They believe that Type 1 diabetes is due to a combination of genetic and environmental factors that are beyond the individual's control. Researchers are working to identify these factors and to stop the autoimmune process that leads to Type 1 diabetes.

Type 2 diabetes mellitus (T2DM), formerly called adult-onset diabetes, is the most common form of the disease. People can develop it at any age, even during childhood. A progressive disease, Type 2 diabetes usually begins with insulin resistance, a condition in which muscle, liver and fat cells do not use insulin properly. At first, the pancreas keeps up with the added demand by producing more insulin. Over time, however, the pancreas loses its ability to secrete enough insulin in response to meals or to even control the glucose level overnight or during periods of fasting. Managing Type 2 diabetes includes lifestyle changes such as making healthy food choices and getting regular physical activity. In addition, people with T2DM may take insulin and/or other glucose-lowering medications to control their diabetes. In the past, T2DM used to be found mainly in overweight or obese adults ages 40 or older. Now, as more children and adolescents have become overweight and inactive, T2DM is occurring in young people.

The symptoms of T2DM in children may be similar to those of Type 1 diabetes. A child or teen may feel very tired or thirsty and have to urinate often due to high blood glucose levels. Other symptoms include weight loss, blurred vision, frequent infections and slow-healing wounds. High blood pressure or elevated blood lipids (cholesterol) are associated with insulin resistance. In addition, physical signs of insulin resistance may appear, such as acanthosis nigricans, a condition in which the skin around the neck, armpits or groin looks dark, thick and velvety. Often, this condition is mistaken for poor hygiene. Some children or adolescents (and adults) with T2DM may have no recognized symptoms when they are diagnosed. For that reason, it is important for the parents/guardian to talk to their health care providers about screening children or teens who are at high risk for T2DM.

The risk factors of T2DM are being overweight, having a family member who has T2DM and being African American, Hispanic/Latino, American Indian, Alaska Native, Asian American or

Pacific Islander, including Native Hawaiian. Other risk factors include having a mother who has had diabetes during her pregnancy (gestational diabetes), having high blood pressure, high cholesterol, abnormal lipid levels, polycystic ovary syndrome and being inactive.

For children and teens at risk, health care professionals can encourage, support and educate the entire family to make lifestyle changes that may delay – or prevent – the onset of Type 2 diabetes. Changes include making healthy food choices, reaching and maintaining a healthy weight and engaging in regular physical activity.

Gestational diabetes develops during pregnancy and is caused by the hormones of pregnancy. These hormones can cause insulin resistance or a shortage of insulin. Although gestational diabetes usually goes away after the baby is born, a woman who has had it is at increased risk for developing diabetes for the rest of her life. In addition, the offspring of that pregnancy is at increased risk for obesity and developing T2DM.

LIVING WITH DIABETES

'Being diagnosed with diabetes, or knowing someone who is diagnosed with the condition, may throw up many questions about how it fits into your daily life, from how it makes you feel, to managing diabetes at work, or while you are driving. 'The practicalities of living with diabetes can be stressful, but you needn't put your life on hold' (Diabetes UK, 2017). Qualitative studies have been carried out suggesting that this description is accurate. One Swedish study even suggests that diabetes is a 'marginal problem': 'Diabetes in the shadow of daily life: factors that make diabetes a marginal problem' is one of a relatively small number of studies offering the patient perspective of what it is like living with diabetes (Ågård et al., 2016). The sample consisted of 24 patients (15 male) with diabetes mellitus. They were recruited from a medical outpatient clinic in western Sweden, in an area with a high incidence of immigrants and low socio-economic status. One main interview question was formulated: '*Can you describe what living with diabetes means to you?*' Content analysis placed the responses into meaning units that were categorized into four main themes and eight sub-themes. The following sections discuss these themes using quotes from the study.

Theme 1: 'A lifelong follower but not a real problem'

Sub-theme 1A: 'No big deal'. The authors reported that respondents did not feel that diabetes was a severe disease but it was perceived as a minor issue, with practical problems such as needing an increased focus on food and medicines, but life in general went on as usual. Those who had had diabetes for a long time had incorporated diabetes management into the routines of their everyday life.

Sub-theme 1B: 'Symptoms, not blood sugar levels, matter'. Another reason for not ascribing diabetes great importance was the lack of symptoms associated with high blood glucose levels. As a result, some respondents felt that they did not bother about complications at the moment, although they knew they could occur in the future.

Theme 2: 'A trifle in relation to the daily struggle with difficulties'

Sub-theme 2A: 'Burdening circumstances'. Many said their perception of living with diabetes was dependent to a great extent on 'burdening circumstances and troubles in life'. One middle-aged man felt unable to manage his diabetes because a work project had failed. Another patient mentioned worries about the future when asked about living with diabetes.

Sub-theme 2B: 'Less important compared with other diseases and symptoms'. Apart from diabetes, respondents could have a combination of other diseases. Medical conditions such as cardiac diseases, high blood pressure, inflammations, chronic obstructive pulmonary disease and depression tended to overshadow the importance of having diabetes. Moreover, symptoms (e.g., sleeping problems) and treatment (e.g., for tuberculosis or leukaemia) related to these diseases were perceived as barriers to the control of diabetes.

Theme 3: 'Something out of one's own control'

Sub-theme 3A: 'Diabetes as a predetermined condition'. Some felt that it had been predetermined for them to get diabetes or because they were a victim of circumstances such as stress, fate, a difficult childhood, conflicts, having lived under a death threat, war and homesickness. Diabetes was 'something evil' that 'through no fault of their own, had affected them'. As a result, they felt little incentive to adhere to lifestyle advice.

Sub-theme 3B: 'No use trying'. A sense of helplessness and lack of responsibility in coping with diabetes led to a sense of resignation.

Theme 4: 'Not worth giving up the good things in life for'

Sub-theme 4A: 'Preference for a good life rather than living right'. The majority had received nutritional advice and knew what they should eat and drink. However, some reported not being willing to refrain from tasty food and alcohol to any great extent. The social and enjoyable dimensions of eating were more important than eating the right food. Some felt that their prescribed diet, apart from not being very tasty, made cooking more complicated and meals more boring.

Sub-theme 4B: 'Reasons for not exercising'. Similarly, the majority were quite aware of the positive effects of physical activity, yet some took almost no exercise at all. They said that they were lazy, unwilling to exercise or felt that exercise was boring. It was more convenient to remain on the couch or sit in front of a computer. Other excuses for not exercising were pain, fatigue, depression, sleep problems, lack of experience, financial problems and/or potentially harmful to the heart.

The findings of the Ågård et al. study illustrate the value of qualitative research in providing insight into patients' attitudes, health beliefs, reasons for adherence or non-adherence, and their ability or willingness to practise self-management skills and knowledge. Data from focus group discussions, together with other kinds of data, can be helpful in understanding patient experience.

A systematic review of qualitative research studies was carried out by Wilkinson et al. (2014). In 37 studies, the main issues impacting on individual self-care were 'communication', 'education', 'personal factors', 'provider issues' and 'support'. Multiple barriers were suggested as influencing the day-to-day management of diabetes, including poor communication with health care providers. The findings suggested the need for an education programme that allows for incremental knowledge gain and also experiential and vicarious learning and the provision of culturally sensitive care. The authors concluded that people living with diabetes face many issues in their day-to-day management of the disease, compounded by vulnerability to wider situational, cultural and social issues. Self-care ability is a 'dynamic, evolutionary process', it was concluded, 'that varies from person to person and involves moving from a disease focused existence to maximising life' (Wilkinson et al., 2014: 111).

As we have seen in earlier chapters, health-related stigma has been strongly associated with both obesity and HIV/AIDS, but it has been less studied with diabetes. Browne et al. (2013) explored the social experiences of Australian adults living with T2DM, with a particular focus on the perception and experience of diabetes-related stigma. They audiorecorded semi-structured interviews, which they subjected to thematic analysis. This study took place in non-clinical settings in metropolitan and regional areas in Victoria. A total of 25 adults with T2DM participated (12 women, median age 61 years, median diabetes duration 5 years); 21 participants (84%) indicated that they believed T2DM was stigmatized, or reported evidence of stigmatization. Specific themes were feeling blamed by others for causing their own condition, experiencing negative stereotyping, being discriminated against or having restricted opportunities in life. Sources of stigma included the media, health care professionals, friends, family and colleagues. Themes relating to the consequences of this stigma were evident, including participants' unwillingness to disclose their condition to others and psychological distress. Participants believed that people with T1DM do not experience similar stigmatization.

The long-term complications of diabetes can be severe, as a visit to the general surgical wards of any metropolitan hospital will prove. The complications include cardiovascular disease, retinopathy (a disease of the retina which results in impairment or loss of vision), nephropathy, which is damage to the kidneys, and diabetic neuropathy, where nerve fibres are damaged as a result of high blood sugar, most often in the legs and feet. The latter can result in the amputation of one, two or possibly more limbs. People living with diabetes can take steps to prevent the development of long-term complications (see Box 23.1).

BOX 23.1

Preventing complications

There are eight steps that help to prevent complications:

1. Regular check-ups with a health care team – at least once a year.
2. Long-term checks on the diabetes, such as an HbA1c test.
3. Testing blood glucose levels at home regularly, and recording the results, aiming for between 4mmol/l and 8mmol/l* before meals and less than 10mmol/l two hours after meals for most of the time.
4. Achieving and maintaining a healthy body weight.
5. Keeping blood pressure and blood fats (e.g., cholesterol) under control.
6. Eating a healthy balanced diet.
7. Increasing physical activity.
8. Not smoking.

Source: Diabetes UK (2017)

An important trial carried out in the USA, the 'Diabetes Control and Complications Trial' (DCCT), assigned patients to conventional or intensive therapy from 1983 to 1993. Participants were randomly assigned to receive either the experimental or standard therapy. The experimental therapy involved the use of an intensive insulin regimen designed to maintain near-normal glycaemic levels in the absence of severe hypoglycaemia. The standard treatment was designed to maintain patients free of clinical symptoms related to hyper- or hypoglycaemia while receiving up to two insulin injections daily. Since 1993 the DCCT has been observational, and intensive therapy was recommended for all patients. Clinical treatment goals of T1DM were changed since the Diabetes Control and Complications Trial demonstrated reduced long-term complications with intensive diabetes therapy.

Nathan et al. (2009) provided an analysis of the incidence of long-term complications. Their study was performed after 30 years of observing the DCCT cohort of 1,441 patients and a sub-set of another relevant cohort (EDC) of 161 patients. The cumulative incidences of proliferative retinopathy, nephropathy and cardiovascular disease were 50%, 25% and 14%, respectively, in the DCCT conventional treatment group, and 47%, 17% and 14%, respectively, in the EDC cohort. However, the DCCT intensive therapy group had substantially lower cumulative inci-dences (21%, 9% and 9%) and fewer than 1% became blind, required kidney replacement, or had an amputation because of diabetes during that time. These results are important in showing that the frequencies of serious complications in patients with T1DM, especially when treated intensively, are lower than that reported historically.

INTERVENTIONS FOR DIABETES PATIENTS

Primary Health Care

The Chronic Care Model (CCM) has been influential in the organization of primary health care and continuity of care between patients, families and professionals. The American Diabetes Association's (ADA) *Standards of Medical Care in Diabetes* is updated annually. These 'Standards' provide the most current evidence-based recommendations for diagnosing and treating adults and children with all forms of diabetes. Recommendations in the 2015 ADA Standards state that: 'Patient-centered communication that incorporates patient preferences, assesses literacy and numeracy, and addresses cultural barriers to care should be used. Care should be aligned with components of the Chronic Care Model (CCM) to ensure productive interactions between a prepared proactive practice team and an informed activated patient' (Chronic Care Model, 2015: 97).

In making lifestyle changes that are crucial to self-care, 'an informed activated patient's' autonomous motivation to self-regulate health-relevant behaviours is important. Koponen et al. (2017) investigated six dimensions of primary health care that are strongly associated with autonomous motivation (self-regulation) for effective diabetes self-management. The study comprised 2,866 patients with T2DM. The six characteristics were access to care, continuity of care, diabetes counselling, trust, patient-centred care and 'autonomy support' from one's physi-cian. Koponen et al.'s study showed that of these six quality dimensions of primary health care, autonomy support from one's physician was most strongly associated with self-regulation for effective diabetes self-management. However, the authors suggest that overall support received from friends, family members, other patients with diabetes and health care professionals may play an even greater role.

Baptista et al. (2016) systematically reviewed studies that evaluated different elements of the CCM in patients with Type 2 diabetes mellitus. They assessed the influence of the CCM on different clinical outcomes. Studies were eligible for inclusion if they compared usual care with interventions that used one or more elements of the CCM. Six out of the twelve studies included in the review showed evidence of the effectiveness of the CCM for diabetes management in primary care as well as significant improvements in clinical outcomes. In six other studies, no improvements regarding clinical outcomes were observed with CCM. The authors concluded that greater benefits could be obtained through combining all elements of CCM.

Lifestyle changes

Some risk factors for T2DM are potentially reversible, e.g., elevated plasma glucose concentrations in the fasting state and after an oral glucose load, overweight and a sedentary lifestyle. One group of investigators hypothesized that modifying these factors with a lifestyle-intervention programme or the administration of metformin would prevent or delay the development of diabetes. The Diabetes Prevention Program Research Group (2002) randomly assigned 3,234 non-diabetic persons with elevated fasting and post-load plasma glucose concentrations to placebo, metformin (850 mg twice daily) or a lifestyle-modification programme with the goals of at least a 7% weight loss and at least 150 minutes of physical activity per week. Metformin hydrochloride lowers blood sugar levels by increasing the sensitivity of muscle cells to insulin, reducing the amount of sugar produced in the liver and delaying the absorption of sugar from the intestines after eating so that there is less of a spike in blood sugar levels after meals. The lifestyle intervention consisted of a 16-lesson curriculum covering diet, exercise and behaviour modification to help the participants achieve the set goals. The participants averaged 51 years of age, and had a mean BMI of 34.0. Two-thirds of the sample were women, and 45% were members of minority groups. The average follow-up was 2.8 years.

The incidence of diabetes was 11.0, 7.8 and 4.8 cases per 100 person-years in the placebo, metformin and lifestyle groups, respectively. The lifestyle intervention reduced the incidence by 58% (95% confidence interval, 48–66%) and metformin by 31% (95% confidence interval, 17–43%), as compared with placebo. The lifestyle intervention was significantly more effective than metformin. The results showed that to prevent one case of diabetes during a period of three years, 6.9 persons would have to participate in the lifestyle-intervention programme and 13.9 would have to receive metformin. While lifestyle changes and treatment with metformin both reduced the incidence of diabetes in persons at high risk, the lifestyle intervention was more effective than metformin.

Diabetes self-management education

Diabetes self-management education (DSME) involves the process of facilitating knowledge, skill and ability necessary for diabetes self-care. Diabetes self-management support (DSMS) is the support that is required for implementing and sustaining coping skills and behaviours needed to self-manage on an ongoing basis. The American Diabetes Association and many other diabetes associations worldwide recommend that all individuals with diabetes receive DSME/S at diagnosis and as needed on an ongoing basis thereafter. The goals of self-management education are to optimize metabolic control, prevent acute and chronic complications and optimize quality of life, while keeping costs acceptable.

Recent studies estimate that of those newly diagnosed with diabetes, fewer than 7% of individuals have private insurance and fewer than 5% of those covered by Medicare participate in DSME. Thus, although the systematic review by Norris et al. (2001) indicated that DSME resulted in clinical improvement, DSME remains under-utilized in diabetes care (Chrvala et al., 2016).

Yet research has revealed significant knowledge and skill gaps in 50–80% among patients with diabetes (Clement, 1995), and ideal glycaemic control (HbA1c <7.0%) is achieved in fewer than half of people with T2DM (Harris et al., 1999). Educational techniques used in

DSME have shifted away from purely didactic presentations to interventions involving patient 'empowerment' with participation and collaboration (Norris et al., 2001).

Norris et al. (2001) systematically reviewed the effectiveness of self-management training in T2DM. They searched for studies between 1980 and 1999 that were original articles reporting the results of RCTs on the effectiveness of self-management training in people with T2DM. A total of 72 studies were identified. Self-management training was observed to have positive effects on knowledge, frequency and accuracy of self-monitoring of blood glucose, self-reported dietary habits, and glycaemic control in studies with short follow-up at six months. Effects of interventions on lipids, physical activity, weight and blood pressure were less definite. With longer follow-up, interventions using regular reinforcement were sometimes effective in improving glycaemic control. The results suggested that interventions involving patient engagement may be more effective than didactic interventions in improving glycaemic control, weight and lipid profiles. Performance, selection, attrition and detection bias were common in the studies reviewed, and external generalizability was often limited. The evidence from the Norris et al. review supports the effectiveness of self-management training in T2DM, particularly in the short term. Larger studies with long-term follow up are needed to confirm the value of DSME.

A new modality for DSME is the smartphone. El-Gayar et al. (2013) reviewed whether diabetes smartphone apps are capable of helping patients with Type 1 or Type 2 diabetes mellitus to self-manage their condition, and identified issues for large-scale adoption. The review covered apps available at the Apple App Store and articles published from January 1995 to August 2012. Findings suggested that apps can support self-management tasks such as physical exercise, insulin dosage or medication, blood glucose testing and diet. Other ancillary tasks included decision support, notification/alert, tagging of input data and integration with social media. The analysis suggested that app usage can improve attitudes favourable to diabetes self-management. However, relatively few people with T2DM are currently making use of the technology due to a perceived lack of additional benefits and ease of use (Scheibe et al., 2015). Improved usability, perceived usefulness and adoption of the technology are necessary for the future adoption of this technology.

DEPRESSION

Depression is common among patients with diabetes, who have a higher risk of diabetes-related complications such as diabetic retinopathy, nephropathy, neuropathy and macrovascular complications. Ali et al. (2006) conducted a systematic literature review consisting of ten randomized controlled trials and 51,331 patients to estimate the prevalence of clinical depression in adults with Type 2 diabetes compared with those without Type 2 diabetes. The prevalence of depression in Type 2 diabetes patients was 9% higher than in those without diabetes.

More recently, Bogle and Kanapathy (2017) carried out a systematic review to determine whether CBT is effective in reducing depressive symptoms and improving glycaemic control among depressed diabetic patients. The results revealed diverse applications of CBT, in which CBT had a positive impact on depressive symptoms, with three studies also finding an improvement in HbA1c, and one also demonstrated improved self-efficacy and self-concept related to successful diabetes management. There is a need for controlled studies with larger sample sizes and follow-up periods of more than six months.

CARING FOR A PERSON WITH DIABETES

Diabetes places a substantial care burden on elderly individuals, their families and society, both through the resulting disability and the substantial periods of time that informal caregivers spend helping to address the associated functional limitations.

Langa et al. (2002) obtained nationally representative estimates of the time, and associated cost, of informal caregiving provided to elderly individuals with diabetes, and determined the diabetes complications that contributed to the need for informal care. Data came from a nationally representative survey of people aged 70 or older ($n = 7,443$). Those without diabetes received an average of 6.1 hours per week of informal care, while those with diabetes but taking no medication received 10.5 hours and those with diabetes who were taking oral medication received 10.1 hours, and those taking insulin received 14.4 hours of care. Disabilities from heart disease, stroke and visual impairment were predictors of diabetes-related informal care. The total cost of informal caregiving for elderly individuals with diabetes in the USA was estimated to be between $3 and $6 billion per year, similar to previous estimates of the annual paid long-term care costs attributable to diabetes. That figure will have increased to at least $4–8 billion in 2018 prices.

The toll on parents of children with T1DM has been described as 'relentless'. Night-time caregiving with nocturnal blood glucose monitoring (NBGM) tends to increase parents' anxiety and stress. Monaghan et al. (2009) invited 71 parents of children with T1DM ages 2–6 to complete questionnaires designed to assess the frequency of NBGM, illness characteristics and health outcomes, and parental concern. Approximately one-third reported regularly monitoring their child's blood glucose level after their child was asleep, suggesting that parents' nighttime caregiving practices and sleep loss needed clinical attention.

Continuous glucose monitoring (CGM) involves a subcutaneously implanted enzyme electrode that senses interstitial fluid as a proxy for blood glucose levels. The relationship between glucose concentrations in interstitial fluid and blood has generated great interest due to the possibility of gaining up to 288 glucose level readings a day without having to do finger pricks. Pickup et al. (2015) analysed narratives about experiences of using CGM in people with T1DM and their caregivers from an online survey. Questions included duration of CGM, frequency of sensor wear, funding, and a free narrative about experiences or views about CGM.

Pickup et al. identified four themes: (1) metabolic control, (2) living with CGM (work and school, sleep, exercise, nutrition, frequency of self-monitoring of blood glucose [SMBG]), (3) psychological issues and patient/caregiver attitudes, and (4) barriers to CGM use (technical issues, financial issues, attitudes of health care professionals towards CGM). The narratives suggested that the experiences were overwhelmingly positive, with improved glycaemic control, diet and exercise management, quality of life, and physical and psychological well-being, as well as reduced frequency of SMBG. The authors concluded that patients and caregivers both view CGM as a valuable addition to caring for many people with T1DM.

ME/CFS

What is ME/CFS?

Myalgic encephalomyelitis (ME) or chronic fatigue syndrome (CFS) is one of the most controversial and hotly debated topics in the history of medicine. Even the correct label for the condition is under dispute, as is the nature of the condition itself and everything else to do with it. The condition has also been named 'Systematic Exertion Intolerance Disease' (SEID), 'Post-Viral Fatigue Syndrome' (PVFS) and 'Chronic Fatigue Immune Dysfunction Syndrome' (CFIDS). In this chapter, we use the label 'ME/CFS'. This condition has been characterized by different authorities and organizations in many diverse ways. ME/CFS is a label for a condition that involves prolonged muscle weakness after minor exertion (accompanied by muscle pain) and neurological symptoms indicative of cerebral dysfunction, such as sleep disturbances, headaches and cognitive problems.

The severity of ME/CFS varies from patient to patient, with some people able to maintain fairly active lives. For many patients, however, ME/CFS places significant limitations on their work, school and family activities, and the pattern of symptoms can be unpredictable. According to the International Consensus Criteria (ICC) for ME/CFS, actual fatigue is not a requirement for diagnosis (Carruthers et al., 2011). The ICC report stated:

> The label 'chronic fatigue syndrome' (CFS) has persisted for many years because of the lack of knowledge of the aetiological agents and the disease process. In view of more recent research and clinical experience that strongly point to widespread inflammation and multisystemic neuropathology, it is more appropriate and correct to use the term 'myalgic encephalomyelitis' (ME) because it indicates an underlying pathophysiology. (Carruthers et al., 2011: 327)

Chronic fatigue can accompany many long-term illnesses. Patients with illnesses such as depression and cancer may be misdiagnosed with ME/CFS. Case definitions for ME/CFS vary between the broad Oxford criteria (Sharpe et al., 1991) and the more specific Fukuda criteria (Fukuda et al., 1994).

CFS can affect adults, children and adolescents. Between 0.2% and 2.3% of children or adolescents suffer from CFS. In children, particularly adolescents, CFS is more likely to develop after an acute flu-like or mononucleosis-like illness, but gradual onset of illness may occur (CDC, 2017b).

Unfortunately, many patients with ME/CFS find the medical health care they receive insufficient. Patients' negative reactions might be explained by the types of intervention offered by health care services to patients with ME/CFS (see Box 23.2).

BOX 23.2

'No one chooses to have ME – everything changed when I became ill'

I first became ill at 16. Before becoming ill, I lived a very active life. I participated in whatever sport was going – soccer, table tennis, life-saving, tennis, cricket and cross-country running. I was also naturally academic and managed to get good results while still enjoying lots of extra-curricular activities.

All that changed when I became ill with ME.

I can remember how it happened. I developed an infection the day before going on a school trip. I decided to still go. We went to an adventure centre in the west of Ireland

(Continued)

---

canoeing, hill-walking, abseiling and orienteering. It was February and it was cold and rainy throughout the trip – not the place to be when you're unwell. I was ill for some days after I came home.

I was never the same after that. Anytime I tried to play sports I felt ill afterwards. I found I was struggling to get my homework done.

I struggled on at school and then university for another four years living a hermit-like existence. I had some natural ability (I came sixth in Ireland in the Irish National Maths Contest in sixth year in school) which helped, but found I had virtually no energy for a rounded life.

I went to an orthopaedic surgeon who recommended exercise, so I started going to a swimming pool three or four times a week. I kept appearing to strain muscles so I'd have to try different strokes like back stroke with only one arm. I had over 100 physiotherapy appointments trying to deal with all the muscle and tendon strains I appeared to have. I was desperate to get back to my previous life. I thought that all I needed to do was get fit and my life could go back to normal. Things took a turn for the worse in college. A couple of hours after an exam, my throat swelled up and I could barely swallow. I developed flu-like symptoms and a high temperature.

Looking back, I'd recognise that as a relapse from the mental exertion of the exam. When I tried to go back to exercising a few weeks later, my reaction was much more severe. Even a few lengths of slow swimming led to high levels of pain the next day. I switched to walking, but developed shin splints. I developed tennis elbow in my right arm and tendonitis in my right hand. My body was falling apart. I started trying to write with my left hand but soon developed tendonitis in that. I took a year out hoping I could get back to functioning.

Unfortunately, it was not to be. I developed an almost constant sore throat. By May, I developed pain in my lower stomach, and diarrhoea.

I was referred to a gastroenterologist who after a colonoscopy diagnosed irritable bowel syndrome. This is quite common in ME but I just thought I was very unlucky to have lots of separate health issues.

Finally, by August, I started having difficulty walking short distances. I would get out of breath even from slow walking. My GP referred me to a consultant in the Blackrock Clinic, the late Prof Austin Darragh who sadly passed away earlier this month. After doing some blood tests, he diagnosed me with ME, or post-viral chronic fatigue syndrome, saying I was a classic case.

Source: Kindlon (2015). Reproduced by permission

Not a single, specific cause of ME/CFS has yet been identified. It could well be that ME/CFS has multiple causes or there could be one single cause yet to be identified. The problem is that nobody knows. Conditions that have been suggested as causes or triggers of ME/CFS include infections, immune disorders, stress, trauma and toxins. The controversies around the definition, the cause and the treatment have been hugely emotive and have involved patients, patient organizations, health care and medical organizations, medical, psychiatric and psychology journals, government departments, insurance companies, and even legal tribunals in hotly debated disputes.

LIVING WITH ME/CFS

Difficulties with diagnosis

Uncertainties around diagnosis is one of the major problems for patients, families and their medical advisers. For doctors, diagnosing ME/CFS is complicated because:

1. There is no lab test or biomarker for ME/CFS.

2. Fatigue and other symptoms of CFS are common to many illnesses.

3. For some ME/CFS patients, it may not be obvious to doctors that they are ill.

4. The illness has a pattern of remission and relapse.

5. Symptoms vary from person to person in type, number and severity.

These factors have contributed to a low diagnosis rate. The CDC (2017b) suggests that of the 1–4 million Americans who have ME/CFS, less than 20% have been diagnosed. However, early diagnosis and treatment of ME/CFS increase the likelihood of improvement. The patient who thinks she/he may have ME/CFS may find it difficult to talk to their doctor or other health care professional about their condition.

ME/CFS can resemble many other illnesses, including mononucleosis, Lyme disease, lupus, multiple sclerosis, fibromyalgia, primary sleep disorders and major depressive disorder. Also, medication can cause side effects that mimic the symptoms of ME/CFS. People may mistakenly assume that they have ME/CFS when they have another illness. An ME/CFS diagnosis can be made only after other conditions have been excluded.

A major, substantive review of the qualitative literature on the lived experiences of ME/CFS patients was published by Anderson et al. (2012). Anderson et al. reviewed and synthesized findings across 34 qualitative studies of people living with ME/CFS. Their analyses included a multi-perspective (e.g., individual, physician, familial) examination of ME/CFS, as well as a comparative analysis of ME/CFS versus other chronic conditions. For patients, illness development influenced identity, reductions in functioning and coping. We base the following description of the living experience with ME/CFS on the findings of Anderson et al. (2012).

Identity changes

People with ME/CFS experience a change in identity throughout the course of their illness, which can lead to a shift in body–mind relationships. They experience a disruption in and reconstruction of their identity and also a loss of confidence and self-esteem. Identity disruption is often related to transformations of family roles (e.g., children taking on additional responsibilities).

Fennell (1995) proposed a four-phase theory of ME/CFS illness experience that included periods of crisis, stabilization, resolution and integration. People with ME/CFS go through cycles of health and unhealthiness that can be transformative. Chronicity contributes to the cycle of being overwhelmed by and eventually learning to live with the illness. ME/CFS patients are made accountable for the cause of their illness due to the contested nature of the illness. Shifting accountability from the medical system to the individual patients is one way in which the societal response blames the victim.

Reductions in functioning

Reductions in functioning across occupational, education, personal or social domains are a characteristic part of living with ME/CFS. Social and economic reductions, personal losses and disruptions, in addition to the physical reductions experienced in everyday life are all commonly experienced. Economic and occupational reductions can be profound as well as multiple losses concerning their jobs and finances, including major disruptions to their careers and financial instability, and, in many cases, unemployment.

The loss of social roles and major disruptions in personal relationships are inevitable for most patients. People with ME/CFS describe reductions in the form of a loss of stamina and ability to develop future plans and changes in relationships, activities and social networks because of the illness.

Coping and balancing activity

The emotional and coping responses tend to vary according to which symptoms are present and the severity of the symptoms. For example, people who develope ME/CFS can use coping mechanisms such as seeking support from others, religion and using selective comparisons ('there are other people worse off than me') to deal with their new illness. It was common for people with ME/CFS to use alternative medications and therapies.

Ray et al. (1993) described four coping strategies that may be used to manage ME/CFS: (1) maintenance of activity, (2) accommodating to the illness, (3) focusing on symptoms, and (4) information seeking. The most common of these themes across the studies reviewed by Anderson et al. (2012) was patient efforts to balance activity. Conflicting suggestions have been made about what is best for patients when it comes to balancing activity as a treatment or coping mechanism. Some patients say that they are able to control symptoms by reducing activity. Many people with ME/CFS practice 'living within [their] limits' by monitoring and/or self-initiating the restriction of activities, including role constriction in employment.

Pacing oneself seems crucial to many patients. ME/CFS can hinder one's ability to perform activities or cause the person to avoid activities altogether, which may in turn reinforce ME/CFS symptoms. The idea of balancing activity is supported by the **envelope theory** (Jason et al., 1999, 2010), which proposes that people with ME/CFS should try to balance their perceived and expended energy levels, thus staying within their 'energy envelope'.

INTERVENTIONS FOR ME/CFS

Interventions for ME/CFS are based on theories of the processes that are responsible for the perpetuation of the symptoms. These theories are highly contested and have caused major controversies that have divided patients from doctors and psychiatrists.

Cognitive behavioural theories of ME/CFS assert that cognitions and behaviours perpetuate the fatigue and impairment of individuals with ME/CFS (Wessely et al., 1989, 1991). This assumption is contested by many patients and patient organizations. Vercoulen et al. (1998) developed a cognitive behavioural model of ME/CFS based on these assumptions. However, findings by Song and Jason (2005) suggested that the model was an inaccurate fit for individuals with ME/CFS, although the model fitted individuals with chronic fatigue in psychiatric conditions. In spite of the evidence against it, the socio-cognitive model continues to be cited as evidence supporting cognitive behavioural and graded exercise therapies for individuals with ME/CFS (e.g., White et al., 2011).

Sunnquist (2016) re-examined the behavioural pathway of the Vercoulen et al. (1998) model, which is characterized by causal attribution for symptoms, activity level, and fatigue and impairment, and found no support in the data for the Vercoulen et al. (1998) model. Sunnquist's study suggested that activity level is an indicator of general illness severity, along with impairment and fatigue, and that individuals do not reduce their activity level due to illness beliefs. As the Vercoulen et al. model has provided the theoretical rationale for cognitive behavioural and graded exercise treatments for ME/CFS, these failed replication attempts support patient concerns about the lack of efficacy of these treatments, and their doubtful theoretical basis.

THE PACE TRIAL: A CATALOGUE OF ERRORS

Rarely in the history of clinical medicine have doctors and patients been placed so bitterly at loggerheads. The dispute has been a long time coming. Thirty years ago, a group of psychiatrists offered a hypothesis based on the biopsychosocial model (BPSM) in which ME/CFS is constructed as a psychosocial illness. According to their theory, ME/CFS patients are alleged to have 'unhelpful cognitions' and 'dysfunctional beliefs' that their symptoms are caused by an organic disease. The Dysfunctional Belief Theory (DBT) assumes that there is no pathology causing the symptoms; patients are being 'hypervigilant to normal bodily sensations' (Wessely et al., 1989, 1991). The physical symptoms are presumed to be the result of 'deconditioning' or 'dysregulation' caused by sedentary behaviour, accompanied by disrupted sleep cycles and stress. Counteracting deconditioning involves normalizing sleep cycles, reducing anxiety levels and increasing physical exertion. To put it bluntly, the DBT asserts that ME/CFS is 'all in the mind'. Small wonder that patient groups have been expressing anger and resentment in their droves.

The PACE Trial is a textbook example of the top-down research approach with its hierarchical organization of personnel, duties and skill-sets (see Chapter 8). Unless carefully managed, the top-down approach creates a self-fulfilling prophecy with confirmation biases at multiple levels. At the top of the research pyramid sits Professor Sir Simon Wessely, originator of the DBT. The principal investigators (PIs) for the PACE Trial, Professors White, Chalder and Sharpe, are themselves advocates of the DBT, with connections both to the Department of Work and Pensions and to insurance companies.

The objective for the PACE Trial was to demonstrate that two interventions based on the DBT, cognitive behavioural therapy (CBT) and graded exercise therapy (GET) help ME/CFS patients to recover. According to critics, the PACE Trial team were operating within a closed system or **groupthink** in which they 'know' their theory is correct and, with every twist and turn, are able to confirm their theory with **subjective validation** and **confirmation bias**. *Groupthink* occurs when a *group* makes faulty decisions because *group* pressures lead to a deterioration of 'mental efficiency, reality testing, and moral judgment' (Janis, 1972).

Given this context, the investigators' impartiality has been challenged with allegations of many potential conflicts of interest (Lubet, 2017). Furthermore, critical analysis suggests that the PACE investigators involved themselves in manipulating protocols midway through the trial, selecting confirming data, omitting disconfirming data and publishing biased reports of findings, which created a catalogue of errors. The outcome of the PACE Trial has been termed a 'travesty of science', while sufferers of ME/CFS continue to be offered unhelpful or harmful treatments and are basically told to 'pull themselves together'. One commentator has asserted that the situation for ME patients in the UK is 'The 3 Ts – Travesty of Science; Tragedy for Patients and Tantamount to Fraud' (Professor Malcolm Hooper, quoted by Williams, 2017: 1).

Critics suggest that the claimed benefits of GET and CBT for patient recovery are spurious. Serious errors in the design, the protocol and the procedures of the PACE Trial are evident. The catalogue of errors is summarized in Box 23.3.

BOX 23.3

The PACE Trial: A catalogue of errors

Critics suggest that the claimed benefits of GET and CBT for patient recovery have been exaggerated. Sir Simon, we respectfully suggest, got this one badly wrong. The explanation lies in a sequence of serious errors in the design, the changed protocol and the procedures of the largest trial, known as the PACE Trial. The PACE Trial investigators neglected or bypassed many accepted scientific procedures for a randomized controlled trial, as follows:

Table 23.1

Error	Category of error	Description of error
1	Ethical issue: Applying for ethical approval and funding for a long-term trial when the PIs already knew CBT effects on ME/CFS were short-lived	On 3 November 2000, Sharpe confirmed: 'There is a tendency for the difference between those receiving CBT and those receiving the comparison treatment to diminish with time due to a tendency to relapse in the former' (www.cfs.inform/dk). Wessely stated in 2001 that CBT is 'not remotely curative' and that 'These interventions are not the answer to CFS' (Editorial: *JAMA* 19 September 2001 286(11)) (Williams, 2016)
2	Ethical issue: Failure to declare conflicts of interest to Joint Trial Steering Committee	Undeclared conflicts of interest by the three PIs in the Minutes of the Joint Trial Steering Committee and Data Monitoring Committee held on 27 September 2004
3	Ethical issue: Failure to obtain fully informed consent after non-disclosure of conflicts of interest	Failing to declare their vested financial interests to PACE participants, in particular that they worked for the PHI industry, advising claims handlers that no payments should be made until applicants had undergone CBT and GET
4	Use of their own discredited 'Oxford' criteria for entry to the trial	Patients with ME would have been screened out of the PACE Trial even though ME/CFS has been classified by the WHO as a neurological disease since 1969 (ICD-10 G93.3)
5	Inadequate outcome measures: Using only subjective outcome measures	The original protocol included the collection of actigraphy data as an objective outcome measure. However, after the trial started, the decision was taken that no post-intervention actigraphy data should be obtained

Error	Category of error	Description of error
6	Changing the primary outcomes of the trial after receiving the raw data	Altering outcome measures mid-trial in a manner which gave improved outcomes
7	Changing entry criteria midway through the trial	Altering the inclusion criteria for trial entry after the main outcome measures were lowered so that some participants (13%) met recovery criteria at the trial entry point
8	The statistical analysis plan was published two years after selective results had been published	The redefinition of 'recovery' was not specified in the statistical analysis plan
9	Inadequate control	Sending participants newsletters promoting one treatment arm over another, thus contaminating the trial
10	Inadequate control	Lack of comparable placebo/control groups with inexperienced occupational therapists providing a control treatment and experienced therapists providing CBT
11	Inadequate control	Repeatedly informing participants in the GET and CBT groups that the therapies could help them get better
12	Inadequate control	Giving patients in the CBT and GET arms more sessions than those in the control group
13	Inadequate control	Allowing therapists from different arms to communicate with each other about how patients were doing
14	Lack of transparency	Blocking the release of the raw data for five years, preventing independent analysis by external experts

Blocking the release of the raw data for five years and preventing independent analysis by external experts was tantamount to a cover-up of the true findings (Geraghty, 2016). ME/CFS patient associations were suspicious of the recovery claims concerning the GET arm of the trial because of their own experiences of intense fatigue after ordinary levels of activity, which were inconsistent with the recovery claims of the PACE Trial reports. For many sufferers even moderate exercise results in long 'wipe-outs', in which they are almost immobilized by muscle weakness and joint pain. In the USA, post-exertional relapse has been recognized as the defining criterion of the illness by the Centers for Disease Control and Prevention, the National Institutes of Health and the Institute of Medicine. For the PACE investigators, however, the announced recovery results validated their conviction that psychotherapy and exercise provided the key to reversing ME/CFS.

When Alem Matthees, a ME/CFS patient, sought the original data under the Freedom of Information Act and a British Freedom of Information tribunal ordered the PACE team to disclose their raw data, some of the data were re-analysed according to the original protocols. The so-called 'recovery' under CBT and GET all but disappeared (Wilshire et al., 2017). The recovery rate for CBT fell to 7% and the rate for GET fell to 4%, which were statistically indistinguishable from the 3% rate for the untreated controls.

In light of the re-analyses of the PACE Trial, the DBT appears to be dead in the water. There is an urgent need for new theoretical approaches and scientifically based treatments for ME/CFS patients. Meanwhile, there is repair work to be done to rebuild patient trust in the medical profession after this misplaced attempt to apply the BPSM to the unexplained syndrome of ME/CFS.

The envelope theory of Jason et al. (1999, 2010, 2016) proposes that people with ME/CFS need to balance their perceived and expended energy levels and provides one way forward, pending further research. Ultimately, we are waiting for an organic account of ME/CFS that is competent to explain the symptoms and to open the door to effective treatments. Patients have a right to nothing less. Recent studies indicate that ME/CFS patients may have systemic abnormalities in cellular energy transduction, particularly when cells are put under mitochondrial stress (Tomas et al., 2017). It seems likely that a physical explanation for ME/CFS will eventually be found, leading to effective treatments.

CARING FOR A PERSON WITH ME/CFS

The lack of effective treatments and training for doctors about ME/CFS makes caring for a person with ME/CFS a challenging task. Fluctuating symptoms, restricted mobility and uncertain prognosis can all take a toll on the family carer. There is a paucity of studies about caring for people with ME/CFS. Experiences of parents with sons or daughters with severe ME/CFS are rarely presented in the scholarly literature. Haig-Ferguson (2014) investigated the impact of having a child with ME/CFS on family relationships from the parents' perspective. Semi-structured interviews explored 18 parents' experiences of having a child with ME/CFS and the impact of this on family relationships. Haig-Ferguson identified five main themes: 'Long and difficult journey', 'Uncertainty', 'Isolation and restriction', 'Focus on the unwell person at the expense of family life' and 'Parental roles'.

In another study, narratives of parent-carers were analysed using interpretative phenomenological analysis (Mihelicova et al., 2015). Results revealed themes of identity change, guilt, feeling like outsiders, uncertainty, changing perceptions of time, coping mechanisms and improvement/symptom management.

Siblings are also likely to experience distress. Velleman et al. (2016) invited 34 siblings to complete questionnaires measuring depression (HADS), anxiety (HADS and Spence Children's Anxiety Scale: SCAS) and European Quality-of-life-Youth (EQ-5D-Y). The scores were compared with scores from normative samples. The results indicated that siblings had higher levels of anxiety on the SCAS than adolescents of the same age from a normative sample, although depression and quality-of-life were similar. Interviews with nine siblings of children with ME/CFS suggested restrictions on family life, 'not knowing' and lack of communication as negative impacts on their family, and change of role/focus, emotional reactions and social stigma as negative impacts on themselves. However, they described positive communication, social support and extra activities as protective factors.

FUTURE RESEARCH

1. Further research is needed on developing applications of the biopsychosocial model to long-term conditions that are acceptable to patients.

2. Self-care ability in people living with diabetes and ME/CFS warrants further in-depth research.

3.   Jason's envelope theory provides a possible basis for ME/CFS treatment, pending further research.

4.   Further research on stigma prevention in relation to both diabetes and ME/CFS is necessary.

SUMMARY

1. Chronic illnesses can strike at any age but more often in middle and older age groups and, while they can be fatal, most people diagnosed with a chronic illness live for many years with the condition.
2. Management of chronic diseases is a principal feature in the lives of 10–15% of the population. This huge amount of informal care occurs almost invisibly to outsiders, with little recognition or financial support from society at large.
3. Chronic illness involves restrictions on activities of daily living and increases in pain and fatigue. 'Juggling' relationships with health professionals, family and friends requires many adaptations and adjustments. Patients may have views about their care and treatment that differ from those of the professionals.
4. Type 2 diabetes mellitus is the most common form of the disease. People can develop it at any age, even during childhood.
5. Stigmatization can occur with long-term conditions and may be experienced by people with diabetes or ME/CFS. This is an extra burden for patients and informal carers to carry. Sources of stigma include the media, health care professionals, friends, family and colleagues.
6. The practicalities of living with diabetes or ME/CFS can be highly stressful, but people with diabetes or ME/CFS do not need to put their lives on hold.
7. For ME/CFS, pacing one's activity seems crucial to many patients. ME/CFS can hinder one's ability to perform activities or cause the person to avoid activities altogether, which may in turn reinforce ME/CFS symptoms. The idea of pacing or balancing activity is supported by Jason's envelope theory.
8. The Dysfunctional Beliefs Theory of ME/CFS assumes that patients have unhelpful cognitions and dysfunctional beliefs that their symptoms are caused by an organic disease when no pathology is present. The theory is unsupported by empirical evidence, but remains the main basis for treatment in the UK.
9. Parents of children with ME/CFS tend to feel that life is a constant struggle with exhaustion, uncertainty, isolation and restrictions. They may feel as if family life is focused on their unwell child, such that some express a need to escape from the situation.
10. More in-depth training of medical and nursing students concerning ME/CFS and more effective treatments based on scientific evidence are urgently needed.

END-OF-LIFE CARE, DYING AND DEATH

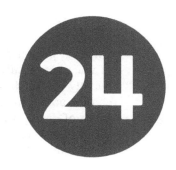

'The art of living well and dying well are one.'

Epicurus

'Death is one of the attributes you were created with; death is part of you. Your life's continual task is to build your death.'

Montaigne

'Goodbye to all my dear friends and family that I love. Today is the day I have chosen to pass away with dignity in the face of my terminal illness, this terrible brain cancer that has taken so much from me ... but would have taken so much more.'

Brittany Maynard (psychologist and right-to-die activist, 2014)

OUTLINE

In this final chapter, we review recent research on the psychological aspects of end-of-life care, dying and death. We consider the concepts of a 'good death' and the 'quality of death and dying' and examine how these constructs can be quantified. We review the growing literature on palliative and end-of-life care, which is insufficiently available and varies in quality. We review recent trends towards legalisation of physician-assisted care and physician-assisted suicide and the use of suffering as a criterion. Finally, we discuss brain death and organ donation.

DYING AND DEATH

Unless a person dies of sudden cardiac arrest in their sleep, the end of life can be a time of uncertainty, suffering and caregiver travail. In the UK, unexplained sudden death is frequently recorded as due to death from 'natural causes'. Many such deaths are due to sudden cardiac arrest, the largest cause of natural death. Old age is not a scientifically recognized cause of death. A more direct cause is sought, although it may not be established in certain cases. Deaths caused by active intervention or 'unnatural' causes are usually from accidents, misadventure (accident following a wilful and dangerous risk), suicide or homicide. A person's death is recorded on his/her death certificate, which is completed by a doctor. In the vast majority of cases, the cause of a person's death is known and can be recorded with adequate certainty.

Improvements in living and working conditions, and in health care, have led to improved survivorship of potentially fatal conditions and increased life expectancy. The 'greying' of society means that many more people are living with varying degrees of illness, suffering and disablement for long periods of time. Families are experiencing increasingly long periods of caring and can face a daunting array of decisions serving as a proxy for their dying loved ones. As a consequence, **palliative care** and **end-of-life (EOL)** care, the **hospice movement**, and even requests for **physician-assisted death (PAD)** or physician-assisted suicide (PAS) are becoming integral parts of the health care industry. These trends also have led to a significant line of research on the **quality of dying and death (QoDD)**. This chapter reviews the current state of the art of dying 'a good death'.

Outside religious dogma and poetry, there has been little in the way of advice. An influential theory by Elisabeth Kübler-Ross (1997) received much publicity but unfortunately has little empirical support. Based on the ideas of Bowlby (1961) and Parkes (1965), Kübler-Ross constructed a five-stage theory of death and dying, of which death is 'the final stage of growth'. She defined five stages experienced when terminally ill patients face their own deaths: denial–dissociation–isolation, anger, bargaining, depression and acceptance. Psychological and medical thinking about death and dying drew inspiration from Kübler-Ross's (1969) work. Although widely cited, Kübler-Ross's five-stage model is gradually fading as an approach to the care of the dying.

Numerous studies have highlighted the poor quality of EOL care, with many hospitalized patients dying in pain and distress while receiving life-sustaining treatments that they did not actually ask for, and with grieving families carrying great emotional stress and, especially in the USA, financial burdens. There are basic preferences and needs that should be met if individual QoDD is to be maximized. Yet basic needs for a high QoDD are unlikely to be met in any modern technology-based, efficiency-driven hospital. As far as possible, decisions about health and social care must always remain with the individual person. However, to an increasing extent the control over an individual's care inevitably passes to medical and nursing staff and to the patient's family. This prospect is especially likely when the person's cognitive abilities suffer deterioration because of illnesses such as stroke, heart failure, dementia or neurological conditions.

Troubling ethical issues are raised on an everyday basis, and family and relatives are thrown into sensitive, emotionally charged, life-changing scenarios for which they may be ill-prepared. Important practical decisions that have to be made on behalf of an incapacitated patient include:

- diet, hydration, and personal hygiene;

- treatment, including pain relief;

- visits by family members;

- transfer to a care or nursing home;

- transfer to a hospital;

- transfer to a hospice;

- do-not-resuscitate (DNR) decisions;

- physician-aided dying.

The complexity of the EOL scenario can often overwhelm an already upset friend or family member and can greatly influence the dying person's QoL and QoDD. Understandably, for the young and able-bodied reader these aspects of health care may seem remote and abstract. Exactly where, when and how we die is unknown. That one will definitely die is the only certain prediction one can make. It is well to reflect on Montaigne's statement: *Your life's continual task is to build your death.*

BUILDING A 'GOOD DEATH'

A good death is what any thinking person wishes for – a good, long, fulfilling life followed by a good death. But what exactly would a good death be like? To answer this question, we must try to define what is meant by the **quality of dying and death (QoDD)**. Specifying the QoDD has been attempted by several investigators and research groups. Defining the QoDD is curiously complex – for the obvious reason that the real experts die before they can give the scientist their opinions! Those self-proclaimed mediums – every one of them a quack – who purport to communicate with the 'spirit world' have failed to deliver one scintilla of data that is useful to science. Nevertheless, ways and means to decipher the nature of a good death are available (Curtis et al., 2002), and listening to 'spirit' mediums is not one of them. The views of loved ones, family members, nurses and other health care professionals can all go into the 'mix' to generate working hypotheses.

A few psychometric questionnaires are available for the evaluation of the quality of death and dying. A systematic review by Kupeli et al. (2016) included measures for assessing quality of death and dying and/or quality of care and satisfaction with care at the very end of life. The measures *Quality of Death and Dying* (Patrick et al., 2001; Curtis et al., 2002, see Box 24.1) and *FAMCARE* (Kristjanson, 1986) have both been validated in a variety of cultural settings and participant groups.

In light of the above items, a good death is much more than freedom from pain, although that can be a positive feature, and death should not necessarily be sudden. People may wish to achieve many different tasks during the process of dying. Three themes that emerged in a debate about ageing and dying were control, **autonomy** and independence (Debate of the Age Health and Care Study Group, 1999). The authors of the debate report identified 12 principles of a good death (see Box 24.2).

BOX 24.1

Items for measuring the Quality of Dying and Death (QoDD)

Each item is asked with the following leader: 'How would you rate this aspect of (patient's name) dying experience?' The response scale is from 0 to 10 where 0 is a 'terrible experience' and 10 an 'almost perfect experience'.

1. Having pain under control.
2. Having control of event.
3. Being able to feed oneself.
4. Having control of bladder, bowels.
5. Being able to breathe comfortably.
6. Having energy to do things one wants to do.
7. Spend time with your children as much as you want (or I have no children).
8. Spend time with your friends and other family as much as you want.
9. Spend time alone.
10. Be touched and hugged by loved ones.
11. Say goodbye to your loved ones.
12. Have the means to end your life if you need to.
13. Discuss your wishes for end-of-life care with your doctor and others.
14. Feel at peace with dying.
15. Avoid worry about strain on your loved ones.
16. Be unafraid of dying.
17. Find meaning and purpose in your life.
18. Die with dignity and respect.
19. Laugh and smile.
20. Avoid being on dialysis or mechanical ventilation.
21. Location of death (home, hospice, hospital).
22. Die with/without loved ones present.
23. State at moment of death (awake, asleep).
24. Have a visit from a religious or spiritual advisor.
25. Have a spiritual service or ceremony.
26. Have health care costs provided.
27. Have funeral arrangements in order.
28. Spend time with spouse, partner. (or I have no spouse, partner)
29. Spend time with pets. (or I have no pets)
30. Clear up bad feelings. (or there were no bad feelings to clear up)
31. Attend important events. (or there were no important events to attend)

Source: Curtis et al. (2002). Reproduced with permission

BOX 24.2

Twelve principles of a good death

To know when death is coming, and to understand what can be expected

To be able to retain control of what happens

To be afforded dignity and privacy

To have control over pain relief and other symptom control

To have choice and control over where death occurs (at home or elsewhere)

To have access to information and expertise of whatever kind is necessary

To have access to any spiritual or emotional support required

To have access to hospice care in any location, not only in hospital

To have control over who is present and who shares the end

To be able to issue advance directives which ensure wishes are respected

To have time to say goodbye, and control over other aspects of timing

To be able to leave when it is time to go, and not to have life prolonged pointlessly

Source: Debate of the Age Health and Care Study Group (1999). Reproduced by permission

---

To have choice and control over where death occurs is one of the key principles. Understandably, most patients wish to die at home. Family members and friends are vital to the support of patients at home. A survey of 57 health care providers found that the most common attributes associated with a 'good death' were being pain free, having family present, and sudden or peaceful death. Severe pain or discomfort were the most commonly reported attributes of a 'bad death' (Najafi et al., 2014).

HOSPICE CARE

Thirty years ago, Wallston et al. (1988) compared the quality of death (QoD) for hospice and non-hospice patients and found that the QoD scores were higher for terminally ill patients in hospices, either at home or hospital-based, than for similar patients who received conventional care. Fourteen years later, Miller et al. (2002) compared analgesic management of daily pain for two cohorts of dying nursing home residents enrolled or not enrolled in a hospice. A retrospective, comparative cohort design was utilized. Over 800 nursing homes in Kansas, Maine, Mississippi, New York and South Dakota contributed a subset of residents who were suffering daily pain near the end of life: 709 hospice and 1,326 non-hospice residents. Detailed drug use data before death were used to examine analgesic management of daily pain. The data showed that 15% of hospice residents and 23% of non-hospice residents in daily pain received no analgesics, and 51% of hospice residents and 33% of non-hospice residents received regular treatment for daily pain. Controlling for clinical confounders, hospice residents were twice as likely as non-hospice residents to receive regular treatment for daily pain (adjusted odds ratio 2.08). These findings suggest that analgesic management of daily pain was better for nursing home residents enrolled in hospice than for those not enrolled in hospice. Worryingly, many dying nursing home residents in daily pain were receiving no analgesic treatment or were receiving analgesic treatment inconsistent with pain management guidelines.

The hospice movement is growing in momentum internationally and the numbers of people who spend their last months of life in nursing homes and hospices are increasing rapidly (Najafi et al., 2014). The percentage of older people in the USA who received hospice care in the last 30 days of life increased from 19% in 1999 to 43% in 2009. The percentage who died at home increased from 15% in 1999 to 24% in 2009. In the next section, we review research on the merits of EOL care.

END-OF-LIFE CARE

It has been apparent for many decades that EOL care is not best left to care homes and hospitals. These environments are not compatible with high-quality EOL care, which requires quiet, unpressurized, sensitive care that is tailored to each individual and his/her family. The vast majority of people want to die at home, but circumstances beyond their control often make this impossible. Cultural and language differences are also important considerations in EOL care.

Gysels et al. (2012) explored cultural issues that shape EOL care in seven European countries. They reviewed 868 papers using the following themes: setting, caregivers, communication, medical EOL decisions, minority ethnic groups, and knowledge of, attitudes towards and values of death and care. They inferred evidence of clearly distinguishable national cultures of EOL care, with differences in meaning, priorities and expertise in each country. The diverse ways in which EOL care is practised should inform future improvements of EOL care.

High-quality EOL care should ideally reflect each individual patient's values and wishes, promote compassionate communication and provide family-oriented care. It should lead to a reduction of non-beneficial, unnecessary and aggressive physical care and avoid prolongation of dying, prevent patient suffering and allow less wastage of precious intensive care unit (ICU) resources.

A 'Study to Understand Prognoses and Preferences for Outcomes and Risks of Treatments' (SUPPORT) investigated how to improve EOL care and reduce the frequency of a 'mechanically supported, painful, and prolonged process of dying' (Conners et al., 1995: 1591). In this highly cited, large-scale study in five US teaching hospitals, Conners et al. made a two-year prospective observational study (phase I) with 4,301 patients followed by a two-year controlled clinical trial (phase II) with 4,804 patients and their physicians randomized to the intervention group ($n = 2,652$) or control group ($n = 2,152$). The patients were hospitalized with one or more of nine life-threatening diagnoses, having a six-month mortality rate of 47%.

A specially trained nurse had multiple contacts with the patient, family, physician and hospital staff to elicit preferences, improve understanding of outcomes, encourage attention to pain control, and facilitate advance care planning and patient–physician communication. Physicians in the intervention group received estimates of the likelihood of six-month survival for every day up to six months, outcomes of cardiopulmonary resuscitation (CPR) and functional disability at two months. Phase I observations found many concerning issues in communication, the frequency of aggressive treatment and the characteristics of hospital deaths. Less than half

(47%) of physicians knew when their patients preferred to avoid CPR; 46% of do-not-resuscitate (DNR) orders were written within two days of death; 38% of patients who died spent at least ten days in an intensive care unit (ICU); and for 50% of conscious patients who died in the hospital, family members reported moderate to severe pain at least half the time.

During the phase II intervention, patients experienced no improvement in patient–physician communication (e.g., 37% of control patients and 40% of intervention patients discussed CPR preferences) or in the five targeted outcomes. Thus, SUPPORT suggested that enhanced opportunities for more patient–physician communication may be inadequate to change established practices. The study authors concluded: 'To improve the experience of seriously ill and dying patients, greater individual and societal commitment and more proactive and forceful measures may be needed' (Conners et al., 1995: 1591).

Over two decades later, is there any solid evidence that the low QoDD observed in 1990s hospitalized patients is changing? Or that hospital physicians are more 'teachable' about practices conducive to raising QoDD? Sadly, the evidence suggests they may not be. Curtis et al. (2011) evaluated an intervention into ICU EOL care in 12 US community hospitals in Washington. The intervention was based on self-efficacy theory: changes in clinician performance were facilitated by increasing knowledge, enhancing attitudes and modelling appropriate behaviours. Unfortunately, the primary outcome, family-QoDD, showed no change with the intervention. Also, no change occurred in family satisfaction or nurse-QoDD.

Care of the dying and support for family members losing a loved one is a role requiring specialist knowledge, experience and training. EOL care appears to be another 'weak link' in medical training, along with communication skills and psychosocial issues more generally. Specialist palliative care has two main client groups: the majority with a diagnosis of cancer and a minority with other critical illnesses. In order to provide better patient care, it is helpful to go back to first principles and work with direct knowledge of people's beliefs about what makes a 'good death'. Steinhauser et al. (2000) researched descriptions of what makes a good death from patients, families and providers, using focus group discussions and interviews. The participants identified six components of a good death:

- pain and symptom management;
- clear decision-making;
- preparation for death;
- completion;
- contributing to others;
- affirmation of the whole person.

Unsurprisingly, Steinhauser et al. found that physicians held a more biomedical perspective than other people, while patients and families felt that psychosocial and spiritual issues are as important as physiological concerns.

Bingley et al. (2006) reviewed narratives by people facing death from cancer and other diseases. The search identified 148 narratives since 1950 from which a sub-sample of 63 narratives could be reviewed. Bingley et al. found that the therapeutic benefits of writing were generally viewed as *a way of making sense of dying, together with a strong sense of purpose in sharing the story*. Common themes were changes in body image, an awareness of social needs when dying, communication with medical staff, symptom control, realities of suffering and spiritual aspects of dying. Writing about cancer in comparison to other illnesses showed differences in content and style. The authors suggested that: 'The narrative acts as companion and witness to the encroaching disability and debility, as well as charting the changes in relationships with loved ones, oneself and one's body image' (Bingley et al., 2006: 194).

Harding and Higginson (2003) reviewed interventions to support caregivers in cancer and palliative care. They made the usual criticisms of psychosocial intervention research: poor designs and methodology, a lack of outcome evaluation, small sample sizes and a reliance on intervention descriptions and formative evaluations in the literature. They suggested that alternatives to 'pure' RCTs would need to be considered in carrying out evaluation research in this domain. As was the case in reviewing interventions for obesity, drinking and smoking (Chapters 10–12), it is apparent that larger-scale studies of higher quality are needed to reach definitive conclusions about the effectiveness of psychosocial interventions. This statement has become a desperate refrain in our textbook of health psychology.

Spiritual aspects are often missing in studies of EOL care. Williams (2006) summarized the qualitative literature on spirituality at the end of life. The majority of participants in 11 relevant studies had a diagnosis of cancer, but those with AIDS, cardiovascular disease and amyotrophic lateral sclerosis were also represented. The studies suggested three main themes within spiritual perspectives at the end of life:

- spiritual despair – alienation, loss of self, dissonance;
- spiritual work – forgiveness, self-exploration, search for balance;
- spiritual well-being – connection, self-actualization, consonance.

Qualitative studies have explored the quality of care from a patient perspective. Singer et al. (1999) used in-depth, open-ended, face-to-face interviews and content analysis in Toronto, Ontario, with 48 dialysis patients, 40 people with HIV infection and 38 residents of a long-term care facility. They identified five domains of quality EOL care: receiving adequate pain and symptom management, avoiding inappropriate prolongation of dying, achieving a sense of control, relieving burden, and strengthening relationships with loved ones.

One of the main determinants of family satisfaction with EOL care is where the death happens – at home or in hospital. Little data exist addressing satisfaction with EOL care among hospitalized patients, as they and their family members are systematically excluded from routine satisfaction surveys. It is imperative that we closely examine patient and institution factors associated with quality EOL care and determine high-priority target areas for quality improvement.

Sadler et al. (2014) mailed a Bereavement Questionnaire to the next of kin of recently deceased inpatients to study factors associated with satisfaction with EOL care in Canada. The primary outcome measure was the global rating of satisfaction. Overall, 67.4% of respondents were very or completely satisfied with the overall quality of care their relative received. A common death location was the intensive care unit (45.7%); however, this was not the preferred location of death for 47.6% of such patients. In total, 71.4% of respondents who thought their relative did not die in their preferred location favoured an out-of-hospital location of death. Respondents who believed their relative died in their preferred location were 1.7 times more likely to be satisfied with the EOL care that was provided ($p = 0.001$). Nearly three-quarters of recently deceased inpatients would have preferred an out-of-hospital death. The authors concluded that improved communication regarding EOL care preferences should be a high-priority quality-improvement target.

Palliative care

Palliative care focuses on relief of suffering and psychosocial support in patients who are suffering pain and/or distress and, in a dying patient, can help bring closure near the end of life. Palliative care should be available to anyone with serious illness experiencing pain, other distressing symptoms or emotional or psychological distress, at any stage of illness, including in conjunction with 'disease-modifying' treatments (Dixon et al., 2015). In the UK, palliative care is delivered by specialist professionals with accredited training, usually working as part of multidisciplinary teams, and by generalists such as GPs, district nurses, hospital doctors, ward nurses, allied health professionals, staff in care homes, social care staff, social workers, chaplains and others.

Some groups are less likely to receive the care they need than others. For example, people with conditions other than cancer receive only 20% of referrals to specialist palliative care, much less than the 70% of people who die from non-cancer conditions each year. People aged 85 or over also receive little specialist palliative care, accounting for 39% of deaths but just 16% of specialist referrals. People from minority groups are as likely as people of white ethnicity to die at home. However, they report receiving poorer quality of care, rate care from care homes particularly poorly, and are more likely to die in hospital than in a care home. People living in more deprived areas have less access to community-based services, are less satisfied with the care they receive, are less likely to feel treated with dignity by all of the professionals involved in their care and also more frequently die in hospital.

Dixon et al. also reported that people without a spouse or partner are less likely to receive home-based services, to die at home, have their pain well controlled or receive care that their families consider to be high quality. It is likely that spouses or partners can help to ensure high-quality care by informally coordinating the care of different professionals, by acting as advocates and by providing care directly (e.g., administering medications).

Investment is needed to extend palliative care provision to everyone who would benefit from it, especially to meet the growing demand for palliative care from an ageing population. Dixon et al. suggest that good-quality palliative care may even provide annual net savings, with studies suggesting that these might amount to more that £37 million in the UK. Similar trends are evident in palliative care in the USA.

Temel et al. (2010) conducted an RCT of early palliative care in addition to standard oncology care for patients with newly diagnosed metastatic non-small-cell lung cancer. Compared with the standard care group, the intervention group had better quality of life, lower rates of depression, and a 2.7-month survival benefit. The results suggest that palliative care is appropriate and potentially beneficial when introduced at the time of diagnosis of a serious or life-limiting illness, at the same time as all other appropriate and beneficial medical therapies are initiated, rather than as a final base type of care when other options have failed. The problem with this idea is the lack of resources in palliative care compared to other types of care that are perceived as 'front-line' services, such as ICUs.

Impact of death on care staff

Stress, anxiety and depression among senior health service staff can run at high levels (Caplan, 1994). A systematic review by Imo (2016) examined the prevalence and associated factors of burnout and stress-related psychiatric disorders among UK doctors. Prevalence of psychiatric morbidity ranged from 17% to 52%, burnout scores ranged from 31% to 54.3%, depersonalization from 17.4% to 44.5% and low personal accomplishment from 6% to 39.6%. General practitioners and consultants had the highest scores. The prevalence of burnout and psychiatric morbidity was found to be associated with low job satisfaction, overload, increased hours worked and neuroticism.

How do hospital doctors learn to cope with dying and death? Granek et al. (2016) interviewed 22 oncologists from three adult oncology centres. Oncologists were at different stages of their careers and varied in their sub-specialties, gender, and personal and professional backgrounds. The analysis revealed different ways of coping with patient death:

- cognitive – accepting and normalizing death and focusing on the positive, and on successes in the practice of oncology;

- behavioural – sports, hobbies, entertainment, and taking vacations;

- relational – accessing social support from family, friends and colleagues;

- professional – focusing on work, withdrawing from patients at end of life, and compartmentalization;

- spiritual coping strategies – turning to faith and religious coping.

The oncologists also reported challenges and barriers in coping effectively with patient deaths, including challenges in accessing social support, challenges that were related to gender and expression of emotion, and challenges in maintaining emotional boundaries when patients died. Granek et al. (2016) concluded that oncologists use diverse coping strategies in dealing with patient death, but obstacles to accessing this support were reported. They recommended that targeted interventions were needed for managing and coping with grief related to patient death in their emotionally difficult work.

The same research group (Granek et al., 2017) found that high burnout scores are associated with negative attitudes towards expressing emotion in coping with patient death. Higher burnout scores were associated with higher negative attitudes towards perceived expressed emotion ($r = .25$) among those who viewed affect as a sign of weakness and unprofessionalism. Interventions that enable oncologists to express emotion about patient death are recommended.

A particularly demanding task is notification of the patient's family that their loved one has died. The death notification process can affect family grief and bereavement and also the well-being of physicians who carry it out. There is no standardized process for making death-notification phone calls. In many cases this task is given to the most junior doctors, and residents are unlikely to be prepared before and to be troubled afterwards. Ombres et al. (2017) investigated death notification practices to develop an evidence-based template for standardizing this process. They developed a survey regarding resident training and experience in death-notification by phone and invited all internal medicine residents at their institution to complete the survey. Of responders, 87% reported involvement in a death that required notification by phone. In all, 80% of residents felt inadequately trained for this task, with over 25% reporting that calls went poorly. Primary care physicians, nurses and chaplains were not involved. Respondents never delayed notification of death until the family arrived at the hospital. There was no consistent approach to rehearsing or making the call, advising families about safe travel to the hospital, greeting families upon arrival, or following up with expressions of condolence. The authors concluded that poor communication skills during death notification may contribute to complicated grief for surviving relatives and stress among physicians. It is clear that more training is needed. Ombres et al. suggested that this training could be combined with training in disclosure of medical error.

DEATH WITH DIGNITY: PHYSICIAN-ASSISTED DEATH

In 1973 in the Netherlands, in the Postma case, a physician helped her mother to end her life upon her explicit, repeated request. The court judged that the physician had committed murder, but gave her only a suspended sentence while acknowledging that it is not in all circumstances the physician's duty to prolong their patient's life. Increasing interest in physician-assisted death (PAD) has occurred since its legalization in 1997 by Oregon's Death with Dignity Act. Four other states, Washington, Montana, Vermont and California, have passed similar laws. PAD may also sometimes be labelled 'physician-assisted suicide' (PAS). The Netherlands, Belgium, Luxembourg, Colombia and Canada (Quebec since 2014, nationally as of June 2016) also permit euthanasia. Euthanasia and physician-assisted suicide are increasingly being legalized, remain relatively rare, and primarily involve patients with cancer (Emanuel et al., 2016).

Since 1988 in Zurich, Switzerland, an organization called 'Dignitas' has helped people with terminal illnesses and severe physical and mental conditions to die assisted by qualified doctors and nurses. Dignitas has helped over 1,000 people die in suicide clinics in Zurich. Additionally, Dignitas provides assisted suicide for people who are deemed to be of sound judgement and submit to an in-depth medical report prepared by a psychiatrist that establishes the patient's condition. In Oregon, until 2012, 1,050 people have received prescriptions for lethal medication and 673 have died after making the choice to take the drugs (Oregon Public Health Division, 2014).

Emanuel et al. (2016) reviewed the legal status of euthanasia and physician-assisted suicide and the available data on attitudes and practices for the period 1947–2016. Public support for euthanasia and PAS in the USA has plateaued since the 1990s (with a range of 47% to 69%). In Western Europe, an increasing and strong public support for euthanasia and PAS has been reported, but in Central and Eastern Europe support is decreasing. In the USA, less than 20% of physicians report receiving requests for euthanasia or PAS, and 5% or less have complied. In Oregon and Washington, less than 1% of physicians write prescriptions for PAS per year. In the Netherlands and Belgium, half or more of physicians reported ever having received a request, with 60% of Dutch physicians having ever granted such requests. Between 0.3% and 4.6% of all deaths are reported as euthanasia or PAS in jurisdictions where they are legal, with the frequency increasing after legalization. More than 70% involve patients with cancer. Typical patients are older, white and well-educated. Pain is mostly not reported as the primary motivation. A large proportion of PAS patients in Oregon and Washington reported being enrolled in hospice or palliative care, as did patients in Belgium. In no jurisdiction was there any evidence that vulnerable patients have been receiving euthanasia or PAS at rates higher than those in the general population.

Active euthanasia is currently not legal in many countries, such as the UK, France, Spain, Italy and Germany. The Suicide Act 1961 makes it an offence to encourage or assist a suicide or a suicide attempt in England and Wales. Anyone doing so could face up to 14 years in prison. It is only legal in Belgium, Holland and Luxembourg. Under the laws in these countries, a person's life can be deliberately ended by their doctor or other health care professional. The person is usually given an overdose of muscle relaxants or sedatives. This causes a coma and then death. Euthanasia is only legal if the following three criteria are met:

1. The person has made an active and voluntary request to end their life.

2. They are considered to have sufficient mental capacity to make an informed decision regarding their care.

3. It is agreed that the person is suffering unbearably and there is no prospect for an improvement in their condition.

'Suffering' is a central concept in the right-to-die movement. A Canadian study by Karsoho et al. (2016) asked how proponents of PAD articulate suffering at the end of life within the decriminalization/legalization debate. They drew upon empirical data from their study of *Carter vs. Canada*, the landmark court case that decriminalized PAD in Canada in 2015, and analysed the different ways proponents constructed relationships between suffering, mainstream curative medicine, palliative care and assisted dying. Karsoho et al. suggest that proponents view curative medicine as 'complicit in the production of suffering at the end of life … [and] … lament a cultural context wherein life-prolongation is the moral imperative of physicians who are paternalistic and death-denying' (Karsoho et al., 2016: 188). Proponents question whether palliative care has the ability to alleviate suffering at the end of life and claim that, in some instances, palliative care produces suffering. However, in spite of such misgivings, the authors reported that proponents insist on the involvement of physicians in assisted dying. They suggest that 'a request for PAD can set in motion an interactive therapeutic process that alleviates suffering at the end of life'. Furthermore, they argue that the 'proponents' articulation of suffering with the role of medicine at the end of life should be understood as a discourse through which one configuration of end-of-life care comes to be accepted and another rejected, a discourse that ultimately does not challenge, but makes productive use of the larger framework of the medicalization of dying' (Karsoho et al., 2016: 188).

The wave of new state laws on PAD is leaving physicians feeling under-prepared and unsupported in how to provide the best possible care to dying patients seeking assistance to die. Some professional organizations, such as the American College of Physicians, American Medical Association and American Osteopathic Association, are refusing to provide clinical guidance on the care of patients actively seeking PAD/PAS (Frye and Youngner, 2016). Other organizations, such as the California Medical Association and the American Academy of Hospice and Palliative Medicine, have dropped their traditional opposition and are taking a 'stance of studied neutrality', a hands-off position chosen to recognize the diversity of views and foster discussion. Frye and Youngner (2016) argue that professional organizations should engage neutrally and take responsibility to minimize or avoid potential harms of PAS.

To determine whether there is a difference in the quality of the dying experience, from the perspective of family members, Smith et al. (2011) surveyed 52 Oregonians who received lethal prescriptions, 34 who requested but did not receive lethal prescriptions, and 63 who did not pursue PAD. Family members retrospectively rated the dying experience of their loved one with the 33-item QoDD (Curtis et al., 2002). Differences were reported in nine of the 33 items, but few significant differences were noted in items that measured domains of connectedness, transcendence and overall quality of death. Those who had received PAD prescriptions had higher quality ratings on items measuring symptom control (e.g., control over surroundings and control of bowels/bladder) and better preparedness for death scores (saying goodbye to loved ones and possession of a means to end life if desired) than those who did not pursue PAD or, in some cases, those who requested but did not receive a lethal prescription. The authors concluded that the quality of death experienced by those who received lethal prescriptions is no worse than those not pursuing PAD, and in some areas it is rated by family members as better.

The Royal College of General Practitioners (RCGP) in the UK rejected the newly proposed Assisted Dying Bill. Consultation with RCGP members (n = 1,700) showed that 77% were in favour of supporting the group's opposition to changing the law (Baker, 2014). On the other hand, the *British Medical Journal* (*BMJ*) supported the bill, stating that 'people should be able to exercise choice over their lives, which should include how and when they die, when death is imminent' (Delamothe et al., 2014: 4349). While the right to exercise choice is one of the main arguments presented by those who support the bill, choice may not be an option for all. As McCartney (2014: 4502) argued:

> … our death is always potentially imminent, and we clearly do not enjoy omnipotent choice over our lives; otherwise, people in poorer areas would live just as long, with as much money and power as those more comfortably off. Indeed, 'choice' in healthcare is often proffered as a consumer interest, pandering to the profit motive in our dissolving NHS. The choices that affect our lives most – income, status, employment – have more to do with the luck of the environment we grow up in than with personal volition. Why should 'choice' over death remain uninfluenced by the bad luck of our environment? And if such choice is paramount, why doesn't the BMJ argue for assisted suicide at any other point in life, not just in terminal illness? Also, we can't be sure that the law will be properly followed. … The care of dying people is already difficult. It makes me uncomfortable when articulate, middle-class people want more so-called choice, when they may hardly know of the stresses and vulnerabilities of others.

Issues were also raised concerning the conceptualization of 'mental capacity', upon which the proposed bill relies. Price et al. (2014) explored how the experts presenting evidence to the Commission on Assisted Dying conceptualized the 'mental capacity' of patients requesting assistance for their death. Findings from this qualitative study suggest that 'mental capacity' was considered as a central safeguard in the proposed bill. However, its conceptualization remained inconsistent. While 'mental capacity' could be defined within the legal 'cognitive' definition of capacity (i.e., a person will be considered mentally capable unless significantly cognitively impaired), it can also be defined within the grounds of autonomy, rationality, voluntariness and motivation. The authors argued that more work is needed to establish consensus as to what constitutes 'mental capacity'. Furthermore, frameworks need to be in place to support professionals in determining 'mental capacity' in practice.

In a systematic review examining the attitudes of health professionals, patients, carers and the public on assisted dying in dementia, Tomlinson and Stott (2014) found that health professionals held more restrictive views towards assisted dying than the public, patients and carers. However, these opinions varied depending on the severity of a patient's condition and capacity. Age, ethnicity, gender and religion also appeared to influence people's attitudes towards assisted dying. Similarly, a systematic review by Vezina-Im et al. (2014) compared physicians' and nurses' motivations to participate in assisted dying. A total of 27 studies were included in the review. Findings suggest that physicians and nurses showed motivation to practise voluntary euthanasia when they were already familiar with this process. However, motivation may vary according to medical speciality. This can also be influenced by patients' prognosis and depressive symptoms.

In a qualitative study in New Zealand, Malpas et al. (2014) presented reasons as to why some older adults would oppose physician-assisted dying. Findings suggest that participants' personal experiences of good death strengthened their views that speeding the dying process is unnecessary. Religious reasoning and beliefs also contributed to their attitudes. 'Slippery slope' worries too were raised that reflected concerns about the potential risk of making this practice the norm in the future. Additionally, there were concerns about potential abuses if this process were legalized. As a participant recalled from a conversation with a family member: 'She thought that I should be euthanized. If I was overseas, Holland, or somewhere they would put me out of my misery. And she actually said to me, "If you were my dog, I would shoot you to put you out of your misery" (Malpas et al., 2014: 356).

The taken-for-granted assumption that underlies arguments for assisted dying is the belief that the quality of life for such individuals is so severely reduced that it makes it unendurable and is bound up with a rhetoric of the moral imperative to relieve suffering. The entrenched disablement prejudices held by health care professionals result in unsupported assumptions that the quality of life of people with disabilities is diminished in such a way that it makes it more unendurable, more hopeless and more limited than that of people for whom other factors have diminished their quality of life (e.g., someone whose family has been killed and finds life unbearable without them). However, as suggested in a study by Terrill et al. (2014), resilience can mitigate the impact of secondary symptoms (e.g., pain and fatigue) on the quality of life of people with long-term physical disablement.

In addition, assisting certain disabled people to die would not be countenanced. For example, it is unlikely that assisting the survivors of genocide to die would be countenanced, despite them enduring extreme suffering, pain, disablement and distress. There are a number of forms of 'assisted-dying', including a person ending their own life by their choice using a tool supplied by someone else; someone else ending a person's life with their consent; someone else ending a person's life without their consent; and withholding life-sustaining treatment (with or without that person's consent). All of these forms of 'assisted-dying' have been applied to disabled people. That 'assisted-dying' can refer to the act without the consent of the person who dies is particularly worrying. It has been suggested that many disabled people fear that episodes of illness may be viewed as an opportunity to 'allow' them 'merciful' release (Marks, 1999), and there may be some basis for this. In states and countries where assisted suicide has been legalized, people with physical and psychiatric disabilities have been helped to die both with and without their consent. One cannot doubt that physician-assisted dying happens unofficially on a daily basis in hospitals and homes everywhere.

BRAIN DEATH AND TAKING ORGANS FOR TRANSPLANTATION

Brain death is irreversible brain damage causing the end of independent respiration and is regarded as indicative of death. When a person is brain dead, the brain can no longer function. The brain will not recover function and the person is considered dead. The doctors can support the heart with medication and also provide oxygen through a ventilator, or breathing machine. The person's body can be supported for days and, sometimes, even weeks. However, without a functioning brain, the person can no longer be considered as living. A brain death diagnosis is final and cannot be reversed. A person with brain death never awakens.

There is a gap between the number of organ donors and patients on waiting lists for transplantation. Vital organ transplantation is premised on 'the dead donor rule': prior to the harvesting of organs, donors must be declared dead according to medical and legal criteria. Donors are also required to give their informed consent to the taking of their vital organs. Doubts can arise about whether individuals diagnosed as 'brain dead' are really dead in accordance with a biological conception of death – *the irreversible cessation of the functioning of the organism as a whole*. A basic understanding of brain death is required in giving and obtaining valid, informed consent to serve as an organ donor. There is a need for reliable empirical data on public understanding of brain death and vital organ transplantation.

There is a need for increasing awareness of the potential for organ donation in EOL care. In Sweden, Nolin et al. (2017) reported that the number of organ donations after brain death (DBD) per million population (pmp) was 14.9, with an almost 10-fold variation from 4.3 to 40.6 DBD pmp between counties. Women were 60% more likely to become donors compared to men. An EOL decision was found in only 50.9% of possible organ donors.

Shah et al. (2015) reviewed evidence on public attitudes to brain death and vital organ transplantation. They identified 43 articles with approximately 18,603 study participants. The data suggested that people generally do not understand three key issues: (1) uncontested biological facts about brain death, (2) the legal status of brain death, and (3) that organs are procured from brain-dead patients while their hearts are still beating and before their removal.

Discussion about death, especially one's own, is a delicate subject and even tabooed. Yet plans and recorded decisions are necessary if viable organs for transplantation are to be obtained to save the lives of others. Families need to discuss personal wishes about organ donation in advance in case brain death should be an issue in the future. Unsurprisingly, family members dealing with a brain-dead loved one who is supported on a ventilator are often unable to carry out the person's expressed wishes to donate organs (Bresnahan, 2015).

To facilitate clear communications about brain death, Bresnahan and Zhuang (2016) published the *Communicating with Family about Brain Death Scale*, which assesses the willingness of individuals to communicate about brain-dead organ donation with their family members. This scale is one step towards facilitating more open discussions about organ donation, and it could help save the lives of more people waiting for transplants.

In some countries, informed consent is not obtained prior to harvesting of organs. It is estimated that more than 90% of the organs transplanted in China before 2010 were procured from prisoners. Paul et al. (2017) reported a continued prevalence in China of organ procurement without consent from prisoners or their families, as well as procurement of organs from incompletely executed, still-living prisoners. This practice violates international ethics standards and fundamental human rights.

FUTURE RESEARCH

1. More research on the quality of dying and death should incorporate the voice of families and relatives.
2. Research is needed in determining ways in which more people can obtain their preference to die at home.

(Continued)

3. Large-scale studies on the characteristics of high-quality end of life are needed to inform improvements.

4. The auditing of medical and nurse training to reveal knowledge and skills gaps relevant to death and dying is needed.

SUMMARY

1. Kübler-Ross (1997) constructed a five-stage theory of death and dying experienced when terminally ill patients face their own deaths: denial–dissociation–isolation, anger, bargaining, depression and acceptance. This theory receives little empirical support.

2. Attempts to define a 'good death' suggest that people may wish to achieve many different tasks during the process of dying. Three themes about dying and death are control, autonomy and independence.

3. The quality of death is higher for terminally ill patients receiving hospice care than for similar patients receiving conventional care.

4. High-quality EOL care aims to reflect each individual patient's values and wishes, promote compassionate communication and provide family-oriented care.

5. End-of-life care leads to a reduction of non-beneficial, unnecessary and aggressive physical care, avoids prolongation of dying, prevents patient suffering and allows less wastage of precious intensive care unit resources.

6. Many people who need EOL or palliative care are not receiving them. EOL and palliative care need to be improved and made more accessible, which requires a greater allocation of resources.

7. Oncologists and other staff dealing on a day-to-day basis with dying patients face challenges and barriers in trying to cope, in accessing social support and in gender-related expression of emotion. Targeted interventions are needed for staff on managing and coping with grief.

8. Increasing interest in physician-assisted death has been occurring since its legalization in 1997 by Oregon's Death with Dignity Act. Although euthanasia and physician-assisted suicide are increasingly being legalized, they remain relatively rare, and primarily involve patients with cancer.

9. Research on public attitudes to brain death and vital organ transplantation suggests that people generally do not understand (1) the biological facts about brain death, (2) the legal status of brain death, and (3) that organs are procured from brain-dead patients while their hearts are still beating and before their removal.

10. Education programmes are needed to increase clarity and reduce confusion about brain death and organ donation in an attempt to increase the availability of much-needed organs.

GLOSSARY

ACE (angiotensin converting enzyme) inhibitor   a drug that is important in the regulation of blood pressure.

Acquisition   the process of learning a response or taking up a specific behaviour through association or conditioning.

Action research   a type of research concerned with the process of change and what else happens when change occurs. Action research is particularly suitable for organizations or systems requiring improvement or change.

Action stage   one of the stages proposed by the *transtheoretical model of change (TMC)* in which a person takes specific actions with the aim of changing unwanted behaviour, bringing positive benefits to well-being.

Acute   the early stages of a condition; normally defined as a condition that lasts for less than six months.

Acute pain   pain that lasts for less than six months.

Addiction   a term used to describe a person's physical and psychological dependency on an activity, drink or drug, seemingly beyond conscious control. Addiction is said to occur when there is: a strong desire to engage in the particular behaviour (especially when the opportunity to engage in such behaviour is not available); an impaired capacity to control the behaviour; discomfort and/or distress when the behaviour is prevented or ceased; persistence of the behaviour despite clear evidence that it is leading to problems.

Addiction theories   theories based on the construct of addiction used to explain alcoholism and other excessive behaviours (e.g., gambling, shopping, drug use, over-eating).

Adipose tissue   tissue in the body in which fat is stored as an energy reserve and which in excess leads to obesity.

Affluenza   the combination of affluence and influenza and referring to the negative psychological consequences of the restless pursuit of more in the consumerist era.

Agency   the capacity to take action in pursuit of intentions and goals.

AIDS (acquired immune deficiency syndrome)   an advanced HIV infection which generally occurs when the CD4 count is below 200/ml. It is characterized by the appearance of opportunistic infections which take advantage of the weakened immune system and include: pneumocystis carinii pneumonia; toxoplasmosis; tuberculosis; extreme weight loss and wasting; being exacerbated by diarrhoea; meningitis and other brain infections; fungal infections; syphilis; and malignancies such as lymphoma, cervical cancer and Kaposi's sarcoma.

Alcohol dependence syndrome   a psychophysiological disorder characterized by increased tolerance of alcohol, withdrawal symptoms following reduced consumption, a persistent desire, or unsuccessful efforts to reduce or control drinking.

Anchoring   the process whereby unfamiliar concepts are given meaning by connecting them with more familiar concepts.

Angina pectoris   the most common form of coronary heart disease. It is characterized by a heavy or tight pain in the centre of the chest that may spread to the arms, necks, jaw, face, back or stomach. Angina symptoms occur when the arteries become so narrow from the *atheroma* that insufficient oxygen-containing blood can be supplied to the heart muscle when its demands are high, such as during exercise.

Angina Plan   a psychological intervention for angina patients; it consists of a patient-held booklet and an audio-taped relaxation programme.

Antibodies   blood proteins produced in response to and counteracting a specific antigen. Antibodies combine chemically with substances which the body recognizes as alien, such as bacteria, viruses, and foreign substances in the blood.

Anticipated regret   the anxiety about the outcome of making a decision.

Anticoagulant drugs   drugs that prevent the clotting of blood.

Anti-essentialist view of human sexuality   the view of human sexuality as a set of potentialities which may or may not be realized within differing social, cultural and historical contexts.

Antigen   a molecule that is capable of binding to an antibody or to an antigen receptor on a T cell, especially one that induces an immune response.

Aromatherapy   a type of complementary medicine that involves the use of essential oils from plant extracts for therapeutic purposes.

Arrhythmia   a condition in which the heart beats with an irregular or abnormal rhythm.

Artefact   an uncontrolled and possibly unknown variable or factor causing a misleading, spurious finding in a study.

Asexual   an individual who does not experience sexual feelings.

Assessment   a procedure through which a patient, client, participant or situation can be evaluated against a benchmark or criterion enabling further actions or interventions to be administered, interpreted or understood.

Assigned sex   the sex that is assigned to an infant at birth based on the child's visible sex organs, including genitalia and other physical characteristics.

Atheroma   furring-up of an artery by deposits, mainly of cholesterol, within its walls. Associated with atherosclerosis, atheroma has the effect of narrowing the lumen (channel) of the artery, thus restricting blood flow. This predisposes a person to a number of conditions, including thrombosis, angina, and stroke.

Atherosclerosis   a disease of the arteries characterized by the deposition of fatty material on their inner walls.

Attachment   the bond that forms between parent and child, which can have life-long consequences.

Attachment styles   Mary Ainsworth identified three main attachment styles: secure (type B), insecure avoidant (type A) and insecure ambivalent/resistant (type C). These attachment styles are the result of early interactions with the mother.

Attitudes   the sum of beliefs about a particular behaviour weighted by evaluations of these beliefs.

Attribution bias   the tendency to attribute positive things to oneself and negative things to others.

Attribution theory   theory of lay causal explanations of events and behaviours.

Attributions   perceived or reported causes of actions, feelings or events.

Authoritarian doctor   a personality type or leadership style favouring obedience rather than freedom of expression.

Autoimmunity   the system of immune responses of an organism against its own healthy cells and tissues. Any disease that results from such an aberrant immune response is termed an autoimmune disease.

Autonomic nervous system   the part of the nervous system responsible for control of bodily functions that are not consciously directed, such as breathing, the heartbeat, and digestive processes.

Autonomy   the ability to act without reference to others.

B cells (otherwise known as '**B lymphocytes**')   lymphocytes (a subtype of white blood cell) that have antigen-binding antibody molecules on the surface, that comprise the antibody-secreting plasma cells when mature, and that in mammals differentiate in the bone marrow. Compare with *T cell*.

Behaviour   actions in response to internal or external events.

Behaviour change technique (BCT)   an approach to health promotion that targets behaviour change in individual members of the population.

Behaviour genetics   a field in which variation among individuals is separated into genetic versus environmental components. The most common research methodologies are family studies, twin studies, adoption studies and genome-wide association studies.

Behaviour(al) setting   the social and physical setting within which a certain behaviour is expected.

Benign tumour   a growth that is not cancerous.

Beta-blockers   drugs that block the actions of the hormone adrenaline (epinephrine), which makes the heart beat faster and more vigorously.

Between groups design   a research design involving two or more matched groups of participants that receive different conditions, for example an intervention versus a control condition.

Biological reductionism   the assumption that all human experience can be directly traced to and explained with reference to its biological basis.

Biological sex   anatomical, physiological, genetic or physical attributes that define whether a person is male, female or intersex. These include genitalia, gonads, hormone levels, hormone receptors, chromosomes, genes and secondary sex characteristics.

Biological therapy   the use of living organisms, substances derived from living organisms, or laboratory-produced versions of such substances to treat disease.

Biomedical model   The traditional approach of medicine to a model's focus on the physical processes of a disease, not taking into account the role of social or psychological factors.

Biomedicine   a health system that identifies the cause of agreed diseases and symptoms as lying in certain physiological processes.

Biopsychosocial model   the view that health and illness are produced by a combination of physical, psychological and cultural factors (Engel, 1977).

Bisexual (otherwise known as 'bi')   a person who experiences romantic, emotional or sexual attraction to the same gender and other genders, whether to equal degrees or to varying degrees.

Black box   a device, system or object used in models which can be viewed in terms of its inputs and outputs without any knowledge of its internal workings.

Black Report   a report on health inequalities published in the UK in 1980, named after the chairman of the committee who produced the report, Sir Douglas Black.

Body image a person's perception of the physical character of their body.

Body mass index (BMI) the body weight in kilograms divided by the square of the height in metres; has a normal range of 20 to 25. An invalid indicator of clinically significant levels of visceral fat.

Bottom-up approach listening to people about what they perceive their needs to be and acting upon that information together in an attempt to meet those needs.

Buddhist a person who practises the religion of Buddhism; living in the present.

Built environment the physical human-made objects in the everyday world.

Bupropion (otherwise known as Zyban) initially employed as an antidepressant, used in smoking cessation.

Burden of disease a concept referring to the overall costs associated with a disease measured by the economic, social and psychological resources that are expended during care, treatment and rehabilitation.

Calorie the energy needed to increase the temperature of 1 kg of water by 1°C, which is about 4.184 kJ. Fat contributes 9 calories per gram, alcohol 7 calories per gram and carbohydrates 4 calories per gram.

Carcinogens substances, radionuclides and radiation that act directly or indirectly in causing cancer.

Cardiovascular diseases conditions that involve narrowed or blocked blood vessels that can lead to a heart attack, chest pain (angina) or stroke. Other heart conditions, such as those that affect the heart's muscle, valves or rhythm, are also considered forms of heart disease.

Case study a retrospective written report on individuals, groups or systems.

Case-control study an epidemiological study in which exposure of patients to factors that may cause their disease (cases) is compared to the exposure to the same factors of participants who do not have the disease (controls).

Catastrophizing the tendency to become emotional and pessimistic about symptoms, illness or difficulties.

Causal ontologies of suffering causal frameworks for explaining illness and suffering.

Central circadian pacemaker a cluster of neurons, the activity of which fluctuates in ± 24-hour cycles; it resides in the pineal gland.

Cerebellum a large portion of the brain, containing 80% of the brain's neurones, serving to coordinate voluntary movements, posture and balance, at the back of and below the cerebrum, and consisting of two lateral lobes and a central lobe.

Cessation   the process of stopping (ceasing) a specific behaviour, habit or activity; one possible outcome of the *action stage* in the *transtheoretical model of change (TMC)*.

Chemotherapy (CT)   the treatment of disease by the use of chemical substances, especially the treatment of cancer by cytotoxic and other drugs.

Chlamydia   a common sexually transmitted infection (STI) caused by the bacterium *Chlamydia trachomatis*, which can damage a woman's reproductive organs. Even though symptoms of chlamydia are usually mild or absent, serious complications that cause irreversible damage, including infertility, can occur 'silently' before a woman recognizes a problem. Chlamydia also can cause discharge from the penis of an infected man.

Cholesterol   a lipid produced in the body from acetyl-CoA and present in the diet.

Chromosomes   thread-like structures located inside the nucleus of animal and plant cells. Each chromosome is made of protein and a single molecule of deoxyribonucleic acid (DNA). Passed from parents to offspring, DNA contains the specific instructions that make each type of living creature unique.

Chronic   any condition that continues for at least six months.

Chronic fatigue syndrome (CFS)   a syndrome identified in Nevada, USA, in 1984, characterized by severe fatigue and other symptoms suggesting a viral infection and persisting over long periods of time. There is much current controversy as to whether it is a *psychosomatic disorder* or caused by an as-yet unidentified virus. CFS is thought to be identical to *myalgic encephalomyelitis* (*ME*).

Chronic pain   pain that lasts longer than six months; whether mild or excruciating, episodic or continuous, merely inconvenient or totally incapacitating, it takes a physical and emotional toll on a person.

Circadian clock   a biochemical oscillator that oscillates with a stable phase relationship to solar time.

Classical conditioning   a learning process whereby a previously neutral stimulus (*conditioned stimulus*, CS) comes to evoke a certain response (unconditioned response, UCR) as a result of repeated previous pairings with a stimulus (*unconditioned stimulus*, UCS) that naturally evokes the response.

Clinical health psychology   the application of psychological theory and research to the prevention and treatment of illness and the identification of aetiologic and diagnostic correlates of health and illness and related dysfunctions.

Closeted   a person who is not open about their sexual orientation or gender identity, or an ally who is not open about their support for people who are LGBTQ.

Cognitions   thoughts, beliefs and images forming the elements of a person's knowledge concerning the physical and psychosocial environment.

Cognitive behavioural therapy (CBT) modification of thoughts, images, feelings and behaviour using the principles of *classical* and *operant conditioning* combined with cognitive techniques concerned with the control of mental states.

Combination antiretroviral therapy (cART) (otherwise known as 'HAART' or 'ART') a treatment for people infected with human immunodeficiency virus (HIV) using anti-HIV drugs. The standard treatment consists of a combination of at least three drugs that suppress HIV replication.

Communication styles different approaches to verbal interaction that are characterized by particular linguistic and rhetorical techniques and strategies such as listening or question asking.

Communicative event a joint achievement that is the product of participants' strategic deployment of culturally available discursive resources.

Communitarian an approach that focuses on the whole community rather than individuals, working towards social justice and reducing inequities.

Community development approach an approach to health promotion that recognizes the close relationship between individual health and socio-economic factors. It aims to remove the socio-economic and environmental causes of ill health through the collective organization of members of the community.

Community health psychology advancing theory, research and social action to promote positive well-being, increase empowerment, and prevent the development of problems of communities, groups and individuals.

Compensatory conditioned response model an influential model put forward by Siegel (1975) to account for the phenomena of addiction, such as tolerance, dependence and withdrawal, using the principles of *classical conditioning*.

Complementary and alternative medicine (CAM) forms of health care that are not controlled by professional medicine and are based on non-orthodox systems of healing.

Compliance (or adherence) the extent to which a person's behaviour changes as a direct consequence of specific social influence, e.g., a measure of the extent to which patients (or doctors) follow a prescribed treatment plan.

Concordance a model of the physician–patient relationship based upon mutual respect and involvement in treatment.

Conditioned stimulus (CS) a stimulus that, because of pairing with another stimulus (*unconditioned stimulus, UCS*) that naturally evokes a reflex response, is eventually able to evoke that response (see *classical conditioning*). The acquisition is believed to occur when there is a positive contingency between two events such that event A is more likely in the presence of event B than in the absence of B.

Conditioning processes of associating stimuli and responses (see *classical conditioning* and *operant conditioning*) producing learning and experience.

Confidence interval   an interval around the mean of a sample that one can state with a known probability contains the mean of the population.

Confirmation bias or **confirmatory bias**   is the tendency to search for, interpret, favour and recall information in a way that confirms one's pre-existing beliefs or hypotheses.

Conflicts of interest   financial or other gains that an investigator may make from an investigation and its findings.

Confucianism   a Chinese philosophy which views human suffering as a result of destiny or *ming*.

Conscientiousness   one of the five factors of personality proposed by McCrae and Costa in their influential theory, which was originally developed in 1985. The other four factors are openness to experience, extraversion, agreeableness and neuroticism.

Consumerist   style of health care that emphasizes opportunities for patient choice.

Contemplation stage   the stage of intending to change at some as-yet unspecified time in the future. It is one of the stages of the *transtheoretical model of change (TMC)*.

Control group   a group of participants assigned to a condition that does not include the specific treatment being evaluated; used for comparative purposes.

COPE   a questionnaire devised by Carver et al. (1989) to assess the individual's predominant coping strategies in response to stress.

Coronary angiogram   an X-ray of the arteries to help to see whether any of the arteries are blocked by *atheroma*.

Coronary artery bypass graft (CABG)   an operation that enables a blocked area of the coronary artery to be bypassed so that blood flow can be restored to heart tissue that has been deprived of blood because of coronary heart disease (CHD). During CABG, a healthy artery or vein is taken from the leg, arm or chest and transferred to the outside of the heart. The new healthy artery or vein then carries the oxygenated blood around the blockage in the coronary artery.

Coronary heart disease (CHD)   a restriction of the blood flow to the coronary arteries, which is often evidenced by chest pains (angina) and which may result in a heart attack.

Correlational study   a study that explores the statistical associations between variables; can never be used to discover causal relationships.

Cortisol   a steroid hormone in the glucocorticoid class of hormones. It is a crucial hormone to protect overall health and well-being; it affects many different bodily functions, e.g., blood sugar levels, metabolism, reducing inflammation and assisting with memory formulation.

Cost-effectiveness   a method of economic analysis that takes account of both the effectiveness and the cost of an intervention.

COVID-19 a disease caused by a new strain of coronavirus. 'CO' stands for corona, 'VI' for virus, and 'D' for disease. Formerly, this disease was referred to as '2019 novel coronavirus' or '2019-nCoV', Also referred to as '(SARS-CoV-2)'.

Critical consciousness (*conscientização*) a concept developed by Paulo Freire referring to the ability to perceive social, political and economic oppression and to take action against oppressive elements of society.

Critical health psychology analyses how power and macro-social processes influence health, health care and social issues, and studies the implications for the theory and practice of health psychology.

Cross-cultural psychology compares and contrasts samples of populations said to be from different cultures in terms of attitudes, beliefs, values and behaviours that are viewed as stable and essential characteristics of particular cultures.

Cross-over or within-participants design a research design in which participants are placed in two or more conditions; in theory, participants 'act as their own controls'. However, there are sequence effects, practice effects and other issues that make this design more complicated.

Cross-sectional design involves obtaining responses from a sample of respondents on one occasion only. With appropriate randomized sampling methods, the sample can be assumed to be a representative cross-section of the population(s) under study and it will be possible to make comparisons between different sub-groups, e.g., males vs. females, older vs. younger, etc.

Cross-sectional study a type of observational study that analyses data collected from a population, or a representative sample, at a specific point in time.

Cues to action reminders or prompts to take action consistent with an intention; cues may be internal (e.g., feeling fatigued can trigger actions to take time out or relax) or external (e.g., seeing health promotion leaflets or posters).

Cultural competence a set of competencies that involve cultural sensitivity and appropriateness of staff and health systems.

Cultural psychology the study of human conduct as a form of meaning-making, according to the approach of Valsiner (2013) and others.

Culture a system of meanings and symbols that defines a worldview that frames the way people locate themselves within the world, perceive the world, and find meaning within it.

Cytokines a large group of proteins, peptides or glycoproteins that are secreted by specific cells of the immune system; they mediate and regulate immunity, inflammation and hematopoiesis.

Death gradient the variation in mortality that occurs across a population when the population is segmented according to socio-economic status such that the mortality rate is higher among those groups which have lower socio-economic status.

Decisional balance   weighing the pros and cons of behaviour change.

Deficit mode   the absence of something which is valued.

Deficit model   an explanation used by health care professionals to account for low compliance, e.g., women who do not use a screening service may be characterized as lacking in knowledge and concern about their health.

Denialism   refusing to admit the truth of a concept or proposition that is supported by the majority of scientific or historical evidence.

Deoxyribonucleic acid (DNA)   is the hereditary material in humans and almost all other organisms. Nearly every cell in a person's body has the same DNA. Most DNA is located in the cell nucleus (where it is called nuclear DNA), but a small amount of DNA can also be found in the mitochondria (where it is called mitochondrial DNA or mtDNA). The information in DNA is stored as a code made up of four chemical bases: adenine (A), guanine (G), cytosine (C) and thymine (T). Human DNA consists of about 3 billion bases, and more than 99% of those bases are the same in all people.

Deviant patient   a perspective on doctor–patient communication focusing on the characteristics of the patient as creating problems for the doctor.

Diary techniques   any data-collection method in which the data are linked to the passage of time. They often involve self-report but may also contain information about observations of others.

Direct observation   directly observing behaviour in a relevant setting, e.g., patients waiting for treatment in a doctor's surgery or clinic. The observation may be accompanied by recordings in written, oral, auditory or visual form. It includes casual observation, formal observation and participant observation.

Disability   (1) 'A physical or mental impairment that substantially limits one or more major life activities, a record of such impairment, or a perception of such impairment.' (2) 'Any physical and/or mental impairment that substantially limits one or more of the major life activities (caring for one's self, walking, seeing, hearing, and the like)' (The Americans with Disabilities Act, 1990).

Disability culture   a group identity, a common history of oppression and a common bond of resilience held with pride and consisting of art, music, literature and other expressions of the experience of disability.

Disability-adjusted life year (DALY)   the total amount of healthy life lost, to all causes, whether from premature mortality or from some degree of disability during a period of time. The DALY is the sum of years of life lost from premature mortality plus years of life with disability, adjusted for severity of disability from all causes, both physical and mental (Murray and Lopez, 1997).

Discourse   talk or text embedded in social interaction presenting an account of the constitution of subjects and objects; an opinion or position concerning a particular subject.

Discourse analysis a set of procedures for analysing language as used in speech or texts. It has links with ethnomethodology, conversation analysis and the study of meaning (semiology).

Discourse of risk ways of talking and practices that attribute ill health to personal characteristics and construct an 'at-risk' status as a state in between health and illness.

Disease prototype a cognitive construct or model of a representative case of a specific disease.

Disease theories the idea that the loss of control of behaviour, such as alcohol consumption or eating, is a disease based on personal or inherited characteristics that predispose particular individuals to the condition (e.g., alcoholism or obesity).

Doctor-centred communication style a communication style that primarily makes use of the doctor's expertise by keeping control of the interview agenda.

Dopamine a neurotransmitter in the brain thought to be responsible for sensations of pleasure triggered by events or by the intake of substances such as tobacco or alcohol.

Double-blind control a procedure used in randomized controlled trials to prevent bias, in which neither the participant not the investigator knows the condition or group that a participant has been allocated to.

Dual energy X-ray absorptiometry (DXA) originally used to measure bone density and total body composition; it can also be used to determine abdominal fat mass.

Dual processing model the idea that cognitive representations of danger (e.g., illness threat) are processed independently of the emotional processing.

Ecological approach a model or theory about health and behaviour that emphasizes environmental influences.

Ecological validity the extent to which the environment within which behaviour or experience is studied captures the relevant features of the real-world environment.

Effect size the size of an observed effect measured in standard deviation units.

Effort–reward balance the balance between the workload of a job and the pay received.

e-health the application of information and communication technology to health or health care.

Electrocardiogram (ECG) a physiological measure used to examine the electrical activity of the heart.

Emotional liability a personal characteristic referring to an unstable, variable pattern in a person's responses to events.

Emotions   feelings associated with facial, bodily and verbal expressive behaviour, and internal, visceral activity and thoughts, when affected by interpersonal and environmental events; examples include love, joy, pleasure, ecstasy, pride, lust, greed, envy, jealousy, sadness, fear, worry, anger, disgust, distress or hate; also referred to as positive or negative 'affect'.

Empathy   the ability to understand and share the feelings of another; trying to sense, perceive, share or conceptualize how another person is experiencing the world.

Empowerment   any process by which people, groups or communities exercise increased control or sense of control over aspects of their everyday lives, including their physical and social environments.

End-of-life (EOL) care   support for people in the last months or years of their life.

Energy balance equation (EBE)   an equation relating energy intake to internal heat produced by food, external work and energy storage as follows: energy intake = internal heat produced + external work + energy stored.

Energy envelope theory   a theory developed by Leonard Jason that recommends that patients to learn to pace activities and stay within an energy envelope appears to have favourable outcomes for patients with ME/CFS.

Energy expenditure   use by the body of chemical energy from food and drink or from body stores during the processes of metabolism that is dissipated as heat, including heat generated by muscular activity. The day's total energy expenditure is measured in calories of heat lost.

Energy intake   the chemical energy in food and drink that can be metabolized to produce energy in the body. The day's total energy intake is measured in calories supplied by all food and drink consumed.

Energy Surfeit Theory (EST)   the theory that energy gained due to consumption of foods relative to loss of energy due to exercise causes the body to gain weight.

Environmental foundations   key elements of the working environment relevant to the occupational health and well-being of employees.

Epidemiological transition   in middle- and low-income countries, the time at which non-communicable disease prevalence equals and overtakes the prevalence of communicable diseases.

Epidemiology   the study of associations between patterns of disease in populations and environmental, lifestyle and genetic factors.

Epigenetics   the study of changes in organisms caused by modification of gene expression rather than alteration of the genetic code itself.

Epigenome   a multitude of chemical compounds that can tell the genome what to do. It consists of a record of the chemical changes to the DNA and histone proteins of an organism;

these changes can be passed down to an organism's offspring via transgenerational epigenetic inheritance.

Equity theory   the tendency of individuals to balance the effort invested in a role with the rewards obtained from the role in return.

Ethical approval   the requirement of any research project to present before a panel of experts on ethical issues, and have the panel's explicit approval of the aims, design, sample size and power analysis, participants and how they will be chosen, information provided to the participants, method of consent used, methods of data analysis, nature and timing of the debriefing of participants, and methods of dissemination.

Ethnicity   pertaining to ethnic group or race.

Ethnocentrism   a bias in perception, thinking or principles stemming from membership of a particular ethnic or cultural group.

Ethnographic methods   seek to build a systematic understanding of a culture from the viewpoint of the insider. Ethnographic methods are multiple attempts to describe the shared beliefs, practices, artefacts, knowledge and behaviours of an intact cultural group. They attempt to represent the totality of a phenomenon in its complete context and naturalistic setting. The methods include autoethnography, combining autobiography with ethnography.

Eudaimonic   refers to self-realization; it defines well-being in terms of the degree to which a person's life activities mesh with deeply held values and are fully engaged in authentic personal expression.

Eugenics   a discredited set of beliefs and practices based on the assumption that the genetic quality of the human population varies between population groups and races.

Eugenics   the belief that controlling breeding should be used to increase the occurrence of desirable heritable characteristics in a population.

Evaluation   the assessment of the efficacy or effectiveness of an intervention, project or programme in terms of processes and/or outcomes.

Evidence-based practice (EBP)   a policy of using only techniques and procedures that have a solid empirical foundation, i.e., the procedures have been demonstrated to benefit the service user.

Exercise tolerance test (ETT)   the recording of the heart's electrical activity while it is under the stress of increased physical demand.

Extrinsic motives   motives based on external factors, such as appearance, conformity or norms.

False positive   a result of a medical test that incorrectly identifies the person as having a certain condition.

Fat *triglycerides* that are either solid (e.g., butter, lard) or liquid (e.g., vegetable or fish oil) at room temperature.

Fat balance equation states that the rate of change of fat stores equals the rate of fat intake minus the rate of fat oxidation.

Female orgasmic disorder persistent or recurrent delay in, or absence of, orgasm following a 'normal' sexual excitement phase.

Flowchart model a diagrammatic representation of the relationships between processes and/ or variables that are believed to be related to each other.

Focus groups one or more group discussions in which participants focus collectively upon a topic or issue usually presented to them as a group of questions (or other stimuli) leading to the generation of interactive data.

Foetal alcohol syndrome an abnormality found in children whose mothers drink heavily during pregnancy; it is characterized by facial abnormalities, mental impairment and stunted growth.

Foetal Origins Hypothesis (or Barker's hypothesis) postulates that foetal conditions, most likely nutritional conditions, 'programme' the foetus for the development of chronic diseases in adulthood.

Food reward theory the theory that suggests that the overconsumption of food, which may lead to overweight and obesity, is a consequence of the activation of pleasure centres in the brain and the reinforcement of eating as a learned behaviour.

Framework a general representation for conceptualizing a research field or question.

Gain-framed messages information about a health behaviour that emphasizes the benefits of taking action.

Galenic medicine a health system derived from Greek and Arabic health beliefs.

Gametes an organism's reproductive cells, also referred to as 'sex cells'. Female gametes are called oocytes, ova or egg cells, and male gametes are called sperm. Gametes are haploid cells, with each cell carrying only one copy of each chromosome.

Gate control theory a theory that views pain as a perceptual experience, in which ascending physiological inputs and descending psychological inputs are equally involved. It posits a gating mechanism in the dorsal horn of the spinal cord that permits or inhibits the transmission of pain impulses to the brain.

Gay the adjective used to describe people who are emotionally, romantically or physically attracted to people of the same gender.

Gender a set of social, psychological or emotional traits, often influenced by societal expectations, that classify an individual as male, female, a mixture of both, or neither.

Gender Nonconforming (GNC)   a person whose identified gender is expansive beyond the binary of male or female.

General adaptation syndrome (GAS)   an influential three-stage model of the physiological response to stress put forward by Hans Selye but no longer thought to be valid.

Genome   the genetic material of an organism. It consists of DNA (or RNA in RNA viruses). The genome includes the genes (the coding regions), the noncoding DNA and the genetic material of the mitochondria and chloroplasts.

Genome-wide association study (GWAS) (otherwise known as the whole genome association study)   an examination of a genome-wide set of genetic variants in different individuals to see whether any variant is associated with a trait.

Genotype   the DNA sequence of the genetic makeup of a cell, organism or individual that determines a specific characteristic (phenotype) of that cell, organism or individual.

Germ theory   a theory of disease that focuses on identifying specific germs or pathogens as the primary cause of disease.

Gestational diabetes   high blood sugar that develops during pregnancy and usually disappears after giving birth. It can occur at any stage of pregnancy, but is more common in the second half. It occurs if your body cannot produce enough insulin (a hormone that helps control blood sugar levels) to meet the extra needs in pregnancy.

Glial cell   sometimes called 'neuroglia' or simply 'glia', this is a non-neuronal cell that maintains homeostasis, forms myelin and provides support and protection for neurones in the central and peripheral nervous systems.

Global burden of disease (GBD)   the universal totality of the economic, social and psychological costs of a disease attributable to both morbidity and mortality over a fixed interval of time.

Globalization   the process by which businesses or other organizations develop international influence or start operating on an international scale.

Glucocorticoids   any of a group of corticosteroids (e.g. hydrocortisone) that are involved in the metabolism of carbohydrates, proteins and fats and have anti-inflammatory activity.

Glycaemic index   a measure of the rise in the blood glucose/sugar level produced by a food.

Glycated haemoglobin (HbA1c) test   this is used to show how well diabetes is being controlled. The HbA1c test gives an average blood glucose level over the previous two to three months.

Gonorrhoea   a sexually transmitted infection (STI) caused by *Neisseria gonorrhoeae*, a bacterium that can grow and multiply easily in the warm, moist areas of the reproductive tract, including the cervix (opening to the womb), uterus (womb) and fallopian tubes (egg canals) in women, and in the urethra (urine canal) in women and men. The bacterium can also grow in the mouth, throat, eyes and anus.

Gradient of reinforcement   a principle applied mainly to *operant conditioning* whereby the acquisition of a learned response occurs more quickly the more rapidly a reward follows the occurrence of the response.

Grassroots   a movement founded in groups of local people working cooperatively to achieve greater well-being.

Gross domestic product (GDP)   the value of the goods and services produced by all sectors of the economy: agriculture, manufacturing, energy, construction, the service sector and government.

Gross national income (GNI)   the total net value of all goods and services produced within a nation over a specified period of time, representing the sum of wages, profits, rents, interest and pension payments to residents of the nation.

Grounded theory analysis   an analysis of transcripts, involving coding, followed by the generation of categories using constant comparative analysis within and between interview transcripts. This is followed by memo-writing, which requires the researcher to expand upon the meaning of the broader conceptual categories. This, in turn, can lead to further data generation through theoretical sampling.

Groupthink   a phenomenon that occurs within a group of people in which the desire for harmony or conformity in the group results in an irrational or dysfunctional decision-making outcome.

Hardiness   a personality trait first proposed by Kobasa (1979) and consisting of a high level of commitment, a sense of control and a willingness to confront challenges. Hardiness may protect the individual against the effects of stress.

Hassles scale   life events stress scale designed by Kanner (1981) and associates and focusing on everyday events that cause annoyance or frustration. See also *uplifts scale*.

Health   a state of well-being with satisfaction of physical, cultural, psychosocial, economic and spiritual needs, not simply the absence of illness.

Health belief model (HBM)   a psychological model that posits that health behaviour is a function of a combination of factors, including the perceived benefits of and barriers to treatment and the perceived susceptibility to and seriousness of the health problem.

Health belief system   ways of thinking about the causes of health and illness.

Health communication   the field of study concerned with the ways in which communication can contribute to the promotion of health.

Health education   the process by which individuals' knowledge about the causes of health and illness is increased.

Health gradient the relationship between *socio-economic status (SES)* and mortality or morbidity that normally shows a monotonic increase as SES changes from low to high.

Health habits routine behaviours acquired by learning or conditioning that protect health or put health at risk.

Health literacy the ability to read and understand about health and health care, enabling an individual to take decisions about treatment and prevention.

Health promotion any event, process or activity that facilitates the protection or improvement of the health of individuals, groups, communities or populations.

Health psychology an interdisciplinary field concerned with the application of psychological knowledge and techniques to health, illness and health care.

Healthism an ideology that situates health and disease as the personal responsibility of the individual; it can lead to the 'medicalization' of everyday life. Healthist ideas can be used as a form of social control.

Healthy living centres local organizations designed to promote health and reduce health inequalities.

Heart attack a sudden occurrence of coronary thrombosis, typically resulting in the death of part of a heart muscle and sometimes fatal.

Heart failure severe failure of the heart to function properly; a cause of death.

Herbal medicine a type of complementary medicine that involves the use of plants and plant extracts to treat illnesses or to promote well-being.

Heritability a statistic (H^2) used in genetics that estimates how much variation in a phenotypic trait in a population is due to genetic variation among individuals in that population. Other causes of measured variation in a trait are characterized as environmental factors, including measurement error.

Hermeneutic phenomenology the study of personal meanings underpinning everyday reality.

Hierarchy of needs a concept developed by Abraham Maslow in his 1943 theory of motivation, in which human needs are alleged to be in a fixed order, starting with physiological need satisfaction and ending with self-actualization.

Histone any of a group of basic proteins found in chromatin.

Histone modification a covalent post-translational modification (PTM) to histone proteins that includes methylation, phosphorylation, acetylation, ubiquitylation and sumoylation. The PTMs made to histones can impact gene expression by altering chromatin structure or recruiting histone modifiers.

Historical analysis   the use of data produced from memory, historical sources or artefacts.

HIV (human immunodeficiency virus)   the virus that causes acquired immune deficiency syndrome (AIDS); it replicates in and kills the helper T cells. The virus is passed from one person to another through blood-to-blood transmission and sexual contact. In addition, infected pregnant women can pass HIV infection to their baby during pregnancy or delivery, as well as through breast-feeding.

Homeopathy   a form of *complementary and alternative medicine (CAM)* which involves the use of highly diluted substances to trigger the body's natural healing system.

Homeostasis   a fundamental principle of living things which entails continuous adjustment towards a set point or optimum level of functioning; the tendency towards a relatively stable equilibrium between interdependent elements.

Homophobia   an aversion to lesbian or gay people that manifests itself in the form of discrimination, prejudice or bias.

Hormone   any member of a class of signalling molecules produced by glands in multicellular organisms that are transported by the circulatory system to target distant organs to regulate physiology and behaviour.

Hospice movement   a movement started by Dame Cicely Mary Saunders who pioneered St Christopher's Hospice in London in 1967, created as a medical, teaching and research facility dedicated to the physical, emotional and spiritual care of the dying. In hospices multi-disciplinary teams strive to offer dignity, peace and calm at the end of life.

Human sexual response cycle   a sequence of stages of sexual arousal taking the individual from initial excitement to a plateau phase, through orgasm, to resolution of sexual tension.

Humours (doctrine of the four humours)   dating back to the physicians of ancient Greece, the belief that the body is essentially composed of four constituents or humours (blood, phlegm, and black and yellow bile), and that diseases and psychological characteristics are attributable to an excess or shortage of one or more of the four.

Hypothalamo-pituitary-adrenal (HPA) axis   a complex of three endocrine glands: the hypothalamus, the pituitary gland and the adrenal glands.

Hysteria (conversion hysteria)   physical symptoms that appear to indicate organic disease but where there is no clinical evidence of disease. Nowadays this term is often replaced by *psychosomatic (or somatoform) disorder*.

Iatrogenesis   health problems caused by medical or health care interventions, including accidents, inappropriate treatments, incorrect diagnoses, drug side effects and other problems.

Identity control   a term used to describe the process by which a person deliberately attempts to control the image they present to others.

Illness perceptions   beliefs about illness.

Illness representations   organized mental models of the character of illness.

Immunization   a medical procedure designed to protect susceptible individuals from communicable diseases by the administration of a vaccine. This procedure is aimed at both immediate protection of individuals and immunity across the whole community where the uptake rate is high.

Immunodeficiency   a state in which the immune system's ability to fight infectious disease and cancer is compromised or entirely absent.

Immunomodulator   a chemical agent that modifies the immune response or the functioning of the immune system (e.g., by the stimulation of antibody formation or the inhibition of white blood cell activity).

Immunosenescence   the gradual deterioration of the immune system brought on by natural age advancement. It involves both the host's capacity to respond to infections and the development of long-term immune memory, especially by vaccination.

Implementation intentions   specific plans about how intentions to change a certain behaviour will actually be successfully implemented.

Incidence   the rate at which new cases of a disease occur in a population during a specified period. In the simplest terms, for example, 'The incidence of STIs in 2008 was 200 cases per 10,000 people per year in Newtown compared with 150 cases per 10,000 people per year in Oldtown'.

Income distribution   the distribution of income across the population. It can be measured in terms of the percentage share of national income earned by the best-off or worst-off proportions of the population; e.g., in the USA in 1991 the highest 20% of the population received 41.9% of the total national income while the worst-off 20% received 4.7%.

Indigenous   belonging to a particular culture, race or tribal group.

Individualism   a cultural value that enshrines the personal control and responsibility of the individual.

Inequality   a difference in life opportunities that is correlated with social position or status, ethnicity, gender, age or any other way of grouping people (see also *social inequality*).

Inequity   a lack of fairness or justice between different social groups.

Inflammation   part of the complex biological response of body tissues to harmful stimuli, which strives to eliminate the initial cause of cell injury, clear out necrotic cells and tissue damaged from the original insult and the inflammatory process, and to initiate tissue repair. The classical signs of inflammation are heat, pain, redness, swelling and loss of function.

Insulin   a hormone produced in the pancreas by the islets of Langerhans, which regulate the amount of glucose in the blood. An animal-derived or synthetic form of insulin is used to treat diabetes.

Insulin theory   the theory that obesity is caused by a chronic elevation in insulin in a diet that contains too much carbohydrate (Taubes, 2007, 2009).

Interaction analysis system (IAS)   an observation instrument that identifies, categorizes and quantifies features of the doctor–patient encounter.

Interactive dyad   a focus on communication between two people.

Intergenerational transmission   the transfer of individual abilities, traits, behaviors and outcomes from parents to their children.

Internal validity   the degree to which the results of a study can be attributed to the manipulations of the researchers and are likely to be free of bias.

Interpretative phenomenological analysis (IPA)   a technique for analysing qualitative data that seeks the meaning of experience.

Interpretative repertoire   a series of linguistic devices that people draw upon in constructing their accounts of events.

Intervention   the intentional and systematic manipulation of variables with the aim of improving health outcomes.

Interviews (structured or semi-structured)   a structured interview schedule is a prepared standard set of questions which are asked in person, or perhaps by telephone, of a person or group of persons concerning a particular research issue or question. A semi-structured interview is much more open-ended and allows the interviewee scope to address the issues which he/she feels to be relevant to the topics being raised by the investigator.

Intrinsic motives   motives based on feelings of pleasure, pride or enjoyment brought about by participating in an activity.

Inverse care law   the observation that the highest access to care is available to those who need it least (e.g., the more educated, articulate, affluent members of society), while the lowest access to care is available to those who need it most.

Job satisfaction   a positive emotional state resulting from work experience.

Job security   holding an employed position that has a high probability of long-term continuation.

Job strain or demand-control model   the idea that employee well-being depends upon the interaction of role demand and control, as proposed by Karasek and Theorell (1990).

Karotype   the number and visual appearance of the chromosomes in the cell nuclei of an organism or species.

Ketosis   a metabolic state in which some of the body's energy supply comes from ketone bodies in the blood.

Latent benefits   the less tangible benefits of employment, e.g., satisfaction of psychological needs.

LBGTQ   an acronym that collectively refers to individuals who are lesbian, gay, bisexual or transgender, with 'Q' representing queer or questioning. It is sometimes stated as 'GLBT' (gay, lesbian, bi and transgender) or 'LBGT'.

Lesbian   a woman who is emotionally, romantically and/or physically attracted to other women.

Leukocytes   (or leucocytes) the white blood cells of the immune system that are involved in protecting the body against both infectious disease and foreign invaders, derived from multi-potent cells in the bone marrow.

Liberation psychology   draws inspiration from the liberation theology developed by the worker-priest movement in Latin America during the 1950s and 1960s. This movement argues that it is the duty of Catholics to fight against social injustice and to adopt a 'preferential option for the poor'. These ideas were practised by Salvadorian Jesuit psychologist Ignacio Martín-Baró.

Life events and difficulties schedule (LEDS)   a psychological measurement of the stressfulness of life events, created by Brown and Harris in 1978. The schedule is based upon an interview which discusses the contextual information around the event.

Lifestyle sports   sports associated with a particular lifestyle, e.g., snowboarding, surfing.

Literature search   'combing through' or 'mining' the literature relevant to a review or a new study.

Liver cirrhosis   a frequently fatal form of liver damage, usually found among long-term heavy drinkers. Initially, fat accumulates on the liver, enlarging it; this restricts blood flow, causing damage to cells, and scar tissue develops, preventing the liver from functioning normally.

Locus of control   personality traits first proposed by social psychologists and then adapted by health psychologists to distinguish between those who attribute their state of health to themselves, powerful others or chance.

Longitudinal designs   involve measuring responses of a single sample on more than one occasion. These measurements may be prospective or retrospective, but prospective longitudinal designs allow greater control over the sample, the variables measured and the times when the measurements take place.

Loss-framed messages   information about a health behaviour that emphasizes the costs of failing to take action.

Lymph nodes (aka lymph glands)   small, bean-shaped organs located throughout the lymphatic system. The lymph nodes store special cells that can trap cancer cells or bacteria that are traveling through the body in lymph.

Lymphatic system   part of the circulatory system and a vital part of the immune system, comprising a network of lymphatic vessels that carry a clear fluid called lymph (from Latin *lympha*, meaning 'water') directionally towards the heart.

Lymphocytes   a type of white blood cell that is part of the immune system. There are two main types of lymphocytes: *B cells* and *T cells*.

Machismo   a strong and exaggerated sense of masculinity emphasizing physical attributes.

Macronutrient   an environmental substance used for energy, growth and bodily functions, which is needed in large amounts by humans: carbohydrates (sugar), lipids (fats) and proteins.

Macrophages   large white blood cells that are an integral part of our immune system. Their job is to locate microscopic foreign bodies and to 'eat' them.

Macro-social   large-scale social, economic, political and cultural forces that influence the life course of masses of people simultaneously.

Maintenance stage   the continued practice of or adherence to a specific health-promoting behaviour, e.g., abstinence from smoking. It is one of the stages in the *transtheoretical model of change (TMC)*.

Mammography   a method for imaging breast tissue of women using radiography for detecting early signs of breast cancer.

Manifest benefits   the concrete benefits of employment (e.g., income).

Meaning   having purpose or value.

ME/CFS   a complex, complicated and misunderstood disorder characterized by extreme fatigue that currently cannot be explained by any underlying medical condition. The fatigue may worsen with physical or mental activity, but doesn't improve with rest. The term 'ME' was first used in the UK, and 'CFS' in the USA, and both terms have been used to describe the same problem. The NHS in England currently uses the joint term, CFS/ME, but is moving towards using the term ME/CFS.

Medical error   errors in medical diagnosis and treatment.

Medical model   a way of thinking about health and illness that assumes all health and illness phenomena are physiological in nature. According to this model, health, illness and treatments have a purely biological or biochemical basis.

Medical silence   a reluctance of the medical profession to publicly acknowledge or report errors.

Medicalization   the process by which experiences and practices that do not match those defined as 'natural' and 'healthy' are pathologized and treated as dysfunctional.

Meta-analysis   a quantitative literature review that combines the evidence from relevant previous studies, taking account of criteria for quality and allowing high statistical power.

Metastasis   the spread of cancer cells to secondary sites in the body.

Methylation   a process by which methyl groups are added to the DNA molecule that change the activity of a DNA segment without changing the sequence. When located in a gene promoter, DNA methylation typically acts to repress gene transcription.

Microbiota   the microorganisms of a particular site (e.g. the gut), habitat or geological period.

Microglial cell   the endogenous brain defence and immune system responsible for central nervous system (CNS) protection against various types of pathogenic factors.

Mindfulness   a heavily hyped Buddhist concept, developed from 1979 and popularized in many publications by Jon Kabat-Zinn; paying attention to one's thoughts, feelings and actions; an acute awareness of the conscious flow of experience.

Mindfulness-based relapse prevention (MBRP)   the application of the methods of *mindfulness-based stress reduction (MBSR)* to the treatment of alcohol and substance use disorders; it was first proposed by Witkiewitz et al. (2005).

Mindfulness-based stress reduction (MBSR)   a method of stress management based on the concept of *mindfulness*.

Mitochondria   structures within cells that convert the energy from food into a usable form.

Mobile health or m-health   the delivery of health care services via mobile communication devices. It overlaps with e-health, the electronic technology that supports the functions and delivery of health care.

Model   an abstract representation of relationships between processes believed to influence each other.

Moral discourses of suffering   a language derived from moral principles that is used to describe and explain health and illness.

Motivational interviewing (or **motivation enhancement therapy**)   a brief intervention developed by W.R. Miller for the treatment of alcohol and drug problems. It aims to boost the clients' self-esteem and motivation to change, in contrast to traditional confrontational approaches.

Multidimensional Health Locus of Control (MHLC) scale   a popular scale for assessing a person's attributions of experience as internally or externally controlled, controlled by powerful others, or the consequence of chance.

Multiple regression   a statistical technique based on correlations between variables that enables predictions to be made about dependent variables using a combination of two or more independent variables.

Myalgic encephalomyelitis (ME)   a syndrome first observed in an epidemic at the Royal Free Hospital, London, in 1955, now usually thought to be identical to *chronic fatigue syndrome* and controversial for the same reasons.

Myelin   a mixture of proteins and phospholipids forming a whitish insulating sheath around many nerve fibres, which increases the speed at which impulses are conducted.

Myocardial infarction (MI)   a form of *coronary heart disease (CHD)* or 'heart attack' that occurs when one of the coronary arteries becomes blocked by a blood clot and part of the heart is starved of oxygen. It usually causes severe chest pain. MI is often the first sign of CHD in many people.

Narrative   a structured discourse that connects agents and events over time in the form of a story.

Narrative approaches   seek insight and meaning through the acquisition of data in the form of stories concerning personal experiences (Murray, 1997). These approaches assume that human beings are natural storytellers and that the principal task of the psychologist is to explore the different stories being told.

Narrative synthesis   a systematic descriptive form of integrating findings (see the Economic and Social Research Council Research Methods Programme general framework for narrative synthesis; Popay et al., 2006).

Natural killer cells (otherwise known as as 'NK cells', 'K cells' and '**killer cells**')   a type of *lymphocyte* and a component of the innate immune system. NK cells play a major role in the host-rejection of both tumours and virally infected cells.

Necessity-Concerns Framework   adherence is influenced by implicit judgements of personal need for the treatment (necessity beliefs) and concerns about the potential adverse consequences of taking it.

Need satisfaction   the attainment of physical health, agency and autonomy; the satisfaction of all physical, cultural, psychosocial, economic and spiritual needs. It is necessary for health and well-being.

Neoadjuvant treatment   treatment given as a first step to shrink a tumour before the main treatment, which is usually surgery. Examples of neoadjuvant therapy include chemotherapy, radiation therapy and hormone therapy.

Neo-material explanations   income inequality is caused by political processes that influence individual economic resources and impact community resources such as schooling, health care, social welfare, and working conditions.

Neuromodulator   a subset of a *neurotransmitter*. Unlike neurotransmitters, the release of neuromodulators occurs in a diffuse manner ('volume transmission') so that an entire neural tissue may be subject to the neuromodulator's action due to exposure.

Neurone (otherwise known as a **neuron** or **nerve cell**)   an electrically excitable cell that processes and transmits information through electrical and chemical signals.

Neurotransmitter   a chemical that enables the transmission of signals from one neurone to the next across synapses. These are also found at the axon endings of motor neurones, where they stimulate the muscle fibres. They and their close relatives are also produced by some glands, such as the pituitary and adrenal glands.

Nicotine   a chemical found in tobacco that acts as a stimulant. It can be fatal in large amounts and is largely responsible for the addictive properties of tobacco. It is also used as an insecticide.

Nicotine paradox   nicotine is a stimulant, yet smokers experience relaxation when they smoke.

Nicotine replacement therapy (NRT)   a pharmaceutical treatment for smoking cessation that has obtained marginally superior results to a placebo in trials sponsored and hyped by the pharmaceutical industry and its consultants. The method should definitely be avoided in pregnancy and adolescence. Real-world studies in the general population show a lack of effectiveness.

Nucleotides (otherwise known as **phosphate nucleotides**)   the building blocks of nucleic acids. They are composed of three sub-unit molecules: a nitrogenous base, a five-carbon sugar (ribose or deoxyribose), and at least one phosphate group. A nucleoside is a nitrogenous base and a five-carbon sugar.

Obesity   a stigmatised condition that is not itself an illness, involving an excessive accumulation of body fat, usually defined as a *body mass index (BMI)* greater than 30. Obesity is a risk factor for illnesses such as diabetes, metabolic syndrome, heart disease and cancer.

Obesogenic   an environment that exposes the population to a large number of foods and drinks that have a high percentage of fats and sugars.

Objectification   the process whereby a more abstract concept acquires meaning through association with everyday phenomena. The process transforms an abstract concept into a concrete image.

Observational studies   studies that are designed to evaluate the effectiveness of interventions that, for whatever reason, cannot or do not use a randomized controlled design.

Obstructive sleep apnoea (OSA)   the temporary cessation of breathing during sleep caused by a physical block to airflow despite respiratory effort. It can be worsened by being overweight and obese, and is associated with snoring.

Occupational stress   psychological, emotional or physical strain resulting from workplace demands and environment.

Oocyte   a cell in an ovary which may undergo meiotic division to form an ovum.

Operant conditioning   a learning process whereby a normally voluntary form of behaviour comes to occur with increasing frequency in a particular situation, or in the presence of a particular stimulus, as a result of previously and repeatedly having been rewarded in similar circumstances.

Operationism   the use of rules or a method of measurement to define an object or quality.

Opportunistic intervention   an attempt to modify health-hazardous behaviour, such as smoking or heavy drinking, by a health professional, frequently a doctor, who has been consulted for other reasons.

Optimistic bias   the mistaken belief that one's chances of experiencing a negative event are lower (or a positive event higher) than that of one's peers.

Outcome evaluation   an assessment of an intervention that examines the objective outcome in a controlled investigation of the effects or impact of the intervention.

Outreach programme   an intervention that aims to achieve sub-cultural change among hard-to-reach target constituencies in order to improve health outcomes.

Palliative care   care for the terminally ill and their families provided by an organized health service.

Palliative treatment   designed to relieve symptoms, and improve quality of life. It can be used at any stage of an illness if there are troubling symptoms, such as pain or sickness. It can also be used to reduce or control the side effects of cancer treatments.

Pansexual (or 'pan')   a person who experiences romantic, emotional or sexual attraction to persons of all gender identities or sexes.

Pap test   a medical procedure for conducting cervical screening examinations.

Parasympathetic nervous system   part of the involuntary nervous system that serves to slow the heart rate, increase intestinal and glandular activity, and relax the sphincter muscles. Together with the *sympathetic nervous system*, it constitutes the *autonomic nervous system*.

Participatory action research (PAR)   a form of action research that deliberately seeks to provoke some form of social or community change in which the instigator/investigator works collaboratively with stakeholders by taking actions to bring about desired change in a step-by-step process.

Participatory learning   the full participation of people in the processes of learning about their needs and opportunities, and in the action required to address them.

Patient informatics   a programme that aims to enable patients to make better use of information and communication technology for health and health care.

Patient safety   the prevention of avoidable errors and adverse effects on patients associated with health care.

Patient satisfaction   a measure of the extent to which patients' expectations of what a medical encounter ought to provide have been met (as judged by the patients).

Patient-centred communication style   a doctor's communication style which mobilizes the patient's knowledge, experience and involvement through techniques such as silence, listening and reflection.

Peer pressure   influence from members of one's peer group.

Peptide   a compound containing two or more amino acids in which the carboxyl group of one acid is linked to the amino group of the other.

Perceived behavioural control   the feeling of having control over one's actions in response to others and the environment.

Percutaneous coronary intervention (PCI)   a procedure that unblocks narrowed coronary arteries without performing surgery. This may be done with either a balloon catheter to push the *atheroma* to the side of the artery or a stent inserted to keep the artery open.

Pessimistic explanatory style   the tendency of some individuals to blame themselves for everything that goes wrong in their lives; it is believed to be associated with poor physical health.

P-hacking (aka data dredging, data fishing or data snooping)   is the use of data mining to uncover patterns in data that can be presented as statistically significant, without any advanced hypothesis as to the underlying causality.

Phenomenology   the study of the participant's perspective of the world.

Phenotype   the set of observable characteristics of an individual resulting from the interaction of the individual's genotype with the environment.

Phosphodiesterase type 5 (PDE5) inhibitor   a drug used to block the degradative action of cGMP-specific phosphodiesterase type 5 (PDE5) on cyclic GMP in the smooth muscle cells lining the blood vessels supplying the corpus cavernosum of the penis.

Physical activity   bodily movement produced by skeletal muscles that requires energy expenditure.

Physical dependency   the experience of unpleasant physical symptoms when a person stops using or reduces consumption of a drug, tobacco or alcohol.

Physical education   the systematic instruction in sports and physical activity given as part of school or college education.

Physical side effects   the unwanted physiological effects that accompany medication.

Physician-assisted death (PAD)   intentionally providing a person with the knowledge or means or both required to commit suicide, including counselling about lethal doses of drugs, prescribing such lethal doses or supplying the drugs.

Placebo   an inert substance or treatment that lacks any specific effect but which may induce the perception of benefit.

Placebo control   a control condition that appears similar to a treatment when in fact it is completely general.

Placebo effect   an effect from a placebo drug or treatment that cannot be attributed to the properties of the placebo itself.

Population pyramid   a graphical method of representing the age distribution of populations at different time points. It shows the number of people in each differently coloured age band, as indicated by the width of the band, with younger age groups at the base and older age groups at the top, and with males on one side and females on the other.

Positivism   the epistemological position that places scientific method as the sole source of reliable knowledge.

Post-traumatic growth (PTG) (aka benefit finding)   is positive psychological change experienced as a result of adversity and other challenges in order to rise to a higher level of functioning.

Post-traumatic stress disorder (PTSD)   the long-term psychological and physiological effects of exposure to traumatic stress, including insomnia, nightmares, flashbacks, problems of memory and concentration, acting or feeling as if the event is recurring and a greatly increased sensitivity to new stressful events.

Poverty   the level of income below which people cannot afford a minimum, nutritionally adequate diet and essential non-food requirements.

Power analysis   a method for deciding how large a sample is needed to enable a statistical judgement that is accurate and reliable, and how likely it is that the particular statistical test to be used will be able to detect effects of a given size in a particular situation; e.g., how big a sample is necessary to have an 8 probability of detecting a difference at the .05 level of significance.

Pre-contemplation stage   the stage of knowing that a habit or behaviour is hazardous but without any intention to change it in the foreseeable future. It is one of the stages in the *transtheoretical model of change (TMC)*.

Pre-exposure prophylaxis (otherwise known as 'PrEP')   applies to people at very high risk for HIV who take HIV medicines daily to lower their chances of becoming infected.

Preparation stage   the stage at which a person intends to take action in the immediate future, having developed a specific plan of action. It is one of the stages in the *transtheoretical model of change (TMC)*.

Prevalence   the number of people with a disease or behaviour shown as a proportion of the population or sub-population at any point in time.

Preventive health behaviours   behaviours people choose to engage in with the aim of protecting and/or improving their health status.

Process evaluation   an assessment of how well an intervention is implemented in terms of the activities that occur, who is conducting the activities, who is being reached, what inputs or resources have been allocated, and what the strengths, weaknesses and areas are that need improvement.

Prospect theory   the theory that proposes that people consider their 'prospects' (i.e., potential gains and losses) when making a decision. It is a theory that has influenced message framing in health promotion.

Prospective study   a longitudinal cohort study that follows over time a group of similar individuals (cohorts) who differ with respect to certain factors under study, to determine how these factors affect rates of a certain outcome.

Protein leverage hypothesis   the hypothesis that humans prioritize protein when regulating food intake (Simpson and Raubenheimer, 2012).

Psychological dependency   a state associated with repeated activity or consumption of a drug or drink, which leads to negative affect following reduced consumption or abstinence and a persistent desire or unsuccessful efforts to cut down or control the activity.

Psychological homeostasis   refers to the psychological need to reach and maintain a state of equilibrium.

Psychoneuroimmunology (PNI)   the study of the effects of psychological variables, and especially stress, on the immune system.

Psycho-oncology   the psychological aspects of cancer care and treatment.

Psychosocial explanations   accounts of events and experiences based on theories and research from psychology and the social sciences.

Psychosomatic (or somatoform) disorders   physical ailments believed to be psychologically caused, including *hysteria* and some conditions that have organic features, such as ulcers and asthma.

Psychosomatic medicine   a precursor of modern health psychology which flourished from the 1930s to the 1950s. Its proponents, including Alexander (1950), believed that psychoanalytic theories about unconscious conflicts could be extended to explain susceptibility to various organic diseases.

Public health psychology   the application of psychological theory, research and technologies towards the improvement of the health of the population.

Punishment circuit   this functions by means of acetylcholine, which stimulates the secretion of adrenal cortico-trophic hormone (ACTH). ACTH in turn stimulates the adrenal glands to release adrenalin to prepare the body's organs for fight or flight. Stimulation of the punishment circuit can inhibit the reward circuit, so that fear and punishment can eliminate pleasure.

Qualitative research methods   methods that are intended to provide an improved understanding of the meanings, purposes and intentions of behaviour, not its amount or quantity.

Quality of dying and death (QoDD)   the degree to which a person's preferences for dying and the moment of death agree with observations of how the person actually died, as reported by others.

Quality of life (QoL)   the general well-being of a person or society, defined in terms of physical health and mental well-being, including happiness and autonomy, and not necessarily wealth.

Quasi-experimental design   a comparison of two or more treatments in as controlled a manner as possible but without the possibility of manipulating an independent variable or randomly allocating participants.

Questionnaires   many constructs in health psychology are measured using questionnaires consisting of a standard set of items with accompanying instructions. Ideally, a questionnare will have been demonstrated to be both a reliable and valid measure of the construct(s) it purports to measure.

Quit For Life (QFL) Programme   a psychological therapy using cognitive behavioural principles enabling smokers to quit (Marks, 1993, 2005).

Racism   discrimination on the basis of race or skin colour.

Radiotherapy (RT)   this uses ionizing radiation, generally as part of cancer treatment to control or kill malignant cells, normally delivered by a linear accelerator.

Randomized controlled trials (RCTs)   these involve the systematic comparison of interventions employing a fully controlled application of one or more interventions or 'treatments' using a random allocation of participants to the different treatment groups.

Rasch analysis   an approach of mathematical modelling based on a latent trait, which accomplishes stochastic (probabilistic) conjoint additivity (conjoint means the measurement of persons and items on the same scale and additivity is the equal-interval property of the scale).

Reactance theory   a theory concerning the tendency to resist attempts by others to control one's behaviour.

Reflexology a type of complementary medicine that involves the application of pressure and massage to specific reflex areas in the body.

Relapse going back to consumption of tobacco, alcohol or a drug after a period of voluntary abstinence.

Relapse prevention therapy strategies and procedures for reducing the likelihood of *relapse.*

Replication the attempt by an investigator to repeat a study to determine whether the original findings can be repeated.

Responsible consumer a consumer who takes a measured, rational, evidence-based approach to his or her consumption of foods, beverages and other potentially hazardous products, such as tobacco.

Restenosis a coronary artery blockage that occurs following *percutaneous coronary intervention (PCI).*

Revascularization a term that describes surgical and catheter procedures that are used to restore blood flow to the heart.

Reward circuit the reward pathway in the brain consisting principally of the mesolimbic dopamine system.

Ribonucleic acid (RNA) a linear molecule composed of four types of smaller molecules called ribonucleotide bases: adenine (A), cytosine (C), guanine (G) and uracil (U). RNA is often compared to a copy from a reference book, or a template, because it carries the same information as its DNA template but is not used for long-term storage.

Risk compensation a theory which suggests that people typically adjust their behaviour in response to the perceived level of risk, becoming more careful where they sense greater risk and less careful if they feel more protected.

Role ambiguity the lack of information necessary to conduct the role, and information deficiency regarding expected role behaviours, role objectives and responsibilities.

Role conflict incompatible role demands placed upon an individual.

Role demand the expectations placed upon a person within a role.

Safer sex practices sexual practices that do not involve the exchange of bodily fluids that may contain the human immunodeficiency virus (HIV). Such bodily fluids are blood, semen and vaginal fluids.

Screening a procedure for the identification of the presence of certain diseases, conditions or behaviours in a community. Those sections of the population who are most at risk of developing a particular disease are examined to see whether they have any early indications. The rationale behind this strategy is that the earlier the disease is identified and treated, the less likely it is to develop into a fatal condition.

Second-hand smoke   smoke exhaled by smokers, polluting the environment of others, whether 'smokers' or 'non-smokers', which they are forced to inhale.

Sedentary   the absence of physical activity.

Self-actualization   the realization or fulfilment of one's talents and potentialities, especially considered as a drive or need (Maslow).

Self-concept   a sense of who you are.

Self-determination   engaging in activities for one's enjoyment or intrinsic motivation.

Self-efficacy   the belief that one will be able to carry out one's plans successfully; a term proposed by Bandura (1977) and thought to be associated with positive health behaviours.

Self-esteem   a personality trait consisting of positive self-regard, originally proposed by Rosenberg (1965).

Self-regulation   the process by which individuals monitor and adjust their medication on an ongoing basis.

Self-regulatory model   this model suggests that health-related practices or coping responses are influenced by patients' beliefs or representations of the illness. These illness representations have a certain structure.

Sensation seeking   a personality trait or type that is characterized by a strong desire for new sensations.

Sense of coherence   a personality trait originally proposed by Antonovsky (1979) to characterize people who see their world as essentially meaningful and manageable. It is associated with coping with stress.

Sense of community   a feeling that one belongs to a group located in space and time with a common identity, history and culture.

Sex survey   a large-scale, questionnaire-based instrument that aims to provide quantifiable, descriptive data about a population's sexual habits.

Sexology   the scientific study of human sexual behaviour.

Sexual behaviour   any activity that stimulates sexual arousal for pleasure or procreation.

Sexual dimorphism   differences in appearance between males and females, such as shape, size and structure, that are caused by the inheritance of one or the other sexual pattern in the genetic material.

Sexual meanings the significance that is attributed to sexual practices as a result of the application of socio-historically and culturally variable and changing interpretative frames.

Sexuality those aspects of human experience which are influenced by and/or expressive of sexual desire and/or practice.

Sexually transmitted infections (STIs) infections that can be transferred from one person to another through sexual contact via vaginal or anal intercourse, kissing, oral–genital contact, and the use of sexual 'toys' such as vibrators.

Single case experimental design an investigation of a series of experimental manipulations on a single research participant.

Single nucleotide polymorphisms frequently called SNPs (pronounced 'snips'), the most common type of genetic variation among people. Each SNP represents a difference in a single nucleotide. For example, a SNP may replace the nucleotide cytosine (C) with the nucleotide thymine (T) in a certain stretch of DNA. SNPs occur normally throughout a person's DNA. They occur once in every 300 nucleotides on average, which means there are roughly 10 million SNPs in the human genome. Most commonly, these variations are found in the DNA between genes. When SNPs occur within a gene or in a regulatory region near a gene, they may play a more direct role in disease by affecting the gene's function.

Skin fold thickness a method of determining body composition and body fat percentage using calipers at different positions on a persons's body.

Social capital the institutions, relationships and norms that shape the quality and quantity of a society's social interactions. Social capital is not just the sum of the institutions that underpin a society, it is the glue that holds them together.

Social cognition a cognitive model of social knowledge.

Social cognition models (SCMs) theories about the relationship between social cognitions, such as beliefs and attitudes, and behaviour, which aim accurately to predict behaviour or behavioural intentions.

Social constructionism (1) the philosophical belief that there is no single, fixed 'reality' but a multiplicity of descriptions, each with its own unique pattern of meanings; (2) 'many potential worlds of meaning that can be imaginatively entered and celebrated, in ways which are constantly changing to give richness and value to human experience' (Mulkay, 1991: 27–8).

Social Darwinism the concept that competition drives social evolution.

Social inequality being treated differently as a consequence of age, race, gender, disability, sexual preference or other attribute (see also *inequality*).

Social justice the process of treating a person, group or community fairly and equally.

Social marketing   the application of consumer-oriented marketing techniques in the design, implementation and evaluation of programmes aimed towards influencing behaviour change. Social marketing draws upon concepts from behavioural theory, persuasion psychology and marketing science.

Social Readjustment Rating Scale (SRRS)   measurement scale for life events stress developed by Holmes and Rahe and widely used in research on life events stress and illness (see also *hassles scale* and *uplifts scale*).

Social representation theory   a system of ideas, values and practices specific to a particular community which enables individuals to orient themselves in the world and communicate with each other.

Social support   informal and formal supportive relationships.

Socio-economic status (SES)   position or class based on occupation, education or income.

Somatic nervous system (otherwise known as the 'voluntary nervous system')   the part of the peripheral nervous system that is associated with skeletal muscular voluntary control of body movements and afferent or sensory nerves.

Spirituality   the quality or state of being spiritual, with or without religious beliefs.

Stages of change   the stages of pre-contemplation, contemplation, preparation, action, maintenance and termination in the *transtheoretical model of change (TMC)*.

Statins   drugs used to reduce cholesterol levels.

Steroid   any of a large class of organic compounds with a characteristic molecular structure containing four rings of carbon atoms (three six-membered and one five-membered), including many hormones, alkaloids and vitamins.

Stigma   the process of marginalizing a group or class of people by labelling them as different and understanding them in terms of stereotypes. This results in a loss of social status and discrimination, affecting many areas of life.

Stigmatization   being treated as an object of derision and shame purely as a consequence of others' ignorance and prejudice.

Stress   an ambiguous term, sometimes used to refer to environmental pressure and sometimes to a particular type of response to pressure. Currently, it is often used to describe an inner state that can occur when either real or perceived demands exceed either the real or perceived capacity to cope with them.

Stress inoculation training (SIT)   a cognitive behavioural method for stress management devised by Meichenbaum (1985), focusing on changing the way in which participants appraise situations as stressful and cope with stressful events.

Stress-management workshop a training programme in stress management usually delivered to groups, frequently lasting for a whole day or a weekend, and focusing on changing the way in which participants appraise situations as stressful and cope with stressful events.

Subjective norms the beliefs of other people about the importance of carrying out a behaviour.

Subjective validation (or personal validation) a cognitive bias by which a person will consider a statement or another piece of information to be correct if it has any personal meaning or significance to them.

Subjective well-being (SWB) a concept that, in plain English, would be called 'happiness'. The adjective 'subjective' is necessary because well-being cannot be inferred from outward appearances or the objective characteristics of the person.

Sudden infant death syndrome (SIDS) the unexplained death of infants while lying in a crib or cot.

Survey a systematic method for determining how a defined sample of participants respond to a set of standard questions attempting to assess their feelings, attitudes, beliefs or knowledge at one or more particular times.

Symmetry rule a tendency to search for a label for bodily symptoms and to expect symptoms if we have an illness label.

Sympathetic nervous system part of the involuntary nervous system that serves to accelerate the heart rate, constrict blood vessels and raise blood pressure. Together with the *parasympathetic nervous system*, it constitutes the *autonomic nervous system*.

Synaptic connection as neurotransmitters activate receptors across the synaptic cleft, the connection between the two neurones is strengthened when both neurones are active at the same time, as a result of the receptor's signalling mechanisms.

Syphilis a chronic infectious disease caused by a spirochete (*Treponema pallidum*), transmitted by direct contact, usually in sexual intercourse, or passed from mother to child *in utero*. The disease progresses through three stages characterized, respectively, by the local formation of chancres, ulcerous skin eruptions and systemic infection leading to general paresis.

Systematic review a review of the empirical literature concerning the efficacy or effectiveness of an intervention that considers all relevant studies, taking account of quality criteria.

Systems theory approach a theory concerned with the contextual structures, processes or relationships within communities, groups or families.

T cells (otherwise known as 'T lymphocytes') a type of *lymphocyte* (a sub-type of white blood cell) that plays a central role in cell-mediated immunity. T cells can be distinguished from other lymphocytes, such as B cells and natural killer cells, by the presence of a T-cell receptor on the cell surface. Compare with *B cells*.

Taoism   a Chinese philosophy which views the universe as being governed by the two basic powers of yin and yang.

Tautology   an empty statement consisting of simpler statements that make it logically true whether the simpler statements are true or false, e.g., *Either I will wear a condom the next time I have sexual intercourse or I will not.*

Taxonomy   a system for the description, identification, nomenclature and classification of objects, organisms or interventions.

Teleworking   working outside the traditional workplace, using information technology and telecommunication systems.

Temperance societies   originating in the USA in the nineteenth century, these societies, of which Alcoholics Anonymous is an example, are dedicated to counteracting the harmful effects of drinking, usually advocating teetotalism.

Tension reduction hypothesis   the hypothesis that people enjoy alcohol primarily because it reduces tension (anxiety, stress), rather than as a drug which directly produces positive moods.

Theory   a general account of relationships between processes believed to influence, cause changes in, or control a phenomenon.

Theory of planned behaviour (TPB)   a theoretical model which argues that behavioural intention is controlled by attitudes, subjective norms and perceived control.

Theory of reasoned action (TRA)   a theoretical model which argues that behavioural intention is controlled by attitudes and subjective norms.

Therapeutic alliance   the relationship between a mental health practitioner and his or her client.

Thin ideal   the concept of the ideally slim female body. The common perception of this ideal is that of a slender, feminine physique with a small waist and little body fat.

(To) legitimate   to justify one's position in the face of stigma, illness or invalidity.

Top-down   controlled, directed or organized from the top using a preconceived theory or model about the processes that are expected to occur.

Total body irradiation (TBI)   a form of radiotherapy used primarily as part of the preparative regimen for haematopoietic stem cell (or bone marrow) transplantation.

Toxic environment   environmental and social conditions that promote disease, disorder and death.

Transgender (otherwise known as 'trans')   a person whose self-identified gender does not fully align with their physical sex as assigned at birth, and who may choose to take steps to medically alter the gendered features of their body.

Transparency   a description of a method or procedure that is detailed and explicit, enabling replication by another investigator.

Transtheoretical model of change (TTM)   a model of behaviour change, developed by DiClementi, Prochaska and others, which attempts to identify universal processes or stages of change, specified as *pre-contemplation, contemplation, preparation, action, maintenance* and *termination.*

Triangulation   collecting evidence using different methods to provide complementary perspectives.

Triglyceride   the main component of dietary fats and oils and the principal form in which fat is stored in the body. It is composed of three fatty acids attached to a glycerol molecule: saturated, mono-unsaturated and polyunsaturated.

Tumour (benign or malignant)   an abnormal new mass of tissue that serves no purpose; a tumour may be malignant or non-malignant depending on whether it is life-threatening or not.

Twelve-step facilitation programme   a theraputic regime which attempts to change thinking and behaviour in a series of 12 steps, as advocated by Alcoholics Anonymous.

Type 1 diabetes mellitus (T1DM) (otherwise known as juvenile diabetes or insulin-dependent diabetes)   a chronic condition in which the pancreas produces little or no insulin, a hormone needed to allow sugar (glucose) to enter cells to produce energy. The far more common Type 2 diabetes occurs when the body becomes resistant to insulin or doesn't make enough insulin.

Type 2 diabetes mellitus (T2DM) (otherwise known as adult-onset or noninsulin-dependent diabetes)   a chronic condition that affects the way the body metabolizes sugar (glucose), the body's source of fuel. In Type 2 diabetes, the body either resists the effects of insulin (a hormone that regulates the movement of sugar into cells) or fails to produce enough insulin to maintain a normal glucose level. More common in adults, T2DM increasingly affects children as childhood obesity is becoming more prevalent.

Type A/B personality   the Type A personality, in contrast to the Type B personality, is characterized by intense achievement motivation, time urgency and hostility.

Unconditioned stimulus (UCS)   a stimulus that evokes a response or reflex without training; e.g., a loud sound will naturally evoke a startle response.

Uncontrolled variable   a background variable that remains uncontrolled by the investigator and that may affect or bias the results of a study.

Uplifts scale   a life events scale designed by Kanner and associates (1981) to assess desirable events, in contrast to their *hassles scale.*

Varenicline (also known as Champix)   used in smoking cessation to prevent craving and withdrawal symptoms.

Vegan   a plant-based diet that excludes all animal-based foods.

Vegetarian   a diet that includes eggs and/or dairy but no other foods derived from animal sources.

Viral challenge studies   a method of studying the relationship between stress and susceptibility to infectious disease in which volunteers are deliberately exposed to minor viruses, usually colds or flu, to determine whether those who have experienced higher levels of stress prior to exposure are more likely to contract the infection.

Visceral fat   fat that accumulates in organs such as the liver that causes insulin resistance and multiple sclerosis (MS).

Vitamin D   a fat-soluble vitamin that is naturally present in very few foods, is added to others, and is available as a dietary supplement. It is produced when ultraviolet rays from sunlight strike the skin and trigger vitamin D synthesis.

Waist circumference   a measure of central adiposity or body fat.

Well-being   the state of 'wellness'; the general state of health of an individual.

Wernicke–Korsakoff syndrome   a form of irreversible brain damage sometimes found among long-term heavy drinkers, its symptoms include extremely impaired short-term memory, confusion and visual disorders.

Withdrawal symptoms   unpleasant symptoms and craving accompanying cessation of tobacco or other drug use, e.g., uncontrolled sweating, palpitations, depression, fear or anxiety.

World Health Organization (WHO)   the directing and coordinating authority for health within the United Nations. The Director-General of the WHO is Dr Tedros Adhanom Ghebreyesus, from Ethiopia.

REFERENCES

Abraham, C. and Michie, S. (2008). A taxonomy of behavior change techniques used in interventions. *Health Psychology*, 27: 379–87.

Abraham, C. and Sheeran, P. (2004). Deciding to exercise: the role of anticipated regret. *British Journal of Health Psychology*, 9: 269–78.

Academy of Medical Sciences. (2004). *Calling Time: The Nation's Drinking as a Major Health Issue*. London: Academy of Medical Sciences.

Acheson, D. (1998). Inequalities in health: Report on inequalities in health did give priority for steps to be tackled. *British Medical Journal* (Clinical Research Edition), 317 (7173): 1659.

Ackerson, K. and Preston, S.D. (2009). A decision theory perspective on why women do or do not decide to have cancer screening: systematic review. *Journal of Advanced Nursing*, 65: 1130–40.

Action on Smoking and Health (ASH). (2010). *Tobacco Explained: The Truth about the Tobacco Industry ... in its Own Words*. Available: http://ash.org.uk/files/documents/ASH_599.pdf [accessed 5 December 2014].

Action on Smoking and Health (ASH). (2014). *Smoking Statistics*. Available: http://ash.org.uk/files/documents/ASH_106.pdf [accessed 5 December 2014].

Adler, N.E. and Matthews K.A. (1994). Health psychology: Why do some people get sick and some stay well? *Annual Review of Psychology*, 45: 229–59.

Adonis, L., Paramanund, J., Basu, D. and Luiz, J. (2016). Framing preventive care messaging and cervical cancer screening in a health-insured population in South Africa: Implications for population-based communication? *Journal of Health Psychology*. doi:10.1177/1359105316628735.

Adwan, L. and Zawia, N.H. (2013). Epigenetics: a novel therapeutic approach for the treatment of Alzheimer's disease. *Pharmacology & Therapeutics*, 139 (1): 41–50.

Ågård, A., Ranjbar, V. and Strang, S. (2016). Diabetes in the shadow of daily life: factors that make diabetes a marginal problem. *Practical Diabetes*, 33 (2): 49–53.

Ahern, A.L., Bennett, K.M., Kelly, M. and Hetherington, M.M. (2011). A qualitative exploration of young women's attitudes towards the Thin Ideal. *Journal of Health Psychology*, 16: 70–9.

Ainsworth, M.D.S., Blehar, M.C., Waters, E. and Wall, S. (1978). *Patterns of Attachment: A Psychological Study of the Strange Situation*. Hillsdale, NJ: Lawrence Erlbaum.

Aitken-Swan, J. and Easson, E.C. (1959). Reactions of cancer patients on being told their diagnosis. *British Medical Journal*, 1 (5124): 779.

Ajzen, I. (1985). From intention to actions: a theory of planned behavior. In J. Kuhl and J. Beckmann (eds.), *Action-Control: From Cognition to Behavior*. Heidelberg: Springer. pp. 11–39.

Ajzen, I. (1991). The theory of planned behavior. *Organizational Behavior and Human Decision Processes*, 50: 179–211.

Ajzen, I. (2002). *The Theory of Planned Behaviour*. Available: www.people.umass.edu/aizen.

Ajzen, I. (2014). The theory of planned behaviour is alive and well, and not ready to retire: a commentary on Sniehotta, Presseau, and Araújo-Soares. *Health Psychology Review*, 9(2): 131–7.

Ajzen, I. and Fishbein, M. (1980). *Understanding Attitudes and Predicting Social Behavior*. Englewood Cliffs, NJ: Prentice Hall.

Albarracín, D., Johnson, B.T., Fishbein, M. and Muellerleile, P.A. (2001). Theories of reasoned action and planned behavior as models of condom use: a meta-analysis. *Psychological Bulletin*, 127: 142–61.

Aldaz, B.E., Treharne, G.J., Knight, R.G., Conner, T.S. and Perez, D. (2016). 'It gets into your head as well as your body': the experiences of patients with cancer during oncology treatment with curative intent. *Journal of Health Psychology*. doi:10.1177/1359105316671185.

Aldwin, C.M. and Park, C.L. (2004). Coping and physical health outcomes: an overview. *Psychology & Health*, 19: 277–81.

Alexander, F. (1950). *Psychosomatic Medicine*. New York: Norton.

Ali, S., Stone, M., Peters, J.L., Davies, M.J. and Khunti, K. (2006). The prevalence of co-morbid depression in adults with Type 2 diabetes: a systematic review and meta-analysis. *Diabetic Medicine*, 23 (11): 1165–73.

Allison, P.J., Edgar, L., Nicolau, B., Archer, J., Black, M. and Hier, M. (2004). Results of a feasibility study for a psycho-educational intervention in head and neck cancer. *Psycho-Oncology*, 13: 482–85. doi:10.1002/pon.816.

Almeida, J., Johnson, R.M., Corliss, H.L., Molnar, B.E. and Azrael, D. (2009). Emotional distress among LGBT youth: the influence of perceived discrimination based on sexual orientation. *Journal of Youth and Adolescence*, 38 (7): 1001–14.

AL-Qezweny, M.N.A., Utens, E.M.W.J., Dulfer, K., Hazemeijer, B.A.F., van Geuns, R.J., Daemen, J. and van Domburg, R. (2016). The association between Type D personality, and depression and anxiety ten years after PCI. *Netherlands Heart Journal*, 24 (9): 538–43.

Alsaiari, A., Joury, A., Aljuaid, M., Wazzan, M. and Pines, J.M. (2017). The content and quality of health information on the internet for patients and families on adult kidney cancer. *Journal of Cancer Education*, 32 (4): 878–84.

Al-Smadi, A.M., Tawalbeh, L.I., Gammoh, O.S., Ashour, A., Tayfur, M. and Attarian, H. (2017). The prevalence and the predictors of insomnia among refugees. *Journal of Health Psychology*. doi:10.1177/1359105316687631.

Altin, S.V., Finke, I., Kautz-Freimuth, S. and Stock, S. (2014). The evolution of health literacy assessment tools: a systematic review. *BMC Public Health*, 14 (1): 1–24. doi:10.1186/1471-2458-14-1207.

American Cancer Society. (2009). *Cancer Facts & Figures*. Atlanta, GA: American Cancer Society.

American Congress of Obstetricians and Gynecologists. (2015). Statement on Teen Pregnancy and Contraception. Available: https://www.acog.org/About-ACOG/News-Room/Statements/2015/ACOG-Statement-on-Teen-Pregnancy-and-Contraceptionwww.acog.org/About-ACOG/News-Room/Statements/2015/ACOG-Statement-on-Teen-Pregnancy-and-Contraception

American Psychiatric Association. (1980). *Diagnostic and Statistical Manual of Mental Disorders*, 3rd edn (DSM-III). Washington, DC: American Psychiatric Association.

American Psychiatric Association. (1994). *Diagnostic and Statistical Manual of Mental Disorders*, 4th edn (DSM-IV). Washington, DC: American Psychiatric Association.

American Psychiatric Association. (2000) *Diagnostic and Statistical Manual of Mental Disorders*, 4th edn, text revision (DSM-IV-TR). Washington, DC: American Psychiatric Association.

Ammassari, A., Murri, R., Pezzotti, P., Trotta, M.P., Ravasio, L., De Longis, P., et al. (2001). Self-reported symptoms and medication side effects influence adherence to highly active antiretroviral therapy in persons with HIV infection. *JAIDS: Journal of Acquired Immune Deficiency Syndromes*, 28 (5): 445–9.

Amnesty International (2017) *The State of the World's Human Rights*. Available: https://www.amnesty.org/en/documents/pol10/4800/2017/en/

Anand, S. and Sen, A. (2000). Human development and economic sustainability. *World Development*, 28: 2029–49.

Anastasi, N. and Lusher, J. (2017). The impact of breast cancer awareness interventions on breast screening uptake among women in the United Kingdom: a systematic review. *Journal of Health Psychology*, 23. doi:10.1177/1359105317697812.

Andersen A.M.N., Andersen, P.K., Olsen, J., Gronbaek, M. and Strandberg-Larsen, K. (2012). Moderate alcohol intake during pregnancy and risk of fetal death. *International Journal of Epidemiology*, 41: 405–13.

Andersen, B.L., Anderson, B. and deProsse, C. (1989). Controlled prospective longitudinal study of women with cancer: II. Psychological outcomes. *Journal of Consulting and Clinical Psychology*, 57: 692–7.

Anderson, C.S., Linto, J. and Stewart-Wynne, E.G. (1995). A population-based assessment of the impact and burden of caregiving for long-term stroke survivors. *Stroke*, 26 (5): 843–9.

Anderson, I., Crengle, S., Kamaka, M.L., Chen, T., Palafox, N. and Jackson-Pulver, L. (2006). Indigenous health in Australia, New Zealand, and the Pacific. *The Lancet*, 367: 1775–85.

Anderson, K.F. (2013). Diagnosing discrimination: stress from perceived racism and the mental and physical health effects. *Sociological Inquiry*, 83: 55–81.

Anderson, L., Oldridge, N., Thompson, D.R., Zwisler, A.D., Rees, K., Martin, N. and Taylor, R.S. (2016). Exercise-based cardiac rehabilitation for coronary heart disease: Cochrane systematic review and meta-analysis. *Journal of the American College of Cardiology*, 67 (1): 1–12.

Anderson, P. and Baumberg, B. (2006). *Alcohol in Europe: A Public Health Perspective – A Report for the European Commission*. London: Institute of Alcohol Studies.

Anderson, V.R., Jason, L.A., Hlavaty, L.E., Porter, N. and Cudia, J. (2012). A review and meta-synthesis of qualitative studies on myalgic encephalomyelitis/chronic fatigue syndrome. *Patient Education and Counseling*, 86 (2): 147–55.

Andreouli, E., Howarth, C. and Sonn, C. (2014). The role of schools in promoting inclusive communities in contexts of diversity. *Journal of Health Psychology*, 19: 16–21.

Andrews, F.M. and Withey, S.B. (1976). *Social Indicators of Well-being: Americans' Perceptions of Life Quality*. New York: Plenum.

Anjana, R.M., Ali, M.K., Pradeepa, R., Deepa, M., Datta, M., Unnikrishnan, R. et al. (2011). The need for obtaining accurate nationwide estimates of diabetes prevalence in India – rationale for a national study on diabetes. *Indian Journal of Medical Research* [online], 133: 369–80. Available: www.ijmr.org.in/text.asp?2011/133/4/369/80127 [accessed 10 August 2014].

Ansell, N. (2014). Challenging empowerment: AIDS-affected southern African children and the need for a multi-level relational approach. *Journal of Health Psychology*, 19: 22–33.

Anthony, J.C. and Echeagaray-Wagner, F. (2013). Epidemiologic analysis of alcohol and tobacco use – patterns of co-occurring consumption and dependence in the United States. *Alcohol Research & Health*, 24: 201–8.

Antonovsky, A. (1979). *Health, Stress, and Coping: New Perspectives on Mental and Physical Well-being*. San Francisco, CA: Jossey-Bass.

Appley, M.H. and Trumbull, R. (1986). Development of the stress concept. In M.H. Appley and R. Trumbull (eds.), *Dynamics of Stress*. The Plenum Series on Stress and Coping. Boston, MA: Springer. pp. 3–18.

Arena, R. (2015). The case for cardiac rehabilitation post-PCI and why we aren't meeting our goal. *American College of Cardiology*. Available: www.acc.org/latest-incardiology/articles/2015/08/13/14/10/the-casefor-cardiac-rehabilitation-post-pci [accessed 22 October 2015].

Armitage, C.J. (2009). Is there utility in the transtheoretical model? *British Journal of Health Psychology*, 14: 195–210.

Armstrong, N. (2007). Discourse and the individual in cervical cancer screening. *Health (London)*, 11: 69–85.

Arno, P., Levine, C. and Memmott, M. (1999). The economic value of informal caregiving. *Health Affairs*, 18: 182–8.

Arrey, A.E., Bilsen, J., Lacor, P. and Deschepper, R. (2015). 'It's My Secret': fear of disclosure among sub-Saharan African migrant women living with HIV/AIDS in Belgium. *PLoS One*, 10 (3): e0119653.

Arthur, H.M., Daniels, C., McKelvie, R., Hirsh, J. and Rush, B. (2000). Effect of a preoperative intervention on preoperative and postoperative outcomes in low-risk patients awaiting elective coronary artery bypass graft surgery: a randomized, controlled trial. *Annals of Internal Medicine*, 133: 253–62.

Asmundson G.J.G., Norton, P.J. and Norton, G.R. (1999). Beyond pain: the role of fear and avoidance in chronicity. *Clinical Psychological Review*, 19: 97–119.

Asmundson, G.J.G., McMillan, K.A. and Carleton, R.N. (2011).Understanding and managing clinically significant pain in patients with an anxiety disorder. *Focus*, 9 (3): 264–72.

Aspinwall, L.G. and MacNamara, A. (2005). Taking positive changes seriously: toward a positive psychology of cancer survivorship and resilience. *Cancer*, 104: 2549–56. doi:10.1002/cncr.21244.

Astin, J.A. (1998). Why patients use alternative medicine: results of a national study. *JAMA*, 279: 1548–53.

Aujla, N., Walker, M., Sprigg, N., Abrams, K., Massey, A. and Vedhara, K. (2016). Can illness beliefs, from the common-sense model, prospectively predict adherence to self-management behaviours? A systematic review and meta-analysis. *Psychology & Health*, 31: 1–28.

Australian Bureau of Statistics. (2014). *Australian Aboriginal and Torres Strait Islander Health Survey: First Results, Australia, 2012–13*. Canberra: Australian Bureau of Statistics. Available: www.abs.gov.au/ausstats/abs@.nsf/Lookup/3D7CEBB5503A110ECA257C2F00145AB4?opendocument.

Aveling, E. and Jovchelovitch, S. (2014). Partnerships as knowledge encounters: a psychosocial theory of partnerships for health and community development. *Journal of Health Psychology*, 19 (1): 34–45.

Avenell, A., Sattar, N. and Lean, M. (2006). Management: Part I – behaviour change, diet, and activity. *British Medical Journal*, 333: 740–3.

Avlund, K., Osler, M., Damsgaard, M.T., Christensen, U. and Schroll, M. (2000). The relations between musculoskeletal diseases and mobility among old people: are they influenced by socio-economic, psychosocial and behavioural factors? *International Journal of Behavioural Medicine*, 7: 322–39.

Ayers, J.W., Westmaas, J.L., Leas, E.C., Benton, A., Chen, Y., Dredze, M. and Althouse, B.M. (2016). Leveraging big data to improve health awareness campaigns: a novel evaluation of the Great American Smokeout. *JMIR Public Health and Surveillance*, 2 (1): e16.

Ayo, N. (2012). Understanding health promotion in a neoliberal climate and the making of health conscious citizens. *Critical Public Health*, 22: 99–105.

Babor, T.F. and Winstanley, E.L. (2008). The world of drinking: national alcohol control experiences in 18 countries. *Addiction*, 103: 721–5.

Babor, T.F., Caetano, R., Casswell, S., Edwards, G., Giesbrecht, N., Graham, K. et al. (Alcohol & Public Policy Group) (2003). *Alcohol: No Ordinary Commodity – Research and Public Policy*. Oxford: Oxford University Press.

Baker, M. (2014). RCGP consultation on assisted dying was comprehensive and conclusively in favour of no change to the law. *British Medical Journal* (Clinical Research Edition), 349: g4003.

Baker, S. (2002). Bardot, Britney, bodies and breasts. *Perfect Beat*, 6: 18–32.

Balarajan, R. and Soni Raleigh, V. (1993). *Ethnicity and Health: A Guide for the NHS*. London: Department of Health.

Balbach, E.D., Smith, E.A. and Malone, R.E. (2006). How the health belief model helps the tobacco industry: individuals, choice, and 'information'. *Tobacco Control*, 15: 37–43.

Baldwin, A.S., Bruce, C.M. and Tiro, J.A. (2012). Understanding how mothers of adolescent girls obtain information about the human papillomavirus vaccine: associations between mothers' health beliefs, information seeking, and vaccination intentions in an ethnically diverse sample. *Journal of Health Psychology*, 18 (7): 926–38.

Balshem, M. (1991). Cancer, control, and causality: talking about cancer in a working-class community. *American Ethnologist*, 18 (1): 152–72.

Bandura, A. (1977). Self-efficacy: towards a unifying theory of behavioural change. *Psychological Review*, 84: 191–215.

Bandura, A. (1986). *Social Foundations of Thought and Action: A Social Cognitive Theory*. Englewood Cliffs, NJ: Prentice Hall.

Bandura, A. (1994). Self-efficacy. In V.S. Ramachaudran (ed.), *Encyclopedia of Human Behavior* (Vol. 4). New York: Academic Press. pp. 71–81.

Bandura, A. (ed.) (1995). *Self-efficacy in Changing Societies*. Cambridge: Cambridge University Press.

Bandura, A. (1997). Social cognitive theory: an agentic perspective. *Annual Review of Psychology*, 52: 1–26.

Bandura, A. (2001). Social cognitive theory: an agentic perspective. *Annual Review of Psychology*, 52: 1–26.

Bangsberg, D.R., Perry, S., Charlebois, E.D., Clark, R.A., Roberston, M., Zolopa, A.R. and Moss, A. (2001). Non-adherence to highly active antiretroviral therapy predicts progression to AIDS. *AIDS*, 15 (9): 1181–3.

Bantum, E.O.C., Albright, C.L., White, K.K., Berenberg, J.L., Layi, G., Ritter, P.L. and Lorig, K. (2014). Surviving and thriving with cancer using a web-based health behavior change intervention: randomized controlled trial. *Journal of Medical Internet Research*, 16 (2): e54.

Baptista, D.R., Wiens, A., Pontarolo, R., Regis, L., Reis, W.C. and Correr, C. J. (2016). The chronic care model for type 2 diabetes: a systematic review. *Diabetology and Metabolic Syndrome*, 8: 7.

Barak, A. and Fisher, W.A. (2001). Toward an internet-driven, theoretically-based innovative approach to sex education. *Journal of Sex Research*, 38: 324–32.

Barbour, K.E., Helmick, C.G., Theis, K.A., Murphy, L.B., Hootman, J.M., Brady, T.J. et al. (2013). Prevalence of doctor-diagnosed arthritis and arthritis-attributable activity limitation – United States, 2010–2012. *Morbidity and Mortality Weekly Report*, 62 (14): 869–73. Available: www.cdc.gov/mmwr/preview/mmwrhtml/mm6244a1.htm [accessed 13 March 2014].

Barg, W., Medrala, W. and Wolanczyk-Medrala, A. (2011). Exercise-induced anaphylaxis: an update on diagnosis and treatment. *Current Allergy and Asthma Reports*, 11: 45. doi:10.1007/s11882-010-0150-y.

Barker, D. (2013). The developmental origins of chronic disease. In N.S. Lansdale, S.M. McHale and A. Booth (eds.), *Families and Child Health*. New York: Springer. pp. 3–12.

Barker, D.J. (1990). The foetal and infant origins of adult disease. *British Medical Journal*, 301: 1111.

Barker, D.J. (1998). In utero programming of chronic disease. *Clinical Science (London)*, 95: 115–28.

Barker, D.J.P. (2007). The origins of the developmental origins theory. *Journal of Internal Medicine*, 261: 412–17.

Barraclough, J., Pinder, P., Cruddas, M., Osmand, C., Taylor, I. and Perry, M. (1992). Life events and breast cancer prognosis. *British Medical Journal*, 304: 1078–81.

Barrett, A.E. (2003). Socioeconomic status and age identity: the role of dimensions of health in the subjective construction of age. *Journal of Gerontology, Series B: Psychological Sciences and Social Sciences*, 58: S101–9.

Bartels, R.M., Harkins, L. and Beech, A.R. (2017). The influence of fantasy proneness, dissociation, and vividness of mental imagery on male's aggressive sexual fantasies. *Journal of Interpersonal Violence*. Available: www.researchgate.net/publication/313684256_The_Influence_of_Fantasy_Proneness_Dissociation_and_Vividness_of_Mental_Imagery_on_Male%27s_Aggressive_Sexual_Fantasies?citedPub=18426957 [accessed 18 March 2017].

Barth, R., Scarborough, A., Lloyd, E.C., Losby, J.L., Casanueva, C.E. and Mann, T. (2008). *Developmental Status and Early Intervention Service Needs of Maltreated Children*. Washington, DC: U.S. Department of Health and Human Services, Office of the Assistant Secretary for Planning and Evaluation.

Barth, J. and Lannen, P. (2011). Efficacy of communication skills training courses in oncology: a systematic review and meta-analysis. *Annals of Oncology: Official Journal of the European Society for Medical Oncology/ESMO*, 22: 1030–40.

Barth, J., Schneider, S. and von Känel, R. (2010). Lack of social support in the etiology and the prognosis of coronary heart disease: a systematic review and meta-analysis. *Psychosomatic Medicine*, 72 (3): 229–38.

Bartlett, D. (1998). *Stress: Perspectives and Processes*. London: Open University Press.

Bassett, R.A., Osterhoudt, K. and Brabazon, T. (2014). Nicotine poisoning in an infant. *The New England Journal of Medicine*, 7 May.

Bassett-Gunter, R., Martin Ginis, K.A. and Latimer-Cheung, A. (2013). Do you want the good news or the bad news? Gain- versus loss-framed messages following health risk information: the effects on leisure time physical activity beliefs and cognitions. *Health Psychology*, 32: 1188–98.

Batt-Rawden, S.A., Chisolm, M.S., Anton, B. and Flickinger, T.E. (2013). Teaching empathy to medical students: an updated, systematic review. *Academic Medicine*, 88 (8): 1171–7.

Bauld, L., Bell, K., McCullough, L., Richardson, L. and Greaves, L. (2009). The effectiveness of NHS smoking cessation services: a systematic review. *Journal of Public Health*, 31: 1–12.

Baum, F. (2000). Social capital, economic capital and power: further issues for a public health agenda. *Journal of Epidemiology & Community Health*, 54: 409–10.

Baumeister, R.F. and Vohs, K.D. (2002). The pursuit of meaningfullness in life. In C.R. Snyder and S.J. Lopez (eds.), *Handbook of Positive Psychology*. New York: Oxford University Press. pp. 608–19.

Beals, J., Spicer, P., Mitchell, C.M., Novins, D.K., Manson, S.M., The AI-SUPERPFP Team et al. (2003). Racial disparities in alcohol use: comparison of two American Indian reservation populations with national data. *American Journal of Public Health*, 93: 1683–5.

Beccuti, G. and Pannain, S. (2011). Sleep and obesity. *Current Opinion in Clinical Nutrition & Metabolic Care*, 14: 402–12.

Beck, F., Gillison, F. and Standage, M. (2010). A theoretical investigation of the development of physical activity habits in retirement. *British Journal of Health Psychology*, 15: 663–79.

Beck, U. (1992) *Risk Society: Towards a New Modernity*. London: Sage.

Becker, M.H. (1974). The Health Belief Model and personal health behavior. *Health Education Monographs*, 2: 324–508.

Becker, A. (2012). Health economics of interdisciplinary rehabilitation for chronic pain: Does it support or invalidate the outcomes research of these programs? *Current Pain & Headache Reports*, 16: 127–32.

Beekers, N., Husson, O., Mols, F., van Eenbergen, M. and van de Poll-Franse, L.V. (2015). Symptoms of anxiety and depression are associated with satisfaction with information provision and internet use among 3080 cancer survivors: results of the PROFILES Registry. *Cancer Nursing*, 38 (5): 335–42.

Beitchman, J.H., Zucker, K.J., Hood, J.E., DaCosta, G.A., Akman, D. and Cassavia, E. (1992). A review of the long-term effects of child sexual abuse. *Child Abuse & Neglect*, 16 (1): 101–18.

Bell, T.R., Langhinrichsen-Rohling, J. and Selwyn, C.N. (2020). Conservation of resources and suicide proneness after oilrig disaster. *Death Studies*, 44(1): 48–57.

Benoist, J. and Cathebras, P. (1993). The body: from immateriality to another. *Social Science & Medicine*, 36: 857–65.

Benson, H. and Wallace, R.K. (1972). Decreased drug abuse with Transcendental Meditation: a study of 1,862 subjects. In J.D. Zarafonetis (ed.), *Drug Abuse: Proceedings of the International Conference*. Philadelphia, PA: Lee and Febiger. pp. 369–76.

Bent, S. (2008). Herbal medicine in the United States: review of efficacy, safety, and regulation. *Journal of General Internal Medicine*, 23: 854–9.

Bent, S. and Ko, R. (2004). Commonly used herbal medicines in the United States: a review. *American Journal of Medicine*, 116: 478–85.

Berghom, I., Svensson, C., Berggren, E. and Kamsula, M. (1999). Patients' and relatives' opinions and feelings about diaries kept by nurses in an intensive care unit: a pilot study. *Intensive & Critical Care Nursing*, 15: 185–91.

Berkhof, M., van Rijssen, H.J., Schellart, A.J., Anema, J.R. and van der Beek, A.J. (2011). Effective training strategies for teaching communication skills to physicians: an overview of systematic reviews. *Patient Education and Counseling*, 84: 152–62.

Berkman, L.F., Blumenthal, J., Burg, M., Carney, R.M., Catellier, D., Cowan, M.J. et al. (2003). Effects of treating depression and low perceived social support on clinical events after myocardial infarction: the Enhancing Recovery in Coronary Heart Disease Patients (ENRICHD) randomized trial. *Journal of the American Medical Association*, 289: 3106–16.

Berkman, N.D., Sheridan, S.L., Donahue, K.E., Halpern, D.J. and Crotty, K. (2011). Low health literacy and health outcomes: an updated systematic review. *Annals of Internal Medicine*, 155: 97–107.

Bermudez-Millan, A., Schumann, K.P., Feinn, R., Tennen, H. and Wagner, J. (2016). Behavioral reactivity to acute stress among black and white women with Type 2 diabetes: the roles of income and racial discrimination. *Journal of Health Psychology*, 21 (9): 2085–97. doi:10.1177/1359105315571776.

Bernard, C. (1865). *Introduction à l'étude de la médecine expérimentale*. Paris: Éditions Garnier-Flammarion.

Berners-Lee, M., Hoolohan, C., Cammack, H. and Hewitt, C.N. (2012). The relative greenhouse gas impacts of realistic dietary choices. *Energy Policy*, 43: 184–90.

Bero, L. (2013). Industry sponsorship and research outcome: a Cochrane Review. *Journal of the American Medical Association Internal Medicine*, 173: 580–1.

Bertholet, N., Daeppen, J.B., Wietlisbach, V., Fleming, M. and Burnard, B. (2005). Reduction of alcohol consumption by brief alcohol intervention in primary care: systematic review and meta-analysis. *Archives of Internal Medicine*, 165: 986–95.

Betsch, C. and Sachse, K. (2013). Debunking vaccination myths: strong risk negations can increase perceived vaccination risks. *Health Psychology*, 32: 146–55.

Betsch, C., Renkewitz, F., Betsch, T. and Ulshöfer, C. (2010). The influence of vaccine-critical websites on perceiving vaccination risks. *Journal of Health Psychology*, 15 (3): 446–55.

Bianconi, E., Piovesan, A., Facchin, F., Beraudi, A., Casadei, R., Frabetti, F. et al. (2013). An estimation of the number of cells in the human body. *Annals of Human Biology*, 40 (6): 463–71.

Bingley, A.F., McDermott, E., Thomas, C., Payne, S., Seymour, J.E. and Clark, D. (2006). Making sense of dying: a review of narratives written since 1950 by people facing death from cancer and other diseases. *Palliative Medicine*, 20: 183–95.

Birks, J. and Grimley Evans, J. (2009). Ginkgo biloba for cognitive impairment and dementia. *Cochrane Database of Systematic Reviews*, 1 (CD003120).

Birnie, K., Speca, M. and Carlson, L.E. (2010). Exploring self-compassion and empathy in the context of mindfulness-based stress reduction (MBSR). *Stress and Health*, 26 (5): 359–71.

Bjørnskov, C. and Sønderskov, K.M. (2013). Is social capital a good concept? *Social Indicators Research*, 114 (3): 1225–42.

Blair, C., Berry, D.J. and FLP Investigators (2017). Moderate within-person variability in cortisol is related to executive function in early childhood. *Psychoneuroendocrinology*, 81: 88–95.

Blaxter, M. (1990). *Health and Lifestyles*. London: Routledge.

Bliss, T.V. and Lømo, T. (1973). Long-lasting potentiation of synaptic transmission in the dentate area of the anaesthetized rabbit following stimulation of the perforant path. *The Journal of Physiology*, 232 (2): 331–56.

Blume, S. (2006). Anti-vaccination movements and their interpretations. *Social Science & Medicine*, 62: 628–42.

Blumhagen, D. (1980). Hyper-tension: a folk illness with a medical name. *Culture, Medicine & Psychiatry*, 4: 197–227.

Boehm, J.K. and Kubzansky, L.D. (2012). The heart's content: the association between positive psychological wellbeing and cardiovascular health. *Psychological Bulletin*, 138: 655–91.

Boepple, L., and Thompson, J. K. (2014). A content analysis of healthy living blogs: Evidence of content thematically consistent with dysfunctional eating attitudes and behaviors. *International Journal of Eating Disorders*, 47 (4): 362–7.

Boersma, K., Carstens-Söderstrand, J. and Linton, S.J. (2014). From acute pain to chronic disability: psychosocial processes in the development of chronic musculoskeletal pain and disability. In R.J. Gatchel and I.Z. Schultz (eds.), *Handbook of Musculoskeletal Pain and Disability Disorders in the Workplace*. New York: Springer. pp. 205–17.

Bogart, K.R. (2015). 'People are all about appearances': a focus group of teenagers with Moebius Syndrome. *Journal of Health Psychology*, 20 (12): 1579–88.

Bogart, L.M., Wagner, G.J., Galvan, F.H., Landrine, H., Klein, D.J. and Sticklor, L.A. (2011). Perceived discrimination and mental health symptoms among black men with HIV. *Cultural Diversity & Ethnic Minority Psychology*, 17 (3): 295–302.

Bogg, T. and Roberts, B.W. (2004). Conscientiousness and health-related behaviors: a meta-analysis of the leading behavioral contributors to mortality. *Psychological Bulletin*, 130: 887–919.

Bogle, V. and Kanapathy, J. (2017). The effectiveness of cognitive behaviour therapy for depressed patients with diabetes: a systematic review. *Journal of Health Psychology*. doi:10.1177/1359105317713360.

Bojorquez, I., Unikel, C., Mendoza, M.E. and de Lachica, F. (2013). Another body project: the thin ideal, motherhood and body dissatisfaction among Mexican women. *Journal of Health Psychology*, 19: 1120–31.

Bond, L., Lauby, J. and Batson, H. (2005). HIV testing and the role of individual- and structural-level barriers and facilitators. *AIDS Care*, 17 (2): 125–40.

Bond, M., Garside, R. and Hyde, C. (2015). A crisis of visibility: The psychological consequences of false-positive screening mammograms, an interview study. *British Journal of Health Psychology*, 20: 792–806.

Bonica, J.J. (1990). *The Management of Pain* (2nd edn). Philadelphia, PA: Lea and Febiger.

Borrelli, B. (2011). The assessment, monitoring, and enhancement of treatment fidelity in public health clinical trials. *Journal of Public Health Dentistry*, 71 (s1): S52–63.

Bosy, D., Etlin, D., Corey, D. and Lee, J.W. (2010). An interdisciplinary pain rehabilitation programme: description and evaluation of outcomes. *Physiotherapy Canada*, 62: 316–26.

Bouillon, R., Okamura, W.H. and Norman, A.W. (1995). Structure-function relationships in the vitamin D endocrine system. *Endocrine Reviews*, 16 (2): 200–57.

Bourdieu, P. (1984). *Distinction: A Social Critique of the Judgement of Taste*. London: Routledge & Kegan Paul.

Bowen, S., Witkiewitz, K., Clifasefi, S.L., Grow, J., Chawla, N., Hsu, S.H. et al. (2014). Relative efficacy of mindfulness-based relapse prevention, standard relapse prevention, and treatment as usual for substance use disorders: a randomized clinical trial. *Journal of the American Medical Association – Psychiatry*, 71: 547–56.

Bowers, M.E. and Yehuda, R. (2016). Intergenerational transmission of stress in humans. *Neuropsychopharmacology*, 41 (1): 232–44.

Bowlby, J. (1961). Processes of mourning. *International Journal of Psychoanalysis*, 42: 317–39.

Bowlby, J. (1969). *Attachment and Loss: Attachment*. New York: Basic Books.

Bowlby, J. (1973). *Attachment and Loss: Separation, Anxiety and Anger*. New York: Basic Books.

Bowlby, J. (1980). *Attachment and Loss: Sadness and Depression*. New York: Basic Books.

Bowling, A. (2001). *Measuring Disease*. London: McGraw-Hill Education.

Bowling, A. (2004). *Measuring Health*. London: McGraw-Hill Education.

Boylan, S., Louie, J.C.Y. and Gill, T.P. (2013). Consumer response to healthy eating, physical activity and weight-related recommendations: a systematic review. *Obesity Reviews*, 13: 606–17.

Brandes, K. and Mullan, B. (2014). Can the commonsense model predict adherence in chronically ill patients? A meta-analysis. *Health Psychology Review*, 8: 129–53.

Braun, F. and Fisher, M. (2013). Why behavioural health promotion endures despite its failure to reduce health inequities. *Sociology of Health & Illness*, 36: 213–25.

Brawley, L.R., Martin, K. and Gyurcsik, N.C. (1998). Problems in assessing perceived barriers to exercise: confusing obstacles with attributions and excuses. In J.L. Duda (ed.), *Advances in Sport and Exercise Psychology Measurement*. Morgantown, WV: Fitness Information Technology. pp. 337–50.

Bray, G.A. (2003). Obesity is a chronic, relapsing neurochemical disease. *International Journal of Obesity*, 28: 34–8.

Bray, S.R., Gyurcsik, N.C., Culos-Reed, S.N., Dawson, K.A. and Martin, K.A. (2001). An exploratory investigation of the relationship between proxy efficacy, self-efficacy and exercise attendance. *Journal of Health Psychology*, 6: 425–34.

Brazier, J., Roberts, J. and Deverill, M. (2002). The estimation of a preference-based measure of health from the SF-36. *Journal of Health Economics*, 21 (2): 271–92.

Brehm, B.J., Seeley, R.J., Daniels, S.R. and D'Alessio, D.A. (2003). A randomized trial comparing a very low carbohydrate diet and a calorie-restricted low fat diet on body weight and cardiovascular risk factors in healthy women. *The Journal of Clinical Endocrinology & Metabolism*, 88 (4): 1617–23.

Breiding, M.J. (2014). Prevalence and characteristics of sexual violence, stalking, and intimate partner violence victimization – National Intimate Partner and Sexual Violence Survey, United States, 2011. *Morbidity and Mortality Weekly Report: Surveillance Summaries*, 63 (8): 1.

Breiding, M.J., Chen, J. and Black, M.C. (2014). *Intimate Partner Violence in the United States – 2010*. Atlanta, GA: National Center for Injury Prevention and Control, Centers for Disease Control and Prevention.

Breivik, H., Collett, B., Ventafridda, V., Cohen, R. and Gallacher, D. (2006). Survey of chronic pain in Europe: prevalence, impact on daily life, and treatment. *European Journal of Pain*, 10 (4): 287–333.

Bresnahan, M. and Zhuang, J. (2016). Development and validation of the Communicating with Family about Brain Death Scale. *Journal of Health Psychology*, 21 (7): 1207–15.

Brett, J. and Austoker, J. (2001). Women who are recalled for further investigation for breast screening: psychological consequences three years after recall and factors affecting re-attendance. *Journal of Public Health Medicine*, 23: 292–300.

Brewer, N.T., Chapman, G.B., Gibbons, F.X., Gerrard, M., McCaul, D. and Weinstein, N. (2007). Meta-analysis of the relationship between risk perception and health behavior: the example of vaccination. *Health Psychology*, 26: 136–45.

Brien, S.E., Ronksley, P.E., Turner, B.J., Mukamal, K.J. and Ghali, W.A. (2011). Effect of alcohol consumption on biological markers associated with risk of coronary heart disease: systematic review and meta-analysis of interventional studies. *British Medical Journal*, 342: d636.

Britto, P.R., Lye, S.J., Proulx, K., Yousafzai, A.K., Matthews, S.G., Vaivada, T. et al. (2017). Nurturing care: promoting early childhood development. *The Lancet*, 389 (10064): 91–102.

Broadbent, E., Wilkes, C., Koschwanez, H., Weinman, J., Norton, S. and Petrie, K.J. (2015). A systematic review and meta-analysis of the brief illness perception questionnaire. *Psychology & Health*, 30 (11): 1361–85.

Broadstock, M., Michie, S. and Marteau, T. (2000). Psychological consequences of predictive genetic testing: a systematic literature review. *European Journal of Human Genetics*, 8: 731–8.

Brochu, P.M. and Esses, V.M. (2011). What's in a name? The effects of the labels 'fat' and 'overweight' on weight bias. *Journal of Applied Social Psychology*, 41: 1981–2008.

Brodersen, J. and Siersma, V.D. (2013). Long-term psychosocial consequences of false-positive screening mammography. *Annals of Family Medicine*, 11: 106–15.

Bronfenbrenner, U. (1979). *The Ecology of Human Development*. Cambridge, MA: Harvard University Press.

Brown, D. (2007). Herbal medicine. In A.D. Cumming, K.R. Simpson and D. Brown (eds.), *Complementary and Alternative Medicine: An Illustrated Color Text*. Edinburgh: Elsevier. pp. 52–6.

Brown, K.W. and Ryan, R.M. (2003). The benefits of being present: mindfulness and its role in psychological well-being. *Journal of Personality & Social Psychology*, 84: 822.

Brown, L., Macintyre, K. and Trujillo, L. (2003). Interventions to reduce HIV/AIDS stigma: What have we learned? *AIDS Education and Prevention*, 15 (1): 49–69.

Brown, S.L. and Whiting, D. (2014). The ethics of distress: toward a framework for determining the ethical acceptability of distressing health promotion advertising. *International Journal of Psychology*, 49: 89–97.

Browne, J.L., Ventura, A., Mosely, K. and Speight, J. (2013). 'I call it the blame and shame disease': a qualitative study about perceptions of social stigma surrounding Type 2 diabetes. *BMJ Open*, 3 (11): e003384.

Brownell, K.D. (1992). Dieting and the search for the perfect body: where physiology and culture collide. *Behavior Therapy*, 22: 1–12.

Brownell, K.D. (1994). Get slim with higher taxes. *New York Times*, 15: A29.

Brownell, K.D. and Fairburn, C.G. (1995). *Eating Disorders and Obesity: A Comprehensive Handbook*. New York: Guilford Press.

Brudzynski, L. and Ebben, W.P. (2010). Body image as a motivator and barrier to exercise participation. *International Journal of Exercise Science*, 3 (1): 14–24.

Brydon-Miller, M. (2004). Using participatory action research to address community health issues. In M. Murray (ed.), *Critical Health Psychology*. London: Palgrave. pp. 187–202.

Buckley, T.M. and Schatzberg, A.F. (2005). On the interactions of the hypothalamic-pituitary-adrenal (HPA) axis and sleep: normal HPA axis activity and circadian rhythm, exemplary sleep disorders. *Journal of Clinical Endocrinology and Metabolism*, 90: 3106–14.

Bui, L., Mullan, B. and McCaffery, K. (2013). Protection motivation theory and physical activity in the general population: a systematic literature review. *Psychology, Health & Medicine*, 18 (5): 522–42.

Bunke, S., Apitzsch, E. and Backstrom, M. (2013). The impact of social influence on physical activity among adolescents – a longitudinal study. *European Journal of Sport Science*, 13: 86–95.

Burg, M.M., Benedetto, M.C., Rosenberg, R. and Soufer, R. (2003). Presurgical depression predicts medical morbidity six months after coronary artery bypass graft surgery. *Psychosomatic Medicine*, 65: 111–18.

Burnham, B.E. (1995). Garlic as a possible risk for postoperative bleeding. *Plastic and Reconstructive Surgery*, 95: 213.

Burton, A.E., Shaw, R.L. and Gibson, J.M. (2015). Living together with age-related macular degeneration: an interpretative phenomenological analysis of sense-making within a dyadic relationship. *Journal of Health Psychology*, 20 (10): 1285–95.

Butland, B., Jebb, S., Kopelman, P., McPherson, K., Thomas, S., Mardell, J. and Parry, V. (2007). *Foresight. Tackling Obesities: Future Choices – Project Report*. London: Government Office for Science.

Butler, L. and Pilkington, K. (2013). Chinese herbal medicine and depression: the research evidence. *Evidence-Based Complementary & Alternative Medicine (eCAM)*, Article ID 739716: 1–14.

Buxon, O.M., Spiegel, K. and Van Cauter, E. (2002). Modulation of endocrine function and metabolism by sleep and sleep loss. In T.L. Lee-Chiong, M.J. Sateia and M.A. Carskadon (eds.), *Sleep Medicine*. Philadelphia, PA: Hanley and Belfus. pp. 59–69.

Byrne, D.G. and Espnes, G.A. (2008). Occupational stress and cardiovascular disease. *Stress & Health*, 24: 231–8.

Byrne, P.S. and Long, B.E.L. (1976). *Doctors Talking to Patients*. London: HMSO.

Cahill, K., Stevens, S., Perera, R. and Lancaster, T. (2013). Pharmacological interventions for smoking cessation: an overview and network meta-analysis. *Cochrane Database of Systematic Reviews*, 5: 5.

Cairn, R.L., Stoneking, M. and Wilson, A.C. (1987). Mitochondrial DNA and human evolution. *Nature*, 325 (3): 31–6.

Cajita, M.I., Cajita, T.R. and Han, H. (2016). Health literacy and heart failure: a systematic review. *The Journal of Cardiovascular Nursing*, 31 (2): 121–30. doi:10.1097/JCN.0000000000000229.

Calder, P.C. (2013). Feeding the immune system. *Proceedings of the Nutrition Society*, 72 (3): 299–309.

Calnan, M. and Williams, S. (1991). Style of life and the salience of health: an exploratory study of health related practices in households from differing socio-economic circumstances. *Sociology of Health & Illness*, 13: 506–29.

Cameron, L.D. and Reeve, J. (2006). Risk perceptions, worry, and attitudes about genetic testing for breast cancer susceptibility. *Psychology and Health*, 21: 211–30.

Camic, P.M., Hulbert, S. and Kimmel, J. (2017). Museum object handling: a health-promoting community-based activity for dementia care. *Journal of Health Psychology*. doi:10.1177/1359105316685899.

Campbell, A. and Hausenblas, H.A. (2009). Effects of exercise interventions on body image: a meta-analysis. *Journal of Health Psychology*, 14: 780–93.

Campbell, C. (2004). Health psychology and community action. In M. Murray (ed.), *Critical Health Psychology*. London: Palgrave. pp. 203–21.

Campbell, C. (2014). Community mobilisation in the 21st century: updating our theory of social change? *Journal of Health Psychology*, 19: 46–59.

Campbell, C. (2015). Health beliefs of community dwelling older adults in the United Arab Emirates: a qualitative study. *Ageing International*, 40 (1): 13–28.

Campbell, C. and Cornish, F. (2014). Reimagining community health psychology: maps, journeys and new terrains. *Journal of Health Psychology*, 19: 3–15.

Campbell, C. and Murray, M. (2004). Community health psychology: promoting analysis and action for social change. *Journal of Health Psychology*, 9: 187–95.

Campbell, C., Cornish, F., Gibbs, A. and Scott, K. (2010). Heeding the push from below: How do social movements persuade the rich to listen to the poor? *Journal of Health Psychology*, 15 (7): 962–71.

Campbell, R. (2008). The psychological impact of rape victims. *American Psychologist*, 63 (8): 702.

Cancer Research UK (2013). *Breast Cancer Statistics*. Available: www.cancerresearchuk.org/cancer-info/cancerstats/types/breast/.

Cane, J., O'Connor, D. and Michie, S. (2012). Validation of the theoretical domains framework for use in behaviour change and implementation research. *Implementation Science*, 7: 37.

Cannon, W.B. (1915). *Bodily Changes in Pain, Hunger, Fear, and Rage*. New York: Appleton & Company.

Cannon, W. B. (1932). *The Wisdom of the Body*. New York: W.W. Norton and Company.

Cao-Lei, L., Massart, R., Suderman, M.J., Machnes, Z., Elgbeili, G., Laplante, D.P. et al. (2014). DNA methylation signatures triggered by prenatal maternal stress exposure to a natural disaster: project ice storm. *PLoS One*, 9 (9): e107653.

Caplan, R.P. (1994). Stress, anxiety, and depression in hospital consultants, general practitioners, and senior health service managers. *British Medical Journal*, 309 (6964): 1261–3.

Carlbring, P., Bohman, S., Brunt, S., Buhrman, M., Westling, B.E., Ekselius, L. et al. (2006). Remote treatment of panic disorder: a randomized trial of internet-based cognitive behavior therapy supplemented with telephone calls. *American Journal of Psychiatry*, 163 (12): 2119–25.

Carlson, J.A., Sallis, J.F., Conway, T.L., Saelens, B.E., Frank, L.D., Kerr, J. et al. (2012). Interactions between psychosocial and built environment factors in explaining older adults' physical activity. *Preventive Medicine*, 54: 68–73.

Carruthers, B.M., van de Sande, M.I., De Meirleir, K.L. et al. (2011). Myalgic encephalomyelitis: International Consensus Criteria. *Journal of Internal Medicine*, 270 (4): 327–38.

Carter, S.M., Rychetnik, L., Lloyd, B., Kerridge, I.H., Baur, L., Bauman, A. et al. (2011). Evidence, ethics, and values: a framework for health promotion. *American Journal of Public Health*, 101: 465–72.

Carver, C., Posse, C., Harris, S., Noriega, V., Scheir, M., Robinson, D. et al. (1993). How coping mediates the effect of optimism on distress. *Health Psychology*, 12: 375–90.

Carver, C.S. and Scheier, M.F. (1982). Control theory: a useful conceptual framework for personality, social, clinical and health psychology. *Psychological Bulletin*, 92: 111–35.

Carver, C.S., Scheier, M.F. and Weintraub, J.K. (1989). Assessing coping strategies: a theoretically based approach. *Journal of Personality & Social Psychology*, 56: 267–83.

Casey, M.M., Eime, R.M., Payne, W.R. and Harvey, J.T. (2009). Using a socioecological approach to examine participation in sport and physical activity among rural adolescent girls. *Qualitative Health Research*, 19: 881–93.

Cassidy, B., Braxter, B., Charron-Prochownik, D. and Schlenk, E.A. (2014). A quality improvement initiative to increase HPV vaccine rates using an educational and reminder strategy with parents of preteen girls. *Journal of Pediatric Health Care*, 28 (2): 155–64.

Centers for Disease Control and Prevention. (2010). *A Public Health Approach for Advancing Sexual Health in the United States: Rationale and Options for Implementation, Meeting Report of an External Consultation*. Atlanta, GA: Centers for Disease Control and Prevention.

Centers for Disease Control and Prevention. (2012). *National Healthcare Disparities Report*. Available: www.ahrq.gov/research/findings/nhqrdr/nhdr12/chap2.html.

Centers for Disease Control and Prevention. Campaign, General Awareness (2013). *Act Against AIDS*. Available: https://content.govdelivery.com/accounts/USCDC/bulletins/945b8b

Centers for Disease Control and Prevention. (2013a). Death and mortality. *NCHS FastStats*. Atlanta, GA: Centers for Disease Control and Prevention. Available: www.cdc.gov/nchs/fastats/deaths.htm [accessed 20 December 2013].

Centers for Disease Control and Prevention. (2013b). *NCHS Obesity Data*. Atlanta, GA: Centers for Disease Control and Prevention. Available: www.cdc.gov/nchs/data/factsheets/factsheet_obesity.htm [accessed 20 December 2013].

Centers for Disease Control and Prevention. (2013c). *Make a Difference at Your School*. Chronic Disease. Paper 31.

Centers for Disease Control and Prevention. (2016a). *Fact Sheet – Current Cigarette Smoking among Adults in the United States*. Atlanta, GA: Centers for Disease Control and Prevention. Available: www.cdc.gov/tobacco/data [accessed 24 February 2017].

Centers for Disease Control and Prevention. (2016b). *HIV/AIDS*. Atlanta, GA: Centers for Disease Control and Prevention. Available: www.cdc.gov/hiv/basics/prep.html [accessed 24 February 2017].

Centers for Disease Control and Prevention. (2017b). *Act against AIDS*. Atlanta, GA: Centers for Disease Control and Prevention. Available: www.cdc.gov/actagainstaids [accessed 24 February 2017].

Centers for Disease Control and Prevention. (2017c). *Sexual Violence: Definitions*. Atlanta, GA: Centers for Disease Control and Prevention. Available: www.cdc.gov/violencepreven tion/sexualviolence/definitions.html [accessed 27 February 2017].

Cermakian, N., Lange, T., Golombek, D., Sarkar, D., Nakao, A., Shibata, S. et al. (2013). Crosstalk between the circadian clock circuitry and the immune system. *Chronobiology International*, 30 (7): 870–88.

Chaiton, M., Sabiston, C., O'Loughlin, J., McGrath, J.J., Maximova, K. and Lambert, M. (2009). A structural equation model relating adiposity, psychosocial indicators of body image and depressive symptoms among adolescents. *International Journal of Obesity*, 33: 588–96.

Chambers, L.A., Rueda, S., Baker, D.N., Wilson, M.G., Deutsch, R., Raeifar, E., Rourke, S.B. and Sigma Review Team (2015). Stigma, HIV and health: a qualitative synthesis. *BMC Public Health*, 15: 848.

Chan, C.W., Goldman, S., Ilstrup, D.M., Kunselman, A.R. and O'Neill, P.I. (1993). The pain drawing and Waddell's nonorganic physical signs in chronic low-back pain. *Spine*, 18: 1717–22.

Chang, F.-C., Chiu, C.-H., Miao, N.-F., Chen, P.-H., Lee, C.-M. and Chiang, J.-T. (2014). Predictors of unwanted exposure to online pornography and online sexual solicitation of youth. *Journal of Health Psychology*, 21 (6): 1107–18.

Chapin, J. (2001). It won't happen to me: the role of optimistic bias in African American teens' risky sexual practices. *Howard Journal of Communication*, 12 (1): 49–59.

Chapman, G.B. and Coups, E.J. (2006). Emotions and preventive health behaviour: worry, regret, and influenza vaccination. *Health Psychology*, 25: 82–90.

Chapman, S. and MacKenzie, R. (2010). The global research neglect of unassisted smoking cessation: causes and consequences. *PLoS Medicine*, 7 (2): e1000216.

Charmaz, K. (2003). Grounded theory. In J.A. Smith (ed.), *Qualitative Psychology: A Practical Guide to Research Methods*. London: Sage. pp. 81–110.

Chauvet-Gelinier, J.C. and Bonin, B. (2017). Stress, anxiety and depression in heart disease patients: a major challenge for cardiac rehabilitation. *Annals of Physical and Rehabilitation Medicine*, 60 (1): 6–12.

Chen, J., Choi, Y.C., Mori, K., Sawada, Y. and Sugano, S. (2012). Recession, unemployment, and suicide in Japan. *Japan Labor Review*, 9: 75–92.

Chen, W.C., Rosner, B., Hankinson, S.E., Colditz, G.A. and Willett, W.C. (2011). Moderate alcohol consumption during adult life, drinking patterns, and breast cancer risk. *Journal of the American Medical Association*, 306: 1884–90.

Chen, X.K., Wen, S.W., Fleming, N., Demissie, K., Rhoads, G.G. and Walker, M. (2007). Teenage pregnancy and adverse birth outcomes: a large population based retrospective cohort study. *International Journal of Epidemiology*, 36 (2): 368–73.

Cheng, Y.H. (1997). Explaining disablement in modern times: hand-injured workers' accounts of their injuries in Hong Kong. *Social Science & Medicine*, 45: 739–50.

Chervin, C., Clift, J., Woods, L., Krause, E. and Lee, K. (2012). Health literacy in adult education: a natural partnership for health equity. *Health Promotion Practice*, 13: 738–46.

Chesler, M.A. and Parry, C. (2001). Gender roles and/or styles in crisis: an integrative analysis of the experiences of fathers of children with cancer. *Qualitative Health Research*, 11: 363–84.

Chesney, M.A., Chambers, D.B., Taylor, J.M., Johnson, L.M. and Folkman, S. (2003). Coping effectiveness training for men living with HIV: results from a randomised clinical trial testing a group-based intervention. *Psychosomatic Medicine*, 65: 1038–46.

Chigwedere, P., Seage III, G.R., Gruskin, S., Lee, T.H. and Essex, M. (2008). Estimating the lost benefits of antiretroviral drug use in South Africa. *JAIDS: Journal of Acquired Immune Deficiency Syndromes*, 49: 410–15.

Chiu, Y. and Hsieh, Y. (2013). Communication online with fellow cancer patients: writing to be remembered, gain strength, and find survivors. *Journal of Health Psychology*, 18 (12): 1572–81.

Chow, E., Tsao, M.N. and Harth, T. (2004). Does psychosocial intervention improve survival in cancer? A meta-analysis. *Palliative Medicine*, 18: 25–31.

Christakis, N.A. and Fowler, J.H. (2007). The spread of obesity in a large social network over 32 years. *The New England Journal of Medicine*, 357: 370–9.

Chronic Care Model. (2015). Standards of medical care in diabetes – 2015 abridged for primary care providers. *Diabetes Care*, 38 (1): S1–94.

Chrvala, C.A., Sherr, D. and Lipman, R.D. (2016). Diabetes self-management education for adults with Type 2 diabetes mellitus: a systematic review of the effect on glycemic control. *Patient Education and Counseling*, 99 (6): 926–43.

Ciccone, D.S., Weissman, L. and Natelson, B.H. (2008). Chronic fatigue syndrome in male Gulf War Veterans and civilians: a further test of the single syndrome hypothesis. *Journal of Health Psychology*, 13: 529–36.

Ciesla, J.A. and Roberts, J.E. (2001). Meta-analysis of the relationship between HIV infection and risk for depressive disorders. *The American Journal of Psychiatry*, 158 (5): 725–30.

Clark, H.R., Goyder, E., Bissell, P., Blank, L. and Peters, J. (2007). How do parents' child-feeding behaviours influence child weight? Implications for childhood obesity policy. *Public Health*, 29: 132–41.

Clark, R., Anderson, N.B., Clark, V.R. and Williams, D.R. (1999). Racism as a stressor for African Americans: a biopsychosocial model. *American Psychologist*, 54 (10): 805.

Clark, W. (2008). Treatment of substance abuse disorders among Latinos. Invited address presented at the 14th Annual Latino Behavioral Health Institute Conference, Los Angeles, CA.

Clark-Carter, D. (1997). *Doing Quantitative Psychological Research: From Design to Report*. Hove: Psychology Press.

Clark-Carter, D. and Marks, D.F. (2004). Intervention studies: design and analysis. In D.F. Marks and L. Yardley (eds.), *Research Methods for Clinical and Health Psychology*. London: Sage. pp. 166–84.

Clarke, P. and Eves, F. (1997). Applying the transtheoretical model to the study of exercise on prescription. *Journal of Health Psychology*, 2: 195–207.

Clement, S. (1995). Diabetes self-management education. *Diabetes Care*, 18: 1204–14.

Coalter, F. (2007). *A Wider Social Role for Sport: Who's Keeping the Score?* London: Routledge.

Cochrane, T., Davey, R.C., Gidlow, C., Smith, G.R., Fairburn, J., Armitage, C.J. et al. (2009). Small area and individual level predictors of physical activity in urban communities: a multi-level study in Stoke-on-Trent, England. *International Journal of Environmental Research & Public Health*, 6: 654–77.

Cockburn, C. and Clarke, G. (2002). 'Everybody's looking at you!' Girls negotiating the 'femininity deficit' they incur in physical education. *Women's Studies International Forum*, 25: 651–65.

Coghill, R.C., McHaffie, J.G. and Yen, Y.-F. (2003). Neural correlates of interindividual differences in the subjective experience of pain. *Proceedings of the National Academy of Science*, 100: 8538–42.

Cohen, J. (1973). Brief notes: Statistical power analysis and research results. *American Educational Research Journal*, 10 (3): 225–9.

Cohen, J. (1988). *Statistical Power Analysis for the Behavioral Sciences* (2nd edn). Hillsdale, NJ: Lawrence Erlbaum.

Cohen, J. (1994). The earth is round (*p* < .05). *American Psychologist*, 49: 997.

Cohen, J. (1995). The earth is round (*p* < .05): rejoinder. *American Psychologist*, 50 (12): 1103.

Cohen, S. (2004). Social relationships and health. *American Psychologist*, 59 (special issue): 676–84.

Cohen, S. and Williamson, G.M. (1991). Stress and infectious disease in humans. *Psychological Bulletin*, 109: 5–24.

Cohen, S., Gianaros, P.J. and Manuck, S.B. (2016). A stage model of stress and disease. *Perspectives on Psychological Science*, 11 (4): 456–63.

Cohen, S., Janicki-Deverts, D. and Miller, G.E. (2007). Psychological stress and disease. *Journal of the American Medical Association*, 298: 1685–7.

Cohen, S.D. and Goldstein, I. (2016). Diagnosis and management of female orgasmic disorder. In L.I. Lipshultz, A.W. Pastuszak, A.T. Goldstein, A. Giraldi and M.A. Perelman (eds.) *Management of Sexual Dysfunction in Men and Women*. New York: Springer. pp. 261–71.

Coleman, L., Cox, L. and Roker, D. (2008). Girls and young women's participation in physical activity: psychological and social influences. *Health Education Research*, 23: 633–47.

Collingridge, G.L. and Singer, W. (1990). Excitatory amino acid receptors and synaptic plasticity. *Trends in Pharmacological Sciences*, 11 (7): 290–6.

Collins, R.L. and Bradizza, C.M. (2001). Social and cognitive learning processes. In N. Heather, T.J. Peters and T. Stockwell (eds.), *International Handbook of Alcohol Dependence and Problems*. London: Wiley. pp. 317–37.

Compton, W.C., Smith, M.L., Cornish, K.A. and Qualls, D.L. (1996). Factor structure of mental health measures. *Journal of Personality and Social Psychology*, 71: 406.

Connell, R. (2005). *Masculinities* (2nd edn). Cambridge: Polity Press.

Conner, M. and Armitage, C. (1998). Extending the theory of planned behavior: a review and avenues for further research. *Journal of Applied Social Psychology*, 28: 1429–64.

Connors, A.F., Dawson, N.V., Desbiens, N.A., Fulkerson, W.J., Goldman, L., Knaus, W.A., Lynn, J. et al. (1995). A controlled trial to improve care for seriously ill hospitalized patients:

the study to understand prognoses and preferences for outcomes and risks of treatments (SUPPORT). *Journal of the American Medical Association*, 274 (20): 1591–8.

Conroy, D. and de Visser, R. (2013). 'Man up!' Discursive constructions of non-drinkers among UK undergraduates. *Journal of Health Psychology*, 18: 1432–44.

Cook, C.C.H. and Gurling, H.M.D. (2001). Genetic predisposition to alcohol dependence and problems. In N. Heather, T.J. Peters and T. Stockwell (eds.), *International Handbook of Alcohol Dependence and Problems*. London: Wiley. pp. 257–80.

Cooke, R. and French, D.P. (2008). How well do the theory of reasoned action and theory of planned behaviour predict intentions and attendance at screening programmes? A meta-analysis. *Psychology & Health*, 23 (7): 745–65.

Cookson, C. (2002). Benefit and risk of vaccination as seen by the general public and the media. *Vaccine*, 20: S85–8.

Cooper, A., Delmonico, D.L. and Burg, R. (2000). Cybersex users, abusers, and compulsives: new findings and implications. *Sexual Addiction & Compulsivity: The Journal of Treatment and Prevention*, 7 (1–2): 5–29.

Cooper, D.M., Radom-Aizik, S., Schwindt, C.D. and Zaldivar Jr, F. (2007). Dangerous exercise: lessons learned from dysregulated inflammatory responses to physical activity. *Journal of Applied Physiology*, 103: 700–9.

Cooper, E.B., Fenigstein, A. and Fauber, R.L. (2014). The faking orgasm scale for women: psychometric properties. *Archives of Sexual Behavior*, 43 (3): 423–35.

Cornish, F., Montenegro, C., van Reisen, K., Zaka, F. and Sevitt, J. (2014). Trust the process: community health psychology after occupy. *Journal of Health Psychology*, 19 (1): 60–71.

Coroiu, A., Körner, A., Burke, S., Meterissian, S. and Sabiston, C.M. (2016). Stress and post-traumatic growth among survivors of breast cancer: a test of curvilinear effects. *International Journal of Stress Management*, 23 (1): 84.

Costa, R.M. and Brody, S. (2007). Women's relationship quality is associated with specifically penile–vaginal intercourse orgasm and frequency. *Journal of Sex & Marital Therapy*, 33 (4): 319–27.

Coughlin, S.S. (2008). Surviving cancer or other serious illness: a review of individual and community resources. *CA: A Cancer Journal for Clinicians*, 58: 60–4. doi:10.3322/CA.2007.0001.

Courtenay, W.H. (2000). Constructions of masculinity and their influence on men's well-being: a theory of gender and health. *Social Science & Medicine*, 50: 1385–401.

Cox, T. (1978). *Stress*. London: Macmillan.

Coyne, J.C. and Kok, R. N. (2014). Salvaging psychotherapy research: a manifesto. *Journal of Evidence-Based Psychotherapies*, 14 (2): 105.

Coyne, J.C. and Tennen, H. (2010). Positive psychology in cancer care: bad science, exaggerated claims, and unproven medicine. *Annals of Behavioural Medicine*, 39: 16–26.

Coyne, J.C., Stefanek, M. and Palmer, S.C. (2007). Psychotherapy and survival in cancer: The conflict between hope and evidence. *Psychological Bulletin*, 133: 367–94.

Craig, P., Dieppe, P., Macintyre, S., Michie, S., Nazareth, I. and Petticrew, M. (2013). Developing and evaluating complex interventions: the new Medical Research Council guidance. *International Journal of Nursing Studies*, 50 (5): 587–92. doi:10.1016/j.ijnurstu.2012.09.009

Craig, R. and Mindell, J. (eds) (2013) *Health Survey for England 2012*. Leeds: Health and Social Care Information Centre.

Crawford, R. (1980). Healthism and the medicalization of everyday life. *International Journal of Health Services*, 10 (3): 365–88.

Crepaz, N., Hart, T.A. and Marks, G. (2004). Highly active antiretroviral therapy and sexual risk behavior: a meta-analytic review. *JAMA*, 292 (2): 224–36.

Creswell, J.W. and Clark, V.L.P. (2007). Designing and conducting mixed methods research. *Wiley Online Library*, 3 (4): 388. doi:10.1111/j.1753-6405.2007.00096.

Crombez, G., Bijttebier, P., Eccleston, C., Mascagni, T., Mertens, G., Goubert, L. and Verstraeten, K. (2003). The child version of the Pain Catastrophizing Scale (PCS-C): a preliminary validation. *Pain*, 104: 639–46.

Crombez, G., Eccleston, C., Van Damme, S., Vlaeyen, J.W. and Karoly, P. (2012). Fear-avoidance model of chronic pain: the next generation. *Clinical Journal of Pain*, 28: 475–83.

Cromby, J. (2012). Beyond belief. *Journal of Health Psychology*, 17: 943–57.

Cropley, M., Ayers, S. and Nokes, L. (2003). People don't exercise because they can't think of reasons to exercise: an examination of causal reasoning with the Transtheoretical Model. *Psychology, Health & Medicine*, 8: 409–14.

Crossley, M.L. (2003). 'Would you consider yourself a healthy person?' Using focus groups to explore health as a moral phenomenon. *Journal of Health Psychology*, 8: 501–14.

Crowe, F.L., Appleby, P.N., Allen, N.E. and Key, T.J. (2011). Diet and risk of diverticular disease in Oxford cohort of European Prospective Investigation into Cancer and Nutrition (EPIC): prospective study of British vegetarians and non-vegetarians. *British Medical Journal*, 343: d4131.

Crowe, F.L., Appleby, P.N., Travis, R.C. and Key, T.J. (2013). Risk of hospitalization or death from ischemic heart disease among British vegetarians and nonvegetarians: results from the EPIC-Oxford cohort study. *American Journal of Clinical Nutrition*, 97: 597–603.

Csikszentmihalyi, M. (1997). *Finding Flow: The Psychology of Engagement with Everyday Life*. New York: Basic Books.

Cummins, R.A. (1998). The second approximation to an international standard of life satisfaction. *Social Indicators Research*, 43: 307–34.

Cummins, R.A. (2010). Subjective wellbeing, homeostatically protected mood and depression: a synthesis. *Journal of Happiness Studies*, 11 (1): 1–17.

Cummins, R.A. (2013). Limitations to positive psychology predicted by subjective well-being homeostasis. In M.L. Wehmeyer (ed.), *The Oxford Handbook of Positive Psychology and Disability* (Oxford Library of Psychology). Oxford: Oxford University Press. pp. 509–26

Cummins, R.A. (2016). The theory of subjective wellbeing homeostasis: a contribution to understanding life quality. In F. Maggino (ed.), *A Life Devoted to Quality of Life* (Social Indicators Research Series, 60). Switzerland: Springer International Publishing. pp. 61–79.

Curry, A. (2017). Our 9,000-year love affair with booze. *National Geographic Magazine*, February.

Curtis, J. and White, P. (1992). Toward a better understanding of the sport practices of Francophone and Anglophone Canadians. *Sociology of Sport Journal*, 9: 403–22.

Curtis, J.R., Nielsen, E.L., Treece, P.D., Downey, L., Dotolo, D., Shannon, S.E. et al. (2011). Effect of a quality-improvement intervention on end-of-life care in the intensive care unit: a randomized trial. *American Journal of Respiratory Critical Care Medicine*, 183: 348–55.

Curtis, J.R., Patrick, D.L., Engelberg, R.A., Norris, K., Asp, C. and Byock, I. (2002). A measure of the quality of dying and death: initial validation using after-death interviews with family members. *Journal of Pain Symptoms Management*, 24: 17–31.

Cusack, K., Jonas, D.E., Forneris, C.A., Wines, C., Sonis, J., Middleton, J.C. et al. (2016). Psychological treatments for adults with posttraumatic stress disorder: a systematic review and meta-analysis. *Clinical Psychology Review*, 43: 128–41.

Dahlgren, G. and Whitehead, M. (1991). *Policies and Strategies to Promote Equity and Health*. Stockholm: Institute for Future Studies.

Daley, A.J., Copeland, R.J., Wright, N.P. and Wales, J.K.H. (2008). 'I can actually exercise if I want to. It isn't as hard as I thought': a qualitative study of the experiences and views of obese adolescents participating in an exercise therapy intervention. *Journal of Health Psychology*, 13: 810–19.

Daley, E.M., Vamos, C.A., Buhi, E.R., Kolar, S.K., McDermott, R.J., Hernandez, N. and Fuhrmann, H.J. (2010). Influences on human papillomavirus vaccination status among female college students. *Journal of Women's Health*, 19: 1885–91.

Dalton, J.A., Feuerstein, M., Carlson, J. and Roghman, K. (1994). Biobehavioral pain profile: development and psychometric properties. *Pain*, 57 (1): 95–107.

Damman, O.C., Bogaerts, N.M.M., Dongen, D., Timmermans, D.R.M. and van Dongen, D. (2016). Barriers in using cardiometabolic risk information among consumers with low health literacy. *British Journal of Health Psychology*, 21 (1): 135–56.

Daniels, N., Kennedy, B. and Kawachi, I. (2000). Justice is good for our health: how greater economic equality would promote public health. *Boston Review*, February/March: 25.

Dannetun, E., Tegnell, A. and Giesecke, J. (2007). Parents' attitudes towards hepatitis B vaccination for their children. A survey comparing paper and web questionnaires, Sweden 2005. *BMC Public Health*, 7: 86. https://doi.org/10.1186/1471-2458-7-86

Dante, G., Pedrielli, G., Annessi, E. and Facchinetti, F. (2013). Herb remedies during pregnancy: a systematic review of controlled clinical trials. *Journal of Maternal-Fetal & Neonatal Medicine*, 26: 306–12.

Dar, R., Stronguin, F. and Etter, J.F. (2005). Assigned versus perceived placebo effects in nicotine replacement therapy for smoking reduction in Swiss smokers. *Journal of Consulting & Clinical Psychology*, 73: 350–3.

Darwin, C. (1888). *The Descent of Man, and Selection in Relation to Sex* (Vol. 1). London: John Murray.

Daskalopoulou, M., George, J., Walters, K., Osborn, D.P., Batty, G.D., Stogiannis, D. et al. (2016). Depression as a risk factor for the initial presentation of twelve cardiac, cerebrovascular, and peripheral arterial diseases: data linkage study of 1.9 million women and men. *PLoS One*, 11 (4): e0153838.

Datta, J. and Petticrew, M. (2013). Challenges to evaluating complex interventions: a content analysis of published papers. *BMC Public Health*, 13: 568–82.

Davidson, K.W., Goldstein, M., Kaplan, R.M., Kaufmann, P.G., Knatterund, G.L., Orleans, C.T. et al. (2003). Evidence-based behavioral medicine: What is it and how do we achieve it? *Annals of Behavioral Medicine*, 26: 161–71.

Davis, P., Chapman, S. and Leask, J. (2002).Antivaccination activists on the World Wide Web. *Archives of Disease in Childhood*, 87 (1): 22–5.

Davis, O.I. (2011). (Re)framing health literacy: transforming the culture of health in the black barbershop. *Western Journal of Black Studies*, 35: 176–86.

Davison, C., Macintyre, S. and Davey Smith, G. (1994). The potential social impact of predictive genetic testing for susceptibility to common chronic diseases: a review and proposed research agenda. *Sociology of Health & Illness*, 16: 340–71.

De Jong, K. and Kleber, R.J. (2007). Emergency conflict-related psychosocial interventions in Sierra Leone and Uganda: lessons from Médecins Sans Frontières. *Journal of Health Psychology*, 12: 485–97.

DeSteno, D., Gross, J.J., Kubzansky, L. (2013). Affective science and health: the importance of emotion and emotion regulation. *Health Psychology*, 32 (5): 474–86.

de la Vega, R., Roset, R., Galán, S. and Miró, J. (2016). Fibroline: a mobile app for improving the quality of life of young people with fibromyalgia. *Journal of Health Psychology*. doi:10.1177/1359105316650509.

De Molina, A.F. and Hunsperger, R.W. (1962). Organization of the subcortical system governing defence and flight reactions in the cat. *The Journal of Physiology*, 160 (2): 200–13.

De Ridder, D. and Schreurs, K. (1996). Coping, social support and chronic disease: a research agenda. *Psychology, Health and Medicine*, 1 (1): 71–82.

De Ridder, D., De Vet, E., Stok, M., Adriaanse, M. and De Wit, J. (2013). Obesity, overconsumption and self-regulation failure: the unsung role of eating appropriateness standards. *Health Psychology Review*, 7: 146–65.

De Vadder, F., Kovatcheva-Datchary, P., Goncalves, D., Vinera, J., Zitoun, C., Duchampt, A. et al. (2014). Microbiota-generated metabolites promote metabolic benefits via gut-brain neural circuits. *Cell*, 156: 84–96.

de Visser, R. and Smith, J.A. (2006). Mister in-between: a case study of masculine identity and health-related behaviour. *Journal of Health Psychology*, 11 (5): 685–95.

Dean, A.G., Sullivan, K.M. and Soe, M.M. (2014). *OpenEpi: Open Source Epidemiologic Statistics for Public Health, Version 2.3.1*. Available: www.scienceopen.com/document?vid=61cdd360-9883-4330-8c18-3f0341b0f715 [accessed 29 August 2017].

Debate of the Age Health and Care Study Group (1999). *The Future of Health and Care of Older People: The Best is Yet to Come*. London: Age Concern.

Deci, E.L. and Ryan, R.M. (1985). *Intrinsic Motivation and Self-determination in Human Behavior*. New York: Plenum Press.

Dedert, E.A., Calhoun, P.S., Watkins, L.L., Sherwood, A. and Beckham, J.C. (2010). Posttraumatic stress disorder, cardiovascular and metabolic disease: a review of the evidence. *Annals of Behavioural Medicine*, 39: 61–78.

Dela Llagas, L. and Portus, L.M. (2016). Promoting health communication and empowerment: intervention towards malaria mosquito control. *International Journal of Health, Wellness & Society*, 6 (3): 61–75.

Delamothe, T., Snow, R. and Godlee, F. (2014). Why the assisted dying bill should become law in England and Wales: it's the right thing to do, and most people want it. *British Medical Journal*, 348 (7965): g4349-2.

Delgado-Morales, R. and Esteller, M. (2017). Opening up the DNA methylome of dementia. *Molecular Psychiatry*, 22 (4): 485–96.

DeMarco, J.N., Cheevers, C., Davidson, J., Bogaerts, S., Pace, U., Aiken, M. et al. (2017). Digital dangers and cyber-victimisation: a study of European adolescent online risky behaviour for sexual exploitation. *Clinical Neuropsychiatry*, 14 (1): 104–12.

DeMatteo, D., Harrison, C., Arneson, C., Salter Goldie, R., Lefebvre, A., Read, S.E. and King, S.M. (2002). Disclosing HIV/AIDS to children: the paths families take to truthtelling. *Psychology, Health & Medicine*, 7: 339–56.

Dempsey, J.A., Veasey, S.C., Morgan, B.J. and O'Donnell, C.P. (2010). Pathophysiology of sleep apnea. *Physiological Review*, 90: 47–112.

Denison, J., Varcoe, C. and Browne, A.J. (2014). Aboriginal women's experiences of accessing health care when state apprehension of children is being threatened. *Journal of Advanced Nursing*, 70: 1105–16.

Denollet, J., Sys, S.U., Stroobant, N., Rombouts, H., Gillebert, T.C. and Brutsaert, D.L. (1996). Personality as independent predictor of long-term mortality in patients with coronary heart disease. *The Lancet*, 347: 417–21.

Department of Health. (2008). *Ambitions for Health: A Strategic Framework for Maximising the Potential of Social Marketing and Health-related Behaviour*. London: NHS. Available: www.dh.gov.uk/prod_consum_dh/groups/dh_digitalassets/documents/digitalasset/dh_086289.pdf. [accessed 16 January 2010].

Department of Health. (2011). *Start Active, Stay Active: A Report on Physical Activity from the Four Home Countries' Chief Medical Officers*. London: Department of Health.

Derogatis, L.R., Morrow, G.R., Fetting, J., Penman, D., Piasetsky, S., Schmale, A.M. et al. (1983). The prevalence of psychiatric disorders among cancer patients. *JAMA*, 249 (6): 751–7.

Des Jarlais, D.C., Lyles, C. and Crepaz, N. (2004). Improving the reporting quality of nonrandomized evaluations of behavioral and public health interventions: the TREND statement. *American Journal of Public Health*, 94: 361–6.

Devi, R., Powell, J. and Singh, S. (2014). A web-based program improves physical activity outcomes in a primary care angina population: randomized controlled trial. *Journal of Medical Internet Research*, 16 (9): e186.

de Visser, R. and Smith, J.A. (2006). Mister in-between: a case study of masculine identity and health-related behaviour. *Journal of Health Psychology*, 11 (5): 685–95.

Dew, K. (1999). Epidemics, panic and power: representations of measles and measles vaccine. *Health*, 3: 379–98.

Diabetes Prevention Program Research Group (2002). Reduction in the incidence of Type 2 diabetes with lifestyle intervention or metformin. *The New England Journal of Medicine*, 346: 393–403.

Diabetes UK (2017). *Life with Diabetes*. Available: www.diabetes.org.uk/Guide-to-diabetes/Life-with-diabetes/ [accessed 28 August 2017].

Dickens, C., Lambert, B.L., Cromwell, T. and Piano, M.R. (2013). Nurse overestimation of patients' health literacy. *Journal of Health Communication*, 18: 62–9.

DiClemente, C.C. (2005). A premature obituary for the transtheoretical model: a response to West (2005). *Addiction*, 100 (8): 1046–48.

DiClemente, R.J. (2016). Validity of self-reported sexual behavior among adolescents: Where do we go from here? *AIDS and Behavior*, 20 (1): 215–7.

Diener, E. (2006). Guidelines for national indicators of subjective well-being and ill-being. *Journal of Happiness Studies*, 7: 397–404.

Diener, E. and Chan, M.Y. (2011). Happy people live longer: subjective well-being contributes to health and longevity. *Applied Psychology: Health and Well-Being*, 3: 1–43.

Diener, E.D., Emmons, R.A., Larsen, R.J. and Griffin, S. (1985). The Satisfaction with Life Scale. *Journal of Personality Assessment*, 49: 71–5.

Dillard, A.J., Ferrer, R.A., Ubel, P.A. and Fagerlin, A. (2012). Risk perception measures' associations with behavior intentions, affect and cognition following colon cancer screening messages. *Health Psychology*, 31: 106–113.

Dillard, A.J., Scherer, L.D., Ubel, P.A., Alexander, S. and Fagerlin, A. (2017). Anxiety symptoms prior to a prostate cancer diagnosis: Associations with knowledge and openness to treatment. *British Journal of Health Psychology*, 22: 151–68.

DiMillo, J., Samson, A., Thériault, A., Lowry, S., Corsini, L., Verma, S. and Tomiak, E. (2015). Genetic testing: when prediction generates stigmatization. *Journal of Health Psychology*, 20 (4): 393–400.

Dinan, T.G. and Cryan, J.F. (2012). Regulation of the stress response by the gut microbiota: implications for psychoneuroendocrinology. *Psychoneuroendocrinology*, 37 (9): 1369–78.

Dishman, R.K. (1986). Exercise compliance: a new view for public health. *Physician & Sports Medicine*, 14: 127–45.

Dixon, J., King, D., Matosevic, T., Clark, M. and Knapp, M. (2015). *Equity in the provision of palliative care in the UK: review of evidence*. London: Personal Social Services Research Unit, London School of Economics and Political Science.

Dixon-Woods, M., Bonas, S., Booth, A., Jones, D.R., Miller, T., Sutton, A.J. et al. (2006). How can systematic reviews incorporate qualitative research? A critical perspective. *Qualitative Research*, 6: 27–44.

Dodge, K.A. and Pettit, G.S. (2003). A biopsychosocial model of the development of chronic conduct problems in adolescence. *Developmental Psychology*, 39 (2): 349.

Dolezal, C., Warne, P., Santamaria, E.K., Elkington, K.S., Benavides, J.M. and Mellins, C.A. (2014). Asking only 'Did you use a condom?' underestimates the prevalence of unprotected sex among perinatally HIV infected and perinatally exposed but uninfected youth. *The Journal of Sex Research*, 51 (5): 599–604.

Dong, M., Anda,R.F.,Felitti, V.J., Dube, S.R., Williamson, D.F., Thompson, T.J., Loo, C.M. and Giles, W.H (2004). The interrelatedness of multiple forms of childhood abuse, neglect, and household dysfunction. *Child Abuse and Neglect*, 28: 771–84. 10.1016/j.chiabu.2004.01.008.

Doran, C.M., Valenti, L., Robinson, M., Britt, H. and Mattick, R.P. (2006). Smoking status of Australian general practice patients and their attempts to quit. *Addictive Behavior*, 31: 758–66.

Dover, G.J. (2009). The Barker hypothesis: how pediatricans will diagnose and prevent common adult-onset diseases. *Transactions of the American Clinical and Climatological Association*, 120: 199–207.

Downs, J.S., Bruin de Bruine, W.D. and Fischhoff, B. (2008). Parents' vaccine comprehension and decisions. *Vaccine*, 26: 1595–607.

Downward, P., Hallmans, K. and Pawlowski, T. (2014). Assessing parental impact on the sports participation of children: a socio-economic analysis of the UK. *European Journal of Sport Science*, 14: 84–90.

Drake, E.B., Henderson, V.W., Stanczyk, F.Z., McCleary, C.A., Brown, W.S., Smith, C.A. et al. (2000). Associations between circulating sex steroid hormones and cognition in normal elderly women. *Neurology*, 54 (3): 599–603.

Druet, C., Stettler, N., Sharp, S., Simmons, R.K., Cooper, C., Davey Smith, G. et al. (2012). Prediction of childhood obesity by infancy weight gain: an individual-level meta-analysis. *Paediatric & Perinatal Epidemiology*, 26: 19–26.

Drummond, D.C., Tiffany, S.T., Glautier, S. and Remington, B. (eds.) (1995). *Addictive Behaviour: Cue Exposure Theory and Practice*. London: Wiley.

DuCharme, K.A. and Brawley, L.R. (1995). Predicting the intentions and behavior of exercise initiates using two forms of self-efficacy. *Journal of Behavioral Medicine*, 18: 479–97.

Duijts, S.F., Zeegers, M.P. and Borne, B.V. (2003). The association between stressful life events and breast cancer risk: a meta-analysis. *International Journal of Cancer*, 107: 1023–9.

Duncan, N., Bowman, B., Naidoo, A., Pillay, J. and Roos, V. (2007). *Community Psychology: Analysis, Context and Action*. Cape Town: UCT Press.

Dunton, G.F. and Vaughan, E. (2008). Anticipated affective consequences of physical activity adoption and maintenance. *Health Psychology*, 27 (6): 703–710.

Dunkel-Schetter, C., Feinstein, L., Taylor, S. and Falke, R. (1992). Patterns of coping with cancer. *Health Psychology*, 11 (2): 79–87.

Dwan, K., Gamble, C., Williamson, P.R., Kirkham, J.J. and The Reporting Bias Group (2013). Systematic review of the empirical evidence of study publication bias and outcome reporting bias – an updated review. *PLoS One*, 8 (7): e66844. doi:10.1371/journal.pone.0066844.

Dwyer, J.J.M., Allison, K.R., Goldberg, E.R., Fein, A.J., Yoshida, K.K. and Boutilier, M.A. (2006). Adolescent girls' perceived barriers to participation in physical activity. *Adolescence*, 41: 75–89.

Eaker, E.D., Sullivan, L.M., Kelly-Hayes, M., D'Agostino, R.B., Sr. and Benjamin, E.J. (2004). Does job strain increase the risk for coronary heart disease or death in men and women? *American Journal of Epidemiology*, 159: 950–8.

Earnshaw, V.A., Bogart, L.M., Poteat, V.P., Reisner, S.L. and Schuster, M.A. (2016a). Bullying among lesbian, gay, bisexual, and transgender youth. *Pediatric Clinics of North America*, 63 (6): 999–1010.

Earnshaw, V.A., Rosenthal, L., Carroll-Scott, A., Santilli, A., Gilstad-Hayden, K. and Ickovics, J.R. (2016b). Everyday discrimination and physical health: exploring mental health processes. *Journal of Health Psychology*, 21 (10): 2218–28. doi:10.1177/1359105315572456.

Earnshaw, V.A., Smith, L.R., Chaudoir, S.R., Amico, K.R. and Copenhaver, M.M. (2013). HIV stigma mechanisms and well-being among PLWH: a test of the HIV stigma framework. *AIDS and Behavior*, 17 (5): 1785–95.

Easton, P., Entwistle, V.A. and Williams, B. (2013). How the stigma of low literacy can impair patient–professional spoken interactions and affect health: insights from a qualitative investigation. *BMC Health Services Research*, 13: 1–12.

Eaton, S.B. and Eaton, S.B. (2003). An evolutionary perspective on human physical activity: implications for health. *Comparative Biochemistry and Physiology – Part A: Molecular and Integrative Physiology*, 136: 153–9.

Ebbeling, C.B., Pawlak, D.B. and Ludwig, D.S. (2002). Childhood obesity: public-health crisis, common sense cure. *The Lancet*, 360: 473–82.

Eccleston, C. (2001). Role of psychology in pain management. *British Journal of Anaesthesia*, 87: 144–52.

Eccleston, C., Morley, S., Williams, A., Yorke, L. and Mastroyannopoulou, K. (2002). Systematic review of randomised controlled trials of psychological therapy for chronic pain in children and adolescents, with a subset meta-analysis of pain relief. *Pain*, 99: 157–65.

Eccleston, Z. and Eccleston, C. (2004). Interdisciplinary management of adolescent chronic pain: developing the role of physiotherapy. *Physiotherapy*, 90: 77–81.

Edgar, L. (2010). *Mastering the Art of Coping in Good Times and Bad*. Oxford: Oxford University Press.

Edgar, L., Rosberger, Z. and Collet, J.-P. (2001). Lessons learned: outcomes and methodology of a coping skills intervention trial comparing individual and group formats for patients with cancer. *The International Journal of Psychiatry in Medicine*, 31: 289–304. doi:10.2190/U0P3-5VPV-YXKF-GRG1.

Edgar, L., Rosberger, Z. and Nowlis, D. (1992). Coping with cancer during the first year after diagnosis: assessment and intervention. *Cancer*, 69: 817–28.

Edwards, A.G., Hailey, S. and Maxwell, M. (2004). Psychological interventions for women with metastatic breast cancer. *Cochrane Database of Systematic Reviews*, 2 (CD004253).

Eggers, S. M., Aarø, L. E., Bos, A. E., Mathews, C., Kaaya, S. F., Onya, H. and de Vries, H. (2016). Sociocognitive predictors of condom use and intentions among adolescents in three sub-Saharan sites. *Archives of Sexual Behavior*, 45: 353–3.

Eisenberg, E., Ognitz, M. and Almog, S. (2014). The pharmacokinetics, efficiency, safety, and ease of use of a novel portable metered-dose cannabis inhaler in patients with chronic neuropathic pain: a phase Ia study. *Journal of Pain and Palliative Care Pharmacotherapy*, 28: 216–25.

Eissa, M.A., Poffenbarger, T. and Portman, R.J. (2001). Comparison of the actigraph versus patients' diary information in defining circadian time periods for analysing ambulatory blood pressure monitoring data. *Blood Pressure Monitoring*, 6: 21–5.

El-Gayar, O., Timsina, P., Nawar, N. and Eid, W. (2013). Mobile applications for diabetes self-management: status and potential. *Journal of Diabetes Science and Technology*, 7 (1): 247–62.

Elmore, J.G., Barton, M.B., Moceri, V.M., Polk, S., Arena, P.J. and Fletcher, S.W. (1998). Ten-year risk of false positive screening mammograms and clinical breast examination. *The New England Journal of Medicine*, 338: 1089–96.

Emanuel, E.J., Onwuteaka-Philipsen, B.D., Urwin, J.W. and Cohen, J. (2016). Attitudes and practices of euthanasia and physician-assisted suicide in the United States, Canada, and Europe. *JAMA*, 316 (1): 79–90.

Engel, G.L. (1977). The need for a new medical model: a challenge for biomedicine, *Science*, 196: 129–36.

Engel, G.L. (1980). The clinical application of the biopsychosocial model. *The American Journal of Psychiatry*, 137: 535–44.

Engels, F. (1845/1958). *The Condition of the Working Class in England in 1844*. London: Lawrence & Wishart.

Epton, T., Harris, P. R., Kane, R., van Koningsbruggen, G. M. and Sheeran, P. (2015). The impact of self-affirmation on health-behavior change: a meta-analysis. *Health Psychology*, 34: 187–96.

Eriksson, M. and Lindström, B. (2006). Antonovsky's Sense of Coherence Scale and the relation with health: a systematic review. *Journal of Epidemiology and Community Health*, 60: 376–81.

Ernst, E. (2012). Homeopathy for eczema: a systematic review of controlled clinical trials. *British Journal of Dermatology*, 166: 1170–2.

Ernst, E. and Pittler, M.H. (2000). Efficacy of ginger for nausea and vomiting: a systematic review of randomized clinical trials. *British Journal of Anaesthesia*, 84: 367–71.

Erwin, H., Fedewa, A., Beighle, A. and Ahn, S. (2012). A quantitative review of physical activity, health, and learning outcomes associated with classroom-based physical activity interventions. *Journal of Applied School Psychology*, 28: 14–36.

Escalante, Y., Backx, K., Saavedra, J.M., García-Hermoso, A. and Domínguez, A.M. (2012). Play area and physical activity in recess in primary schools. *Kinesiology*, 44: 123–9.

Estacio, E.V. and Marks, D.F. (2010). Critical reflections on social injustice and participatory action research: the case of the indigenous Ayta community in the Philippines. *Procedia – Social and Behavioral Sciences*, 5: 548–52.

Estacio, E.V., Whittle, R. and Protheroe, J. (2017). The digital divide: examining socio-demographic factors associated with health literacy, access and use of internet to seek health information. *Journal of Health Psychology*. doi:10.1177/1359105317695429.

European Commission (2014). *Eurobarometer on Sport and Physical Activity*. MEMO/14/207. Available: http://europa.eu/rapid/press-release_MEMO-14-207_en.htm. [accessed 28 August 2017].

Evangeli, M., Pady, K. and Wroe, A.L. (2016). Which psychological factors are related to HIV testing? A quantitative systematic review of global studies. *AIDS and Behavior*, 20 (4): 880–918.

Evans, R.I. (1988). Health promotion – science or ideology? *Health Psychology*, 7: 203–19.

Eysenbach, G. (2003). The impact of the Internet on cancer outcomes. *CA: A Cancer Journal for Clinicians*, 53: 356–71.

Eysenck, H.J., Tarrant, M. and Woolf, M. (1960). Smoking and personality. *British Medical Journal*, 280: 1456–60.

Faber, A. and Dubé, L. (2015). Parental attachment insecurity predicts child and adult high caloric food consumption. *Journal of Health Psychology*, 20 (5): 511–24.

Fadeel, B. and Orrenius, S. (2005). Apoptosis: a basic biological phenomenon with wide-ranging implications in human disease. *Journal of Internal Medicine*, 258: 479–517.

Fallah, R., Akbari, M.E., Azargashb, E. and Khayamzadeh, E. (2016). Incidence and survival in breast cancer patients and stressful life events. *Asian Pacific Journal of Cancer Prevention*, 17 (S3): 245–52.

Fanon, F. (2008) *Concerning Violence*. London: Penguin.

Fashler, S.R., Cooper, L.K., Oosenbrug, E.D., Burns, L.C., Razavi, S., Goldberg, L. and Katz, J. (2016). Systematic review of multidisciplinary chronic pain treatment facilities. *Pain Research and Management*. doi:10.1155/2016/5960987.

Faul, F., Erdfelder, E., Lang, A.G. and Buchner, A. (2007). G*Power 3: a flexible statistical power analysis program for the social, behavioral, and biomedical sciences. *Behavior Research Methods*, 39 (2): 175–91.

Feinman, R.J. and Fine, E.J. (2004). 'A calorie is a calorie' violates the second law of thermodynamics. *Nutrition Journal*, 3: 9.

Fekjær, H.O. (2013). Alcohol – a universal preventive agent? A critical analysis. *Addiction*, 108: 2051–7.

Fennell, P.A. (1995). The four progressive stages of the CFS experience: a coping tool for patients. *Journal of Chronic Fatigue Syndrome*, 1: 69–79.

Ferguson, E. and Chandler, S. (2005). A stage model of blood donor behaviour: Assessing volunteer behaviour. *Journal of Health Psychology*, 10 (3): 359–72.

Ferguson, J., Bauld, L., Chesterman, J. and Judge, K. (2005). The English smoking treatment services: one-year outcomes. *Addiction* (suppl. 2): 59–69.

Ferreira-Neto, J.L. and Henriques, M.A. (2016). Psychologists in public health: historical aspects and current challenges. *Journal of Health Psychology*, 21 (3): 281–90. doi:10.1177/1359105316628760.

Ferrie, J.E. (2004). *Work, Stress and Health: The Whitehall II Study*. London: Cabinet Office. Available: www.ucl.ac.uk/whitehallII/pdf/Whitehallbooklet_1_.pdf [accessed 2 December 2014].

Ferrie, J.E., Shipley, M.J., Stansfeld, S.A. and Marmot, M.G. (2002). Effects of chronic job insecurity and change in job security on self reported health, minor psychiatric morbidity, physiological measures, and health related behaviours in British civil servants: the Whitehall II study. *Journal of Epidemiology & Community Health*, 56 (6): 450–54.

Ferriman, A. (2007). *BMJ* readers choose the 'sanitary revolution' as greatest medical advance since 1840. *British Medical Journal*, 334: 111.

Fillmore, K.M., Stockwell, T., Chikritzhs, T., Bostrom, A. and Kerr, W. (2007). Moderate alcohol use and reduced mortality risk: systematic error in prospective studies and new hypotheses. *Annals of Epidemiology*, 17 (suppl. 5): S16–23.

Fine, E.J. and Feinman, R.D. (2004). Thermodynamics of weight loss diets. *Nutrition & Metabolism*, 1: 15.

Fine, M. and Asch, A. (1982). The question of disability: no easy answers for the women's movement. *Reproductive Rights National Network Newsletter*, 4: 19–20.

Finkelhor, D. (1994). The international epidemiology of child sexual abuse. *Child Abuse & Neglect*, 18 (5): 409–17.

Finkelhor, D. (2008). *Childhood Victimization: Violence, Crime, and Abuse in the Lives of Young People*. Oxford: Oxford University Press.

Finkelhor, D., Shattuck, A., Turner, H.A. and Hamby, S.L. (2014). The lifetime prevalence of child sexual abuse and sexual assault assessed in late adolescence. *Journal of Adolescent Health*, 55 (3): 329–33.

Fiore, M. (2008). *Treating Tobacco Use and Dependence: 2008 Update: Clinical Practice Guideline*. Darby, PA: DIANE Publishing.

Fishbein, M. and Ajzen, I. (1975). *Belief, Attitude, Intention and Behavior: An Introduction to Theory and Research*. Reading, MA: Addison-Wesley.

Fisher, J.D. and Fisher, W.A. (1992). Changing AIDS risk behavior. *Psychological Bulletin*, 111: 455–74.

Fisher, J.D. and Fisher, W.A. (2000). Individual level theories of HIV risk behavior change. In J. Peterson and R. DiClemente (eds.), *Handbook of HIV Prevention*. New York: Plenum. pp. 3–56.

Fisher, J.D., Fisher, W.A., Amico, K.R. and Harman, J.J. (2006). An information-motivation-behavioral skills model of adherence to antiretroviral therapy. *Health Psychology*, 25 (4): 462–73.

Flanagan, J.C. (1978). A research approach to improving our quality of life. *American Psychologist*, 33: 138–47.

Flick, U. (1998). The social construction of individual and public health: contributions of social representations theory to a social science of health. *Social Science Information*, 37: 639–62.

Flowers, P., Davis, M., Lohm, D., Waller, E. and Stephenson, N. (2016). Understanding pandemic influenza behaviour: an exploratory biopsychosocial study. *Journal of Health Psychology*, 21 (5): 759–69.

Flynn, J.R. (2007). *What is Intelligence? Beyond the Flynn Effect*. Cambridge: Cambridge University Press.

Fogarty, L., Roter, D., Larson, S., Burke, J.G., Gillespie, J. and Levy, B. (2002). Patient adherence to HIV medication regimens: a review of published and abstract reports. *Patient Education & Counseling*, 46: 93–108.

Fogel, R. (2004). *The Escape from Premature Hunger and Death, 1700–2100: Europe, America and the Third World*. Cambridge: Cambridge University Press.

Fogelholm, M., Anderssen, S., Gunnarsdottir, I. and Lahti-Koski, M. (2012). Dietary macronutrients and food consumption as determinants of long-term weight change in adult populations: a systematic literature review. *Food & Nutrition Research*, 56. doi:10.3402/fnr.v56i0.19103.

Folkman, S. and Lazarus, R.S. (1988). *Ways of Coping Questionnaire*. Palo Alto, CA: Consulting Psychologists Press.

Folkman, S. and Moskowitz, J.T. (2004). Coping: pitfalls and promise. *Annual Review of Psychology*, 55: 745–74.

Follick, M.J., Smith, T.W. and Ahern, D.K. (1985). The Sickness Impact Profile: a global measure of disability in chronic low back pain. *Pain*, 21: 67–76.

Food and Agriculture Organization (2012, updated 2015). The State of Food Insecurity in the World 2015. Available at: http://www.fao.org/hunger/en/ [accessed 28 August 2017].

Ford, S., Scholz, B. and Lu, V.N. (2015). Social shedding: identification and health of men's sheds users. *Health Psychology*, 34 (7): 775–78. doi:10.1037/hea0000171.

Foresight Report (2007). *Tackling Obesities: Future Choices*. London: Government Office for Science and Department of Health. Available: www.gov.uk/government/collections/tackling-obesities-future-choices [accessed 28 August 2017].

Foucault, M. (1976). *The Birth of the Clinic*. London: Routledge.

Foucault, M. (1980). *Power/Knowledge: Selected Interviews and Other Writings*. New York: Parthenon.

Fox, B.H. (1988). Psychogenic factors in cancer, especially its incidence. In S. Maes, D. Spielberger, P.B. Defares and I.G. Sarason (eds.), *Topics in Health Psychology*. New York: Wiley. pp. 37–55.

Fraser-Thomas, J., Côté, J. and Deakin, J. (2008). Examining adolescent sport dropout and prolonged engagement from a developmental perspective. *Journal of Applied Sport Psychology*, 20: 318–33.

Frazier, P., Tennen, H., Gavian, M., Park, C., Tomich, P. and Tashiro, T. (2009). Does self-reported post-traumatic growth reflect genuine positive change? *Psychological Science*, 20: 912–19.

Fredericks, B., Maynor, P., White, N., English, F.W. and Ehrich, L.C. (2014). Living with the legacy of conquest and culture: social justice leadership in education and the Indigenous peoples of Australia and America. In I. Bogotch and C.M. Shields (eds.), *International Handbook of Educational Leadership and Social (In)Justice*. Amsterdam: Springer. pp. 751–80.

Fredrickson, J., Kremer, P., Swinburn, B., de Silva, A. and McCabe, M. (2015). Weight perception in overweight adolescents. *Journal of Health Psychology*, 20 (6): 774–84.

Freedy, J.R. and Hobfoll, S.E. (1994). Stress inoculation for reduction of burnout: a conservation of resources approach. *Anxiety, Stress and Coping*, 6 (4): 311–25.

Freeman, M. (2000). Narrative foreclosure in later life. In G. Kenyon, E.T. Bohlmeijer, and W.R. Randall (eds.), *Storying Later Life: Issues, Investigations and Interventions in Narrative Gerontology* (pp. 3–19). New York: Oxford University Press.

Freire, P. (1970). *Pedagogy of the Oppressed*. New York: Continuum.

French, D.P. (2013). The role of self-efficacy in changing health-related behavior: cause, effect or spurious association? *British Journal of Health Psychology*, 18: 237–43.

French, D.P., Cooke, R., Mclean, N., Williams, M. and Sutton, S. (2007). What do people think about when they answer Theory of Planned Behaviour questionnaires? *Journal of Health Psychology*, 12: 672–87.

Frew, P.M., Saint-Victor, D., Owens, L.E. and Omer, S.B. (2014). Socioecological and message framing factors influencing maternal influenza immunization among minority women. *Vaccine*, 32: 1736–44.

Friedman, H.S. and Kern, M.L. (2014). Personality, well-being and health. *Annual Review of Psychology*, 65: 719–42.

Friedman, H.S., Martin, L.R., Tucker, J.S., Criqui, M., Kern, M.L. and Reynolds, C. (2008). Stability of physical activity across the life-span. *Journal of Health Psychology*, 13: 966–78.

Friedman, M. and Rosenman, R.H. (1959). Association of specific overt behavior pattern with blood and cardiovascular findings: blood cholesterol level, blood clotting time, incidence of arcus senilis, and clinical coronary artery disease. *JAMA*, 169: 1286–96.

Frye, J. and Youngner, S.J. (2016). A call for a patient-centered response to legalized assisted dying. *Annals of Internal Medicine*, 165 (10): 733–4.

Fugh-Berman, A. (2003). *The 5-minute Herb & Dietary Supplement Consult*. Philadelphia, PA: Lippincott Williams & Wilkins.

Fukuda, K., Straus, S.E., Hickie, I., Sharpe, M.C., Dobbins, J.G., Komaroff, A.L. and The International Chronic Fatigue Syndrome Study Group (1994). The chronic fatigue syndrome: a comprehensive approach to its definition and study. *Annals of Internal Medicine*, 121: 953–9.

Gabarron, E. and Wynn, R. (2016). Use of social media for sexual health promotion: a scoping review. *Global Health Action*, 9. doi:10.3402/gha.v9.32193.

Galindo, R.W. (2004). Fighting hunger in Brazil. [La lucha contra el hambre en Brasil]. *Perspectives in Health*, 9: 26–9.

Gallagher, K. and Updegraff, J. (2012). Health message framing effects on attitudes, intentions, and behavior: a meta-analytic review. *Annals of Behavioral Medicine*, 43: 101–16.

Gallant, S.J., Keita, G.P. and Royak-Schaler, R. (eds.) (1997). *Health Care for Women: Psychological, Social and Behavioral Influences*. Washington, DC: American Psychological Association.

Galvin, R. (2002). Disturbing notions of chronic illness and individual responsibility: towards a geneaology of morals. *Health (London)*, 6: 107–37.

Gamble, K.L., Berry, R., Frank, S.J. and Young, M.E. (2014). Circadian clock control of endocrine factors. *Nature Reviews Endocrinology*, 10 (8): 466–75.

Gamble, T. and Walker, I. (2016). Wearing a bicycle helmet can increase risk taking and sensation seeking in adults. *Psychological Science*, 27 (2): 289–94. doi:10.1177/0956797615620784.

Garbett, K., Harcourt, D. and Buchanan, H. (2016). Using online blogs to explore positive outcomes after burn injuries. *Journal of Health Psychology*. doi:10.1177/1359105316638549.

Garcia-Retamero, R. and Cokely, E.T. (2011). Effective communication of risks to young adults: using message framing and visual aids to increase condom use and STD screening. *Journal of Experimental Psychology – Applied*, 17: 270–87.

Garland, S.M., Kjaer, S.K., Munoz, N., Block, S.L., Brown, D.R., DiNubile, M.J. et al. (2016). Impact and effectiveness of the quadrivalent human papillomavirus vaccine: a systematic review of 10 years of real-world experience. *Clinical Infectious Diseases*, 63: 519–27.

Geertz, C. (1973). *The Interpretation of Culture*. New York: Basic Books.

Geraghty, K.J. (2016). 'PACE-gate': when clinical trial evidence meets open data access. *Journal of Health Psychology*. doi:10.1177/1359105316675213.

Gerend, M.A., Shepherd, M.A. and Shepherd, J.E. (2013). The multidimensional nature of perceived barriers: global versus practical barriers to HPV vaccination. *Health Psychology*, 32: 361–9.

Getrich, C.M., Sussman, A.L., Helitzer, D., Hoffman, R.M., Warner, T.D., Sánchez, V. et al. (2012). Expressions of machismo in colorectal cancer screening among New Mexico Hispanic subpopulations. *Qualitative Health Research*, 22: 546–59.

Ghaemi, S.N. (2009). The rise and fall of the biopsychosocial model. *The British Journal of Psychiatry*, 195: 3–4. doi:10.1192/bjp.bp.109.063859.

Gibson, A.A., Seimon, R.V., Lee, C.M.Y., Ayre, J., Franklin, J., Markovic, T.P. et al. (2015). Do ketogenic diets really suppress appetite? A systematic review and meta-analysis. *Obesity Reviews*, 16 (1): 64–76.

Gifford, S. (1986). The meaning of lumps: a case study of the ambiguities of risk. In C.R. Janes, R. Stall and S.M. Gifford (eds.), *Anthropology and Epidemiology: Interdisciplinary Approaches to the Study of Health and Disease*. Dordrecht: Reidel. pp. 213–46.

Gilbert, K.L., Quinn, S.C., Goodman, R.M., Butler, J. and Wallace, J. (2013). A meta-analysis of social capital and health: a case for needed research. *Journal of Health Psychology*, 18 (11): 1385–99.

Gilbert, W. (1986). Origin of life: The RNA world. *Nature*, 319 (6055).

Giles, M., McClenahan, C., Armour, C., Millar, S., Rae, G., Mallett, J. and Stewart-Knox, B. (2014). Evaluation of a theory of planned behaviour-based breastfeeding intervention in Northern Irish schools using a randomized cluster design. *British Journal of Health Psychology*, 19: 16–35.

Giles-Corti, B. and Donovan, R.J. (2002). The relative influence of individual, social and physical environmental determinants of physical activity. *Social Science & Medicine*, 54: 1793–812.

Gillies, V. and Willig, C. (1997). 'You get the nicotine and that in your blood': constructions of addiction and control in women's accounts of cigarette smoking. *Journal of Community & Applied Social Psychology*, 7: 285–301.

Ginzel, K.H., Maritz, G.S., Marks, D.F., Neuberger, M., Pauly, J.R., Polito, J.R. et al. (2007). Critical review: nicotine for the fetus, the infant and the adolescent? *Journal of Health Psychology*, 12: 215–24.

Girginov, V. and Hills, L. (2008). A sustainable sports legacy: creating a link between the London Olympics and sports participation. *International Journal of Sports History*, 25: 2091–116.

Glanz, K. and Lerman, C. (1992). Psychosocial impact of breast cancer: a critical review. *Annals of Behavioral Medicine*, 14: 204–12.

Glaser, B.G. (1992). *Basics of Grounded Theory Analysis: Emergence Versus Forcing*. Mill Valley, CA: Sociology Press.

Glaser, B.G. and Strauss, A. (1967). *The Discovery of Grounded Theory: Strategies for Qualitative Research*. Chicago, IL: Aldine.

Glasgow, R.E. and Rosen, G.M. (1978). Behavioral bibliotherapy: a review of self-help behavior therapy manuals. *Psychological Bulletin*, 85 (1): 1–23.

Glasgow, R.E., Vogt, T.M. and Boles, S.M. (1999). Evaluating the public health impact of health promotion interventions: the RE-AIM framework. *American Journal of Public Health*, 89 (9): 1322–7.

Gleeson, K. and Frith, H. (2006). (De)constructing body image. *Journal of Health Psychology*, 11: 79–90.

Glynn, T.J. (2014). E-cigarettes and the future of tobacco control. *CA: A Cancer Journal for Clinicians*, 64: 164–8.

Godin, G., Conner, M. and Sheeran, P. (2005). Bridging the intention–behaviour gap: the role of moral norm. *British Journal of Social Psychology*, 44 (4): 497–512.

Goffman, E. (1963). *Stigma: Notes on the Management of Spoiled Identity*. London: Penguin.

Goldacre, M.J. and Roberts, S.E. (2004). Hospital admission for acute pancreatitis in an English population, 1963–98: database study of incidence and mortality. *British Medical Journal*, 328: 1466–9.

Goldberg, A.D., Allis, C.D. and Bernstein, E. (2007). Epigenetics: a landscape takes shape. *Cell*, 128 (4): 635–8.

Goldfield, G.S., Moore, C., Henderson, K., Buchholz, A., Obeid, N. and Flament, M.F. (2010). Body dissatisfaction, dietary restraint, depression, and weight status in adolescents. *Journal of School Health*, 80: 186–92.

Gollwitzer, P.M. (1993). Goal achievement: the role of intentions. *European Review of Social Psychology*, 4 (1): 141–85.

Gollwitzer, P.M. (1999). Implementation intentions: strong effects of simple plans. *American Psychologist*, 54 (7): 493–503.

Gollwitzer, P.M. and Brandstätter, V. (1997). Implementation intentions and effective goal pursuit. *Journal of Personality and Social Psychology*, 73 (1): 186–99.

Gollwitzer, P.M. and Sheeran, P. (2006). Implementation intentions and goal achievement: A meta-analysis of effects and processes. *Advances in Experimental Social Psychology*, 38: 69–119.

Golub, S.A., Kowalczyk, W., Weinberger, C.L. and Parsons, J.T. (2010). Preexposure prophy-laxis and predicted condom use among high-risk men who have sex with men. *JAIDS: Journal of Acquired Immune Deficiency Syndromes*, 54 (5): 548–55.

Gone, J.P. (2013). Redressing First Nations' historical trauma: theorizing mechanisms for indigenous culture as mental health treatment. *Transcultural Psychiatry*, 50 (5): 683–706.

Gooch, C.L., Pracht, E. and Borenstein, A.R. (2017). The burden of neurological disease in the United States: a summary report and call to action. *Annals of Neurology*, 81 (4): 479–84.

Goodman, M.J., Ogdie, A., Kanamori, M.J., Cañar, J. and O'Malley, A.S. (2006). Barriers and facilitators of colorectal cancer screening among mid-Atlantic Latinos: focus group findings. *Ethnicity and Disease*, 16: 255–61.

Goossens, L., Braet, C., Van Durme, K., Decaluwé, V. and Bosmans, G. (2012). The parent–child relationship as predictor of eating pathology and weight gain in preadolescents. *Journal of Clinical Child & Adolescent Psychology*, 41: 445–57.

Gostin, L.O. and Friedman, E.A. (2013). Towards a framework convention on global health: a transformative agenda for global health justice. *Yale Journal of Health Policy, Law, and Ethics*, 13 (1): 1–75.

Gottlieb, S.L., Low, N., Newman, L.M., Bolan, G., Kamb, M. and Broutet, N. (2014). Toward global prevention of sexually transmitted infections (STIs): the need for STI vaccines. *Vaccine*, 32 (14): 1527–35.

Gøtzsche, P.C. (2013). Regular self-examination or clinical examination for early detection of breast cancer. *Cochrane Database of Systematic Reviews*, 2: 1–14.

Gøtzsche P.C. and Jørgensen KJ. (2013). Screening for breast cancer with mammography. *Cochrane Database of Systematic Reviews*, Issue 6. Art. No.: CD001877.

Goyal, M., Singh, S., Sibinga, E.M.S., Gould, N.F., Rowland-Seymour, A., Sharma, R. et al. (2014). Meditation programs for psychological stress and well-being: a systematic review and meta-analysis. *JAMA Internal Medicine*, 174: 357–68.

Graham, H. (1976). Smoking in pregnancy: the attitudes of expectant mothers. *Social Science & Medicine*, 10: 399–405.

Graham, H. (1987). Women's smoking and family health. *Social Science & Medicine*, 25: 47–56.

Graham, K., Treharne, G.J., Ruzibiza, C. and Nicolson, M. (2015). The importance of health(ism): a focus group study of lesbian, gay, bisexual, pansexual, queer and transgender individuals' understandings of health. *Journal of Health Psychology*, 22: 237–47. doi:10.1177/1359105315600236.

Graham, R., Kremer, J. and Wheeler, G. (2008). Physical activity and psychological well-being among people with chronic illness and disability. *Journal of Health Psychology*, 13: 447–58.

Graham, T.M. (2017). Who's left out and who's still on the margins? Social exclusion in community psychology journals. *Journal of Community Psychology*, 45 (2): 193–209. doi:10.1002/jcop.21842.

Grande, G., Romppel, M. and Barth, J. (2012). Association between Type D personality and prognosis in patients with cardiovascular diseases: a systematic review and meta-analysis. *Annals of Behavioral Medicine*, 43: 299–310.

Granek, L., Ariad, S., Shapira, S., Bar-Sela, G. and Ben-David, M. (2016). Barriers and facilitators in coping with patient death in clinical oncology. *Supportive Care in Cancer*, 24 (10): 4219–27.

Granek, L., Ben-David, M., Nakash, O., Cohen, M., Barbera, L., Ariad, S. and Krzyzanowska, M.K. (2017). Oncologists' negative attitudes towards expressing emotion over patient death and burnout. *Supportive Care in Cancer*, 25 (5): 1607–14.

Grant, B.C. (2001). 'You're never too old': beliefs about physical activity and playing sport in later life. *Ageing & Society*, 21: 777–98.

Grant, B.F. and Dawson, D.A. (1997). Age at onset of alcohol use and its association with DSM-IV alcohol abuse and dependence: results from the National Longitudinal Alcohol Epidemiologic Survey. *Journal of Substance Abuse*, 9: 103–10.

Gray, R. and Sinding, C. (2002). *Standing Ovation: Performing Social Science Research about Cancer*. Walnut Creek, CA: Altamira Press.

Gray, R.E., Ivonoffski, V. and Sinding, C. (2001). Making a mess and spreading it around: articulation of an approach to research-based theatre. In A. Bochner and C. Ellis (eds.), *Ethnographically Speaking*. Walnut Creek, CA: Altamira Press. pp. 57–75.

Green, J.G., McLaughlin, K.A., Berglund, P.A., Gruber, M.J., Sampson, N.A., Zaslavsky, A.M. and Kessler, R.C. (2010). Childhood adversities and adult psychiatric disorders in the national comorbidity survey replication I: associations with first onset of DSM-IV disorders. *Archives of General Psychiatry*, 67 (2): 113–23.

Green, L.W. (2014). Closing the chasm between research and practice: evidence of and for change. *Health Promotion Journal of Australia*, 25: 25–9.

Greenwald, B.D., Narcessian, E.J. and Pomeranz, B.A. (1999). Assessment of psychiatrists' knowledge and perspectives on the use of opioids: review of basic concepts for managing chronic pain. *American Journal of Physical Medicine & Rehabilitation*, 78: 408–15.

Greenwood, M.L. and de Leeuw, S.N. (2012). Social determinants of health and the future well-being of Aboriginal children in Canada. *Paediatrics & Child Health*, 17 (7): 381.

Greer, S., Moorey, S., Baruch, J.D.R., Watson, M., Robertson, B.M., Mason, A. et al. (1992). Adjuvant psychological therapy for patients with cancer: a prospective randomised trial. *British Medical Journal*, 304: 675–80.

Gregg, J. and Curry, R.H. (1994). Explanatory models for cancer among African-American women at two Atlanta neighborhood health centers: the implications for a cancer screening program. *Social Science & Medicine*, 39: 519–26.

Griffiths, C., Panteli, N., Brunton, D., Marder, B., & Williamson, H. (2015). Designing and evaluating the acceptability of Realshare: an online support community for teenagers and young adults with cancer. *Journal of Health Psychology*, 20 (12): 1589–601.

Grimshaw, J.M., Eccles, M.P., Lavis, J.N., Hill, S.J. and Squires, J.E. (2012). Knowledge translation of research findings. *Implementation Science*, 7: 50–66.

Gritz, E.R., Carr, C.R. and Marcus, A.C. (1989). Unaided smoking cessation: great American smokeout and New Year's Day quitters. *Journal of Psychosocial Oncology*, 6 (3–4): 217–34.

Grogan, S. (2006). Body image and health: contemporary perspectives. *Journal of Health Psychology*, 11: 523–30.

Grogan, S. and Richards, H. (2002). Body image: focus groups with boys and men. *Men & Masculinities*, 4: 219–32.

Grogan, S., Parlane, V.L. and Buckley, E. (2017). Younger British men's understandings of prostate cancer: a qualitative study. *Journal of Health Psychology*, 22: 743–53.

Grollman, E.A. (2012). Multiple forms of perceived discrimination and health among adolescents and young adults. *Journal of Health and Social Behavior*, 53: 199–214.

Grossardt, B.R., Bower, J.H., Geda, Y.E., Colligan, R.C. and Rocca, W.A. (2009). Pessimistic, anxious, and depressive personality traits predict all-cause mortality: the Mayo Clinic cohort study of personality and aging. *Psychosomatic Medicine*, 71: 491–500.

Grubbs, J.B., Stauner, N., Exline, J.J., Pargament, K.I. and Lindberg, M.J. (2015). Perceived addiction to internet pornography and psychological distress: examining relationships concurrently and over time. *Psychology of Addictive Behaviors*, 29 (4): 1056.

Gu, J., Strauss, C., Bond, R. and Cavanagh, K. (2015). How do mindfulness-based cognitive therapy and mindfulness-based stress reduction improve mental health and wellbeing? A systematic review and meta-analysis of mediation studies. *Clinical Psychology Review*, 37: 1–12.

Gueye, A., Speizer, I.S., Corroon, M. and Okigbo, C.C. (2015). Belief in family planning myths at the individual and community levels and modern contraceptive use in urban Africa. *International Perspectives on Sexual & Reproductive Health*, 41 (4): 191–9. doi:10.1363/4119115.

Gurol-Urganci, I., de Jongh, T., Vodopivec-Jamsek, V., Atun, R. and Car, J. (2013). Mobile phone messaging reminders for attendance at healthcare appointments. *Cochrane Database of Systematic Reviews*, 12.

Gurrieri, L., Previte, J. and Brace-Govan, J. (2013). Women's bodies as sites of control: inadvertent stigma and exclusion in social marketing. *Journal of Macromarketing*, 33: 128–43. doi:10.1177/0276146712469971.

Gutierrez, N., Kindratt, T.B., Pagels, P., Foster, B. and Gimpel, N.E. (2014). Health literacy, health information seeking behaviors and internet use among patients attending a private and public clinic in the same geographic area. *Journal of Community Health*, 39: 83–9.

Guttmacher Institute (2016). Fact Sheet: American Teens' Sexual and Reproductive Health. Available: https://www.guttmacher.org/fact-sheet/american-teens-sexual-and-reproductive-health

Guyenet, S. (2012). The Carbohydrate Hypothesis of obesity: a critical examination. *Whole Health Source*. Available: http://wholehealthsource.blogspot.co.uk/ [accessed 28 August 2017].

Gysels, M., Evans, N., Meñaca, A., Andrew, E., Toscani, F., Finetti, S. et al. (2012). Culture and end of life care: a scoping exercise in seven European countries. *PLoS One*, 7: e34188.

Haaken, J.K. and O'Neill, M. (2014). Moving images: psychoanalytically informed visual methods in documenting the lives of women migrants and asylum seekers. *Journal of Health Psychology*, 19: 79–89.

Hadas, Y., Katz, M.G., Bridges, C.R. and Zangi, L. (2017). Modified mRNA as a therapeutic tool to induce cardiac regeneration in ischemic heart disease. *Wiley Interdisciplinary Reviews: Systems Biology and Medicine*, 9 (1). doi:10.1002/wsbm.1367.

Hadjez-Berrios, E. (2014). A socio-psychological perspective on community participation in health during the Unidad Popular Government: Santiago de Chile, from 1970 to 1973. *Journal of Health Psychology*, 19 (1): 90–6.

Hafekost, K., Lawrence, D., Mitrou, F., O'Sullivan, T.A. and Zubrick, S.R. (2013). Tackling overweight and obesity: does the public health message match the science? *BMC Medicine*, 11: 41.

Hagger, M.S. and Hardcastle, S.J. (2014). Interpersonal style should be included in taxonomies of behavior change techniques. *Frontiers in Psychology*, 5: 254.

Hagger, M.S., Chatzisarantis, N.L.D. and Biddle, S.J.H. (2002). A meta-analytic review of the theories of reasoned action and planned behaviour in physical activity: predictive validity and the contribution of additional variables. *Journal of Sport & Exercise Psychology*, 24: 3–32.

Hagger, M.S., Chatzisarantis, N.L.D., Culverhouse, T. and Biddle, S.J.H. (2003). The processes by which perceived autonomy support in physical education promotes leisure-time physical activity intentions and behavior: a trans-contextual model. *Journal of Educational Psychology*, 95: 784–95.

Haig-Ferguson, A. (2014). The impact of managing a child's chronic fatigue syndrome/myalgic encephalopathy (CFS/ME) on family relationships. Doctoral dissertation, University of the West of England, UK.

Haines, A.P., Imeson, J.D. and Meade, T.W. (1987). Phobic anxiety and ischaemic heart disease. *British Medical Journal* (Clinical Research Edition), 295: 297–9.

Hales, C.N. and Barker, D.J. (1992). Type 2 (non-insulin-dependent) diabetes mellitus: the thrifty phenotype hypothesis. *Diabetologia*, 35 (7): 595–601.

Halfon, M., Phan, O. and Teta, D. (2015). Vitamin D: a review on its effects on muscle strength, the risk of fall, and frailty. *BioMed Research International*. doi:10.1155/2015/953241.

Halim, M.L., Moy, K.H. and Yoshikawa, H. (2017). Perceived ethnic and language-based discrimination and Latina immigrant women's health. *Journal of Health Psychology*, 22 (1): 68–78. doi:10.1177/1359105315595121.

Hall, A. (2008). Brazil's Bolsa Família: a double-edged sword? *Development and Change*, 39 (5): 799–822.

Hall, A. (2012). The last shall be first: political dimensions of conditional cash transfers in Brazil. *Journal of Policy Practice*, 11: 25–41.

Hall, A.M., Ferreira, P.H., Maher, C.G., Latimer, J. and Ferreira, M.L. (2010). The influence of the therapist–patient relationship on treatment outcome in physical rehabilitation: a systematic review. *Physical Therapy*, 90: 1099–110.

Hall, K.D., Sacks, G., Chandramohan, D., Chow, C.C., Wang, Y.C., Gortmaker, S.L. and Swinburn, B.A. (2011). Quantification of the effect of energy imbalance on bodyweight. *The Lancet*, 378 (9793): 826–37.

Hall, M., Grogan, S. and Gough, B. (2016). Bodybuilders' accounts of synthol use: the construction of lay expertise online. *Journal of Health Psychology*, 21 (9): 1939–48. doi:10.1177/1359105314568579.

Hamajima, N., Hirose, K., Rohan, T., Calle, E.E., Heath Jr, C.W., Coates, R.J. et al. (Collaborative Group on Hormonal Factors in Breast Cancer). (2002). Alcohol, tobacco and breast cancer – collaborative reanalysis of individual data from 53 epidemiological studies: including 58,515 women with breast cancer and 95,067 women without the disease. *British Journal of Cancer*, 87: 1234–45.

Hamblen, J. and Barnett, E. (2016). *PTSD in Children and Adolescents*. Washington, DC: US Department of Veterans Affairs: PTSD: National Center for PTSD. Retrieved from: www.ncptsd.org.

Hamilton, C. and Denniss, R. (2010). *Affluenza: When Too Much is Never Enough*. London: Allen & Unwin.

Hamilton, K. and White, K. (2010). Understanding parental physical activity: meanings, habits, and social role influence. *Psychology of Sport and Exercise*, 11: 275–85.

Hamine, S., Gerth-Guyette, E., Faulx, D., Green, B.B. and Ginsburg, A.S. (2015). Impact of mHealth chronic disease management on treatment adherence and patient outcomes: a systematic review. *Journal of Medical Internet Research*, 17 (2): e52. doi:10.2196/jmir.3951.

Hammerness, P., Basch, E., Ulbricht, C., Barrette, E.P., Foppa, I., Basch, S. et al. (2003). St. John's wort: a systematic review of adverse effects and drug interactions for the consultation psychiatrist. *Psychosomatics*, 44: 271–82.

Hampson, S.E., Edmonds, G.W., Goldberg, L.R., Dubanoski, J.P. and Hillier, T.A. (2015). A life-span behavioral mechanism relating childhood conscientiousness to adult clinical health. *Health Psychology*, 34 (9): 887.

Hans, M.B. and Koeppen, A.H. (1989). Huntington's chorea: its impact on the spouse. *Journal of Nervous & Mental Disease*, 168: 209–14.

Harcombe, Z., Baker, J.S. and Davies, B. (2016). Evidence from prospective cohort studies does not support current dietary fat guidelines: a systematic review and meta-analysis. *British Journal of Sports Medicine*, doi:10.1136/bjsports-2016-096550.

Harding, R. and Higginson, I.J. (2003). What is the best way to help caregivers in cancer and palliative care? A systematic literature review of interventions and their effectiveness. *Palliative Medicine*, 17: 63–74.

Hardy, S. and Grogan, S. (2009). Preventing disability through exercise: investigating older adults' influences and motivations to engage in physical activity. *Journal of Health Psychology*, 14: 1036–106.

Hariri, A.A., Oliver, N.S., Johnston, D.G., Stevenson, J.C. and Godsland, I.F. (2013). Adiposity measurements by BMI, skinfolds and dual energy x-ray absorptiometry in relation to risk markers for cardiovascular disease and diabetes in adult males. *Disease Markers*, 35: 753–64.

Harlan, L.C., Bernstein, A.M. and Kessler, L.G. (1991). Cervical cancer screening: Who is not screened and why? *American Journal of Public Health*, 81: 885–90.

Harlow, H.F. (1986). *From Learning to Love: The Selected Papers of HF Harlow*. Westport, CT: Praeger Publishers.

Harper, P.S. (1997). What do we mean by genetic testing? *Journal of Medical Genetics*, 34: 749–52.

Harper, P.S. (2010). *Practical Genetic Counselling* (7th edn). London: CRC Press.

Harrington, M. and Fullagar, S. (2013). Challenges for active living provision in an era of healthism. *Journal of Policy Research in Tourism, Leisure & Events*, 5: 139–57.

Harris, M.I., Eastman, R.C., Cowie, C.C., Flegal, K.M. and Eberhardt, M.S. (1999). Racial and ethnic differences in glycemic control of adults with Type 2 diabetes. *Diabetes Care*, 22: 403–8.

Harris, P., Cooper, K., Relton, C. and Thomas, K. (2012). Prevalence of complementary and alternative medicine (CAM) use by the general population: a systematic review and update. *International Journal of Clinical Practice*, 66: 924–39.

Hart, B. and Risley, T. (1995). *Meaningful Differences in the Everyday Experiences of Young American Children*. Baltimore, MD: Brookes.

Hartman, S.J., Dunsiger, S.I., Marinac, C.R., Marcus, B.H., Rosen, R.K. and Gans, K.M. (2015). Internet-based physical activity intervention for women with a family history of breast cancer. *Health Psychology*, 34: 1296–304. doi:10.1037/hea0000307.

Harvey, A.G. and Bryant, R.A. (2002). Acute stress disorder: a synthesis and critique. *Psychological Bulletin*, 128: 886–902.

Harvey, H., Good, J., Mason, J. and Reissland, N. (2015a). A Q-methodology study of parental understandings of infant immunization: implications for health-care advice. *Journal of Health Psychology*, 20: 1451–62.

Harvey, H., Reissland, N. and Mason, J. (2015b). Parental reminder, recall and educational interventions to improve early childhood immunisation uptake: a systematic review and meta-analysis. *Vaccine*, 33 (25): 2862–80.

Hassed, C., De Lisle, S., Sullivan, G. and Pier, C. (2009). Enhancing the health of medical students: outcomes of an integrated mindfulness and lifestyle program. *Advances in Health Sciences Education*, 14 (3): 387–98.

Hausenblas, H.A. and Fallon, E.A. (2006). Exercise and body image: a meta-analysis. *Psychology & Health*, 21: 33–47.

Hausenblas, H.A., Carron, A.V. and Mack, D.E. (1997). An application of the theories of reasoned action and planned behavior to exercise behavior. *Journal of Sport & Exercise Behavior*, 199: 36–51.

Hayes, P. (2016). Early puberty, medicalisation and the ideology of normality. *Women's Studies International Forum*, 56: 9–18.

Hayes, S.C., Luoma, J.B., Bond, F.W., Masuda, A. and Lillis, J. (2006). Acceptance and commitment therapy model, processes and outcomes. *Behaviour Research and Therapy*, 44: 1–25.

Hayward, R.D., Krause, N., Ironson, G. and Pargament, K.I. (2016). Externalizing religious health beliefs and health and well-being outcomes. *Journal of Behavioral Medicine*, 39 (5): 887–95. doi:10.1007/s10865-016-9761-7.

Headey, B. and Wearing, A. (1989). Personality, life events, and subjective well-being: toward a dynamic equilibrium model. *Journal of Personality and Social Psychology*, 57: 731–9. doi:10.1037/0022-3514.57.4.731.

Healey, J. (ed.) (2006). *Body Image and Self Esteem*. Thirroul, NSW, Australia: Spinney Press.

Health and Social Care Information Centre, Lifestyles Statistics (2008). *Statistics on NHS Stop Smoking Services: England, April 2007 to March 2008*. Leeds: Health and Social Care Information Centre. Available: www.ic.nhs.uk/webfiles/publications/Stop%20smoking%20ANNUAL%20bulletins/SSS0708/SSS%202007-08%20final%20format%20v2.pdf.

Health and Social Care Information Centre. (2013). *Health Survey for England – 2013*. Leeds: Health and Social Care Information Centre.

Heath, A.C. and Madden, P.A.F. (1995). Genetic influences on smoking behavior. In J.R. Turner, L.R. Carden and J.K. Hewitt (eds.), *Behavior Genetic Approaches in Behavioral Medicine*. New York: Plenum Press. pp. 45–66.

Heather, N. and Robertson, I. (1997). *Problem Drinking*. Oxford: Oxford University Press.

Heikkilä, K., Nyberg, S.T., Theorell, T. et al. (2013). Work stress and risk of cancer: meta-analysis of 5700 incident cancer events in 116,000 European men and women. *British Medical Journal*, 346. doi: http://dx.doi.org/10.1136/bmj.f165.

Helgeson, V.S. and Fritz, H.L. (1999). Cognitive adaptation as a predictor of new coronary events after percutaneous transluminal coronary angioplasty. *Psychosomatic Medicine*, 61: 488–95.

Hemingway, H. and Marmot, M. (1999). Psychosocial factors and the aetiology and prognosis of coronary heart disease: systematic review of prospective cohort studies. *British Medical Journal*, 318: 1460–7.

Henderson, K.A. and Ainsworth, B.E. (2003). A synthesis of perceptions about physical activity among older African American and American Indian women. *American Journal of Public Health*, 93: 313–17.

Henderson, L., Millett, C. and Thorogood, N. (2008). Perceptions of childhood immunisation in a minority community: Qualitative study. *Journal of the Royal Society of Medicine*, 101: 244–51.

Herle, M., Fildes, A., Rijsdijk, F., Steinsbekk, S. and Llewellyn, C.H. (2017). The home environment shapes emotional eating. *Child Development*. doi:10.1111/cdev.12799.

Hernandez, D.B. and Kalichman, S. (2017). The impact of HIV stigma on depression among people living with HIV: moderated mediation by social support, alcohol use and food insecurity. Unpublished paper.

Herr, K., Bjoro, K. and Decker, S. (2006). Tools for assessment of pain in nonverbal older adults with dementia: a state-of-the-science review. *Journal of Pain and Symptom Management*, 31: 170–92.

Herzlich, C. (1973). *Health and Illness: A Social Psychological Approach*. London: Academic Press.

Herzlich, C. (2017). A journey in the field of health: from social psychology to multi-disciplinarity. *Journal of Health Psychology*, doi:10.1177/1359105317709474.

Herzlich, C. and Pierret, J. (1987). *Illness and Self in Society*. Baltimore, MD: Johns Hopkins University Press.

Herzog, T.A. (2008). Analyzing the Transtheoretical Model using the framework of Weinstein, Rothman, and Sutton (1998): the example of smoking cessation. *Health Psychology*, 27: 548–56.

Hess, C.B. and Chen, A.M. (2014). Measuring psychosocial functioning in the radiation oncology clinic: a systematic review. *Psycho-Oncology*, 23 (8): 841–54.

Heymann-Mönnikes, I., Arnold, R., Florin, I., Herda, A., Melfsen, S. and Mönnikes, H. (2000). The combination of medical treatment plus multicomponent behavioural therapy is superior to medical treatment alone in the therapy of irritable bowel syndrome. *American Journal of Gastroenterology*, 95: 981–94.

Hilton, C.E. and Johnston, L.H. (2017) Health psychology: it's not what you do, it's the way that you do it. *Health Psychology Open*, 2 (2): doi: https://doi.org/10.1177/2055102917714910

Hilton, L., Hempel, S., Ewing, B.A., Apaydin, E., Xenakis, L., Newberry, S. et al. (2016). Mindfulness meditation for chronic pain: systematic review and meta-analysis. *Annals of Behavioral Medicine*, 51 (2): 199–213.

Hingle, M., Nichter, M., Medeiros, M. and Grace, S. (2013). Texting for health: the use of participatory methods to develop healthy lifestyle messages for teens. *Journal of Nutrition Education and Behavior*, 45: 12–19.

Hittner, J.B. and Kryzanowski, J.J. (2010). Residential status moderates the association between gender and risky sexual behavior. *Journal of Health Psychology*, 15: 634–40.

HLS-EU Consortium (2012). *Comparative Report of Health Literacy in Eight EU Member States: The European Health Literacy Survey (HLS-EU)*. Available: https://oepgk.at/_wissenscenter/the-european-health-literacy-survey-hls-eu/ [accessed 28 August 2017].

Hobfoll, S.E. (1989). Conservation of resources: a new attempt at conceptualizing stress. *American Psychologist*, 44 (3): 513–24.

Hobfoll, S.E. and Freedy, J. (2017). Conservation of resources: a general stress theory applied to burnout. In W.B. Schaufeli, C. Maslach and T. Marek (eds) *Professional Burnout*. London: Routledge. pp. 115–29.

Hodgson, J., Metcalfe, S., Gaff, C., Donath, S., Delatycki, M.B., Winship, I. et al. (2016). Outcomes of a randomised controlled trial of a complex genetic counselling intervention to improve family communication. *European Journal of Human Genetics*, 24 (3): 356–60.

Hofstede, G. and Bond, M.H. (1988). The Confucius connection: from cultural roots to economic growth. *Organizational Dynamics*, 16 (4): 5–21.

Hogben, M., Ford, J., Becasen, J.S. and Brown, K.F. (2015). A systematic review of sexual health interventions for adults: narrative evidence. *Journal of Sex Research*, 52 (4): 444–69.

Holbrook, M.L. (ed.). (1880). *Parturition Without Pain: A Code of Directions for Escaping from the Primal Curse*. ML Holbrook.

Hollis, J.F., Connett, J.E., Stevens, V.J. and Greenlick, M.R. (1990). Stressful life events, Type A behaviour, and the prediction of cardiovascular and total mortality over six years. *Journal of Behavioural Medicine*, 13: 263–81.

Holloway, I.W., Rice, E., Gibbs, J., Winetrobe, H., Dunlap, S. and Rhoades, H. (2014). Acceptability of smartphone application-based HIV prevention among young men who have sex with men. *AIDS and Behavior*, 18: 285–96.

Hollywood, A. and Ogden, J. (2014). Gaining weight after taking orlistat: a qualitative study of patients at 18 months. *Journal of Health Psychology*, 21 (5): 590–8.

Holmes, M.M., Resnick, H.S., Kilpatrick, D.G. and Best, C.L. (1996). Rape-related pregnancy: estimates and descriptive characteristics from a national sample of women. *American Journal of Obstetrics and Gynecology*, 175 (2): 320–5.

Holmes, T.H. and Rahe, R.H. (1967). The social readjustment rating scale. *Journal of Psychosomatic Research*, 11: 213–18.

Holroyd, K.A. and Coyne, J. (1987). Personality and health in the 1980s: psychosomatic medicine revisited? *Journal of Personality*, 55: 359–76.

Homans, H. and Aggleton, P. (1988). Health education, HIV infection and AIDS. In P. Aggleton and H. Homans (eds.), *Social Aspects of AIDS*. London: Falmer Press. pp. 154–76.

Hong, Y., Peña-Purcell, N.C. and Ory, M.G. (2012). Outcomes of online support and resources for cancer survivors: a systematic literature review. *Patient Education & Counseling*, 86: 288–96.

Hooper, L., Abdelhamid, A., Moore, H. J., Douthwaite, W., Skeaff, C. M. and Summerbell, C. D. (2012). Effect of reducing total fat intake on body weight: systematic review and meta-analysis of randomised controlled trials and cohort studies. *British Medical Journal*, 345, e7666.

Hootman, J.M., Brault, M.W., Helmick, C.G., Theis, K.A. and Armour, B.S. (2009). Prevalence and most common causes of disability among adults – United States, 2005. *Morbidity and Mortality Weekly Report*, 58 (16): 421–6. Available: www.cdc.gov/mmwr/preview/mmwrhtml/mm5816a2.htm?s_cid=mm5816a2_e [accessed 23 December 2013].

Horrocks, C. and Johnson, S. (2014). A socially situated approach to inform ways to improve health and wellbeing. *Sociology of Health & Illness*, 36: 175–86.

Hou, S., Charlery, S.R. and Roberson, K. (2014). Systematic literature review of internet interventions across health behaviors. *Health Psychology and Behavioral Medicine*, 2 (1): 455–81.

Hou, W.K., Law, C.C., Yin, J. and Fu, Y.T. (2010). Resource loss, resource gain, and psychological resilience and dysfunction following cancer diagnosis: a growth mixture modeling approach. *Health Psychology*, 29: 484–95. doi:10.1037/a0020809.

Houston, E., Mikrut, C., Guy, A., Fominaya, A.W., Tatum, A.K., Kim, J.H. et al. (2016). Another look at depressive symptoms and antiretroviral therapy adherence: the role of treatment self-efficacy. *Journal of Health Psychology*, 21 (10): 2138–47.

Houtepen, L.C., Vinkers, C.H., Carrillo-Roa, T., Hiemstra, M., van Lier, P.A., Meeus et al. (2016). Genome-wide DNA methylation levels and altered cortisol stress reactivity following childhood trauma in humans. *Nature Communications*, 7 (3): 10967.

Howard, T., Jacobson, K.L. and Kripalani, S. (2013). Doctor talk: physicians' use of clear verbal communication. *Journal of Health Communication*, 18: 991–1001.

Huang, T., Yang, B., Zheng, J., Li, G., Wahlqvist, M.L. and Li, D. (2012). Cardiovascular disease mortality and cancer incidence in vegetarians: a meta-analysis and systematic review. *Annals of Nutrition & Metabolism*, 60: 233–40.

Hudson, J., Day, M. and Oliver, E.J. (2015). A 'new life' study or 'delaying the inevitable'? Exploring older people's narratives during exercise uptake. *Psychology of Sport and Exercise*, 16: 112–20.

Hughes, J., Jelsma, J., Maclean, E., Darder, M. and Tinise, X. (2004). The health-related quality of life of people living with HIV/AIDS. *Disability & Rehabilitation*, 26: 371–6.

Huijg, J.M., Gebhardt, W.A., Crone, M.R., Dusseldorp, E. and Presseau, J. (2014). Discriminant content validity of a theoretical domains framework questionnaire for use in implementation research. *Implementation Science*, 9: 11.

Human Development Report (2000). *Human Rights and Human Development*. New York: Oxford University Press.

Hume, D.J., Yokum, S. and Stice, E. (2016). Low energy intake plus low energy expenditure (low energy flux), not energy surfeit, predicts future body fat gain. *The American Journal of Clinical Nutrition*, 103 (6): 1389–96.

Humpel, N., Owen, N. and Leslie, E. (2002). Environmental factors associated with adults' participation in physical activity: a review. *American Journal of Preventive Medicine*, 22: 188–99.

Hur, M., Lee, M.S., Kim, C. and Ernst, E. (2012). Aromatherapy for treatment of hypertension: a systematic review. *Journal of Evaluation in Clinical Practice*, 18: 37–41.

Husted, M. and Ogden, J. (2014). Emphasising personal investment effects weight loss and hedonic thoughts about food after obesity surgery. *Journal of Obesity*. doi:10.1155/2014/810374.

Hutchison, A.J., Jonhston, L.H. and Breckon, J.D. (2013). A grounded theory of successful long-term physical activity behaviour change. *Qualitative Research in Sport, Exercise and Health*, 5: 109–26.

Huynh, H.P. and Sweeny, K. (2013). Clinician styles of care: transforming patient care at the intersection of leadership and medicine. *Journal of Health Psychology*, doi:10.1177/135 9105313493650.

Huynh, H.P., Sweeny, K. and Miller, T. (2016). Transformational leadership in primary care: clinicians' patterned approaches to care predict patient satisfaction and health expectations. *Journal of Health Psychology*. doi:10.1177/1359105316676330.

Hwang, Y., Cho, H., Sands, L. and Jeong, S. (2012). Effects of gain- and loss-framed messages on the sun safety behavior of adolescents: the moderating role of risk perceptions. *Journal of Health Psychology*, 17: 929–40.

Ikard, F.F., Green, D. and Horn, D. (1969). A scale to differentiate between types of smoking as related to management of affect. *International Journal of the Addictions*, 4: 649–59.

Illich, I. (1976). *Limits to Medicine*. London: Calder & Boyars.

Imo, U.O. (2016). Burnout and psychiatric morbidity among doctors in the UK: a systematic literature review of prevalence and associated factors. *BJPsych Bulletin*. doi:10.1192/pb.bp.116.054247.

Ingledew, D.K., Markland, D. and Medley, A.R. (1998). Exercise motives and stages of change. *Journal of Health Psychology*, 3: 477–89.

Institute of Alcohol Studies (2003). *Crime and Disorder, Binge Drinking and the Licensing Bill*. London: Institute of Alcohol Studies.

Institute of Medicine (2001). *Crossing the Quality Chasm: A New Health System for the 21st Century*. Washington, DC: National Academies Press.

Institute of Medicine (2006). Committee on sleep medicine and research. In H.R. Colten and B.M. Altevogt (eds.), *Sleep Disorders and Sleep Deprivation: An Unmet Public Health Problem*. Washington, DC: National Academy of Sciences.

Institute of Medicine (2007a). *Cancer Care for the Whole Patient: Meeting Psychosocial Health Needs*. Washington, DC: National Academies Press.

Institute of Medicine (2007b). *Implementing Cancer Survivorship Care Planning*. Washington, DC: National Academies Press.

Institute of Medicine (2011). *Report from the Committee on Advancing Pain Research, Care, and Education. Relieving Pain in America: A Blueprint for Transforming Prevention, Care, Education, and Research*. Washington, DC: The National Academies Press.

International Association for the Study of Pain. (2010). *Annual Report*. Seattle, WA: IASP.

International Wellbeing Group (2013). *Personal Wellbeing Index Manual* (5th edn). Available: www.deakin.edu.au/research/acqol/instruments/wellbeing-index/pwi-a-english.pdf. [accessed 28 August 2017].

Jackson, C. (2006). 'Wild' girls? An exploration of 'ladette' cultures in secondary schools. *Gender and Education*, 18 (4): 339–60.

Jacobs, R.J., Lou, J.Q., Ownby, R.L. and Caballero, J. (2016). A systematic review of eHealth interventions to improve health literacy. *Health Informatics Journal*, 22 (2): 81–98. doi:10.1177/1460458214534092.

Jacobsen, P.B. (2009). Promoting evidence-based psychosocial care for cancer patients. *Psycho-Oncology*, 18: 6–13.

Jacobson, R.M., Etta, L.V. and Bahta, L. (2013). The C.A.S.E. approach: guidance for talking to vaccine-hesitant parents. *Minnesota Medicine*, 96 (4): 49–50.

James, C.A., Hadley, D.W., Holtzman, N.A. and Winkelstein, J.A. (2006). How does the mode of inheritance of a genetic condition influence families? A study of guilt, blame, stigma, and understanding of inheritance and reproductive risks in families with X-linked and autosomal recessive diseases. *Genetics in Medicine*, 8 (4): 234–42.

James, D. (2007). *Affluenza: How to be Successful and Stay Sane*. London: Vermillion.

Jamner, L.D. and Tursky, B. (1987). Syndrome specific descriptor profiling: a psychophysiological and psychophysical approach. *Health Psychology*, 6: 417–30.

Janis, I.L. (1972). *Victims of Groupthink*. New York: Houghton Mifflin.

Jarvis, M.J. (2004). Why people smoke. *British Medical Journal*, 328: 277–9.

Jason, L.A., Melrose, H., Lerman, A., Burroughs, V., Lewis, K., King, C.P. et al. (1999). Managing chronic fatigue syndrome: overview and case study. *AAOHN Journal*, 47: 17–21.

Jason, L.A., Roesner, N., Porter, N., Parenti, B., Mortensen, J. and Till, L. (2010). Provision of social support to individuals with chronic fatigue syndrome. *Journal of Clinical Psychology*, 66: 249–58.

Jason, L.A., Sunnquist, M., Brown, A., Evans, M. and Newton, J.L. (2016). Are myalgic encephalomyelitis and chronic fatigue syndrome different illnesses? A preliminary analysis. *Journal of Health Psychology*, 21 (1): 3–15. doi:10.1177/1359105313520335.

Jenkins, C., Arulogun, O.S., Singh, A., Mande, A.T., Ajayi, E., Calys-Tagoe, B. et al. (2016). Stroke Investigative Research and Education Network: community engagement and outreach within phenomics core. *Health Education & Behavior*, 43 (1 suppl.): 82S–92S.

Jensen, M.P., Karoly, P. and Huger, R. (1987). The development and preliminary validation of an instrument to assess patients' attitudes toward pain. *Journal of Psychosomatic Research*, 31: 393–400.

Jernigan, D.H. (2012). Global alcohol producers, science, and policy: the case of the International Center for Alcohol Policies. *American Journal of Public Health*, 102: 80–9.

Jimenez, X.F. (2016). Attachment in medical care: a review of the interpersonal model in chronic disease management. *Chronic Illness*, 13 (1): 14–27.

Jin, L. and Acharya, L. (2016). Cultural beliefs underlying medication adherence in people of Chinese descent in the United States. *Health Communication*, 31 (5): 513–21. doi:10.1080/10410236.2014.974121.

Jin, M., Cai, S., Guo, J., Zhu, Y., Li, M., Yu, Y. et al. (2013). Alcohol drinking and all cancer mortality: a meta-analysis. *Annals of Oncology*, 24: 807–16.

Joffe, H. (1999). *Risk and 'The Other'*. Cambridge: Cambridge University Press.

Joffress, M., Reed, D.M. and Nomura, A.M.Y. (1985). Psychosocial processes and cancer incidence among Japanese men in Hawaii. *American Journal of Epidemiology*, 121: 488–500.

Johns Hopkins University (2020). The Center for Systems Science and Engineering. COVID-19 interactive dashboard. Available: https://arcg.is/0fHmTX.

Johnson, F. and Wardle, J. (2005). Dietary restraint, body dissatisfaction, and psychological distress: a prospective analysis. *Journal of Abnormal Psychology*, 114: 119–25.

Johnson, R.B., Onwuegbuzie, A.J. and Turner, L.A. (2007). Toward a definition of mixed methods research. *Journal of Mixed Methods Research*, 1 (2): 112–33.

Jokela, M., Batty, G.D., Hintsa, T., Elovainio, M., Hakulinen, C. and Kivimäki, M. (2014). Is personality associated with cancer incidence and mortality? An individual–participant meta-analysis of 2156 incident cancer cases among 42 843 men and women. *British Journal of Cancer*, 110 (7): 1820–4.

Jolley, D. and Douglas, K.M. (2014). The effects of anti-vaccine conspiracy theories on vaccination intentions. *PLoS One*, 9 (2): e89177.

Jones, C.J., Smith, H.E. and Llewellyn, C.D. (2014a). Evaluating the effectiveness of health belief model interventions in improving adherence: a systematic review. *Health Psychology Review*, 8 (3): 253–69.

Jones, D.R., Goldblatt, P.O. and Leon, D.A. (1984). Bereavement and cancer: some data on deaths of spouses from the longitudinal study of Office of Population Censuses and Surveys. *British Medical Journal*, 289: 461–4.

Jones, L., Crabb, S., Turnbull, D. and Oxlad, M. (2014b). Barriers and facilitators to effective Type 2 diabetes management in a rural context: a qualitative study with diabetic patients and health professionals. *Journal of Health Psychology*, 19: 441–53.

Jones, C.J., Smith, H.E. and Llewellyn, C.D. (2016). A systematic review of the effectiveness of interventions using the Common Sense Self-Regulatory Model to improve adherence behaviours. *Journal of Health Psychology*, 21 (11): 2709–27.

Joseph, J.J. and Golden, S.H. (2017). Cortisol dysregulation: the bidirectional link between stress, depression, and type 2 diabetes mellitus. *Annals of the New York Academy of Sciences*, 1391 (1): 20–34.

Jumbe, S., Hamlet, C. and Meyrick, J. (2017). Psychological aspects of bariatric surgery as a treatment for obesity. *Current Obesity Reports*, 6 (1): 71–8.

Jylhä, M. (2009). What is self-rated health and why does it predict mortality? Towards a unified conceptual model. *Social Science & Medicine*, 69: 307–16.

Kabat-Zinn, J. (1990). *Full Catastrophe Living: How to Cope with Stress, Pain and Illness Using Mindfulness Meditation*. New York: Bantam Dell.

Kadianaki, I. (2014). The transformative effects of stigma: coping strategies as meaning-making efforts for immigrants living in Greece. *Journal of Community & Applied Social Psychology*, 24 (2): 125–38.

Kagan J. (2016). An overly permissive extension. *Perspective on Psychological Science*, 11: 442–50.

Kaiser Family Foundation (2016). *Sexual Health of Adolescents and Young Adults in the United States*. Available: http://kff.org/womens-health-policy/fact-sheet/sexual-health-of-adolescents-and-young-adults-in-the-united-states/ [accessed 28 August 2017].

Kalichman, S.C. (2009). *Denying AIDS*. New York: Springer.

Kalichman, S.C., Benotsch, E.G., Weinhardt, L., Austin, J., Luke, W. and Cherry, C. (2003). Health-related Internet use, coping, social support, and health indicators in people living with HIV/AIDS: preliminary results from a community survey. *Health Psychology*, 22 (1): 111.

Kalichman, S.C., Ramachandran, B. and Catz, S. (1999). Adherence to combination antiretroviral therapies in HIV patients of low health literacy. *Journal of General Internal Medicine*, 14: 267–73.

Kammann, R. (1979). *Sourcebook for Affectometer 1*. Dunedin: 'Why not?' Foundation.

Kammann, R. and Flett, R. (1983). Affectometer 2: a scale to measure current level of general happiness. *Australian Journal of Psychology*, 35: 259–65.

Kangas, M., Henry, J.L. and Bryant, R.A. (2002). Posttraumatic stress disorder following cancer: a conceptual and empirical review. *Clinical Psychology Review*, 22 (4): 499–524.

Kanner, A.D., Coyne, J.C., Schaefer, C. and Lazarus, R.S. (1981). Comparison of two modes of stress measurement: daily hassles and uplifts versus major life events. *Journal of Behavioral Medicine*, 4: 1–39.

Kaplan, H.S. (1975). *New Sex Therapy: Active Treatment of Sexual Dysfunctions*. New York: Psychology Press.

Karademas, E.C., Bati, A., Karkania, V., Georgiou, V. and Sofokleous, S. (2013). The association between Pandemic Influenza A (H1N1) public perceptions and reactions: a prospective study. *Journal of Health Psychology*, 18: 419–28.

Karasek, R. and Theorell, T. (1990). *Healthy Work: Stress, Productivity, and the Reconstruction of Working Life*. New York: Basic Books.

Karsoho, H., Fishman, J.R., Wright, D.K. and Macdonald, M.E. (2016). Suffering and medicalization at the end of life: the case of physician-assisted dying. *Social Science & Medicine*, 170: 188–96.

Kassavou, A., French, D.P. and Chamberlain, K. (2015). How do environmental factors influence walking in groups? A walk-along study. *Journal of Health Psychology*, 20 (10): 1328–39.

Katsulis, Z., Ergai, A., Leung, W.Y., Schenkel, L., Rai, A., Adelman, J. et al. (2016). Iterative user centered design for development of a patient-centered fall prevention toolkit. *Applied Ergonomics*, 56: 117–26.

Kaufman, M. (1987). The construction of masculinity and the triad of men's violence. In *Beyond Patriarchy: Essays on Pleasure, Power, and Change*. Toronto: Oxford University Press. pp. 1–29.

Kawachi, I., Colditz, G.A., Ascherio, A., Rimm, E.B., Giovannucci, E., Stampfer, M.J. and Willett, W.C. (1994). Prospective study of phobic anxiety and risk of coronary heart disease in men. *Circulation*, 89: 1992–7.

Kawachi, I., Sparrow, D., Spiro, A., Vokonas, P. and Weiss, S.T. (1996). A prospective study of anger and coronary heart disease. *Circulation*, 94 (9): 2090–5.

Keane, V., Stanton, B., Horton, L., Aronson, R., Galbraith, J. and Hughart, N. (1993). Perceptions of vaccine efficacy, illness, and health among inner-city parents. *Clinical Pediatrics*, 32: 2–7.

Kearney, A. (2006). Increasing our understanding of breast self-examination: women talk about cancer, the health care system, and being women. *Qualitative Health Research*, 16: 802–20.

Kearney, A. and Murray, M. (2009). Breast cancer screening recommendations: is mammography the only answer? *Journal of Midwifery and Women's Health*, 54: 393–400.

Kearney, M.S. and Levine, P.B. (2014). Media influences on social outcomes: the impact of MTV's 16 and pregnant on teen childbearing. *The American Economic Review*, 105 (12): 3597–632.

Kearns, R.D., Turk, D.C. and Rudy, T.E. (1985). The West Haven–Yale Multidimensional Pain Inventory (WHYMPI). *Pain*, 23: 345–56.

Keefe, R.J., Hauck, E.R., Egert, J., Rimer, B. and Kornguth, P. (1994). Mammography pain and discomfort: a cognitive behavioural perspective. *Pain*, 56: 247–60.

Keehn, R.J. (1980). Follow-up studies of World War II and Korean conflict prisoners. III: Mortality to January 1, 1976. *American Journal of Epidemiology*, 111: 194–211.

Kelly, Y., Britton, A., Cable, N., Sacker, A. and Watt, R.G. (2016). Drunkenness and heavy drinking among 11year olds: findings from the UK Millennium Cohort Study. *Preventive Medicine*, 90: 139–42.

Kelly, Y., Iacovou, M., Quigley, M., Gray, R., Wolke, D., Kelly, J. and Sacker, A. (2013). Light drinking versus abstinence in pregnancy – behavioural and cognitive outcomes in 7-year-old children: a longitudinal cohort study. *BJOG: An International Journal of Obstetrics and Gynaecology*, 120 (11): 1340–47.

Kelm, Z., Womer, J., Walter, J.K. and Feudtner, C. (2014). Interventions to cultivate physician empathy: a systematic review. *BMC Medical Education*, 14 (1): 219.

Keng, S.L., Smoski, M.J. and Robins, C.J. (2011). Effects of mindfulness on psychological health: a review of empirical studies. *Clinical Psychology Review*, 31: 1041–56.

Kennedy, A., Rogers, A., Blickem, C., Daker-White, G. and Bowen, R. (2014). Developing cartoons for long-term condition self-management information. *BMC Health Services Research*, 14: 1–20.

Kern, M.L. and Friedman, H.S. (2008). Do conscientious individuals live longer? A quantitative review. *Health Psychology*, 27: 505–12.

Kerr, J., Eves, F.F. and Carroll, D. (2001). Getting more people on the stairs: the impact of a new message format. *Journal of Health Psychology*, 6: 495–500.

Key, T.J., Appleby, P.N., Spencer, E.A., Travis, R.C., Allen, N.E., Thorogood, M. and Mann, J.I. (2009). Cancer incidence in British vegetarians. *British Journal of Cancer*, 101: 192–7.

Key, T.J., Fraser, G.E., Thorogood, M., Appleby, P.N., Beral, V., Reeves, G. et al. (1998). Mortality in vegetarians and non-vegetarians: a collaborative analysis of 8,300 deaths among 76,000 men and women in five prospective studies. *Public Health Nutrition*, 1: 33–41.

Khoury, B., Lecomte, T., Fortin, G., Masse, M., Therien, P., Bouchard, V. et al. (2013). Mindfulness-based therapy: a comprehensive meta-analysis. *Clinical Psychology Review*, 33: 763–71.

Kickbusch, I., Wait, S. and Maag, D. (2005). *Navigating Health: The Role of Health Literacy*. Available: www.ilonakickbusch.com/health-literacy/NavigatingHealth.pdf [accessed 29 December 2009].

Kiecolt-Glaser, J. K. and Glaser, R. (1992). Psychoneuroimmunology: Can psychological interventions modulate immunity? *Journal of Consulting and Clinical Psychology*, 60 (4): 569.

Kilby, C.J., Sherman, K. and Wuthrich, V. (2020). How do you think about stress? A qualitative analysis of beliefs about stress. *Journal of Health Psychology*, in press.

Kilfoyle, K.A., Vitko, M., O'Conor, R. and Bailey, S.C. (2016). Health literacy and women's reproductive health: a systematic review. *Journal of Women's Health*, 25 (12): 1237–55. doi:10.1089/jwh.2016.5810.

Kim, K. and Han, H. (2016). Potential links between health literacy and cervical cancer screening behaviors: a systematic review. *Psycho-Oncology*, 25 (2): 122–30. doi:10.1002/pon.3883.

Kim, M.H., Zhou, A., Mazenga, A., Ahmed, S., Markham, C., Zomba, G. et al. (2016). Why did I stop? Barriers and facilitators to uptake and adherence to ART in option B+ HIV care in Lilongwe, Malawi. *PLoS One*, 11: e0149527.

Kim, Y.H., Son, C.G., Ku, B.C., Lee, H.W., Lim, H.S. and Lee, M.S. (2014). Herbal medicines for treating tic disorders: a systematic review of randomised controlled trials. *Chinese Medicine*, 9 (1): 6. https://doi.org/10.1186/1749-8546-9-6

Kim, Y.S. and Joh, T.H. (2006). Microglia, major player in the brain inflammation: their roles in the pathogenesis of Parkinson's disease. *Experimental & Molecular Medicine*, 38 (4): 333.

Kinderman, P. (2017). Psychology is action, not thinking about oneself. *The Psychologist*, 30: 50–5.

Kindlon, T. (2015). No one chooses to have ME – everything changed when I became ill. *Irish Independent*, 30 October.

King, A.C. (1994). Community and public health approaches to the promotion of physical activity. *Medicine & Science in Sports & Exercise*, 26: 1405–12.

King, L.A., Hicks, J.A., Krull, J.L. and Del Gaiso, A.K. (2006). Positive affect and the experience of meaning in life. *Journal of Personality and Social Psychology*, 90: 179–96.

Kingod, N., Cleal, B., Wahlberg, A. and Husted, G.R. (2017). Online peer-to-peer communities in the daily lives of people with chronic illness. *Qualitative Health Research*, 27 (1): 89–99. doi:10.1177/1049732316680203.

Kingsbury, J.H., Gibbons, F.X. and Gerrard, M. (2015). The effects of social and health consequence framing on heavy drinking intentions among college students. *British Journal of Health Psychology*, 20 (1): 212–20. doi:10.1111/bjhp.12100.

Kirsch, I. (2015). Antidepressants and the placebo effect. *Zeitschrift für Psychologie*, 222 (3): 128–34.

Kirsch, I., Jungleblut, A., Jenkins, L. and Kolstad, A. (1993). *Adult Literacy in America: A First Look at the Results of the National Adult Literacy Survey*. Washington, DC: National Center for Education Statistics, US Department of Education.

Kissane, D.W., Grabsch, B., Love, A., Clarke, D.M., Bloch, S. and Smith, G.C. (2004). Psychiatric disorder in women with early stage and advanced breast cancer: a comparative analysis. *Australian and New Zealand Journal of Psychiatry*, 38 (5): 320–6.

Kitson, A., Marshall, A., Bassett, K. and Zeitz, K. (2013). What are the core elements of patient-centred care? A narrative review and synthesis of the literature from health policy, medicine and nursing. *Journal of Advanced Nursing*, 69 (1): 4–15.

Kivimäki, M. and Siegrist, J. (2016). Work stress and cardiovascular disease: reviewing research evidence with a focus on effort-reward imbalance at work. In J. Siegrist and M. Wahrendorf (eds.), *Work Stress and Health in a Globalized Economy*. Cham: Springer. pp. 89–101.

Kivimäki, M., Leino-Arjas, P., Luukkonen, R., Riihimäki, H., Vahtera, J. and Kirjonen, J. (2002). Work stress and risk of cardiovascular mortality: prospective cohort study of industrial employees. *British Medical Journal*, 325: 857–60.

Kivimäki, M., Nyberg, S.T., Batty, G.D., Fransson, I.F., Heikkilä, K., Alfredsson, L. et al. (2012). Job strain as a risk factor for coronary heart disease: a collaborative meta-analysis of individual participant data. *The Lancet*, 380: 1491–7.

Kleinman, A. (1980). *Patients and Healers in the Context of Culture*. Berkeley, CA: University of California Press.

Klenerman, L., Slade, P.D., Stanley, I.M., Pennie, B., Reilly, J.P., Atchinson, L.E. et al. (1995). The prediction of chronicity in patients with an acute attack of low back pain in a general practice setting. *Spine*, 20: 478–84.

Klengel, T. and Binder, E.B. (2015). Epigenetics of stress-related psychiatric disorders and gene × environment interactions. *Neuron*, 86 (6): 1343–57.

Klinner, C., Carter, S.M., Rychetnik, L., Li, V., Daley, M., Zask, A. and Lloyd, B. (2014). Integrating relationship- and research-based approaches in Australian health promotion practice. *Health Promotion International*. doi:10.1093/heapro/dau026.

Knopik, V.S., Maccani, M.A., Francazio, S. and McGeary, J.E. (2012). The epigenetics of maternal cigarette smoking during pregnancy and effects on child development. *Development and Psychopathology*, 24 (4): 1377–90.

Kobasa, S.C. (1979). Stressful life events, personality, and health: an inquiry into hardiness. *Journal of Personality and Social Psychology*, 37 (1): 1.

Kobayashi, L.C., Wardle, J., Wolf, M.S. and von Wagner, C. (2016). Aging and functional health literacy: a systematic review and meta-analysis. *Journals of Gerontology: Series B: Psychological Sciences and Social Sciences*, 71 (3): 445–57.

Kohn, M., Belza, B., Petrescu-Prahova, M. and Miyawaki, C.E. (2016). Beyond strength: participant perspectives on the benefits of an older adult exercise program. *Health Education & Behavior*, 43 (3): 305–12.

Konttinen, H., Haukkala, A. and Uutela, A. (2008). Comparing sense of coherence, depressive symptoms and anxiety, and their relationships with health in a population-based study. *Social Science & Medicine*, 66: 2401–12.

Koponen, A., Simonsen, N. and Suominen, S. (2017). Quality of primary health care and autonomous motivation for effective diabetes self-management among patients with Type 2 diabetes. *Health Psychology Open*, 4 (1). doi:10.1177/2055102917707181

Korn, L., Gonen, E., Shaked, Y. and Golan, M. (2013) Health perceptions, self and body image, physical activity and nutrition among undergraduate students in Israel. *PLoS One*, 8 (3): e58543. Available: https://doi.org/10.1371/journal.pone.0058543

Krahé, B., Berger, A., Vanwesenbeeck, I., Bianchi, G., Chliaoutakis, J., Fernández-Fuertes, A.A. et al. (2015). Prevalence and correlates of young people's sexual aggression perpetration and victimisation in 10 European countries: a multi-level analysis. *Culture, Health & Sexuality*, 17 (6): 682–99.

Krantz, D.S. and McCeney, M.K. (2002). Effects of psychological and social factors on organic disease: a critical assessment of research on coronary heart disease. *Annual Review of Psychology*, 53: 341–69.

Kreibig, S.D. (2010). Autonomic nervous system activity in emotion: a review. *Biological Psychology*, 84 (3): 394–421.

Krieger, N. (1987). Shades of difference: theoretical underpinnings of the medical controversy on black/white differences in the United States, 1830–1970. *International Journal of Health Services*, 17: 259–78.

Krieger, N. and Davey Smith, G. (2004). 'Bodies count', and body counts: social epidemiology and embodying inequality. *Epidemiologic Reviews*, 26: 92–103.

Kristjanson, L.J. (1986). Indicators of quality of palliative care from a family perspective. *Journal of Palliative Care*, 1: 8–17.

Kruger, A.K., Reither, E.N., Peppard, P.E., Krueger, P.K. and Hale, L. (2014). Do sleep-deprived adolescents make less-healthy food choices? *British Journal of Nutrition*, 111: 1898–904.

Kübler-Ross, E. (1969). *On Death and Dying: What the Dying Have to Teach Doctors, Nurses, Clergy and Their Own Families*. New York: Macmillan.

Kübler-Ross, E. (ed.) (1997). *Death*. New York: Simon & Schuster.

Kuenemund, A., Zwick, S., Rief, W. and Exner, C. (2016). (Re-)defining the self – enhanced posttraumatic growth and event centrality in stroke survivors: a mixed-method approach and control comparison study. *Journal of Health Psychology*, 21 (5): 679–89.

Kuhn, T.S. (1970). *The Structure of Scientific Revolutions*. Chicago, IL: University of Chicago Press.

Kuijpers, W., Groen, W.G., Aaronson, N.K. and van Harten, W.H. (2013). A systematic review of web-based interventions for patient empowerment and physical activity in chronic diseases: relevance for cancer survivors. *Journal of Medical Internet Research*, 15 (2): e37.

Kunesh, M.A., Hasbrook, C.A. and Lewthwaite, R. (1992). Physical activity socialization: peer interactions and affective responses among a sample of sixth grade girls. *Sociology of Sport Journal*, 9: 385–96.

Kupeli, N., Candy, B., Vivat, B., Harrington, J., Davis, S., Sampson, E.L. et al. (2016). Which measures assessing quality of death and dying and satisfaction with care at the very end of life have been psychometrically validated? A systematic review. *BMJ Supportive & Palliative Care*, 6 (3): 396.

Kuper, H. and Marmot, M. (2003). Job strain, job demands, decision latitude, and risk of coronary heart disease within the Whitehall II study. *Journal of Epidemiology & Community Health*, 57: 147–53.

Kvikstad, A. and Vatten, L. (1996). Risk and prognosis of cancer in middle-aged women who have experienced the death of a child. *International Journal of Cancer*, 67: 165–9.

Kvikstad, A., Vatten, L. and Tretli, S. (1995). Widowhood and divorce in relation to overall survival among middle-aged Norwegian women with cancer. *British Journal of Cancer*, 71: 1343–7.

Kwan, B.M., Stevens, C.J. and Bryan, A.D. (2017). What to expect when you're exercising: an experimental test of the anticipated affect-exercise relationship. *Health Psychology*, 36: 309–19.

Kwasnicka, D., Dombrowski, S.U., White, M. and Sniehotta, F. (2016). Theoretical explanations for maintenance of behaviour change: a systematic review of behaviour theories. *Health Psychology Review*, 10 (3): 277–96. doi:10.1080/17437199.2016.1151372.

Lamb, S. and Sington, D. (1998). *Earth Story: The Shaping of Our World*. London: British Broadcasting Corporation Books.

Landrine, H. and Corral, I. (2014). Sociocultural correlates of cigarette smoking among African-American men versus women: implications for culturally specific cessation interventions. *Journal of Health Psychology*, 21 (6): 954–61. doi:10.1177/1359105314542821.

Landrine, H., Corral, I., Hall, M.B., Bess, J.J. and Efird, J. (2016). Self-rated health, objective health, and racial discrimination among African-Americans: explaining inconsistent findings and testing health pessimism. *Journal of Health Psychology*, 21 (11): 2514–24. doi:10.1177/1359105315580465.

Lane, H., Porter, K., Estabrooks, P. and Zoellner, J. (2016). A systematic review to assess sugar-sweetened beverage interventions for children and adolescents across the socioecological model. *Journal of the Academy of Nutrition and Dietetics*, 116 (8): 1295–1307.

Langa, K.M., Vijan, S., Hayward, R.A., Chernew, M.E., Blaum, C.S., Kabeto, M.U. et al. (2002). Informal caregiving for diabetes and diabetic complications among elderly Americans. *The Journals of Gerontology Series B: Psychological Sciences and Social Sciences*, 57 (3): S177–86.

Lavie, C.J., Arena, R. and Franklin, B.A. (2016). Cardiac rehabilitation and healthy life-style interventions: rectifying program deficiencies to improve patient outcomes. *Journal of the American College of Cardiology*, 67 (1): 13–15.

Law, G.U., Tolgyesi, C.S. and Howard, R.A. (2014). Illness beliefs and self-management in children and young people with chronic illness: a systematic review. *Health Psychology Review*, 8: 362–80.

Law, M.R., Frost, C.D. and Wald, N.J. (1991). By how much does dietary salt lower blood pressure? I – Analysis of observational data among populations. *British Medical Journal*, 302: 811–15.

Lawrence, W. and Barker, M. (2016). Improving the health of the public: what is the role of health psychologists? *Journal of Health Psychology*, 21 (2): 135–7. doi:10.1177/1359105314528013.

Lawson, J., Reynolds, F., Bryant, W. and Wilson, L. (2014). 'It's like having a day of freedom, a day off from being ill': exploring the experiences of people living with mental health problems who attend a community-based arts project, using interpretative phenomenological analysis. *Journal of Health Psychology*, 19: 765–77.

Lawson, K., Wiggins, S., Green, T., Adam, S., Bloch, M. and Hayden, M.R. (1996). Adverse psychological events occurring in the first year after predictive testing for Huntington's disease. *Journal of Medical Genetics*, 33: 856–62.

Lazarus, R.S. and Folkman, S. (1984). *Stress, Appraisal and Coping*. New York: Springer.

Leachman, S.A. and Merlino, G. (2017) Medicine: the final frontier in cancer diagnosis. *Nature*, 542 (7639): 36–8.

Lee, H., Pollock, G., Lubek, I., Niemi, S., O'Brien, K., Green, M. et al. (2010). Creating new career pathways to reduce poverty, illiteracy and health risks, while transforming and empowering Cambodian women's lives. *Journal of Health Psychology*, 15: 982–92.

Lee, J. and Macdonald, D. (2010). 'Are they just checking our obesity or what?' – The healthism discourse and rural young women. *Sport, Education & Society*, 15: 203–19.

Lee, M.S., Choi, J., Posadzki, P. and Ernst, E. (2012). Aromatherapy for health care: an overview of systematic reviews. *Maturitas*, 71: 257–60.

Leichter, H.M. (1997). Lifestyle correctness and the new secular morality. In A. Brandt and P. Rozin (eds.), *Morality & Health*. New York: Routledge. pp. 359–78.

Leitch, A.M. (1995). Controversies in breast cancer screening. *Cancer*, 76 (S10): 2064–9.

Leitenberg, H. and Henning, K. (1995). Sexual fantasy. *Psychological Bulletin*, 117 (3): 469.

Leng, G. (2014). Gut instinct: body weight homeostasis in health and obesity. *Experimental Physiology*, 99 (9): 1101–3.

Lent, R., Azevedo, F.A., Andrade-Moraes, C.H. and Pinto, A.V. (2012). How many neurons do you have? Some dogmas of quantitative neuroscience under revision. *European Journal of Neuroscience*, 35 (1): 1–9.

Lerman, C. (1997). Psychological aspects of genetic testing: introduction to the special issue. *Health Psychology*, 16: 3–7.

Lerner, W.D. and Fallon, H.J. (1985). The alcohol withdrawal syndrome. *The New England Journal of Medicine*, 313: 951–2.

Leslie, C. (1976). *Asian Medical Systems: A Comparative Study*. Los Angeles, CA: University of California Press.

Lethaby, A., Brown, J., Marjoribanks, J., Kronenberg, F., Roberts, H. and Eden, J. (2007). Phytoestrogens for vasomotor menopausal symptoms. *Cochrane Database of Systematic Reviews*, 4 (7).

Lethem, J., Slade, P.D., Troup, J.D.G. and Bentley, G. (1983). Outline of fear-avoidance model of exag-gerated pain perceptions. *Behavior Research & Therapy*, 21: 401–8.

Lett, H.S., Blumenthal, J.A., Babyak, M.A., Sherwood, A., Strauman, T., Robins, C. and Newman, M.F. (2004). Depression as a risk factor for coronary artery disease: evidence, mechanisms, and treatment. *Psychosomatic Medicine*, 66: 305–15.

Leventhal, H., Meyer, D. and Nerenz, D. (1980). The commonsense representation of illness changes. In S. Rachman (ed.), *Contributions to Medical Psychology* (Vol. 2). Oxford: Pergamon. pp. 17–30.

Leventhal, H., Brissette, I. and Leventhal, E.A. (2003). The common-sense model of self-regulation of health and illness. In L.D. Cameron and H. Leventhal (eds.), *The Self-Regulation of Health and Illness Behaviour*. London: Routledge. pp. 42–65.

Leventhal, H., Phillips, L.A. and Burns, E. (2016). The common-sense model of self-regulation (CSM): a dynamic framework for understanding illness self-management. *Journal of Behavioral Medicine*, 39 (6): 935–46.

Lever, J., Frederick, D.A. and Peplau, L.A. (2006). Does size matter? Men's and women's views on penis size across the lifespan. *Psychology of Men & Masculinity*, 7 (3): 129–43.

Levi, O., Liechtentritt, R. and Savaya, R. (2014). Binary phenomenon of hope: perceptions of traumatized veterans. *Journal of Health Psychology*, 18: 1153–65.

Levine, C. (2000). *Always on Call*. New York: United Hospital Fund.

Levine, C., Kuerbis, A.N., Gould, D.A., Navaie-Waliser, M., Feldman, P.H. and Donelan, K. (2000) *A Survey of Family Caregivers in New York City: Findings and Implications for the Health Care System*. New York: United Hospital Fund.

Lewin, K. (1936). *Principles of Topological Psychology*. New York: McGraw-Hill.

Lewin, K. (1947). Frontiers in group dynamics: II. Channels of group life; social planning and action research. *Human Relations*, 1: 143–53.

Lewin, R.J., Furze, G., Robinson, J., Griffith, K., Wiseman, S., Pye, M. and Boyle, R. (2002). A randomised controlled trial of a self-management plan for patients with newly diagnosed angina. *British Journal of General Practice*, 52: 199–201.

Lewis, J.E., Miguez-Burbano, M.-J. and Malow, R.M. (2009). HIV risk behavior among college students in the United States. *College Student Journal*, 43: 475–91.

Lexchin, J., Bero, L.A., Djulbegovic, B. and Clark, O. (2003). Pharmaceutical industry sponsorship and research outcome and quality: systematic review. *British Medical Journal*, 326: 1167–70.

Ley, C. and Rato Barrio, M. (2013). Evaluation of a psychosocial health programme in the context of violence and conflict. *Journal of Health Psychology*, 18 (10): 1371–81.

Li, X., Han, M., Wang, Y. and Liu, J. (2013). Chinese herbal medicine for gout: a systematic review of randomized clinical trials. *Clinical Rheumatology*, 32: 943–59.

Li, Y., Ju, J., Yang, C., Jiang, H., Xu, J. and Zhang, S. (2014). Oral Chinese herbal medicine for improvement of quality of life in patients with chronic heart failure: a systematic review and meta-analysis. *Quality of Life Research*, 23: 1177–92.

Lichtman, J.H., Bigger, J.T., Blumenthal, J.A., Frasure-Smith, N., Kaufmann, P.G., Lespérance, F. et al. (2008). Depression and coronary heart disease. *Circulation*, 118: 1768–75.

Lie, D., Carter-Pokras, O., Braun, B. and Coleman, C. (2012). What do health literacy and cultural competence have in common? Calling for a collaborative health professional pedagogy. *Journal of Health Communication*, 17: 13–22.

Lieff, J. (2013). *Are Microglia the Most Intelligent Brain Cells?* Available: http://jonlieffmd.com/blog/are-microglia-the-most-intelligent-brain-cells [accessed 28 August 2017].

Liimakka, S. (2014). Healthy appearances–distorted body images? Young adults negotiating body motives. *Journal of Health Psychology*, 19: 230–41.

Lim, H.A., Griva, K., Tan, J.Y.S. and Mahendran, R. (2016). A longitudinal exploration of the psychological resources influencing depression and anxiety in newly diagnosed Asian persons with cancer. *Psycho-Oncology*, 26 (2): 278–81. doi: 10.1002/pon.4110.

Lim, J.N.W. and Ojo, A.A. (2017). Barriers to utilisation of cervical cancer screening in Sub Sahara Africa: a systematic review. *European Journal of Cancer Care*, 26 (1). doi:10.1111/ecc.12444.

Lim, J.S., Mietus-Snyder, M., Valente, A., Schwarz, J.-M. and Lustig, R.M. (2010). The role of fructose in the pathogenesis of NAFLD and the metabolic syndrome. *Nature Reviews Gastroenterology & Hepatology*, 7: 251–64.

Lim, S., Warner, S., Dixon, M., Berg, B., Kim, C. and Newhouse-Bailey, M. (2011). Sport participation across national contexts: a multilevel investigation of individual and systemic influences on adult sport participation. *European Sport Management Quarterly*, 11: 197–224.

Lindberg, L., Santelli, J. and Desai, S. (2016). Understanding the decline in adolescent fertility in the United States, 2007–2012. *Journal of Adolescent Health*, 59 (5): 577–83.

Lindor, K.D., Dickson, E.R., Baldus, W.P., Jorgensen, R.A., Ludwig, J., Murtaugh, P.A. et al. (1994). Ursodeoxycholic acid in the treatment of primary biliary cirrhosis. *Gastroenterology*, 106: 1284–90.

Link, B.G. and Phelan, J. (2014). Stigma power. *Social Science & Medicine*, 103: 24–32.

Linn, A.J., van Weert, J.C., van Dijk, L., Horne, R. and Smit, E.G. (2016). The value of nurses' tailored communication when discussing medicines: exploring the relationship between satisfaction, beliefs and adherence. *Journal of Health Psychology*, 21 (5): 798–807. doi:10.1177/1359105314539529.

Linton, S.J. (1990). Activities of daily living scale for patients with chronic pain. *Perceptual and Motor Skills*, 71: 722.

Linton, S.J., Buer, N., Vlaeyen, J. and Hellsing, A. (2000). Are fear-avoidance behaviours related to the inception of one episode of back pain? A prospective study. *Psychology & Health*, 14: 1051–9.

Linton, S.J. and Shaw, W.S. (2011) Impact of psychological factors in the experience of pain. *Physical Therapy*, 91(5): 700–11.

Litt, I.F. (1993). Health issues for women in the 1990s. In S. Matteo (ed.), *American Women in the Nineties: Today's Critical Issues*. Boston, MA: Northeastern University Press.

Livingston, E.H. (2010). The incidence of bariatric surgery has plateaued in the US. *American Journal of Surgery*, 200: 378–85.

Livingstone, S., Kirwil, L., Ponte, C. and Staksrud, E. (2014). In their own words: What bothers children online? *European Journal of Communication*, 29 (3): 271–88.

Llewellyn, C.H., Trzaskowski, M., Plomin, R. and Wardle, J. (2013). Finding the missing heritability in pediatric obesity: the contribution of genome-wide complex trait analysis. *International Journal of Obesity*, 37 (11): 1506–9.

Locke, A. and Horton-Salway, M. (2010). 'Golden age' versus 'Bad old days': a discursive examination of advice giving in antenatal classes. *Journal of Health Psychology*, 15: 1214–24.

Loewenthal, K.M. and Bradley, C. (1996). Immunization uptake and doctors' perceptions of uptake in a minority group: Implications for interventions. *Psychology, Health & Medicine*, 2: 223–30.

Logan, T., Evans, L., Stevenson, E. and Jordan, C.E. (2005). Barriers to services for rural and urban survivors of rape. *Journal of Interpersonal Violence*, 20: 591–616.

Long, L.C., Fox, M.P., Sauls, C., Evans, D., Sanne, I. and Rosen, S.B. (2016). The high cost of HIV-positive inpatient care at an urban hospital in Johannesburg, South Africa. *PLoS One*, 11 (2): e0148546.

Lorenc, A., Leach, J. and Robinson, N. (2014). Clinical guidelines in the UK: Do they mention complementary and alternative medicine (CAM) – are CAM professional bodies aware? *European Journal of Integrative Medicine*, 6: 164–75.

Lorenc, T., Marrero-Guillamón, I., Llewellyn, A., Aggleton, P., Cooper, C., Lehmann, A. and Lindsay, C. (2011). HIV testing among men who have sex with men (MSM): systematic review of qualitative evidence. *Health Education Research*, 26 (5): 834–46.

Lovallo, W.R. (2013). Early life adversity reduces stress reactivity and enhances impulsive behavior: Implications for health behaviors. *International Journal of Psychophysiology*, 90 (1): 8–16.

Lovell, S.A., Kearns, R.A. and Prince, R. (2014). Neoliberalism and the contract state: exploring innovation and resistance among New Zealand health promoters. *Critical Public Health*, 24 (3): 308–20. doi:10.1080/09581596.2013.808317.

Lovelock, J.E. and Margulis, L. (1974). Atmospheric homeostasis by and for the biosphere: the Gaia hypothesis. *Tellus*, 26: 2–10.

Lowe, M.R. and Fisher Jr, E.B. (1983). Emotional reactivity, emotional eating, and obesity: a naturalistic study. *Journal of Behavioral Medicine*, 6: 135–49.

Lubek, I. (2005). Beer and women: excessive alcohol consumption and risk of HIV/AIDS among Cambodian beer promotion women ('beer girls'). Presentation at the Universiteit van Leiden, 26 January 2005. Available: www.fairtradebeer.com/reportfiles/sirchesi/siem reapnewsletter2008.pdf [accessed 10 December 2009].

Lubek, I., Lee, H., Kros, S., Wong, M.L., Van Merode, T., Liu, J. et al. (2014). HIV/AIDS, beersellers and critical community health psychology in Cambodia: a case study. *Journal of Health Psychology*, 19 (1): 110–16. doi:10.1177/1359105313500253.

Lubek, I., Wong, M.L., Dy, B.C., Kros, S., Pen, S., Chhit, M. et al. (2003). *Only 'Beer Girls', No 'Beer Boys' in Cambodia: Confronting Globalisation and Inequalities in Literacy, Poverty, Employment, and Risk for HIV/AIDS*. Chichester: Wiley-Blackwell.

Lubet, S. (2017). Investigator bias and the PACE trial. *Journal of Health Psychology*, doi:10.1177/1359105317697324.

Lucas, T., Hayman Jr, L.W., Blessman, J.E., Asabigi, K. and Novak, J.M. (2016). Gain versus loss-framed messaging and colorectal cancer screening among African Americans: a preliminary examination of perceived racism and culturally targeted dual messaging. *British Journal of Health Psychology*, 21 (2): 249–67. doi:10.1111/bjhp.12160.

Lucero, J., Wallerstein, N., Duran, B., Alegria, M., Greene-Moton, E., Israel, B. et al. (2016). Development of a mixed methods investigation of process and outcomes of community-based participatory research. *Journal of Mixed Methods Research*. doi:10.1177/1558689816633309.

Luppino, F.S., de Wit, L.M., Bouvy, P.F., Stijnen, T., Cuijpers, P., Penninx, B.W. and Zitman, F.G. (2010). Overweight, obesity, and depression: a systematic review and meta-analysis of longitudinal studies. *Archives of General Psychiatry*, 67: 220–9.

Lupton, D. (1995). *The Imperative of Health*. London: Sage.

Lurie, N., Slater, J., McGovern, P., Ekstrum, J., Quam, L. and Margolis, K. (1993). Preventive care for women: Does the sex of the physician matter? *The New England Journal of Medicine*, 329: 478–82.

Luschen, G., Cockerham, W. and Kunz, G. (1996). The socio-cultural context of sport and health: problems of causal relations and structural interdependence. *Sociology of Sport Journal*, 13: 197–213.

Lustig, R.H. (2013). *Fat Chance: The Hidden Truth about Food, Obesity, and Disease*. London: Fourth Estate.

Lykes, M.B. (2001). Activist participatory research and the arts with rural Mayan women: interculturality and situated meaning making. In D. Tolman and M. Brydon-Miller (eds.), *From Subjects to Subjectivities: A Handbook of Interpretive and Participatory Methods*. New York: New York University Press. pp. 183–97.

Lynch, J.W. and Davey Smith, G. (2002). Commentary: income inequality and health: the end of the story? *Journal of Epidemiology & Community Health*, 31: 549–51.

Lynch, J.W., Davey Smith, G., Harper, S., Hillemeier, M., Ross, N., Kaplan, G.A. and Wolfson, M. (2004). Is income inequality a determinant of population health? Part 1. A systematic review. *Milbank Quarterly*, 82: 5–99.

Lynch, J.W., Davey Smith, G., Kaplan, G.A. and House, J. (2000). Income inequality and mortality: importance to health of individual income, psychosocial environment, or material conditions. *British Medical Journal*, 320: 1200–4.

Lyons, C., Kaufman, A.R. and Rima, B. (2015). Implicit theories of the body among college women: Implications for physical activity. *Journal of Health Psychology*, 20: 1142–53.

MacArtney, J.I. and Wahlberg, A. (2014). The problem of complementary and alternative medicine use today: Eyes half closed? *Qualitative Health Research*, 24: 114–23.

Macinko, J.A., Shi, L., Starfield, B. and Wulu, J.T. (2003). Income inequality and health: a critical review of the literature. *Medical Care Research & Reviews*, 60: 407–52.

Macintyre, S. and Hunt, K. (1997). Socio-economic position, gender and health. *Journal of Health Psychology*, 2: 315–34.

Mackay, S.J. and Parry, O. (2015). Two world views: perspectives on autistic behaviours. *Journal of Health Psychology*, 20 (11): 1416–26.

MackSense Ltd (2014). *Obesity in the UK*. Available: http://MackSense.co.uk/en/research-reports/ [accessed 28 August 2017].

MacLachlan, M. (2000). Cultivating pluralism in health psychology. *Journal of Health Psychology*, 5: 373–82.

Macleod, J. and Davey Smith, G. (2003). Psychosocial factors and public health: a suitable case for treatment? *Journal of Epidemiology & Community Health*, 57: 565–70.

Macleod, J., Davey Smith, G., Heslop, P., Metcalfe, C., Carroll, D. and Hart, C. (2002). Psychological stress and cardiovascular disease: empirical demonstration of bias in a prospective observational study of Scottish men. *British Medical Journal*, 324: 1247–51.

Macmillan (2015) http://www.macmillan.org.uk/_images/macmillan-cancer-support-annual-report-2015_tcm9-287545.pdf

Macmillan Cancer Support (2015). *Routes from Diagnosis*. Available: www.macmillan.org.uk/_images/routesfromdiagnosisreport_tcm9-265651.pdf [accessed 28 August 2017].

Maddux, J.E. (2002). Self-efficacy: the power of believing you can. In C.R. Snyder and S.J. Lopez (eds.), *Handbook of Positive Psychology*. New York: Oxford University Press. pp. 277–87.

Magnus, M.C., Ping, M., Shen, M.M., Bourgeois, J. and Magnus, J.H. (2011). Effectiveness of mammography screening in reducing breast cancer mortality in women aged 39–49 years: a meta-analysis. *Journal of Women's Health*, 20: 845–52.

Maguen, S., Lucenko, B.A., Reger, M.A., Gahm, G.A., Litz, B.T., Seal, K.H. et al. (2010). The impact of reported direct and indirect killing on mental health symptoms in Iraq war veterans. *Journal of Traumatic Stress*, 23 (1): 86–90.

Mahajan, A.P., Sayles, J.N., Patel, V.A., Remien, R., Sawires, S.R., Ortiz, D.J. et al. (2008). Stigma in the HIV/AIDS epidemic: a review of the literature and recommendations for the way forward. *AIDS*, 22 (suppl. 2): S67–79.

Mahendran, R., Lim, H.A., Tan, J.Y., Ng, H.Y., Chua, J., Lim, S.E., et al. (2017). Evaluation of a brief pilot psychoeducational support group intervention for family caregivers of cancer patients: a quasi-experimental mixed-methods study. *Health Qual. Life Outcomes*, 15: 17.

Mahmoodi, N. and Sargeant, S. (2017). Shared decision-making – rhetoric and reality: women's experiences and perceptions of adjuvant treatment decision-making for breast cancer. *Journal of Health Psychology*. doi:10.1177/1359105316689141.

MailOnline (2010). McDonald's, KFC and Pepsi to help write government policy on obesity and diet-related diseases. Available: http://www.dailymail.co.uk/news/article-1329395/ McDonalds-KFC-Pepsi-help-set-government-health-policy-obesity.html

Malinauskaite, I., Slapikas, R., Courvoisier, D., Mach, F. and Gencer, B. (2017). The fear of dying and occurrence of posttraumatic stress symptoms after an acute coronary syndrome: a prospective observational study. *Journal of Health Psychology*, 22 (2): 208–17.

Malpas, P.J., Wilson, M.K.R., Rae, N. and Johnson, M. (2014). Why do older people oppose physician-assisted dying? A qualitative study. *Palliative Medicine*, 28 (4): 353–9.

Mantwill, S., Monestel-Umaña, S. and Schulz, P.J. (2015). The relationship between health literacy and health disparities: a systematic review. *PloS One*, 10 (12): 1–22. doi:10.1371/ journal.pone.0145455.

Mantzari, E., Vogt, F. and Marteau, T.M. (2015). Financial incentives for increasing uptake of HPV vaccination: a randomized controlled trial. *Health Psychology*, 34: 160–71.

Marcus, B.H., Banspach, S.W., Lefebvre, R.L., Rossi, J.S., Carleton, R.A. and Abrams, D.B. (1992). Using the stages of change model to increase the adoption of physical activity among community participants. *American Journal of Health Promotion*, 6: 424–9.

Marcus, B.H., Eaton, C.A., Rossi, J.S. and Harlow, L.L. (1994). Self-efficacy, decision-making and stages of change: an integrative model of physical exercise. *Journal of Applied Social Psychology*, 24: 489–508.

Marcus, D.A. (2000). Treatment of non-malignant chronic pain. *American Family Physician*, 61: 1331–8.

Marcus, K.S., Kerns, R.D., Rosenfeld, B. and Breitbart, W. (2000). HIV/AIDS-related pain as a chronic pain condition: implications of a biopsychosocial model for comprehensive assessment and effective management. *Pain Medicine*, 1: 260–73.

Marcus, M.D., Wing, R.R. and Lamparski, D.M. (1985). Binge eating and dietary restraint in obese patients. *Addictive Behaviors*, 10: 163–8.

Marks, D.F. (1973). Visual imagery differences in the recall of pictures. *British Journal of Psychology*, 64 (1): 17–24.

Marks, D. (1999a). Dimensions of oppression: theorising the embodied subject. *Disability & Society*, 14: 611–26.

Marks, D.F. (1992). Smoking cessation as a testbed for psychological theory: a group cognitive therapy programme with high long-term abstinence rates. *Journal of Smoking-Related Disorders*, 3: 69–78.

Marks, D.F. (1993). *The QUIT FOR LIFE Programme: An Easier Way to Stop Smoking and Not Start Again*. Leicester: The British Psychological Society.

Marks, D.F. (1996). Health psychology in context. *Journal of Health Psychology*, 1: 7–21.

Marks, D.F. (1998). Addiction, smoking and health: developing policy-based interventions. *Psychology, Health & Medicine*, 3: 97–111.

Marks, D.F. (2002a). *The Health Psychology Reader*. London: Sage.

Marks, D.F. (2002b). *Perspectives on Evidence*. London: National Institute for Health and Clinical Excellence. Available: www.nice.org.uk/aboutnice/whoweare/aboutthehda/evidencebase/publichealthevidencesteeringgroupproceedings/perspectives_on_evidence_based_practice.jsp [accessed 28 August 2017].

Marks, D.F. (2002c). *Perspectives on Evidence*. London: National Institute for Health and Clinical Excellence. Available: www.nice.org.uk/aboutnice/whoweare/aboutthehda/evidencebase/publichealthevidencesteeringgroupproceedings/perspectives_on_evidence_based_practice.jsp [accessed 28 August 2017].

Marks, D.F. (2004). Rights to health, freedom from illness: a life and death matter. In M. Murray (ed.), *Critical Health Psychology*. London: Palgrave. pp. 61–82.

Marks, D.F. (2005). *Overcoming Your Smoking Habit*. London: Robinson.

Marks, D.F. (2009). How should psychology interventions be reported? *Journal of Health Psychology*, 14: 475–89.

Marks, D.F. (2010). IQ variations across time, race, and nationality: an artifact of differences in literacy skills. *Psychological Reports*, 106 (3): 643–64.

Marks, D.F. (2013). Health psychology: overview. In A.M. Nezu, C.M. Nezu and P.A. Geller (eds.), *Handbook of Psychology, Vol. 9: Health Psychology*. New York: Wiley. pp. 3–25.

Marks, D.F. (2015). Homeostatic theory of obesity. *Health Psychology Open*, 1.

Marks, D.F. (2016a). Dyshomeostasis, obesity, addiction and chronic stress. *Health Psychology Open*, 3 (1): 2055102916636907.

Marks, D.F. (2016b) *Obesity: Comfort vs. Discontent*. Provence: Yin & Yang Books. Accessible at http://www.smashwords.com/books/view/636290

Marks, D.F. (2017a). *Stop Smoking Now*. London: Little, Brown.

Marks, D.F. (2018). *A General Theory of Behaviour*. London: Sage.

Marks, D. F. (2019). The Hans Eysenck affair: Time to correct the scientific record. *Journal of Health Psychology*, 24 (4): 409–20.

Marks, D.F. and Sykes, C.M. (2002). A randomized controlled trial of cognitive behaviour therapy for smokers living in a deprived part of London. *Psychology, Health & Medicine*, 7: 17–24.

Marks, D.F. and Yardley, L. (2004). *Research Methods for Clinical and Health Psychology*. London: Sage.

Marmot, M. (2013). *Fair society, healthy lives*. The Marmot Review. Straetgic Review of Health Inequalities in England post 2010. London: The Marmot Review. Available: www.ucl.ac.uk/marmotreview

Marmot, M. and Allen, J. (2014). Social determinants of health equity. *American Journal of Public Health*, 104 (suppl. 4): S517–19.

Marmot, M.G. (2016). Empowering communities. *American Journal of Public Health*, 106 (2): 230–1. doi:10.2105/AJPH.2015.302991.

Marmot, M.G., Altman, D.G., Cameron, D.A., Dewar, J.A., Thompson, S.G. and Wilcox, M. (2013). The benefits and harms of breast cancer screening: an independent review. *British Journal of Cancer*, 108 (11): 2205–40.

Marrs, R.W. (1995). A meta-analysis of bibliotherapy studies. *American Journal of Community Psychology*, 23 (6): 843–70.

Marsh, H.W. (1990). A multidimensional, hierarchical self-concept: theoretical and empirical justification. *Educational Psychology Review*, 2: 77–172.

Marsh, H.W., Papaioannou, A. and Theodorakis, Y. (2006). Causal ordering of physical self-concept and exercise behavior: reciprocal effects model and the influence of physical education teachers. *Health Psychology*, 25: 316–28.

Marshall, W.L., Serran, G., Moulden, H., Mulloy, R., Fernandez, Y.M., Mann, R. et al. (2002). Therapist features in sexual offender treatment: their reliable identification and influence on behaviour change. *Clinical Psychology & Psychotherapy*, 9 (6): 395–405.

Marti, A. and Ordovas, J. (2011). Epigenetics lights up the obesity field. *Obesity Facts*, 4 (3): 187–90.

Martin, J.A., Hamilton, B.E., Ventura, S.J., Osterman, M.J.K. and Mathew, T.J. (2014). Births: Final data for 2011. Hyattsville, MD: National Center for Health Statistics.

Martín-Baró, I. (1994). Writings for a liberation psychology. In A. Aron and S. Corne (eds.), *Writings for a Liberation Psychology*. Cambridge, MA: Harvard University Press.

Martinez, S.M., Arredondo, E.M. and Roesch, S. (2013). Physical activity promotion among churchgoing Latinas in San Diego, California: Does neighborhood cohesion matter? *Journal of Health Psychology*, 18 (10): 1319–29.

Martinez Cobo, J. (1987). *Study of the Problem of Discrimination against Indigenous Populations* (Vol. 5). New York: UNESCO.

Maslach, C. and Jackson, S. (1981). The measurement of experienced burnout. *Journal of Occupational Behaviour*, 2: 99–113.

Maslow, A.H. (1943). A theory of human motivation. *Psychological Review*, 50 (4): 370–96.

Mason, J.W. (1971). A re-evaluation of the concept of 'non-specificity' in stress theory. *Journal of Psychiatric Research*, 8: 323–33.

Mason, J.W. (1975). A historical view of the stress field: parts 1 and 2. *Journal of Human Stress*, 1: 6–12, 22–36.

Massaryk, R. and Hatokova, M. (2016). Qualitative inquiry into reasons why vaccination Messages fail. *Journal of Health Psychology*, 23. doi:10.1177/1359105316656770.

Masters, W.H. and Johnson, V.E. (1966). *Human Sexual Response*. Toronto and New York: Bantam Books.

Mataoui, F. and Kennedy, S.L. (2016). Providing culturally appropriate care to American Muslims with cancer. *Clinical Journal of Oncology Nursing*, 20 (1): 11–12.

Mathers, C.D. and Loncar, D. (2006). Projections of global mortality and burden of disease from 2002 to 2030. *PLoS Medicine*, 3: e442.

Mathiowetz, N.A. and Oliker, S. (2005). *The gender gap in caregiving to adults*. Paper presented at the American Time Use Survey Early Results Conference, University of Wisconsin-Milwaukee.

Matias, T., Dominski, F.H. and Marks, D.F. (2020). Human needs in COVID-19 isolation. *Journal of Health Psychology*, 25 (7): 871–82.

Matthew, R.A. (2017). Community engagement: behavioral strategies to enhance the quality of participatory partnerships. *Journal of Community Psychology*, 45 (1): 117–27. doi:10.1002/jcop.21830.

Matthews, D.R., Hosker, J.P., Rudenski, A.S., Naylor, B.A., Treacher, D.F. and Turner, R.C. (1985). Homeostasis model assessment: insulin resistance and β-cell function from fasting plasma glucose and insulin concentrations in man. *Diabetologia*, 28 (7): 412–19.

Mayr, E. and Provine, W.B. (1980). *The Evolutionary Synthesis: Perspectives on the Unification of Biology*. Cambridge, MA: Harvard University Press.

Mazzoni, D. and Cicognani, E. (2014). Sharing experiences and social support requests in an internet forum for patients with systemic lupus erythematosus. *Journal of Health Psychology*, 19 (5): 689–96. doi:10.1177/1359105313477674.

McAllister, M., Payne, K., MacLeod, R., Donnai, D. and Davies, L. (2008a). Developing outcome measures for clinical genetics services: a triangulation approach. *Psychology & Health*, 23: 179–80.

McAllister, M., Payne, K., Macleod, R., Nicholls, S., Donnai, D. and Davies, L. (2008b). Patient empowerment in clinical genetic services. *Journal of Health Psychology*, 13 (7): 895–905.

McAuley, E. and Jacobson, L. (1991). Self-efficacy and exercise participation in adult sedentary females. *American Journal of Health Promotion*, 5: 185–91.

McCabe, M.P. and Althof, S.E. (2014). A systematic review of the psychosocial outcomes associated with erectile dysfunction: Does the impact of erectile dysfunction extend beyond a man's inability to have sex? *The Journal of Sexual Medicine*, 11 (2): 347–63.

McCaffery, A.M., Eisenberg, D.M., Legedza, A.T.R., Davis, R.B. and Phillips, R.A. (2004). Prayer for health concerns: results of a national survey on prevalence and patterns of use. *Archives of Internal Medicine*, 164: 858–62.

McCaffery, K.J., Holmes-Rovner, M., Smith, S.K., Rovner, D., Nutbeam, D., Clayman, M.L. et al. (2013). Addressing health literacy in patient decision aids. *BMC Medical Informatics and Decision Making*, 13 (suppl. 2): S10.

McCaffery, M. and Thorpe, D. (1988). Differences in perception of pain and development of adversarial relationships among health care providers. *Advances in Pain Research & Therapy*, 11: 113–22.

McCambridge, J., Kypri, K., Miller, P., Hawkins, B. and Hastings, G. (2014). Be aware of Drinkaware. *Addiction*, 109: 519–24.

McCarthy, C. and Marks, D.F. (2010). Exploring the health and well-being of refugee and asylum seeking children. *Journal of Health Psychology*, 15 (4): 586–95. doi:10.1177/1359105309353644.

McCartney, G., Collins, C., Walsh, D. and Batty, G.D. (2012). Why the Scots die younger: synthesizing the evidence. *Public Health*, 126: 459–70.

McCartney, M. (2014). *The BMJ* is wrong: doctor assisted dying would overmedicalise death. *British Medical Journal* (Clinical Research Edition), 349: g4502.

McCaul, K.D., Dyche Branstetter, A., Schroeder, D.M. and Glasgow, R.M. (1996). What is the relationship between breast cancer risk and mammography screening? A meta-analytic review. *Health Psychology*, 15: 423–9.

McCaul, K.D., Sandgren, A., King, B., O'Donnell, S., Branstetter, A. and Foreman, G. (1999). Coping and adjustment to breast cancer. *Psycho-Oncology*, 8: 230–36.

McCracken, L.M. and Eccleston, C. (2003). Coping or acceptance: What to do about chronic pain? *Pain*, 105: 197–204.

McCracken, L.M. and Vowles, K.E. (2014). Acceptance and commitment therapy and mindfulness for chronic pain: model, process, and progress. *American Psychologist*, 69: 178–87.

McCracken, L.M., Carson, J.W., Eccleston, C. and Keefe, F.J. (2004a). Acceptance and change in the context of chronic pain. *Pain*, 109: 4–7.

McCracken, L.M., Gauntlett-Gilbert, J. and Vowles, K.E. (2007). The role of mindfulness in a contextual cognitive-behavioral analysis of chronic pain-related suffering and disability. *Pain*, 131: 63–9.

McCracken, L.M., Vowles, K.E. and Eccleston, C. (2004b). Acceptance of chronic pain: component analysis and a revised assessment method. *Pain*, 107: 159–66.

McCracken, L.M., Zayfert, C. and Gross, R.T. (1992). The Pain Anxiety Symptoms Scale: development and validation of a scale to measure fear of pain. *Pain*, 50: 67–73.

McCrae, R.R. and Costa, P.T. (1985). Updating Norman's 'adequate taxonomy': intelligence and personality dimensions in natural language and in questionnaires. *Journal of Personality & Social Psychology*, 49: 710–21.

McCrae, R.R. and Costa, P.T. (2003). *Personality in Adulthood: A Five-Factor Theory Perspective* (2nd edn). New York: Guilford Press.

McDermott, M.S., Oliver, M., Iverson, D. and Sharma, R. (2016). Effective techniques for changing physical activity and healthy eating intentions and behaviour: a systematic review and meta-analysis. *British Journal of Health Psychology*, 21: 827–41.

McEachan, R.R.C., Conner, M., Taylor, N.J. and Lawton, R.J. (2011). Prospective prediction of health-related behaviours with the theory of planned behaviour: a meta-analysis. *Health Psychology Review*, 5: 97–144.

McGee, H.M., Hevey, D. and Horgan, J.H. (1999). Psychosocial outcome assessments for use in cardiac rehabilitation service evaluation: a 10-year systematic review. *Social Science & Medicine*, 48: 1373–93.

McGowan, L.P., Clark-Carter, D.D. and Pitts, M.K. (1998). Chronic pelvic pain: a meta-analytic review. *Psychology & Health*, 13 (5): 937–51.

McKeown, T. (1979). *The Role of Medicine*. Princeton, NJ: Princeton University Press.

McKinley, E.D. (2000). Under Toad days: surviving the uncertainty of cancer recurrence. *Annals of Internal Medicine*, 133: 479–80. doi:10.7326/0003-4819-133-6-200009190-00019.

McMahon, S.B., Cafferty, W.B. and Marchand, F. (2005). Immune and glial cell factors as pain mediators and modulators. *Experimental Neurology*, 192 (2): 444–62.

Mead, N. and Bower, P. (2002). Patient-centred consultations and outcomes in primary care: a review of the literature. *Patient Education and Counseling*, 48: 51–61.

Medeiros, E. (2007). Integrating mental health into post-conflict rehabilitation: the case of Sierra Leonean and Liberian 'child soldiers'. *Journal of Health Psychology*, 12: 498–504.

Medical Research Council. (2000). *A Framework for the Development and Evaluation of RCTs for Complex Interventions to Improve Health*. London: Medical Research Council.

Medical Research Council (2008). *Developing and Evaluating Complex Interventions: New Guidance*. London: Medical Research Council.

Meichenbaum, D. (1985). *Stress Inoculation Training*. New York: Pergamon.

Meichenbaum, D. (1996). Stress inoculation training for coping with stressors. *Clinical Psychologist*, 49: 4–7.

Meichenbaum, D. (2014). Ways to implement interventions in schools in order to make them safer, more inviting and pedagogically more effective. Available: www.melissainstitute.org/documents/Conf18-Meichenbaum-WaysToImplement.pdf.

Melzack, R. (1975). The McGill Pain Questionnaire: major properties and scoring methods. *Pain*, 1: 277–99.

Melzack, R. (1999). From the gate to the neuromatrix. *Pain*, 82 (suppl. 1): S121–6.

Melzack, R. and Katz, J. (2013). McGill Pain Questionnaire. In G.F. Gebhart and R.F. Schmidt (eds.), *Encyclopedia of Pain*. Berlin/Heidelberg: Springer. pp. 1792–4.

Melzack, R. and Katz, J. (2014). The neuromatrix in behavioral medicine. In D.I. Mostofsky (ed.), *The Handbook of Behavioral Medicine*. Chichester: Wiley & Sons. pp. 759–74.

Melzack, R. and Wall, P. (1982/1988). *The Challenge of Pain*. London: Penguin Books.

Melzack, R. and Wall, P. D. (1967). Pain mechanisms: a new theory. *Survey of Anesthesiology*, 11 (2): 89–90.

Mendes, Á., Paneque, M., Sousa, L., Clarke, A. and Sequeiros, J. (2016). How communication of genetic information within the family is addressed in genetic counselling: a systematic review of research evidence. *European Journal of Human Genetics*, 24 (3): 315–25.

Menotti, A., Keys, A., Aravanis, C., Blackburn, H., Dontas, A., Fidanza, F. et al. (1989). Seven countries study first 20-year mortality data in 12 cohorts of six countries. *Annals of Medicine*, 21 (3): 175–9.

Merskey, J. (1996). Classification of chronic pain: descriptions of chronic pain syndromes and definitions of pain terms. *Pain*, 3 (suppl.): S1–225.

Mescher, A.L. (2016). *Junqueira's Basic Histology: Text and Atlas*. New York: McGraw-Hill Education Material.

Messaoudi, M., Lalonde, R. and Violle, N. (2011). Assessment of psychotropic-like properties of a probiotic formulation (*Lactobacillus helveticus* R0052 and *Bifidobacterium longum* R0175) in rates and human subjects. *British Journal of Nutrition*, 105: 755–64.

Meston, C.M., Hull, E., Levin, R.J. and Sipski, M. (2004). Disorders of orgasm in women. *The Journal of Sexual Medicine*, 1 (1): 66–8.

Meszaros, J.R., Asch, D.A., Baron, J., Hershey, J.C., Kunreuther, H. and Schwartz-Buzaglo, J. (1996). Cognitive processes and the decisions of some parents to forego pertussis vaccination for their children. *Journal of Clinical Epidemiology*, 49 (6): 697–703.

Meyer, R. (2016, September). Stigma as a barrier to care, treatment, and prevention of STDs in LGBT individuals. In *2016 National STD Prevention Conference*. Washington, DC: Center of Disease Control and Prevention.

Meyer, T.J. and Mark, M.M. (1995). Effects of psychosocial interventions with adult cancer patients: a meta-analysis of randomized experiments. *Health Psychology*, 14 (2): 101–8.

Meyerowitz, B.E., Richardson, J., Hudson, S. and Leedham, B. (1998). Ethnicity and cancer outcomes: behavioral and psychosocial considerations. *Psychological Bulletin*, 123: 47–70.

Michael, J., Cliff, W., McFarland, J., Modell, H. and Wright, A. (2017). *The Core Concepts of Physiology*. New York: American Physiological Society/Springer.

Michell, J. (1999). *Measurement in Psychology: Critical History of a Methodological Concept*. Cambridge: Cambridge University Press.

Michell, J. (2002). Measurement: a beginner's guide. *Journal of Applied Measurement*, 4: 298–308.

Michell, J. (2003). The quantitative imperative: positivism, naïve realism and the place of qualitative methods in psychology. *Theory & Psychology*, 13: 5–31.

Michell, J. (2008). Is psychometrics pathological science? *Measurement*, 6 (1–2): 7–24.

Michell, J. (2012). 'The constantly recurring argument': inferring quantity from order. *Theory & Psychology*, 22: 255–71.

Michie, S., Johnston, M., Francis, J., Hardeman, W. and Eccles, M. (2008). From theory to intervention: mapping theoretically derived behavioural determinants to behaviour change techniques. *Applied Psychology*, 57 (4): 660–80.

Michie, S. and Wood, C.E. (2015). Health behaviour change techniques. In M. Conner and P. Norman (eds.), *Predicting and Changing Health Behaviour: Research and Practice with Social Cognition Models*. New York: McGraw-Hill. pp. 358–89.

Michie, S., Abraham, C., Eccles, M.P., Francis, J.J., Hardeman, W. and Johnston, M. (2011). Strengthening evaluation and implementation by specifying components of behaviour change interventions: a study protocol. *Implementation Science*, 6: 10.

Michie, S., Johnston, M., Abraham, C., Lawton, R., Parker, D. and Walker, A. (2005). Making psychological theory useful for implementing evidence based practice: a consensus approach. *Quality & Safety in Health Care*, 14 (1): 26–33.

Michie, S., McDonald, V. and Marteau, T. (1996b). Understanding responses to predictive genetic testing: a grounded theory approach. *Psychology & Health*, 11: 455–70.

Mielewczyk, M. and Willig, C. (2007). Old wine and an older look: the case for a radical make-over in health. *Theory & Psychology*, 17: 811–37.

Mihelicova, M., Siegel, Z., Evans, M., Brown, A. and Jason, L. (2015). Caring for people with severe myalgic encephalomyelitis: an interpretative phenomenological analysis of parents' experiences. *Journal of Health Psychology*, 21 (12): 2824–37. doi:10.1177/1359105315587137.

Miles, A. (1981). *The Mentally Ill in Contemporary Society*. Oxford: Martin Robertson.

Miller, A.L., Kaciroti, N., LeBourgeois, M.K., Chen, Y.P., Sturza, J. and Lumeng, J.C.B. (2014). Sleep timing moderates the concurrent sleep duration–body mass index association in low-income preschool-age children. *Academic Pediatrics*, 14: 207–13.

Miller, E.A. and Pole, A. (2010). Diagnosis blog: checking up on health blogs in the blogosphere. *American Journal of Public Health*, 100 (8): 1514–19.

Miller, G., Chen, E. and Cole, S.W. (2009). Health psychology: developing biologically plausible models linking the social world and physical health. *Annual Review of Psychology*, 60: 501–24.

Miller, L.M.S., Zirnstein, M. and Chan, P.K. (2013). Knowledge differentially supports memory for nutrition information in later life. *Journal of Health Psychology*, 18 (9): 1141–52.

Miller, M.J., Abrams, M.A., McClintock, B., Cantrell, M.A., Dossett, C.D., McCleeary, E.M. et al. (2008). Promoting health communication between the community-dwelling well-elderly and pharmacists: the Ask Me 3 program. *Journal of the American Pharmacists' Association*, 48: 784–92.

Miller, S.C., Mor, V., Wu, N., Gozalo, P. and Lapane, K. (2002). Does receipt of hospice care in nursing homes improve the management of pain at the end of life? *Journal of the American Geriatrics Society*, 50 (3): 507–15.

Miller, T.Q., Smith, T.W., Turner, C.W., Guijarro, M.L. and Hallet, A.J. (1996). A meta-analytic review of research on hostility and physical health. *Psychological Bulletin*, 119: 322–48.

Miller, W.R. and Rose, G.S. (2009). Toward a theory of motivational interviewing. *American Psychologist*, 64 (6): 527–37.

Miller, W.R. and Wilbourne, P. (2002). Mesa Grande: a methodological analysis of clinical trials of treatments for alcohol use disorders. *Addiction*, 97: 265–77.

Mills, E., Cooper, C., Seely, D. and Kanfer, I. (2005). African herbal medicines in the treatment of HIV: Hypoxis and Sutherlandia. An overview of evidence and pharmacology. *Nutrition Journal*, 4 (1): 19.

Miovic, M. and Block, S. (2007). Psychiatric disorders in advanced cancer. *Cancer*, 110: 1665–76.

Mission Australia (2010). *National Survey of Young Australians 2010: Key and Emerging Issues*. Australia: Mission Australia.

Mize, S.J.S., Robinson, B.E., Bockting, W.O. and Scheltema, K.E. (2002). Meta-analysis of the effectiveness of HIV prevention interventions for women. *AIDS Care*, 14: 163–80.

Mo, P.K. and Lau, J.T. (2014). Illness representation on H1N1 influenza and preventive behaviors in the Hong Kong general population. *Journal of Health Psychology*, 20 (12): 1523–33.

Modell, H., Cliff, W., Michael, J., McFarland, J., Wenderoth, M.P. and Wright, A. (2015). A physiologist's view of homeostasis. *Advances in Physiology Education*, 39 (4): 259–66.

Modi, N., Murgasova, D., Ruager-Martin, R., Thomas, E.L., Hyde, M.J., Gale, C. et al. (2011). The influence of maternal body mass index on infant adiposity and hepatic lipid content. *Pediatric Research*, 70: 287–91.

Modood, T., Berthoud, R., Lakey, J., Nazroo, J., Smith, P., Virdee, S. and Beishon, S. (1997). *Ethnic Minorities in Britain: Diversity and Disadvantage*. London: Policy Studies Institute.

Moen, P., Robinson, J. and Dempster-McClain, D. (1994). Caregiving and women's well-being (a life course approach). *Journal of Gerontology*, 49: 176–86.

Mohan, A.V., Riley, M.B., Boyington, D.R. and Kripalani, S. (2013). Illustrated medication instructions as a strategy to improve medication management among Latinos: a qualitative analysis. *Journal of Health Psychology*, 18 (2): 187–97.

Moher, D., Schultz, K.F., Altman, D.G. and The CONSORT Group (2001). The CONSORT statement: revised recommendations for improving the quality of reports of parallel-group randomized trials. *The Lancet*, 357: 1191–4.

Mohr, N. (2012). Average and total numbers of animals who died to feed Americans in 2010. Available: https://docs.google.com/file/d/0Bzm1dJXWcgufMjdiNDNmZTItOWMwMy00ZjhjLWE2NGUtNWRkMDM1NmRlNjU3/edit [accessed 28 August 2017].

Molloy, G.J., Dixon, D., Hamer, M. and Sniehotta, F.F. (2010). Social support and regular physical activity: Does planning mediate this link? *British Journal of Health Psychology*, 15: 859–70.

Monaghan, M.C., Hilliard, M.E., Cogen, F.R. and Streisand, R. (2009). Nighttime caregiving behaviors among parents of young children with Type 1 diabetes: associations with illness characteristics and parent functioning. *Families, Systems, & Health*, 27 (1): 28.

Money, J. and Erhardt, A.A. (1972). *Man and Woman, Boy and Girl: The Differentiation and Dimorphism of Gender Identity from Conception to Maturity*. Baltimore, MD: Johns Hopkins University Press.

Monroe, S.M. and Simons, A.D. (1991). Diathesis-stress theories in the context of life stress research: implications for the depressive disorders. *Psychological Bulletin*, 110: 406–25.

Montenegro, R.A. and Stephens, C. (2006). Indigenous health in Latin America and the Caribbean. *The Lancet*, 367: 1859–69.

Moodie, R., Stuckler, D., Monteiro, C., Sheron, N., Neal, B., Thamarangsi, T. et al. (2013). Profits and pandemics: prevention of harmful effects of tobacco, alcohol, and ultra-processed food and drink industries. *The Lancet*, 381: 670–9.

Mookadam, F. and Arthur, H.M. (2004). Social support and its relationship to morbidity and mortality after acute myocardial infarction: systematic overview. *Archives of Internal Medicine*, 164: 1514–18.

Mooney, M., White, T. and Hatsukami, D. (2004). The blind spot in the nicotine replacement therapy literature: assessment of the double-blind in clinical trials. *Addictive Behavior*, 29: 673–84.

Moore, C.L., Grulich, A.E., Prestage, G., Gidding, H.F., Jin, F., Petoumenos, K. et al. (2016). Hospitalization for anxiety and mood disorders in HIV-infected and uninfected gay and bisexual men. *JAIDS: Journal of Acquired Immune Deficiency Syndromes*, 73 (5): 589–97.

Moore, S., Barling, N. and Hood, B. (1998). Predicting testicular and breast self examination: a test of the Theory of Reasoned Action. *Behaviour Change*, 15: 41–9.

Morinis, C.A. and Brilliant, G.E. (1981). Smallpox in northern India: diversity and order in a regional medical culture. *Medical Anthropology*, 5: 341–64.

Morris, G. and Maes, M. (2014). Oxidative and nitrosative stress and immune-inflammatory pathways in patients with myalgic encephalomyelitis (ME)/chronic fatigue syndrome (CFS). *Current Neuropharmacology*, 12 (2): 168–85.

Morris, J.A., Jordan, C.L. and Breedlove, S.M. (2004). Sexual differentiation of the vertebrate nervous system. *Nature Neuroscience*, 7 (10): 1034–9.

Mosavianpour, M., Sarmast, H.H., Kissoon, N. and Collet, J.P. (2016). Theoretical domains framework to assess barriers to change for planning health care quality interventions: a systematic literature review. *Journal of Multidisciplinary Healthcare*, 9: 303–10.

Moscovici, S. (1984). The phenomenon of social representations. In R.M. Farr and S. Moscovici (eds.), *Social Representations*. Cambridge: Cambridge University Press. pp. 3–70.

Moser, D.K. and Dracup, K. (2004). Role of spousal anxiety and depression in patients' psychosocial recovery after a cardiac event. *Psychosomatic Medicine*, 66: 527–32.

Moser, E.M. and Stagnaro-Green, A. (2009). Teaching behavior change concepts and skills during the third-year medicine clerkship. *Academic Medicine*, 84 (7): 851–8.

Mouraux, A., Diukova, A., Lee, M.C., Wise, R.G. and Iannetti, G.D. (2011). A multisensory investigation of the functional significance of the 'pain matrix'. *NeuroImage*, 54: 2237–49.

Moynihan, P.J. and Kelly, S.A.M. (2014). Effect on caries of restricting sugars intake: systematic review to inform WHO guidelines. *Journal of Dental Research*, 93: 8–18.

Mozaffarian, D., Hao, T., Rimm, E.B., Willett, W.C. and Hu, F.B. (2011). Changes in diet and lifestyle and long-term weight gain in women and men. *The New England Journal of Medicine*, 364: 2392–404.

Mulkay, M. (1991). *Sociology of Science: A Sociological Pilgrimage*. Milton Keynes: Open University Press.

Murray, M. (2007). 'It's in the blood and you're not going to change it': fish harvesters' narrative accounts of injuries and disability. *Work*, 28: 165–74.

Murray, M. (2009). Telling stories and making sense of cancer. *International Journal of Narrative Practice*, 1: 25–36.

Murray, M. (2012b). Critical health psychology and the scholar-activist tradition. In C. Horrocks and S. Johnson (eds.), *Advances in Health Psychology: Critical Approaches*. London: Palgrave Macmillan. pp. 29–43.

Murgatroyd, C. and Spengler, D. (2011). Epigenetic programming of the HPA axis: early life decides. *Stress*, 14 (6): 581–9.

Muris, P., Merckelbach, H., Schmidt, H., Gadet, B. and Bogie, N. (2001). Anxiety and depression as correlates of self-reported behavioural inhibition in normal adolescents. *Behaviour Research and Therapy*, 39 (9): 1051–61.

Murphy, D.J. and Hall, C.A. (2011). Energy return on investment, peak oil, and the end of economic growth. *Annals of the New York Academy of Sciences*, 1219 (1): 52–72.

Murray, C.J.L. and Lopez, A.D. (1997). Alternative projections of mortality and disability by cause 1990–2020: Global Burden of Disease Study. *The Lancet*, 349: 1498–504.

Murray, M. (1997). A narrative approach to health psychology: background and potential. *Journal of Health Psychology*, 2: 9–20.

Murray, M. (2012). Social and political health psychology in action. In M. Forshaw and D. Sheffield (eds.), *Health Psychology in Action*. London: Wiley-Blackwell. pp. 128–37.

Murray, M. (2014a). Social history of health psychology: context and textbooks. *Health Psychology Review*, 8: 215–37.

Murray, M. (2014b). *Critical Health Psychology* (2nd edn). London: Palgrave.

Murray, M. and Campbell, C. (2003). Living in a material world: reflecting on some assumptions of health psychology. *Journal of Health Psychology*, 8: 231–6.

Murray, M. and Chamberlain, K. (eds.) (2015). *New Directions in Health Psychology* (Vols I–V). London: Sage.

Murray, M. and McMillan, C. (1993). Health beliefs, locus of control, emotional control and women's cancer screening behaviour. *British Journal of Clinical Psychology*, 32: 87–100.

Murray, M. and Tilley, N. (2004). Developing community health action and research through the arts. In R. Flowers (ed.), *Education and Social Action Conference*. Sydney: University of Technology Sydney. pp. 150–6.

Murray, M. and Ziegler, F. (2015). The narrative psychology of community health workers. *Journal of Health Psychology*, 20 (3): 338–49. doi:10.1177/1359105314566615.

Murray, M., Jarrett, L., Swan, A.V. and Rumun, R. (1988). *Smoking Among Young Adults*. Aldershot: Gower.

Murray, M., Pullman, D. and Heath Rodgers, T. (2003). Social representations of health and illness among 'baby-boomers' in Eastern Canada. *Journal of Health Psychology*, 8: 485–500.

Murray, M., Swan, A.V. and Mattar, N. (1983). The task of nursing and risk of smoking. *Journal of Advanced Nursing*, 8: 131–8.

Mykletun, A., Bjerkeset, O., Dewey, M., Prince, M., Overland, S. and Stewart, R. (2007). Anxiety, depression, and cause-specific mortality: the HUNT study. *Psychosomatic Medicine*, 69: 323–31.

Myrtek, M. (2001). Meta-analyses of prospective studies on coronary heart disease, Type A personality and hostility. *International Journal of Cardiology*, 79: 245–51.

Najafi, S., Lieto, J. and Johnson, L.A. (2014). Physicians' practices and end of life. Available at: http://digitalcommons.hsc.unt.edu/rad/RAD14/Other/28/ [accessed 28 August 2017].

Nakagawa, F., Miners, A., Smith, C.J., Simmons, R., Lodwick, R.K., Cambiano, V. et al. (2015). Projected lifetime healthcare costs associated with HIV infection. *PLoS One*, 10 (4): e0125018.

Nakiwala, A.S. (2016). From recipients to partners: children in malaria education in Uganda. *Health Education*, 116 (2): 202–19.

Nan, C., Guo, B., Warner, C., Fowler, T., Barrett, T., Boomsma, D. et al. (2012). Heritability of body mass index in pre-adolescence, young adulthood and late adulthood. *European Journal of Epidemiology*, 27: 247–53.

Nanni, M.G., Caruso, R., Mitchell, A.J., Meggiolaro, E. and Grassi, L. (2015). Depression in HIV infected patients: a review. *Current Psychiatry Reports*, 17 (1): 530. doi:10.1007/s11920-014-0530-4.

Nathan, D.M., Zinman, B., Cleary, P.A., Backlund, J.Y.C., Genuth, S., Miller, R. et al. (2009). Modern-day clinical course of Type 1 diabetes mellitus after 30 years' duration: the diabetes control and complications trial/epidemiology of diabetes interventions and complications and Pittsburgh epidemiology of diabetes complications experience (1983–2005). *Archives of Internal Medicine*, 169 (14): 1307.

National AIDS Trust. (2011). Available: http://www.nat.org.uk/press-release/one-five-adults-do-not-realise-hiv-transmitted-through-sex-without-condom-between-man.

National Cancer Institute, Breast Cancer Screening Consortium. (1990). Screening mammography: a missed clinical opportunity. *Journal of the American Medical Association*, 264: 54–8.

National Center for Complementary and Alternative Medicine (NCCAM). (2013). Complementary, alternative, or integrative health: What's in a name? Available: http://nccam.nih.gov/health/whatiscam [accessed 7 May 2014].

National Center for Health Statistics. (1994). *Healthy People 2000 Review, 1993*. Hyattsville, MD: Public Health Service.

National Diabetes Education Program. (2017). *Diabetes Primer for School Personnel*. Available: www.niddk.nih.gov/health-information/health-communication-programs/ndep/health-care-professionals/school-guide/Documents/NDEP61_SchoolGuide_01_primer-508.pdf [accessed 10 February 2017].

National Health Service. (2010). *Free Local NHS Stop Smoking Services*. Available: http://smokefree.nhs.uk/what-suits-me/local-nhs-services/ [accessed 5 January 2010].

National Institute of Diabetes and Digestive and Kidney Diseases. (2017). *Overweight and Obesity Statistics*. Available: www.niddk.nih.gov/health-information/health-statistics/Pages/overweight-obesity-statistics.aspx [accessed 28 August 2017].

National Institute of Justice. (2003). *Youth Victimization: Prevalence and Implications*. Washington, DC: National Institute of Justice.

National Institutes of Health. (2017). *What I Need to Know about Erectile Dysfunction*. Available: www.niddk.nih.gov/-/media/99041A12CBB940809A3E668285D1E6C9.ashx [accessed 22 March 2017].

National Institutes of Health/National Human Genome Research Institute. (2017). *Talking Glossary of Genetic Terms*. Available: www.genome.gov/glossary/ [accessed 15 April 2017].

Nayak, A. and Kehily, M.J. (2014). 'Chavs, chavettes and pramface girls': teenage mothers, marginalised young men and the management of stigma. *Journal of Youth Studies*, 17 (10): 1330–45.

Nelson, P., Cox, H., Furze, G., Lewin, R.J., Morton, V., Norris, H. et al. (2013). Participants' experiences of care during a randomized controlled trial comparing a lay-facilitated angina management programme with usual care: a qualitative study using focus groups. *Journal of Advanced Nursing*, 69 (4): 840–50.

Nelson-Coffey, S.K., Fritz, M.M., Lyubomirsky, S. and Cole, S.W. (2017). Kindness in the blood: a randomized controlled trial of the gene regulatory impact of prosocial behavior. *Psychoneuroendocrinology*, 81: 8–13.

Nemutandani, S.M., Hendricks, S.J.H. and Mulaudzi, F. (2015). HIV/AIDS and TB knowledge and beliefs among rural traditional health practitioners in Limpopo province, South Africa. *African Journal for Physical Health Education, Recreation & Dance*, 21 (suppl. 1): 119–34.

Neuman, H., Debelius, J.W., Knight, R. and Koren, O. (2015). Microbial endocrinology: the interplay between the microbiota and the endocrine system. *FEMS Microbiology Review*, 39 (4): 509–21. doi:10.1093/femsre/fuu010.

Neupert, S.D., Lachman, M.E. and Whitbourne, S.B. (2009). Exercise self-efficacy and control beliefs predict exercise behavior after an exercise intervention for older adults. *Journal of Aging and Physical Activity*, 17: 1–16.

New, S.J. and Senior, M. (1991). 'I dont believe in needles': qualitative aspects of study into the update of infant immunisation in two English health authorities. *Social Science & Medicine*, 33: 509–18.

Newell, S.A., Sanson-Fisher, R.W. and Savolainen, N.J. (2002). Systematic review of psychological therapies for cancer patients: overview and recommendations for future research. *Journal of the National Cancer Institute*, 94: 558–84.

Newton, F.J., Ewing, M.T. and Pitt, L.F. (2012). The intra- and inter-personal dynamics associated with consuming sensitive products: understanding the consumption of erectile function aids using dimensional qualitative research. *Psychology & Marketing*, 29 (1): 1–14.

Ng, D.M. and Jeffery, R.W. (2003). Relationships between perceived stress and health behaviours in a sample of working adults. *Health Psychology*, 22: 638–42.

Ng, E.C.W. (2010). Community-building: a strategy to address inequality of health in Australia. *Journal of Health Psychology*, 15 (7): 1020–9.

Ng, S.C., Lam, Y.T., Tsoi, K.K.F., Chan, F.K.L., Sung, J.J.Y. and Wu, J.C.Y. (2013). Systematic review: the efficacy of herbal therapy in inflammatory bowel disease. *Alimentary Pharmacology & Therapeutics*, 38: 854–63.

NHS Choices (2017). *Coping with a Cancer Diagnosis*. Available: www.nhs.uk/Livewell/cancer/Pages/coping-with-cancer-diagnosis.aspx [accessed 28 August 2017].

NHS Digital (2016). *NHS Immunisation Statistics, England – 2015–16*. London: Health and Social Care Information Centre.

Nicholson, A., Kuper, H. and Hemingway, H. (2006). Depression as an aetiologic and prognostic factor in coronary heart disease: a meta-analysis of 6362 events among 146 538 participants in 54 observational studies. *European Heart Journal*, 27: 2763–74.

Nissen, K.G. (2016). Correlates of self-rated attachment in patients with cancer and their caregivers: a systematic review and meta-analysis. *Psycho-Oncology*, 25 (9): 1017–27.

Njau, B., Ostermann, J., Brown, D., Mühlbacher, A., Reddy, E. and Thielman, N. (2014). HIV testing preferences in Tanzania: a qualitative exploration of the importance of confidentiality, accessibility, and quality of service. *BMC Public Health*, 14: 838.

Njor, S.H., Schwartz, W., Blichert-Toft, M. and Lynge, E. (2015). Decline in breast cancer mortality: How much is attributable to screening? *Journal of Medical Screening*, 22: 20–27.

Noar, S.M., Black, H.G. and Pierce, L.B. (2009). Efficacy of computer technology-based HIV prevention interventions: a meta-analysis. *AIDS*, 23: 107–15.

Nolas, S. (2014). Towards a new theory of practice for community health psychology. *Journal of Health Psychology*, 19 (1): 126–36. doi:10.1177/1359105313500252.

Nolin, T., Mårdh, C., Karlström, G. and Walther, S.M. (2017). Identifying opportunities to increase organ donation after brain death: an observational study in Sweden 2009–2014. *Acta Anaesthesiologica Scandinavica*, 61 (1): 73–82.

Norman, P. and Brain, K. (2005). An application of an extended health belief model to the prediction of breast self-examination among women with a family history of breast cancer. *British Journal of Health Psychology*, 10: 1–16.

Norris, S.L., Engelgau, M.M. and Narayan, K.V. (2001). Effectiveness of self-management training in Type 2 diabetes. *Diabetes Care*, 24 (3): 561–87.

Northouse, L., Williams, A.L., Given, B. and McCorkle, R. (2012). Psychosocial care for family caregivers of patients with cancer. *Journal of Clinical Oncology*, 30 (11): 1227–34.

Notcutt, W. (2004). Cannabis in the treatment of chronic pain. In G.W. Guy, B.A. Whittle and P. Robson (eds.), *The Medicinal Uses of Cannabis and Cannabinoids*. London: Pharmaceutical Press. pp. 271–99.

Nutbeam, D. (1998). Health promotion glossary. *Health Promotion International*, 13: 349–64.

Nutbeam, D. (2000). Health literacy as a public health goal: a challenge for contemporary health education and communication strategies into the 21st century. *Health Promotion International*, 15: 259–67.

Nykjaer, C., Alwan, N.A., Greenwood, D.C., Simpson, N.A.B., Hay, A.W.M., White, K.L.M. and Cade, J.E. (2014). Maternal alcohol intake prior to and during pregnancy and risk of adverse birth outcomes: evidence from a British cohort. *Journal of Epidemiology and Community Health*, 68: 542–9.

O'Brien Cousins, S. (2000). 'My heart couldn't take it': older women's beliefs about exercise benefits and risks. *Journals of Gerontology Series B: Psychological Sciences and Social Sciences*, 55: 283–94.

O'Keefe Jr, J.H. and Cordain, L. (2004). Cardiovascular disease resulting from a diet and lifestyle at odds with our Paleolithic genome: how to become a 21st-century hunter-gatherer. *Mayo Clinic Proceedings*, 79 (1): 101–8.

O'Leary, A. and Helgeson, V.S. (1997). Psychosocial factors and women's health: integrating mind, heart, and body. In S.J. Gallant, G.P. Keita and R. Royal-Schaler (eds.), *Health Care for Women: Psychological, Social and Behavioral Influences*. Washington, DC: American Psychological Association. pp. 25–40.

Oberlander, T.F., Weinberg, J., Papsdorf, M., Grunau, R., Misri, S. and Devlin, A.M. (2008). Prenatal exposure to maternal depression, neonatal methylation of human glucocorticoid receptor gene (NR3C1) and infant cortisol stress responses. *Epigenetics*, 3 (2): 97–106.

Ochieng, B.M.N. (2013). Black families' perceptions of barriers to the practice of a healthy lifestyle: a qualitative study in the UK. *Critical Public Health*, 23: 6–16.

Office for National Statistics (2009). *Teen Pregnancy Rates Go Back Up*. London: ONS. Available: http://news.bbc.co.uk/1/hi/uk/7911684.stm [accessed 26 November 2009].

Office for National Statistics (2016). *Conceptions in England and Wales – Office for National Statistics*. London: ONS. Available: www.ons.gov.uk/.../birthsdeathsandmarriages/.../conceptionstatistics/2014 [accessed 28 August 2017].

Ogden, J. (2003). Some problems with social cognition models: a pragmatic and conceptual analysis. *Health Psychology*, 22: 424–8.

Ogden, J. (2016). Celebrating variability and a call to limit systematisation: the example of the behaviour change technique taxonomy and the behaviour change wheel. *Health Psychology Review*, 10 (3): 245–50.

Ohenjo, N., Willis, R., Jackson, D., Nettleton, C., Good, K. and Mugarura, B. (2006). Health of Indigenous people in Africa. *The Lancet*, 367: 1937–76.

Oken, B.S., Storzbach, D.M. and Kaye, J.A. (1998). The efficacy of ginkgo biloba on cognitive function in Alzheimer disease. *Archives of Neurology*, 55: 1409–15.

Okomo, U., Ogugbue, M., Inyang, E. and Meremikwu, M.M. (2017). Sexual counselling for treating or preventing sexual dysfunction in women living with female genital mutilation: a systematic review. *International Journal of Gynecology & Obstetrics*, 136 (S1): 38–42.

Oldridge, N.B., Guyatt, G.H., Fischer, M.E. and Rimm, A.A. (1988). Cardiac rehabilitation after myocardial infarction: combined experience of randomized clinical trials. *JAMA*, 260 (7): 945–50.

Oliveira, V.C., Ferreira, M.L., Pinto, R.Z., Filho, R.F., Refshauge, K. and Ferreira, P.H. (2015). Effectiveness of training clinicians' communication skills on patients' clinical outcomes: a systematic review. *Journal of Manipulative & Physiological Therapeutics*, 38 (8): 601–16. doi:10.1016/j.jmpt.2015.08.002.

Olson, C.M. (2016). Behavioral nutrition interventions using e-and m-health communication technologies: a narrative review. *Annual Review of Nutrition*, 36: 647–64.

Ombres, R., Montemorano, L. and Becker, D. (2017). Death notification: someone needs to call the family. *Journal of Palliative Medicine*, 20 (6): 672–5.

Omran, A.R. (1971). The epidemiological transition: a theory of the epidemiology of population change. *The Milbank Quarterly*, 83: 731–57.

Onyike, C.U., Crum, R.M., Lee, H.B., Lyketsos, C.G. and Eaton, W.W. (2003). Is obesity associated with major depression? Results from the Third National Health and Nutrition Examination Survey. *American Journal of Epidemiology*, 158: 1139–47.

Open Science Collaboration (2015). Estimating the reproducibility of psychological science. *Science*, 349 (6251). doi:10.1126/science.aac4716.

Opp, M.R. and Krueger, J.M. (2015). Sleep and immunity: a growing field with clinical impact. *Brain, Behavior, and Immunity*, 47: 1–3.

Opperman, E., Braun, V., Clarke, V. and Rogers, C. (2014). 'It feels so good it almost hurts': young adults' experiences of orgasm and sexual pleasure. *The Journal of Sex Research*, 51 (5): 503–15.

Oregon Public Health Division (2014). Available: www.ocregister.com/articles/physician-524739-death-oregon.html [accessed 28 August 2017].

Orth-Gomér, K., Rosengren, A. and Wilhelmsen, L. (1993). Lack of social support and incidence of coronary heart disease in middle-aged Swedish men. *Psychosomatic Medicine*, 55 (1): 37–43.

Oster, E. (2013). *Expecting Better*. London: Orion.

Oulton, N. (2012). The wealth and poverty of nations: true PPPs for 141 countries. Centre for Economic Performance Discussion Paper No. 1080. London: LSE.

Owuor, J.O.A., Locke, A., Heyman, B. and Clifton, A. (2016). Concealment, communication and stigma: the perspectives of HIV-positive immigrant black African men and their partners living in the United Kingdom. *Journal of Health Psychology*, 21 (12): 3079–91.

Oygard, L. and Anderssen, N. (1998). Social influences and leisure-time physical activity levels in young people: a twelve-year follow-up study. *Journal of Health Psychology*, 3: 59–69.

Ozer, E.J., Best, S.R., Lipsey, T.L. and Weiss, D.S. (2003). Predictors of posttraumatic stress disorder and symptoms in adults: a meta-analysis. *Psychological Bulletin*, 129: 52–73.

Padez, C., Mourão, I., Moreira, P. and Rosado, V. (2009). Long sleep duration and childhood overweight/obesity and body fat. *American Journal of Human Biology*, 21: 371–6.

Paechter, C. (2003). Power, bodies and identity: how different forms of physical education construct varying masculinities and femininities in secondary schools. *Sex Education*, 3: 47–59.

Pain Australia. (2010). *National Pain Strategy: Pain Management for All Australians*. Tamarama, NSW: Pain Australia.

Palmer, C.K., Thomas, M.C., von Wagner, C. and Raine, R. (2014). Reasons for non-uptake and subsequent participation in the NHS Bowel Cancer Screening Programme: a qualitative study. *British Journal of Cancer*, 110: 1705–11.

Palmer, R.H.C., McGeary, J.E., Francazio, S., Raphael, B.J., Lander, A.D., Heath, A.C. and Knopik, V.S. (2012). The genetics of alcohol dependence: advancing towards systems-based approaches. *Drug and Alcohol Dependence*, 125: 179–91.

Parent, M. and Bradstreet, T. (2017). Sexual orientation, bullying for being labeled gay or bisexual, and steroid use among US adolescent boys. *Journal of Health Psychology*, doi:10.1177/1359105317692144.

Paresce, D.M., Ghosh, R.N. and Maxfield, F.R. (1996). Microglial cells internalize aggregates of the Alzheimer's disease amyloid β-protein via a scavenger receptor. *Neuron*, 17 (3): 553–65.

Park, C.L., Folkman, S. and Bostrom, A. (2001). Appraisals of controllability and coping in caregivers and HIV men: testing the goodness-of-fit hypothesis. *Journal of Consulting & Clinical Psychology*, 69: 481–8.

Parker, I. (1997). Discursive psychology. In D. Fox and I. Prilleltensky (eds.), *Critical Psychology: An Introduction*. London: Sage.

Parker, R. and Aggleton, P. (2003). HIV and AIDS-related stigma and discrimination: a conceptual framework and implications for action. *Social Science & Medicine*, 57 (1): 13–24.

Parkes, C.M. (1965). Bereavement and mental illness, 2: A classification of bereavement reactions. *British Journal of Medical Psychology*, 38: 13–26.

Patel, S.R. and Hu, F.B. (2008). Short sleep duration and weight gain: a systematic review. *Obesity (Silver Spring)*, 16 (3): 643–53.

Patrick, D.L., Engelberg, R.A. and Curtis, J.R. (2001). Evaluating the quality of dying and death. *Journal of Pain and Symptom Management*, 22 (3): 717–26.

Patterson, L., Kee, F., Hughes, C. and O'Reilly, D. (2014). The relationship between BMI and the prescription of anti-obesity medication according to social factors: a population cross-sectional study. *BMC Public Health*, 14: 87.

Paul, N.W., Caplan, A., Shapiro, M.E., Els, C., Allison, K.C. and Li, H. (2017). Human rights violations in organ procurement practice in China. *BMC Medical Ethics*, 18 (1): 11.

Paulson, S. (2005). The social benefits of belonging to a dance exercise group for older people. *Generations Review*, 15: 37–41.

Paulson, S. (2011). The use of ethnography and narrative interviews in a study of 'cultures of dance'. *Journal of Health Psychology*, 16: 148–57.

Pavalko, E.K. and Caputo, J. (2013). Social inequality and health across the life course. *American Behavioral Scientist*, 57 (8): 1040–56.

Paxton, S.J., Neumark-Sztainer, D., Hannan, P.J. and Eisenberg, M.E. (2006). Body dissatisfaction prospectively predicts depressive mood and low self-esteem in adolescent girls and boys. *Journal of Clinical Child and Adolescent Psychology*, 35: 539–49.

Pearce, P.F. (2009). Physical activity: not just for quantitative researchers. *Qualitative Health Research*, 19: 879–80.

Pearl, R.L., Puhl, R.M. and Dovidio, J.F. (2015). Differential effects of weight bias experiences and internalization on exercise among women with overweight and obesity. *Journal of Health Psychology*, 20 (12): 1626–32.

Peckham, E.J., Nelson, E.A., Greenhalgh, J., Cooper, K., Roberts, E.R. and Agrawal, A. (2013). Homeopathy for treatment of irritable bowel syndrome. *Cochrane Database of Systematic Reviews*, 11 (CD009710).

Pellowski, J.A. and Kalichman, S.C. (2016). Health behavior predictors of medication adherence among low health literacy people living with HIV/AIDS. *Journal of Health Psychology*, 21 (9): 1981–91.

Pellowski, J.A., Kalichman, S.C., Matthews, K.A. and Adler, N. (2013). A pandemic of the poor: social disadvantage and the US HIV epidemic. *American Psychologist*, 68: 197–209.

Pelosi, A.J. (2019). Personality and fatal diseases: revisiting a scientific scandal. *Journal of Health Psychology*, 24 (4): 421–39.

Pennebaker, J.W. (1985). Traumatic experience and psychosomatic disease: exploring the roles of behavioural inhibition, obsession, and confiding. *Canadian Psychology/Psychologie Canadienne*, 26 (2): 82–95.

Pennebaker, J.W. (1995). *Emotion, Disclosure, and Health*. Washington, DC: American Psychological Association.

Penninx, B.W., Guralnik, J.M., Pahor, M., Ferrucci, L., Cerhan, J.R., Wallace, R.B. and Havlik, R.J. (1998). Chronically depressed mood and cancer risk in older persons. *Journal of the National Cancer Institute*, 90: 1888–93.

People's Health Movement (2000). *The People's Charter for Health*. Available: http://phmovement.org/ [accessed 16 June 2017].

Pereira-Santos, M., Costa, P.R.F., Assis, A.M.O. and Santos, D.B. (2015). Obesity and vitamin D deficiency: a systematic review and meta-analysis. *Obesity Reviews*, 16 (4): 341–9.

Permut, M. (2016). Psychological sense of community as an example of prefiguration among occupy protesters. *Journal of Social and Political Psychology*, 4 (1): 180–95. doi:10.5964/jspp.v4i1.533.

Perri, M.G., Foreyt, J.P. and Anton, S.D. (2004). Preventing weight regain after weight loss. *Handbook of Obesity: Clinical Applications*, 2: 185–99.

Perrier, M.-J. and Martin Ginis, K.A. (2017). Narrative interventions for health screening behaviours: a systematic review. *Journal of Health Psychology*, 22: 375–93.

Peters, G.Y., Ruiter, R.A.C. and Kok, G. (2014). Threatening communication: a qualitative study of fear appeal effectiveness beliefs among intervention developers, policymakers, politicians, scientists, and advertising professionals. *International Journal of Psychology*, 49 (2): 71–9.

Petrie, K.J., Cameron, L.D., Ellis, C.J., Buick, D. and Weinman, J. (2002). Changing illness perceptions after myocardial infarction: an early intervention randomized controlled trial. *Psychosomatic Medicine*, 64: 580–6.

Pettersen, B.J., Anousheh, R., Fan, J., Jaceldo-Siegl, K. and Fraser, G.E. (2012). Vegetarian diets and blood pressure among white subjects: results from the Adventist Health Study-2 (AHS-2). *Public Health Nutrition*, 15: 1909–16.

Petticrew, M., Bell, R. and Hunter, D. (2002). Influence of psychological coping on survival and recurrence in people with cancer: systematic review. *British Medical Journal*, 325: 1066–9.

Petticrew, M.P., Lee, K. and McKee, M. (2012). Type A behavior pattern and coronary heart disease: Philip Morris's 'Crown Jewel'. *American Journal of Public Health*, 102: 2018–25.

Pfeiffer, D.A. (2013). *Eating Fossil Fuels: Oil, Food and the Coming Crisis in Agriculture*. Gabriola, BC, Canada: New Society Publishers.

PFLAG (2017). www.pflag.org/about

Phillips, D.A. and Shonkoff, J.P. (eds.) (2000). *From Neurons to Neighborhoods: The Science of Early Childhood Development*. Washington, DC: National Academies Press.

Phillips, G., Felix, L., Galli, L., Patel, V. and Edwards, P. (2010). The effectiveness of m-health technologies for improving health and health services: a systematic review protocol. *BMC Research Notes*, 3 (1): 250.

Phua, J., Jin, S. and Hahn, J.M. (2017). Celebrity-endorsed e-cigarette brand Instagram advertisements: effects on young adults' attitudes towards e-cigarettes and smoking intentions. *Journal of Health Psychology*. doi:10.1177/1359105317693912.

Pickup, J.C., Holloway, M.F. and Samsi, K. (2015). Real-time continuous glucose monitoring in Type 1 diabetes: a qualitative framework analysis of patient narratives. *Diabetes Care*, 38 (4): 544–50.

Pierce, J.P. and Gilpin, E.A. (2002). Impact of over-the-counter sales on effectiveness of pharmaceutical aids for smoking cessation. *Journal of the American Medical Association*, 288: 1260–4.

Pincus, T., Griffith, J., Isenberg, D. and Pearce, S. (1997). The well-being questionnaire: testing the structure in groups with rheumatoid arthritis. *British Journal of Health Psychology*, 2: 167–74.

Pinhas, L., Toner, B.B., Ali, A., Garfinkel, G.E. and Stuckless, N. (1998). The effects of the ideal of female beauty on mood and body satisfaction. *International Journal of Eating Disorders*, 25: 223–6.

Pitceathly, C., Watson, M. and Cawthorn, A. (2013). Counseling and specific psychological treatments in common clinical settings: an overview. In T.N. Wise, M. Bondi and A. Constatini (eds.), *Psycho-Oncology*. Arlington, VA: American Psychiatric Publishing. pp. 117–44.

Pittas, A.G., Lau, J., Hu, F.B. and Dawson-Hughes, B. (2007). The role of vitamin D and calcium in Type 2 diabetes: a systematic review and meta-analysis. *The Journal of Clinical Endocrinology & Metabolism*, 92 (6): 2017–29.

Pittler, M.H. and Ernst, E. (2000). Ginkgo biloba extract for the treatment of intermittent claudication: a meta-analysis of randomized trials. *American Journal of Medicine*, 108: 276–81.

Pittler, M.H. and Ernst, E. (2003). Kava extract versus placebo for treating anxiety. *Cochrane Database of Systematic Reviews*, 1 (CD003383).

Plant, M. (2004). Editorial: the alcohol harm reduction strategy for England. *British Medical Journal*, 328: 905–6.

Plant, M. and Plant, M. (2006). *Binge Britain: Alcohol and the National Response*. Oxford: Oxford University Press.

Platt, L., Melendez-Torres, G.J., O'Donnell, A., Bradley, J., Newbury-Birch, D., Kaner, E. and Ashton, C. (2016). How effective are brief interventions in reducing alcohol consumption: do the setting, practitioner group and content matter? Findings from a systematic review and metaregression analysis. *BMJ Open*, 6 (8): e011473.

Poag-DuCharme, K.A. and Brawley, L.R. (1993). Self-efficacy theory: use in the prediction of exercise behavior in the community setting. *Journal of Applied Sport Psychology*, 5: 178–94.

Polderman, T.J., Benyamin, B., De Leeuw, C.A., Sullivan, P.F., Van Bochoven, A., Visscher, P.M. et al. (2015). Meta-analysis of the heritability of human traits based on fifty years of twin studies. *Nature Genetics*, 47 (7): 702–9.

Polito, J.R. (2008). Smoking cessation trials. *Canadian Medical Association Journal*, 179: 10.

Polivy, J., Herman, C.P. and Warsh, S. (1978). Internal and external components of emotionality in restrained and unrestrained eaters. *Journal of Abnormal Psychology*, 87: 497–504.

Pollard, S., Bansback, N. and Bryan, S. (2015). Physician attitudes toward shared decision making: a systematic review. *Patient Education & Counseling*, 98 (9): 1046–57. doi:10.1016/j.pec.2015.05.004.

Pollock, B.D., Chen, W., Harville, E., Zhao, Q. and Bazzano, L. (2016). Abstract P208: anger during young adulthood increases the risk of developing coronary heart disease. *Circulation*, 133 (suppl. 1).

Pomerleau, O.F. (1979). Behavioral factors in the establishment, maintenance, and cessation of smoking. *NIDA Research Monograph*, (26): 47.

Posadzki, P., Alotaibi, A. and Ernst, E. (2012). Adverse effects of homeopathy: a systematic review of published case reports and case series. *International Journal of Clinical Practice*, 66: 1178–88.

Posadzki, P., Watson, L.K., Alotaibi, A. and Ernst, E. (2013a). Prevalence of use of complementary and alternative medicine (CAM) by patients/consumers in the UK: systematic review of surveys. *Clinical Medicine*, 13: 126–31.

Posadzki, P., Watson, L.K., Alotaibi, A. and Ernst, E. (2013b). Prevalence of herbal medicine use by UK patients/consumers: a systematic review of surveys. *Focus on Alternative & Complementary Therapies*, 18: 19–26.

Posluszny, D., Spencer, S. and Baum, A. (2007). Post-traumatic stress disorder. In S. Ayers, A. Baum, C. McManus, S. Newman, K. Wallston, J. Weinman and R. West (eds.), *Cambridge

Handbook of Psychology, Health and Medicine (2nd edn). Cambridge: Cambridge University Press. pp. 814–20.

Potter, J. and Wetherell, M. (1987). *Discourse and Social Psychology*. London: Sage.

Potvin, L., Camirand, J. and Beland, F. (1995). Patterns of health services utilization and mammography use among women aged 50–59 in the Québec Medicare system. *Medical Care*, 33: 515–30.

Pourhabib, S., Chessex, C., Murray, J. and Grace, S.L. (2016). Elements of patient-health-care provider communication related to cardiovascular rehabilitation referral. *Journal of Health Psychology*, 21 (4): 468–82. doi:10.1177/1359105314529319.

Prabhu, A., Obi, K.O. and Rubenstein, J.H. (2014). The synergistic effects of alcohol and tobacco consumption on the risk of esophageal squamous cell carcinoma: a meta-analysis. *American Journal of Gastroenterology*, 109 (6): 822–7.

Prescott-Clarke, P. and Primatesta, P. (eds.) (1998). *Health Survey for England 95–97*. London: The Stationery Office.

Prestwich, A., Conner, M., Hurling, R., Ayres, K. and Morris, B. (2016). An experimental test of control theory-based interventions for physical activity. *British Journal of Health Psychology*, 21: 812–26.

Prestwich, A., Sniehotta, F.F., Whittington, C., Dombrowski, S.U., Rogers, L. and Michie, S. (2014). Does theory influence the effectiveness of health behaviour interventions? Meta analysis. *Health Psychology*, 33: 465–74.

Price, A., McCormack, R., Wiseman, T. and Hotopf, M. (2014). Concepts of mental capacity for patients requesting assisted suicide: a qualitative analysis of expert evidence presented to the commission on assisted dying. *BMC Medical Ethics*, 15: 32.

Priest, J. (2007). The healing balm effect: using a walking group to feel better. *Journal of Health Psychology*, 12: 36–52.

Priest, N., Paradies, Y., Trenerry, B., Truong, M., Karlsen, S. and Kelly, Y. (2013). A systematic review of studies examining the relationship between reported racism and health and wellbeing for children and young people. *Social Science & Medicine*, 95: 115–27.

Prochaska, J.O. (2006). Moving beyond the transtheoretical model. *Addiction*, 101 (6): 768–74.

Prochaska, J.O. and DiClemente, C.C. (1983). Stages and processes of self-change of smoking: toward an integrative model of change. *Journal of Consulting & Clinical Psychology*, 51: 390–5.

Prochaska, J.O. and DiClemente, C.C. (1992). *The Transtheoretical Approach: Crossing the Traditional Boundaries of Therapy*. Homewood, IL: Dow Jones/Irwin.

Prochaska, J.O. and Velicer, W.F. (1997). The transtheoretical model of health behavior change. *American Journal of Health Promotion*, 12 (1): 38–48.

Protheroe, J. and Rowlands, G. (2013). Matching clinical information with levels of patient health literacy. *Nursing Management – UK*, 20 (3): 20–1.

Protheroe, J., Estacio, E.V. and Saidy-Khan, S. (2015). Observational study of patient information materials in GP practices: Are they promoting health literacy? *British Journal of General Practice*, 65 (632): e192–7. doi: 10.3399/bjgp15X684013.

Protheroe, J., Whittle, R., Bartlam, B., Estacio, E.V., Clark, L. and Kurth, J. (2016). Health literacy, associated lifestyle and demographic factors in adult population of an English city: a cross-sectional survey. *Health Expectations: An International Journal of Public Participation in Health Care and Health Policy*. doi:10.1111/hex.12440.

Punyacharoensin, N., Edmunds, W.J., De Angelis, D., Delpech, V., Hart, G., Elford, J. et al. (2016). Effect of pre-exposure prophylaxis and combination HIV prevention for men who have sex with men in the UK: a mathematical modelling study. *The Lancet HIV*, 3 (2): e94–104.

Putnam, R. (2000). *Bowling Alone: The Collapse and Revival of American Community*. New York: Simon & Schuster.

Putnam, R.D., Leonarchi, R. and Nanetti, R.Y. (1993). *Making Democracy Work: Civic Traditions in Modern Italy*. Princeton, NJ: Princeton University Press.

Qureshi, S.U., Pyne, J.M., Magruder, K.M., Schulz, P.E. and Kunik, M.E. (2009). The link between post-traumatic stress disorder and physical comorbidities: a systematic review. *Psychiatric Quarterly*, 80: 87–97.

Ragland, D.R. and Brand, R.J. (1988). Type A behaviour and mortality from coronary heart disease. *The New England Journal of Medicine*, 318: 65–9.

Raistrick, D. (2005). The United Kingdom: alcohol today. *Addiction*, 100: 1212–14.

Rajguru, P., Kolber, M.J., Garcia, A.N., Smith, M.T., Patel, C.K. and Hanney, W.J. (2014). Use of mindfulness meditation in the management of chronic pain: a systematic review of randomized controlled trials. *American Journal of Lifestyle Medicine*, 9 (3): 176–84.

Rakowski, W., Dube, C.E. Marcus, B.H., Prochaska, J.O., Velicer, W.F. and Abrams, D.B. (1992). Assessing elements of women's decisions about mammography. *Health Psychology*, 11: 111–18.

Ramraj, C., Shahidi, F.V., Darity, W., Kawachi, I., Zuberi, D. and Siddiqi, A. (2016). Equally inequitable? A cross-national comparative study of racial health inequalities in the United States and Canada. *Social Science & Medicine*, 161: 19–26.

Ranby, K.W. and Aiken, L.S. (2016). Incorporating husband influences into a model of physical activity among older women. *British Journal of Health Psychology*, 21: 677–93.

Rassool, G. H. (2000). The crescent and Islam: healing, nursing and the spiritual dimension. Some considerations towards an understanding of the Islamic perspectives on caring. *Journal of Advanced Nursing*, 32 (6): 1476–84.

Rathert, C., Mittler, J.N., Banerjee, S. and McDaniel, J. (2017). Patient-centered communication in the era of electronic health records: What does the evidence say? *Patient Education & Counseling*, 100 (1): 50–64. doi:10.1016/j.pec.2016.07.031.

Rathert, C., Wyrwich, M.D. and Boren, S.A. (2013). Patient-centered care and outcomes: a systematic review of the literature. *Medical Care Research & Review*, 70 (4): 351–79. doi:10.1177/1077558712465774.

Rawls, J. (1999). *A Theory of Justice*. Cambridge, MA: Belknap Press.

Ray, C., Weir, W., Stewart, D., Miller, P. and Hyde, G. (1993). Ways of coping with chronic fatigue syndrome: development of an illness management questionnaire. *Social Science & Medicine*, 37: 385–91.

Reed, D.M., LaCroix, A.Z., Karasek, R.A., Miller, D. and MacLean, C.A. (1989). Occupational strain and the incidence of coronary heart disease. *American Journal of Epidemiology*, 129: 495–502.

Rees, G., Lamoureux, E.L., Xie, J., Sturrock, B.A. and Fenwick, E.K. (2015). Using Rasch analysis to evaluate the validity of the diabetes-specific version of the Illness Perception Questionnaire–Revised. *Journal of Health Psychology*, 20 (10): 1340–56.

Rees, K., Bennett, P., West, R., Davey, S.G. and Ebrahim, S. (2004). Psychological interventions for coronary heart disease. *Cochrane Database of Systematic Reviews*, 2 (CD002902).

Reiter, P.L., Brewer, N.T., Gottlieb, S.L., McRee, A.-L. and Smith, J.S. (2009). Parents' health beliefs and HPV vaccination of their adolescent daughters. *Social Science & Medicine*, 69: 475–80.

Renzaho, A.M.N., Romios, P., Crock, C. and Sønderlund, A.L. (2013). The effectiveness of cultural competence programs in ethnic minority patient centered health care: a systematic review of the literature. *International Journal for Quality in Health Care*, 25: 261–9.

Reyna, V.F. (2012). Risk perception and communication in vaccination decisions: a fuzzy-trace theory approach. *Vaccine*, 30: 3790–7.

Rhodes, R.E. and de Bruyn, G.-J. (2013). How big is the physical activity intention–behaviour gap? A meta-analysis using the action control framework. *British Journal of Health Psychology*, 18: 296–309.

Rhodes, R.E., Courneya, K.S., Blanchard, C.M. and Plotnikoff, R.C. (2007). Prediction of leisure-time walking: an integration of social cognitive, perceived environmental, and personality factors. *International Journal of Behavioral Nutrition and Physical Activity*, 4: 51.

Rhodes, R.E. and Dickau, L. (2012) Experimental evidence for the intention-behavior relationship in the physical activity domain: a meta-analysis. *Health Psychology*, 31 (6): 724–7.

Richardson, S., Shaffer, J.A., Falzon, L., Krupka, D., Davidson, K.W. and Edmondson, D. (2012). Meta-analysis of perceived stress and its association with incident coronary heart disease. *American Journal of Cardiology*, 110: 1711–16.

Richter, C. (1942). Total self-regulatory functions in animals and human beings. *Harvey Lecture Series*, 38: 63–103.

Richter, C.P. (1967). Sleep and activity: their relation to the 24-hour clock. *Research Publications: Association for Research in Nervous and Mental Disease*, 45, 8.

Riesen, W.F., Darioli, R. and Noll, G. (2004). Lipid-lowering therapy: strategies for improving compliance. *Current Medical Research & Opinion*, 20: 165–73.

Riess, H., Kelley, J.M., Bailey, R.W., Dunn, E.J. and Phillips, M. (2012). Empathy training for resident physicians: a randomized controlled trial of a neuroscience-informed curriculum. *Journal of General Internal Medicine*, 27 (10): 1280–6.

Riley, B.D., Culver, J.O., Skrzynia, C., Senter, L.A., Peters, J.A., Costalas, J.W. et al. (2012). Essential elements of genetic cancer risk assessment, counseling, and testing: updated recommendations of the National Society of Genetic Counselors. *Journal of Genetic Counseling*, 21 (2): 151–61.

Riley, K.E. and Kalichman, S. (2014). Mindfulness-based stress reduction for people living with HIV/AIDS: preliminary review of intervention trial methodologies and findings. *Health Psychology Review*, 9 (2): 224–43.

Rimal, R.N. (2001). Longitudinal influences of knowledge and self-efficacy on exercise behavior: tests of a mutual reinforcement model. *Journal of Health Psychology*, 6: 31–46.

Rimer, B.K., Keintz, M.K., Kessler, H.B., Engstrom, P.F. and Rosan, J.R. (1989). Why women resist screening mammography: patient-related barriers. *Radiology*, 74: 2034–41.

Riper, H., Blankers, M., Hadiwijaya, H., Cunningham, J., Clarke, S., Wiers, R. et al. (2014). Effectiveness of guided and unguided low-intensity internet interventions for adult alcohol misuse: a meta-analysis. *PLoS One*, 9 (6): e99912.

Riska, E. (2000). The rise and fall of Type A man. *Social Science & Medicine*, 51: 1665–74.

Rivera-Ramos, Z.A. and Buki, L.P. (2011). I will no longer be a man! Manliness and prostate cancer screenings among Latino men. *Psychology of Men and Masculinity*, 12 (1): 13–25.

Rizzo, N.S., Sabate, J., Jaceldo-Siegl, K. and Fraser, G.E. (2011). Vegetarian dietary patterns are associated with a lower risk of the metabolic syndrome: the adventist health study 2. *Diabetes Care*, 34: 1225–7.

Robinson, M., Oddy, W., McLean, N., Jacoby, P., Pennell, C.E., de Klerk, N. et al. (2010). Low–moderate prenatal alcohol exposure and risk to child behavioural development: a prospective cohort study. *British Journal of Obstetrics and Gynaecology*, 117: 1139–52.

Roche, A.M. and Freeman, T. (2004). Brief interventions: good in theory but weak in practice. *Drug & Alcohol Review*, 23: 11–18.

Rochelle, T.L. and Marks, D.F. (2010). Medical pluralism of the Chinese in London: an exploratory study. *British Journal of Health Psychology*, 15: 715–28.

Rodgers, R.F., Salès, P. and Chabrol, H. (2010). Psychological functioning, media pressure and body dissatisfaction among college women. *Revue Européenne de Psychologie Appliquée/European Review of Applied Psychology*, 60: 89–95.

Rodin, J. (1973). Effects of distraction on performance of obese and normal subjects. *Journal of Comparative and Physiological Psychology*, 83: 68–75.

Rodin, G., Mackay, J.A., Zimmermann, C., et al. (2009) Clinician-patient communication: a systematic review. *Support Care Cancer*, 17(6): 627–44.

Roerecke, M. and Rehm, J. (2012). The cardioprotective association of average alcohol consumption and ischaemic heart disease: a systematic review and meta-analysis. *Addiction*, 107: 1246–60.

Rogers, C.R. (1957). The necessary and sufficient conditions of therapeutic personality change. *Journal of Consulting Psychology*, 21 (2): 95–103.

Rogers, R.W. (1975). A protection motivation theory of fear appeals and attitude change. *Journal of Psychology*, 91 (1): 93–114.

Rohleder, P. (2016). Disability and HIV in Africa: breaking the barriers to sexual health care. *Journal of Health Psychology*, first published 18 February. doi:10.1177/1359105316628738.

Rohleder, P. and Flowers, P. (eds.). (2018). Special Issue on Sexual Health Psychology: Exploring new directions. *Journal of Health Psychology*, 23 (2): 143–7.

Rollnick, S. and Miller, W.R. (1995). What is motivational interviewing? *Behavioural and Cognitive Psychotherapy*, 23 (4): 325–34.

Rollnick, S., Heather, N. and Bell, A. (1992). Negotiating behaviour change in medical settings: the development of brief motivational interviewing. *Journal of Mental Health*, 1 (1): 25–37.

Ronksley, P.E., Brien, S.E., Turner, B.J., Mukamal, K.J. and Ghali, W.A. (2011). Association of alcohol consumption with selected cardiovascular disease outcomes: a systematic review and meta-analysis. *British Medical Journal*, 342: d671.

Rootman, I. and Gordon-El-Bihbety, D. (2008). *A Vision for a Health Literate Canada*. Ottawa: CPHA.

Rosberger, Z., Edgar, L., Collet, J.-P. and Fournier, M.A. (2002). Patterns of coping in women completing treatment for breast cancer: a randomized controlled trial of Nucare, a brief psychoeducational workshop. *Journal of Psychosocial Oncology*, 20: 19–37. doi:10.1300/J077v20n03_02.

Roseman, M., Milette, K., Bero, L.A., Coyne, J.C., Lexchin, J., Turner, E.H. and Thombs, B.D. (2011). Reporting of conflicts of interest in meta-analyses of trials of pharmacological treatments. *JAMA*, 305: 1008–17.

Rosen, R.C., Riley, A., Wagner, G., Osterloh, I.H., Kirkpatrick, J. and Mishra, A. (1997). The international index of erectile function (IIEF): a multidimensional scale for assessment of erectile dysfunction. *Urology*, 49 (6): 822–30.

Rosenberg, M. (1965). *Society and the Adolescent Self-Image*. Princeton, NJ: Princeton University Press.

Rosengren, A., Tibblin, G. and Wilhelmsen, L. (1991). Self-perceived psychological stress and incidence of coronary artery disease in middle-aged men. *American Journal of Cardiology*, 68: 1171–5.

Rosenstock, I.M. (1966). Why people use health services. *Milbank Memorial Fund Quarterly*, 44: 94–127.

Rosenthal, L., Earnshaw, V.A., Carroll-Scott, A., Henderson, K.E., Peters, S.M., McCaslin, C. and Ickovics, J.R. (2015). Weight- and race-based bullying: health associations among urban adolescents. *Journal of Health Psychology*, 20 (4): 401–12.

Ross, C.E. (2000). Walking, exercising, and smoking: Does neighborhood matter? *Social Science & Medicine*, 51: 265–74.

Rotblatt, M. and Ziment, I. (2002). *Evidence-Based Herbal Medicine*. Philadelphia, PA: Hanley and Belfus.

Roth, R., Lynch, K., Hyöty, H., Lönnrot, M., Driscoll, K.A., Bennett Johnson, S., and TEDDY Study Group (2019). The association between stressful life events and respiratory infections during the first 4 years of life: The Environmental Determinants of Diabetes in the Young study. *Stress and Health*, 35 (3): 289–303.

Rothman, A.J. and Salovey, P. (1997). Shaping perceptions to motivate healthy behaviour: the role of message framing. *Psychological Bulletin*, 121: 3–19.

Rothman, K. and Keller, A. (1972). The effect of joint exposure to alcohol and tobacco on risk of cancer of the mouth and pharynx. *Journal of Chronic Diseases*, 25: 711–16.

Ruby, M.B., Dunn, E.W., Perrino, A., Gillis, R. and Viel, S. (2011). The invisible benefits of exercise. *Health Psychology*, 38: 67–74.

Rudman, L.A., Glick, P., Marquardt, T. and Fetterolf, J.C. (2016). When women are urged to have casual sex more than men are: perceived risk moderates the sexual advice double standard. *Sex Roles*, 75 (5–6): 1–10. doi:10.1007/s11199-016-0723-x.

Ruiter, R.A.C., Kessels, L.T.E., Peters, G.Y. and Kok, G. (2014). Sixty years of fear appeal research: current state of the evidence. *International Journal of Psychology*, 49 (2): 63–70.

Russell, J.A. (2003). Core affect and the psychological construction of emotion. *Psychological Review*, 110 (1): 145–72.

Rutherford, L., Hinchcliffe, S. and Clarke, C. (eds.) (2013). *Scottish Health Survey 2012*. Edinburgh: ScotCen Social Research.

Rutledge, T., Reis, V.A., Linke, S.E., Greenberg, B.H. and Mills, P.J. (2006). Depression in heart failure – a meta-analytic review of prevalence, intervention effects, and associations with clinical outcomes. *Journal of the American College of Cardiology*, 48: 1527–37.

Ryan, R.M. and Deci, E.L. (2001). On happiness and human potentials: a review of research on hedonic and eudaimonic well-being. *Annual Review of Psychology*, 52 (1): 141–66.

Rytwinski, N.K., Avena, J.S., Echiverri-Cohen, A.M., Zoellner, L.A. and Feeny, N.C. (2014). The relationship between posttraumatic stress disorder severity, depression severity and physical health. *Journal of Health Psychology*, 19: 509–20.

Sabina, C., Wolak, J. and Finkelhor, D. (2008). The nature and dynamics of internet pornography exposure for youth. *CyberPsychology & Behavior*, 11 (6): 691–93.

Sadeghi, S., Brooks, D. and Goldstein, R.S. (2013). Patients' and providers' perceptions of the impact of health literacy on communication in pulmonary rehabilitation. *Chronic Respiratory Disease*, 10 (2): 65–76.

Sadler, E., Hales, B., Henry, B., Xiong, W., Myers, J., Wynnychuk, L. et al. (2014). Factors affecting family satisfaction with inpatient end-of-life care. *PloS One*, 9 (11): e110860.

Saffer, H. and Dave, D. (2002). Alcohol consumption and alcohol advertising bans. *Applied Economics*, 34: 1325–34.

Saha, S., Mundle, M., Ghosh, S., Koley, M. and Sheikh, I.H. (2013). Qualitative systematic review of homeopathic outcome studies in patients with HIV/AIDS. *International Journal of High Dilution Research*, 12: 2–12.

Salisbury, C.M. and Fisher, W.A. (2014). 'Did you come?' A qualitative exploration of gender differences in beliefs, experiences, and concerns regarding female orgasm occurrence during heterosexual sexual interactions. *The Journal of Sex Research*, 51 (6): 616–31.

Sallis, J.F., Bauman, A. and Pratt, M. (1998). Environmental and policy interventions to promote physical activity. *American Journal of Preventive Medicine*, 15: 379–97.

Sallis, J.F., King, A.C., Sirard, J.R. and Albright, C.L. (2007). Perceived environmental predictors of physical activity over six months in adults: activity counseling trial. *Health Psychology*, 26: 701–9.

Salmon, J., Owen, N., Crawford, D., Bauman, A. and Sallis, J.F. (2003). Physical activity and sedentary behavior: a population-based study of barriers, enjoyment, and preference. *Health Psychology*, 22: 178–188.

Samuel, L.J., Commodore-Mensah, Y. and Dennison Himmelfarb, C.R. (2014). Developing behavioral theory with the systematic integration of community social capital concepts. *Health Education & Behavior*, 41 (4): 359–75. doi:10.1177/1090198113504412.

Sánchez, A., Silvestre, C., Campo, N., Grandes, G. and PreDE research group. (2016). Type-2 diabetes primary prevention program implemented in routine primary care: a process evaluation study. *Trials*, 17 (1): 254.

Sandesara, P.B., Lambert, C.T., Gordon, N.F., Fletcher, G.F., Franklin, B.A., Wenger, N.K. and Sperling, L. (2015). Cardiac rehabilitation and risk reduction: time to 'rebrand and reinvigorate'. *Journal of the American College of Cardiology*, 65: 389–95.

Sano, Y., Antabe, R., Atuoye, K.N., Hussey, L.K., Bayne, J., Galaa, S.Z. et al. (2016). Persistent misconceptions about HIV transmission among males and females in Malawi. *BMC International Health & Human Rights*, 16: 1–10. doi:10.1186/s12914-016-0089-8.

Sartre, J.P. (1964). *Les Mots*. Paris: Gallimard.

Savell, E., Fooks, G. and Gilmore, A.B. (2016). How does the alcohol industry attempt to influence marketing regulations? A systematic review. *Addiction*, 111 (1): 18–32.

Sayette, M.A. (2007). Alcohol abuse. In S. Ayers, A. Baum, C. McManus, S. Newman, K. Wallston, J. Weinman and R. West (eds.), *Cambridge Handbook of Psychology, Health and Medicine* (2nd edn). Cambridge: Cambridge University Press. pp. 534–7.

Sayette, M.A. (2017). The effects of alcohol on emotion in social drinkers. *Behaviour Research and Therapy*, 88: 76–89.

Schachter, S. and Rodin, J. (1974). *Obese Humans and Rats*. Hove: Lawrence Erlbaum.

Schaefer Ziemer, K. and Hoffman, M.A. (2013). Beliefs and attitudes regarding human papillomavirus vaccination among college-age women. *Journal of Health Psychology*, 18 (10): 1360–70.

Scheib, H.A. and Lykes, M.B. (2013). African American and Latina community health workers engage PhotoPAR as a resource in a post-disaster context: Katrina at 5 years. *Journal of Health Psychology*, 18: 1069–84.

Scheibe, M., Reichelt, J., Bellmann, M. and Kirch, W. (2015). Acceptance factors of mobile apps for diabetes by patients aged 50 or older: a qualitative study. *Medicine 2.0*, 4 (1): e1.

Schellong, K., Schulz, S., Harder, T. and Plagemann, A. (2012). Birth weight and long-term overweight risk: systematic review and a meta-analysis including 643,902 persons from 66 studies and 26 countries globally. *PLoS One*, 7 (10): e47776.

Schmidt, H.M., Munder, T., Gerger, H., Frühauf, S. and Barth, J. (2014). Combination of psychological intervention and phosphodiesterase-5 inhibitors for erectile dysfunction: a narrative review and meta-analysis. *The Journal of Sexual Medicine*, 11 (6): 1376–91.

Schnoll, R., Harlow, L., Stolbach, L. and Brandt, U. (1998). A structural model of the relationships among stage of disease, age, coping, and psychological adjustment in women with breast cancer. *Psycho-Oncology*, 7: 69–77.

Schober, R. (1997). Complementary and conventional medicines working together. *Canadian Health Psychologist*, 5: 14–18.

Schofield, P.E., Stockler, M.R., Zannino, D., Tebbutt, N.C., Price, T.J., Simes, R.J. et al. (2016). Hope, optimism and survival in a randomised trial of chemotherapy for metastatic colorectal cancer. *Supportive Care in Cancer*, 24 (1): 401–8.

Schulz, P.J. and Nakamoto, K. (2013). Health literacy and patient empowerment in health communication: the importance of separating conjoined twins. *Patient Education and Counseling*, 90 (1): 4–11.

Schumacher, J.R., Hall, A.G., Davis, T.C., Arnold, C.L., Bennett, R.D., Wolf, M.S. and Carden, D.L. (2013). Potentially preventable use of emergency services: the role of low health literacy. *Medical Care*, 51 (8): 654–8.

Schuster, J., Ganapathi, S., Pagunutti, T. et al. (2006). *AIDS, alcohol and violence against women: strategies for reducing workplace health risks to Cambodian beer-selling women*. Paper presented at the XVI International AIDS Conference, Toronto, Canada, 13–18 August 2006.

Schütze, M., Boeing, H., Pischon, T., Rehm, J., Kehoe, T., Gmel, G. et al. (2011). Alcohol attributable burden of incidence of cancer in eight European countries based on results from prospective cohort study. *British Medical Journal*, 342. doi:10.1136/bmj.d1584.

Schwartz, M., Savage, W., George, J. and Emohare, L. (1989). Women's knowledge and experience of cervical screening: a failure of health education and medical organization. *Community Medicine*, 11: 279–89.

Scott, S., Curnock, E., Mitchel, R., Robinson, M., Taulbut, M., Tod, E. and McCartney, G. (2013). *What Would It Take to Eradicate Health Inequalities? Testing the Fundamental Causes Theory of Health Inequalities in Scotland*. Glasgow: NHS Health Scotland.

Scottish Government (2008). *Equally Well*. Report of the Ministerial Task Force on Health Inequalities. Available: www.scotland.gov.uk/Resource/Doc/229649/0062206.pdf [accessed 6 August 2014].

Scott-Sheldon, L.A., Carey, M.P., Carey, K.B., Cain, D., Vermaak, R. and Mthembu, J. (2013). Does perceived life stress mediate the association between HIV status and alcohol use? Evidence from adults living in Cape Town, South Africa. *AIDS Care*, 25: 1026–32.

Scott-Sheldon, L.A.J., Kalichman, S.C., Carey, M.P. and Fielder, R.L. (2008). Stress management interventions for HIV+ adults: a meta-analysis of randomized controlled trials, 1989 to 2006. *Health Psychology*, 27: 129–39.

Seacat, J.D., Dougal, S.C. and Roy, D. (2016). A daily diary assessment of female weight stigmatization. *Journal of Health Psychology*, 21 (2): 228–40.

Searle, A., Haase, A.M., Chalder, M., Fox, K.R., Taylor, A.H., Lewis, G. and Turner, K.M. (2014). Participants' experiences of facilitated physical activity for the management of depression in primary care. *Journal of Health Psychology*, 19 (11): 1430–42.

Sedgh, G., Singh, S. and Hussain, R. (2014). Intended and unintended pregnancies worldwide in 2012 and recent trends. *Studies in Family Planning*, 45 (3): 301–14.

Sedgh, G., Singh, S., Shah, I.H., Åhman, E., Henshaw, S.K. and Bankole, A. (2012). Induced abortion: incidence and trends worldwide from 1995 to 2008. *The Lancet*, 379 (9816): 625–32.

Segar, J. (2012). Complementary and alternative medicine: exploring the gap between evidence and usage. *Health*, 16 (4): 366–81.

Seitz, D.C.M., Besier, T. and Goldbeck, L. (2009). Psychosocial interventions for adolescent cancer patients: a systematic review of the literature. *Psycho-Oncology*, 18: 683–90.

Seligman, M.E. and Csikszentmihalyi, M. (2000). *Positive Psychology: An Introduction*. Washington, DC: American Psychological Association.

Seligman, M.E., Steen, T.A., Park, N. and Peterson, C. (2005). Positive psychology progress: empirical validation of interventions. *American Psychologist*, 60 (5): 410.

Selye, H. (1976). *Stress in Health and Disease*. Reading, MA: Butterworth.

Sen, A. (1999). *Development as Freedom*. Oxford: Oxford University Press.

Shah, N.R. and Braverman, E.R. (2012). Measuring adiposity in patients: the utility of body mass index (BMI), percent body fat, and leptin. *PLoS One*, 10: 1371.

Shah, S.K., Kasper, K. and Miller, F.G. (2015). A narrative review of the empirical evidence on public attitudes on brain death and vital organ transplantation: the need for better data to inform policy. *Journal of Medical Ethics*, 41 (4): 291–6.

Shakespeare, T. (1998). Choices and rights: eugenics, genetics and disability equality. *Disability & Society*, 13: 665–81.

Shamloul, R. and Ghanem, H. (2013). Erectile dysfunction. *The Lancet*, 381 (9861): 153–65.

Shannon, C.E. and Weaver, W. (1949). *The Mathematical Theory of Communication*. Urbana, IL: University of Illinois.

Shaper, A.G., Wannamethee, G. and Walker, M. (1988). Alcohol and mortality in British men: explaining the U-shaped curve. *The Lancet*, 2: 1267–83.

Sharp, D.J., Peter, T.J., Bartholomew, J. and Shaw, A. (1996). Breast screening: a randomised controlled trial in UK general practice of three generations designed to increase uptake. *Journal of Epidemiology and Community Health*, 50: 72–5.

Sharpe, K. and Earle, S. (2002). Feminism, abortion and disability: Irreconcilable differences? *Disability & Society*, 17: 137–45.

Sharpe, M.C., Archard, L.C., Banatvala, J.E., Borysiewicz, L.K., Clare, A.W., David, A. et al. (1991). A report – chronic fatigue syndrome: guidelines for research. *Journal of the Royal Society of Medicine*, 84 (2): 118–21.

Shaw, S. (1979). A critique of the concept of the alcohol dependence syndrome. *British Journal of Addiction*, 74: 339–48.

Sheeran, P., Abraham, C. and Orbell, S. (1999). Psychosocial correlates of heterosexual condom use: a meta-analysis. *Psychological Bulletin*, 125 (1): 90–132.

Sherwin, B.B. (1997). Estrogen effects on cognition in menopausal women. *Neurology*, 48 (5 suppl. 7): S21–6.

Shields, C.A. and Brawley, L.R. (2007). Limiting exercise options: depending on a proxy may inhibit exercise self-management. *Journal of Health Psychology*, 12: 663–71.

Shinya, K., Ebina, M., Yamada, S., Ono, M., Kasai, N. and Kawaoka, Y. (2006). Avian flu: influenza virus receptors in the human airway. *Nature*, 440: 435–6.

Siegel, S. (1975). Conditioned insulin effects. *Journal of Comparative Physiology & Psychology*, 89: 189–99.

Sieverding, M., Matterne, U. and Ciccarello, L. (2010). What role do social norms play in the context of men's cancer screening intention and behavior? Application of an extended theory of planned behavior. *Health Psychology*, 29: 72–81.

Sijtsma, K. (2012). Psychological measurement between physics and statistics. *Theory & Psychology*, 22: 786–809.

Silva, S.A., Pires, A.P., Guerreiro, C. and Cardoso, A. (2013). Balancing motherhood and drug addiction: the transition to parenthood of addicted mothers. *Journal of Health Psychology*, 18: 359–67.

Simpson, C., Griffin, B. and Mazzeo, S. (2017). Psychological and behavioral effects of obesity prevention campaigns. *Journal of Health Psychology*. doi:10.1177/135910531 7693913.

Simpson, S.J. and Raubenheimer, D. (2012). *The Nature of Nutrition: A Unifying Framework*. Princeton, NJ: Princeton University Press.

Sin, N.L., Kumar, A.D., Gehi, A.K. and Whooley, M.A. (2016). Direction of association between depressive symptoms and lifestyle behaviors in patients with coronary heart disease: the Heart and Soul Study. *Annals of Behavioral Medicine*, 50 (4): 523–32.

Sinha, S., Curtis, K., Jayakody, A., Viner, R. and Roberts, H. (2007). 'People make assumptions about our communities': sexual health amongst teenagers from Black and Minority Ethnic backgrounds in East London. *Ethnicity & Health*, 12: 423–41.

Singer, P. (1993). *Practical Ethics*. Cambridge: Cambridge University Press.

Singer, P.A., Martin, D.K. and Kelner, M. (1999). Quality end-of-life care: patients' perspectives. *Journal of the American Medical Association*, 281: 163–8.

Skinner, C. and Spurgeon, P. (2005). Valuing empathy and emotional intelligence in health leadership: a study of empathy, leadership behaviour and outcome effectiveness. *Health Services Management Research*, 18 (1): 1–12.

Skinner, C.S., Champion, V.L., Gonin, R. and Hanna, M. (1997). Do perceived barriers and benefits vary by mammography stage? *Psychology, Health & Medicine*, 2: 65–75.

Skinner, D. and Claassens, M. (2016). It's complicated: Why do tuberculosis patients not initiate or stay adherent to treatment? A qualitative study from South Africa. *BMC Infectious Diseases*, 16: 1–9. doi:10.1186/s12879-016-2054-5.

Skogerbø, Å., Kesmodel, U., Wimberley, T., Støvring, H., Bertrand, J., Landrø, N. and Mortensen, E. (2012). The effects of low to moderate alcohol consumption and binge drinking in early pregnancy on executive function in 5-year-old children. *British Journal of Obstetrics and Gynaecology*, 119: 1201–10.

Slater, A. and Tiggemann, M. (2006). The contribution of physical activity and media UK during childhood and adolescence to adult women's body image. *Journal of Health Psychology*, 11: 553–65.

Sleasman, J.W. and Goodenow, M.M. (2003). HIV-1 infection. *Journal of Allergy & Clinical Immunology*, 111: S582–92.

Slenker, S. and Grant, M. (1989). Attitudes, beliefs and knowledge about mammography among women over forty years of age. *Journal of Cancer Education*, 4: 61–5.

Slenker, S.E. and Spreitzer, E.A. (1988). Public perceptions and behaviors regarding cancer control. *Journal of Cancer Education*, 3: 171–80.

Smedslund, G. (2000). A pragmatic basis for judging models and theories in health psychology: the axiomatic method. *Journal of Health Psychology*, 5: 133–49.

Smee, C., Parsonage, M., Anderson, R. and Duckworth, S. (1992). *Effect of Tobacco Advertising on Tobacco Consumption: A Discussion Document Reviewing the Evidence*. London: Economics and Operational Research Division, Department of Health.

Smith, A. (1759/1976). *The Theory of Moral Sentiments*, D.D. Raphael and A.L. Macfie (eds.). Oxford: Oxford University Press.

Smith, C., Cook, R. and Rohleder, P. (2017). A qualitative investigation into the HIV disclosure process within an intimate partnership: 'The moment I realized that our relationship was developing into something serious, I just had to tell him'. *British Journal of Health Psychology*, 22 (1): 110–27.

Smith, J. (2004). *Building a Safer NHS for Patients: Improving Medication Safety. A Report by the Chief Pharmaceutical Officer*. London: The Stationery Office.

Smith, J.A. and Osborn, M. (2003). Interpretative phenomenological analysis. In J.A. Smith (ed.), *Qualitative Psychology: A Practical Guide to Research Methods*. London: Sage. pp. 51–80.

Smith, J.A., Flowers, P. and Larkin, M. (2009). *Interpretative Phenomenological Analysis: Theory, Method and Research*. London: Sage.

Smith, J.A., Jarman, M. and Osborn, M. (1999). Doing interpretative phenomenological analysis. In M. Murray and K. Chamberlain (eds.), *Qualitative Health Psychology: Theories and Methods*. London: Sage.

Smith, K.A., Goy, E.R., Harvath, T.A. and Ganzini, L. (2011). Quality of death and dying in patients who request physician-assisted death. *Journal of Palliative Medicine*, 14: 445–50.

Smith, P., Haberl, H., Popp, A., Erb, K.H., Lauk, C., Harper, R. et al. (2013). How much land-based greenhouse gas mitigation can be achieved without compromising food security and environmental goals? *Global Change Biology*, 19: 2285–302.

SmithBattle, L.I. (2013). Reducing the stigmatization of teen mothers. *MCN: The American Journal of Maternal/Child Nursing*, 38 (4): 235–41.

Smyth, J.M., Stone, A.A., Hurewitz, A. and Kaell, A. (1999). Effects of writing about stressful experiences on symptom reduction in patients with asthma and rheumatoid arthritis. *Journal of the American Medical Association*, 281: 722–33.

Sniehotta, F.F., Presseau, J. and Araujo-Soanes, V. (2014). Time to retire the theory of planned behaviour. *Health Psychology Review*, 8 (1): 1–7.

Sointu, E. (2013). Complementary and alternative medicines, embodied subjectivity and experiences of healing. *Health*, 17: 530–45.

Somerfield, M.R. (1997). The utility of systems models of stress and coping for applied research: the case of cancer adaptation. *Journal of Health Psychology*, 2: 133–83.

Song, S. and Jason, L.A. (2005). A population-based study of chronic fatigue syndrome (CFS) experienced in differing patient groups: an effort to replicate Vercoulen et al.'s model of CFS. *Journal of Mental Health*, 14: 277–89.

Sonneville, K.R., Calzo, J.P., Horton, N.J., Haines, J., Austin, S.B. and Field, A.E. (2012). Body satisfaction, weight gain and binge eating among overweight adolescent girls. *International Journal of Obesity*, 36: 944–9.

Sorensen, K., Van den Broucke, S., Fullam, J., Doyle, G., Pelikan, J., Slonska, Z. et al. (HLS-EU) Consortium Health Literacy Project European. (2012). Health literacy and public health: a systematic review and integration of definitions and models. *BMC Public Health*, 12: 80. doi:10.1186/1471-2458-12-80.

Soylu, C., Ozaslan, E., Karaca, H. and Ozkan, M. (2015). Psychological distress and loneliness in caregiver of advanced oncological inpatients. *Journal of Health Psychology*, 21 (9): 1896–906.

Spector, N.H. and Korneva, E.A. (1981). Neurophysiology, immunophysiology and neuroimmunomodulation. In R. Ader (ed.), *Psychoneuroimmunology*. New York: Academic Press. pp. 449–73.

Speer, P.W., Tesdahl, E.A. and Ayers, J.F. (2014). Community organizing practices in a globalizing era: building power for health equity at the community level. *Journal of Health Psychology*, 19 (1): 159–69.

Spencer, L., Adams, T.B., Malone, S., Roy, L. and Yost, E. (2006). Applying the transtheoretical model to exercise: a systematic and comprehensive review of the literature. *Health Promotion Practice*, 7: 428–43.

Spiegel, D. (2014). Minding the body: psychotherapy and cancer survival. *British Journal of Health Psychology*, 19 (3): 465–85.

Spiegel, D., Kraemer, H., Bloom, J. and Gottheil, E. (1989). Effect of psychosocial treatment on survival of patients with metastatic breast cancer. *The Lancet*, 334: 888–91.

Stall, R., Mills, T.C., Williamson, J., Hart, T., Greenwood, G., Paul, J. et al. (2003). Association of co-occurring psychosocial health problems and increased vulnerability to HIV/AIDS among urban men who have sex with men. *American Journal of Public Health*, 93 (6): 939–42.

Stam, H.J. (2014). A sound body in a sound mind: a critical historical analysis of health psychology. In M. Murray (ed.), *Critical Health Psychology* (2nd edn). London: Palgrave.

Stansfeld, S., Head, J. and Marmot, M. (2000). *Work Related Factors and Ill Health: The Whitehall II Study*. London: HSE Books.

Stanton, A. and Snider, R. (1993). Coping with a breast cancer diagnosis: a prospective study. *Journal of Personality and Social Psychology*, 46: 489–502.

Stanton, A.L., Rowland, J.H. and Ganz, P.A. (2015). Life after diagnosis and treatment of cancer in adulthood: contributions from psychosocial oncology research. *American Psychologist*, 70 (2): 159.

Stapleton, J.L., Hillhouse, J., Levonyan-Radloff, K. and Manne, S. L. (2017). Review of interventions to reduce ultraviolet tanning: need for treatments targeting excessive tanning, an emerging addictive behavior. *Psychology of addictive behaviors: Journal of the Society of Psychologists in Addictive Behaviors*, 31 (8): 962–78.

Starcevic, V. and Aboujaoude, E. (2017). Internet addiction: Reappraisal of an increasingly inadequate concept. *CNS Spectrums*, 22 (1): 7–13.

Steeg, P.S. (2003). Metastasis suppressors alter the signal transduction of cancer cells. *Nature Reviews Cancer*, 3: 55–63.

Steele, C.M. (1988). The psychology of self-affirmation: Sustaining the integrity of the self. In L. Berkowitz (ed.), *Advances in Experimental Social Psychology* (Vol. 21). New York: Academic Press. pp. 261–302. doi:10.1016/S0065-2601(08)60229-4

Steger, M.F., Frazier, P., Oishi, S. and Kaler, M. (2006). The Meaning in Life Questionnaire: assessing the presence of and search for meaning in life. *Journal of Counseling Psychology*, 53: 80–93.

Stein, J. and Rotheram-Borus, M. (2004). Cross-sectional and longitudinal associations in coping strategies and physical health outcomes among HIV-positive youth. *Psychology & Health*, 19: 321–36.

Steinhauser, K.E., Clipp, E.C., McNeilly, M., Christakis, N.A., McIntyre, L.M. and Tulsky, J.A. (2000). In search of a good death: observations of patients, families, and providers. *Annals of Internal Medicine*, 132: 825–32.

Stenhoff, A.L., Sadreddini, S., Peters, S. and Wearden, A. (2015). Understanding medical students' views of chronic fatigue syndrome: a qualitative study. *Journal of Health Psychology*, 20 (2): 198–209.

Stensland, P. and Malterud, K. (1999). Approaching the locked dialogues of the body: communicating illness through diaries. *Journal of Primary Health Care*, 17: 75–80.

Stephens, C. (2008). *Health Promotion: A Psychosocial Approach*. New York: McGraw-Hill International.

Stephens, C. (2010). Privilege and status in an unequal society: shifting the focus of health promotion research to include the maintenance of advantage. *Journal of Health Psychology*, 15 (7): 993–1000. doi:10.1177/1359105310371554.

Stephens, C. (2014). Beyond the barricades: social movements as participatory practice in health promotion. *Journal of Health Psychology*, 19 (1): 170–5. doi:10.1177/13 59105313500245.

Stevens, S.S. (1951). Mathematics, measurement, and psychophysics. In S.S. Stevens (ed.), *Handbook of Experimental Psychology*. Oxford: Wiley. pp. 1–49.

Stevinson, C., Pittler, M.H. and Ernst, E. (2000). Garlic for treating hypercholesterolemia: a meta-analysis of randomized clinical trials. *Annals of Internal Medicine*, 133: 420–9.

Stewart, D.E., Abbey, S.E., Shnek, Z.M., Irvine, J. and Grace, S.L. (2004). Gender differences in health information needs and decisional preferences in patients recovering from an acute ischemic coronary event. *Psychosomatic Medicine*, 66: 42–8.

Stewart, W.F., Lipton, R.B., Simon, D., Liberman, J. and Von Korff, M. (1999). Validity of an illness severity measure for headache in a population sample of migraine sufferers. *Pain*, 79: 291–301.

Stock, W.E. and Geer, J.H. (1982). A study of fantasy-based sexual arousal in women. *Archives of Sexual Behavior*, 11 (1): 33–47.

Stokols, D. (1992). Establishing and maintaining healthy environments: toward a social ecology of health promotion. *American Psychologist*, 47: 6–22.

Stolerman, I.P. and Jarvis, M.J. (1995). The scientific case that nicotine is addictive. *Psychopharmacology*, 117: 2–10.

Stolte, O. and Hodgetts, D. (2015). Being healthy in unhealthy places: health tactics in a homeless lifeworld. *Journal of Health Psychology*, 20 (2): 144–53.

Stone, D.H. and Stewart, S. (1996). Screening and the new genetics: a public health perspective and the ethical debate. *Journal of Public Health Medicine*, 18: 3–5.

Stone, G.C., Weiss, S.M., Matarazzo, J.D., Miller, N.E. and Rodin, J. (eds.) (1987). *Health Psychology: A Discipline and a Profession*. Chicago, IL: University of Chicago Press.

Stone, S.V. and Costa, P.T. (1990). Disease-prone personality or distress-prone personality? The role of neuroticism in coronary heart disease. In H.S. Friedman (ed.), *Personality and Disease*. London: Wiley. pp. 178–200.

Stone, S.V. and McCrae, R.R. (2007). Personality and health. In S. Ayers, A. Baum, C. McManus, S. Newman, K. Wallston, J. Weinman and R. West (eds.), *Cambridge Handbook of Psychology, Health and Medicine* (2nd edn). Cambridge: Cambridge University Press. pp. 151–5.

Strange, C., Bremner, A., Fisher, C., Howat, P. and Wood, L. (2016). Local community playgroup participation and associations with social capital. *Health Promotion Journal of Australia*. doi:10.1071/HE15134.

Strauss, A.L. (1987). *Qualitative Analysis for Social Scientists*. New York: Cambridge University Press.

Street, R.L., Makoul, G., Arora, N.K. and Epstein, R.M. (2009). How does communication heal? Pathways linking clinician–patient communication to health outcomes. *Patient Education and Counseling*, 74 (3): 295–301.

Stroebe, W. (2000). *Social Psychology and Health* (2nd edn). Buckingham: Open University Press.

Stuckler, D., McKee, M., Ebrahim, S. and Basu, S. (2012). Manufacturing epidemics: the role of global producers in increased consumption of unhealthy commodities including processed foods, alcohol, and tobacco. *PLoS Medicine*, 9 (6): e1001235.

Suls, J. and Bunde, J. (2005). Anger, anxiety and depression as risk factors for cardiovascular disease: the problems and implications of overlapping affective dispositions. *Psychological Bulletin*, 131: 260–300.

Suls, J. and Rittenhouse, J.D. (1990). Models of linkages between personality and disease. In H.S. Friedman (ed.), *Personality & Disease*. London: Wiley. pp. 38–64.

Sulzberger, P. and Marks, D.F. (1977). *The ISIS Smoking Cessation Programme*. Dunedin, NZ: Isis Research Centre.

Sunnquist, M. (2016). A reexamination of the cognitive behavioral model of chronic fatigue syndrome: investigating the cogency of the model's behavioral pathway. *College of Science and Health Theses and Dissertations*, 193.

Surtees, P., Wainwright, N., Luben, R., Khaw, K.T. and Day, N. (2003). Sense of coherence and mortality in men and women in the EPIC-Norfolk United Kingdom prospective cohort study. *American Journal of Epidemiology*, 158 (12): 1202–9.

Sutin, A.R., Ferrucci, L., Zonderman, A.B. and Terracciano, A. (2011). Personality and obesity across the adult life span. *Journal of Personality and Social Psychology*, 101: 579–92.

Sutton, S. (2000a). A critical review of the Transtheoretical Model applied to smoking cessation. In P. Norman, C. Abraham and M. Conner (eds.), *Understanding and Changing Health Behaviour: From Health Beliefs to Self-Regulation*. Amsterdam: Harwood Academic. pp. 207–25.

Sutton, S. (2000b). Interpreting cross-sectional data on stages of change. *Psychology & Health*, 15: 163–71.

Sutton, S., Bickler, G., Aldridge, J. and Saidi, G. (1994). Prospective study of predictors of attendance for breast screening in inner London. *Journal of Epidemiology & Community Health*, 48: 65–73.

Swaab, D.F. (2004). Sexual differentiation of the human brain: relevance for gender identity, transsexualism and sexual orientation. *Gynecological Endocrinology*, 19 (6): 301–12.

Swales, J. (2000). Population advice on salt restriction: the social issues. *American Journal of Hypertension*, 13: 2–7.

Swinburn, B., Egger, G. and Raza, F. (1999). Dissecting obesogenic environments: the development and application of a framework for identifying and prioritizing environmental interventions for obesity. *Preventive Medicine*, 29: 563–70.

Sykes, C.M. and Marks, D.F. (2001). Effectiveness of cognitive behaviour therapy self-help programme for smokers in London, UK. *Health Promotion International*, 16: 255–60.

Sykes, C.M., Willig, C. and Marks, D.F. (2004). Discourses in the European Commission's 1996–2000 Health Promotion Programme. *Journal of Health Psychology*, 9: 131–41.

Symons, C., Polman, R., Moore, M., Borkoles, E., Eime, R., Harvey, J. et al. (2013). The relationship between body image, physical activity, perceived health, and behavioral regulation among Year 7 and Year 11 girls from metropolitan and rural Australia. *Annals of Leisure Research*, 16: 115–29.

Synergy Expert Group. (2016). Implementation intention and planning interventions in health psychology: recommendations from the Synergy Expert Group for research and practice. *Psychology & Health*, 31(7): 814–39.

Syrjala, K.L., Donaldson, G.W., Davis, M.W., Kippes, M.E. and Carr, J.E. (1995). Relaxation and imagery and cognitive-behavioral training reduce pain during cancer treatment: a controlled clinical trial. *Pain*, 63: 189–98.

Szyf, M. (2013). DNA methylation, behavior and early life adversity. *Journal of Genetics and Genomics*, 40: 331–8.

Taku, K., Umegaki, K., Sato, Y., Taki, Y., Endoh, K. and Watanabe, S. (2007). Soy isoflavones lower serum total and LDL cholesterol in humans: a meta-analysis of 11 randomized controlled trials. *American Journal of Clinical Nutrition*, 85: 1148–56.

Tang, M.Y., Shahab, L., Robb, K.A. and Gardner, B. (2014). Are parents more willing to vaccinate their children than themselves? *Journal of Health Psychology*, 21 (5): 781–87.

Tapia, A.H., Moore, K.A. and Johnson, N.J. (2013). Beyond the trustworthy tweet: a deeper understanding of microblogged data use by disaster response and humanitarian relief organizations. In *Proceedings of the 10th International ISCRAM Conference*. Baden-Baden, Germany. pp. 770–78. Available: http://www.iscram.org/taxonomy/term/44 [accessed 28 August 2017].

Tarry-Adkins, J.L. and Ozanne, S.E. (2011). Mechanisms of early life programming: current knowledge and future directions. *The American Journal of Clinical Nutrition*, 94 (suppl. 6): 1765S–71S.

Taubes, G. (2007). *Good Calories, Bad Calories*. New York: Knopf.

Taubes, G. (2009). *The Diet Delusion*. New York: Random House.

Taubes, G. (2012). Treat obesity as physiology, not physics. *Nature*, 492: 155.

Tayefi, M., Shafiee, M., Kazemi-Bajestani, S.M.R., Esmaeili, H., Darroudi, S., Khakpouri, S. et al. (2017). Depression and anxiety both associate with serum level of hs-CRP: a gender-stratified analysis in a population-based study. *Psychoneuroendocrinology*, 81: 63–9.

Taylor, C., Carlos Poston, W.S., Jones, L. and Kraft, M.K. (2006). Environmental justice: obesity, physical activity, and health eating. *Journal of Physical Activity & Health*, 3 (suppl. 1): S30–54.

Taylor, S.E., Repetti, R.L. and Seeman, T. (1997). Health psychology: What is an unhealthy environment and how does it get under the skin? *Annual Review of Psychology*, 48: 411–47.

Te Morenga, L., Mallard, S. and Mann, J. (2013). Dietary sugars and body weight: systematic review and meta-analyses of randomised controlled trials and cohort studies. *British Medical Journal*, 346: e7492.

Tedeschi, R.G. and Calhoun, L.G. (1996). The posttraumatic growth inventory: measuring the positive legacy of trauma. *Journal of Traumatic Stress*, 9 (3): 455–71.

Tedeschi, R.G. and Calhoun, L.G. (2004). 'Posttraumatic growth: Conceptual foundations and empirical evidence'. *Psychological Inquiry*, 15 (1): 1–18.

Teicholz, N. (2015). The scientific report guiding the US dietary guidelines: Is it scientific? *British Medical Journal*, 351. doi: 10.1136/bmj.h4962.

Teixeira, P.J., Carraca, E.V., Markland, D., Silva, M.N. and Ryan, R.M. (2012). Exercise, physical activity, and self-determination theory: a systematic review. *International Journal of Behavioral Nutrition and Physical Activity*, 9: 78.

Temel, J.S., Greer, J.A., Muzikansky, A., Gallagher, E.R., Admane, S., Jackson, V.A. et al. (2010). Early palliative care for patients with metastatic non-small-cell lung cancer. *The New England Journal of Medicine*, 363 (8): 733–42.

Terrill, A.L., Molton, I.R., Ehde, D.M., Amtmann, D., Bombardier, C.H., Smith, A.E. and Jensen, M.P. (2014). Resilience, age, and perceived symptoms in persons with long-term physical disabilities. *Journal of Health Psychology*, 21 (5): 640–9. doi:1177/1359105314532973.

Tessaro, I., Eng, E. and Smith, J. (1994). Breast cancer screening in older African-American women: Qualitative research findings. *American Journal of Health Promotion*, 8: 286–92.

Thaler, J.P., Yi, C.X., Schur, E.A., Guyenet, S.J., Hwang, B.H., Dietrich, M.O. et al. (2012). Obesity is associated with hypothalamic injury in rodents and humans. *Journal of Clinical Investigation*, 122: 153–62.

Thom, B. (2001). A social and political history of alcohol. In N. Heather, T.J. Peters and T. Stockwell (eds.), *International Handbook of Alcohol Dependence and Problems*. London: Wiley. pp. 281–97.

Thomas, E.L., Parkinson, J.R., Frost, G.S., Goldstone, A.P., Doré, C.J., McCarthy, J.P. et al. (2012). The missing risk: MRI and MRS phenotyping of abdominal adiposity and ectopic fat. *Obesity*, 20: 76–87.

Thomas, I. (1979). *The Medusa and the Snail*. New York: Bantam.

Thombs, B.D., Roseman, M., Coyne, J.C., de Jonge, P., Delisle, V.C., Arthurs, E. et al. (2013). Does evidence support the American Heart Association's recommendation to screen patients for depression in cardiovascular care? An updated systematic review. *PLoS One*, 8 (1): e52654.

Thompson, C.M., Crook, B., Love, B., Macpherson, C.F. and Johnson, R. (2016). Understanding how adolescents and young adults with cancer talk about needs in online and face-to-face support groups. *Journal of Health Psychology*, 21 (11): 2636–46. doi:10.1177/1359105315581515.

Thompson, J.K. and Stice, E. (2001). Thin-ideal internalization: mounting evidence for a new risk factor for body-image disturbance and eating pathology. *Current Directions in Psychological Science*, 10: 181–3.

Thompson, S.L., Chenhall, R.D. and Brimblecombe, J.K. (2013). Indigenous perspectives on active living in remote Australia: a qualitative exploration of the socio-cultural link between health, the environment and economics. *BMC Public Health*, 13: 1–11.

Thomson, R. (1982). Side effects and placebo amplification. *The British Journal of Psychiatry*, 140: 64–68.

Thurnham, D.I. (2014). Interactions between nutrition and immune function: using inflammation biomarkers to interpret micronutrient status. *Proceedings of the Nutrition Society*, 73: 1–8.

Tibben, A., Frets, P.G., van de Kamp, J.J., Niermeijer, M.F., Vegter-van der Vlis, M., Roos, R.A. et al. (1993). Presymptomatic DNA testing for Huntington disease: pre-test attitudes and expectations of applicants and their partners in the Dutch program. *American Journal of Medical Genetics*, 48: 10–16.

Tibben, A., Timman, R., Banninck, E.C. and Duinvoorden, H.J. (1997). Three-year follow-up after presymptomatic testing for Huntington's disease in tested individuals and partners. *Health Psychology*, 16: 20–35.

Tickner, S., Leman, P.J. and Woodcock, A. (2007). 'It's just the normal thing to do': exploring parental decision-making about the 'five-in-one' vaccine. *Vaccine*, 25: 7399–409.

Tiffany, S.T. (1990). A cognitive model of drug urges and drug-use behavior: role of automatic and nonautomatic processes. *Psychological Review*, 97 (2): 147–68.

Tileaga, C. (2013). *Political Psychology: Critical Perspectives*. Cambridge: Cambridge University Press.

Timonen, V. (2015). *Beyond Successful and Active Ageing: A Theory of Model Ageing*. Bristol: Policy Press.

Titchener, E.B. (1909/2014). Introspection and empathy. *Dialogues in Philosophy, Mental and Neuro Sciences*, 7 (1): 25–30.

Titmuss, R. M. (1968). Community care: fact or fiction? In R.M. Titmuss (ed.), *Commitment to Welfare*. London: George Allen & Unwin. pp. 104–9.

Tjaden, P. and Thoennes, N. (1998). *Prevalence, Incidence, and Consequences of Violence against Women: Findings from the National Violence against Women Survey*. Washington, DC: Research in Brief, US Department of Justice.

Todd, K.H., Deaton, C., D'Adamo, A.P. and Goe, L. (2000). Ethnicity and analgesic practice. *Annals of Emergency Medicine*, 35: 11–16.

Tomas, C., Brown, A., Strassheim, V., Elson, J., Newton, J. and Manning, P. (2017) Cellular bioenergetics is impaired in patients with chronic fatigue syndrome. *PLoS One* 12 (10): e0186802. https://doi.org/10.1371/journal.pone.0186802.

Tomkins, S.S. (1966). *Affect, Imagery, Consciousness. Vol. 1: The Positive Affects*. New York: Springer.

Tomlinson, A., Ravenscroft, N., Wheaton, B. and Gilchrist, P. (2005). *Lifestyle Sports and National Sport Policy: An Agenda for Research*. Eastbourne: University of Brighton.

Tomlinson, E. and Stott, J. (2014). Assisted dying in dementia: a systematic review of the international literature on the attitudes of health professionals, patients, carers and the public, and the factors associated with these. *International Journal of Geriatric Psychiatry*, 30 (1): 10–20.

Tonstad, S., Butler, T., Yan, R. and Fraser, G.E. (2009). Type of vegetarian diet, bodyweight, and prevalence of Type 2 diabetes. *Diabetes Care*, 32: 791–6.

Tonstad, S., Stewart, K., Oda, K., Batech, M., Herring, R.P. and Fraser, G.E. (2013). Vegetarian diets and incidence of diabetes in the Adventist Health Study-2. *Nutrition, Metabolism & Cardiovascular Diseases*, 23: 292–9.

Torre, R. and Myrskylä, M. (2014). Income inequality and population health: an analysis of panel data for 21 developed countries, 1975–2006. *Population Studies*, 68 (1): 1–13.

Townsend, N., Wickramasinghe, K., Williams, J., Bhatnagar, P. and Rayner, M. (2015). *Physical Activity Statistics 2015*. London: British Heart Foundation.

Townsend, P. and Davidson, N. (1982). *Inequalities in Health: The Black Report*. London: Penguin.

Townsend, P., Davidson, N. and Whitehead, M. (1992). *Inequalities in Health: The Black Report and the Health Divide*. London: Penguin Books.

Trafimow, D. (2009). The theory of reasoned action: a case study of falsification in psychology. *Theory & Psychology*, 19: 501–18.

Trafimow, D., Sheeran, P., Conner, M. and Finlay, K.A. (2002). Evidence that perceived behavioural control is a multidimensional construct: perceived control and perceived difficulty. *British Journal of Social Psychology*, 41: 101–21.

Triandis, H.C. (1995). *Individualism & Collectivism*. Boulder, CO: Westview Press.

True, W.R., Heath, A.C., Scherrer, J.F., Waterman, B., Goldberg, J., Lin, N. et al. (1997). Genetic and environmental contributions to smoking. *Addiction*, 92: 1277–87.

Trumbull, R. and Appley, M.H. (1986). A conceptual model for the understanding of stress dynamics in M.H. Appley and R. Trumbull (eds.), *Dynamics of Stress: Physiological, Psychological and Social Perspectives*. New York: Plenum. pp. 21–45.

Truong, M., Paradies, Y. and Priest, N. (2014). Interventions to improve cultural competency in healthcare: a systematic review of reviews. *BMC Health Services Research*, 14 (1): 1–31.

Tsien, J.Z., Huerta, P.T. and Tonegawa, S. (1996). The essential role of hippocampal CA1 NMDA receptor–dependent synaptic plasticity in spatial memory. *Cell*, 87 (7): 1327–38.

Tucker, I. and Smith, L.A. (2014). Topology and mental distress: self-care in the life spaces of home. *Journal of Health Psychology*, 19: 176–83.

Tudor Hart, J. (1971). The inverse care law. *The Lancet*, 297: 405–12.

Turecki, G. (2014). The molecular bases of the suicidal brain. *Nature Reviews Neuroscience*, 15 (12): 802.

Turk, D.C. and Wilson, H.D. (2013). Chronic pain. In A.M. Nezu (ed.), *Handbook of Psychology* (Vol. 9). Chichester: John Wiley.

Turner, B. (1984). *The Body and Society: Explorations in Social Theory*. Oxford: Blackwell.

Tversky, A. and Kahneman, D. (1981). The framing of decisions and the rationality of choice. *Science*, 221: 453–8.

Tyler, R.E. and Williams, S. (2014). Masculinity in young men's health: exploring health, help-seeking and health service use in an online environment. *Journal of Health Psychology*, 19: 457–70.

Ulbricht, C.E. and Basch, E.M. (2005). *Natural Standard Herb and Supplement Reference: Evidence-Based Clinical Reviews*. Maryland Heights, MO: Mosby.

Ullman, S.E., Filipas, H.H., Townsend, S.M. and Starzynski, L.L. (2005). Trauma exposure, posttraumatic stress disorder and problem drinking in sexual assault survivors. *Journal of Studies on Alcohol*, 66 (5): 610–19.

UNAIDS. (2007). *Policy Brief: Greater Involvement of People Living with HIV (GIPA)*. Geneva: UNAIDS. Available: http://data.unaids.org/pub/BriefingNote/2007/JC1299_Policy_Brief_GIPA.pdf [accessed 15 April 2008].

UNAIDS. (2016). *Get on the Fast Track. The Life-cycle Approach to HIV*. Geneva: UNAIDS. Available: www.unaids.org/sites/default/files/media_asset/Get-on-the-Fast-Track_en.pdf [accessed 28 August 2017].

United Nations. (2009). *State of the World's Indigenous Peoples*. New York: United Nations.

United Nations. (2017). *General Assembly: Draft Resolution on Participation of Indigenous Peoples at the UN*. New York: United Nations. Available: www.un.org/development/desa/indigenouspeoples/ [accessed online 7 February 2017].

United Nations Development Programme. (1995). *Human Development Report*. New York: Oxford University Press.

United Nations General Assembly. (1948). *Universal Declaration of Human Rights*. New York: United Nations. Available: www.un.org/Overview/rights.html [accessed 1 April 2005].

United Nations System Standing Committee on Nutrition. (2006) Report of the Standing Committee on Nutrition at its Thirty-Third Session. Available at: http://www.unscn.org/files/Annual_Sessions/33rd_SCN_Session/33rd_session_REPORT.pdf [accessed on 28 August 2017].

United Nations High Commissioner for Refugees (UNHCR). (2014). *Living in the Shadows: Jordan Home Visits Report 2014*. Available: www.unhcr.org/jordan2014urbanreport/home-visit-report.pdf [accessed 7 February 2017].

Updegraff, J.A. and Rothman, A.J. (2013). Health message framing: moderators, mediators, and mysteries. *Social and Personality Psychology Compass*, 7 (9): 668–79. doi:10.1111/spc3.12056.

Uphoff, E.P., Pickett, K.E., Cabieses, B., Small, N. and Wright, J. (2013). A systematic review of the relationships between social capital and socioeconomic inequalities in health: a contribution to understanding the psychosocial pathway of health inequalities. *International Journal for Equity in Health*, 12 (1): 54–65. doi:10.1186/1475-9276-12-54.

Urban, B.J., France, R.D., Steinberger, E.K., Scott, D.L. and Maltbre, A.A. (1986). Long-term use of narcotic/antidepressant medication in the management of phantom limb pain. *Pain*, 24: 1991–6.

US Department of Health and Human Services. (2004). *The Health Consequences of Smoking: A Report of the Surgeon General*. Atlanta, GA: US Department of Health and Human Services, Centers for Disease Control and Prevention, National Center for Chronic Disease Prevention and Health Promotion, Office on Smoking and Health.

US Department of Health and Human Services' Children's Bureau. (2010). *Child Maltreatment.* Available: www.acf.hhs.gov/cb/resource/child-maltreatment-2010 [accessed 28 August 2017].

US Department of Justice. (2016). *Questions and Answers: The Americans with Disabilities Act and Persons with HIV/AIDS*. Available: www.ada.gov/hiv/ada_q&a_hiv.pdf [accessed 24 February 2017].

US Federal Trade Commission (FTC) (2016). *Cigarette Report for 2014*. Available: www.ftc.gov/system/files/documents/reports/federal-tradecommission-cigarette-report-2014-federal-trade-commission-smokeless-tobacco-report/ftc_cigarette_report_2014.pdf. [accessed 28 August 2017].

US Surgeon General. (1989). *Reducing the Health Consequences of Smoking: 25 Years of Progress: A Report of the Surgeon General*. Bethesda, MD: Center for Chronic Disease Prevention and Health Promotion.

US Surgeon General. (2008). *Treating Tobacco Use and Dependence: 2008 Update*. A report of the Surgeon General. Atlanta GA: USDHHS, CDC, National Center for Chronic Disease Prevention and Health Promotion, Office on Smoking and Health.

US Surgeon General. (2010). *The Surgeon General's Vision for a Healthy and Fit Nation*. Rockville, MD: US Department of Health and Human Services. Public Health Service.

Ussher, J.M., Perz, J., Rose, D., Dowsett, G.W., Chambers, S., Williams, S. et al. (2016). Threat of sexual disqualification: the consequences of erectile dysfunction and other sexual changes for gay and bisexual men with prostate cancer. *Archives of Sexual Behavior*, 1–15.

Ussher, J.M., Tim Wong, W.K. and Perz, J. (2011). A qualitative analysis of changes in relationship dynamics and roles between people with cancer and their primary informal carer. *Health*, 15 (6): 650–67.

Vallabhaneni, S., Li, X., Vittinghoff, E., Donnell, D., Pilcher, C.D. and Buchbinder, S.P. (2012). Seroadaptive practices: association with HIV acquisition among HIV-negative men who have sex with men. *PLoS One*, 7 (10): e45718.

Valsiner, J. (2013). *An Invitation to Cultural Psychology*. New Delhi: Sage.

Vamos, C.A., Lockhart, E., Vázquez-Otero, C., Thompson, E.L., Proctor, S., Wells, K.J. and Daley, E.M. (2016). Abnormal pap tests among women living in a hispanic migrant farmworker community: a narrative of health literacy. *Journal of Health Psychology*. doi:10.1177/1359105316664137.

Van Cauter, E. and Tasali, E. (2011). Endocrine physiology in relation to sleep and sleep disturbances. In M.H. Kryger, T. Roth and W.C. Dement (eds.), *Principles and Practice of Sleep Disorders* (5th edn). Philadelphia, PA: Elsevier and Saunders. pp. 291–311.

Van Dyck, D., Cerin, E., Conway, T.L., De Bourdeaudhuij, I., Owen, N., Kerr, J. et al. (2014). Interacting psychosocial and environmental correlates of leisure-time physical activity: a three-country study. *Health Psychology*, 33: 699–709.

van Melle, J.P., de Jonge, P., Honig, A., Schene, A.H., Kuyper, A.M., Crijns, H.J. et al. (2007). Effects of antidepressant treatment following myocardial infarction. *British Journal of Psychiatry*, 190: 460–66.

Van't Riet, J., Cox, A.D., Cox, D., Zimet, G.D., De Bruijn, G., Van den Putte, B. et al. (2016). Does perceived risk influence the effects of message framing? Revisiting the link between prospect theory and message framing. *Health Psychology Review*, 10 (4): 447–59. doi:10.1080/17437199.2016.1176865.

Vandewalle, J., Moens, E. and Braet, C. (2014). Comprehending emotional eating in obese youngsters: the role of parental rejection and emotion regulation. *International Journal of Obesity*, 38: 525–30.

Vasiljevic, M., Ng, Y.L., Griffin, S.J., Sutton, S. and Marteau, T.M. (2016). Is the intention–behaviour gap greater amongst the more deprived? A meta-analysis of five studies on physical activity, diet, and medication adherence in smoking cessation. *British Journal of Health Psychology*, 21 (1): 11–30. doi:10.1111/bjhp.12152

Vaughan, C. (2014). Participatory research with youth: Idealising safe social spaces or building transformative links in difficult environments? *Journal of Health Psychology*, 19 (1): 184–92.

Veale, D., Miles, S., Bramley, S., Muir, G. and Hodsoll, J. (2015). Am I normal? A systematic review and construction of nomograms for flaccid and erect penis length and circumference in up to 15,521 men. *BJU International*, 115 (6): 978–86.

Velleman, S., Collin, S.M., Beasant, L. and Crawley, E. (2016). Psychological wellbeing and quality-of-life among siblings of paediatric CFS/ME patients: a mixed-methods study. *Clinical Child Psychology and Psychiatry*, 21 (4): 618–33.

Vercoulen, J.H., Swanink, C.M., Galama, J.M. et al. (1998). The persistence of fatigue in chronic fatigue syndrome and multiple sclerosis: development of a model. *J Psychosomatic Research*, 45 (6): 507–17.

Verdino, J. (2017). The third tier in treatment: attending to the growing connection between gut health and emotional well-being. *Health Psychology Open*, 4 (2): doi:2055102917724335.

Verhoef Vézina-Im, L.A., Lavoie, M.J., Love, E.J., Krol, P. and Rose Olivier-D, M.S. (1992). Motivations of physicians and their exercise participation. *Women's Health*, 19: 14–29.

Verhulst, B., Neale, M.C. and Kendler, K.S. (2015). The heritability of alcohol use disorders: a meta-analysis of twin and adoption studies. *Psychological Medicine*, 45 (5): 1061–72.

Vézina-Im, L., Lavoie, M., Krol, P. et al. (2014). Motivations of physicians and nurses to practice voluntary euthanasia: a systematic review. *BMC Palliative Care*, 13(20). https://doi.org/10.1186/1472-684X-13-20.

Vian, T., DeSilva, M.B., Cabral, H.J., Williams, G.C., Gifford, A.L., Zhong, L. et al. (2016). The role of motivation in predicting antiretroviral therapy adherence in China. *Journal of Health Psycholpgy*, doi:10.1177/1359105316672922.

Vilela, L.D., Nicolau, B., Mahmud, S., Edgar, L., Hier, M., Black, M. et al. (2006). Comparison of psychosocial outcomes in head and neck cancer patients receiving a coping strategies intervention and control subjects receiving no intervention. *The Journal of Otolaryngology*, 35: 88.

Virtanen, M., Jokela, M., Nyberg, S.T., Madsen, I.E.H., Lallukka, T., Ahola, K. et al. (2015). Long working hours and alcohol use: systematic review and meta-analysis of published studies and unpublished individual participant data. *BMJ*, 350: g7772.

Vlaeyen, J.W.S. and Linton, S.J. (2000). Fear-avoidance and its consequences in chronic musculoskeletal pain: a state of the art. *Pain*, 85: 317–32.

Vogler, B., Pittler, M. and Ernst, E. (1999). The efficacy of ginseng: a systematic review of randomised clinical trials. *European Journal of Clinical Pharmacology*, 55: 567–75.

Volkow, N.D., Wang, G.J. and Baler, R.D. (2011). Reward, dopamine and the control of food intake: implications for obesity. *Trends in Cognitive Science*, 15: 37–46.

Von Lengerke, T., Vinck, J., Rutten, A., Reitmeir, P., Abel, T., Kannas, L. et al. (2004). Health policy perception and health behaviours: a multilevel analysis and implications for public health psychology. *Journal of Health Psychology*, 9: 157–75.

Von Ruesten, A., Weikert, C., Fietze, I. and Boeing, H. (2012). Association of sleep duration with chronic diseases in the European Prospective Investigation into Cancer and Nutrition (EPIC)-Potsdam study. *PloS One*, 7 (1): e30972.

Von Wagner, C., Baio, G., Raine, R., Snowball, J., Morris, S., Atkin, W. et al. (2011). Inequalities in participation in an organized national colorectal cancer screening programme: results from the first 2.6 million invitations in England. *International Journal of Epidemiology*, 40 (3): 712–18.

Vowles, K.E., Witkiewitz, K., Sowden, G. and Ashworth, J. (2014). Acceptance and commitment therapy for chronic pain: evidence of mediation and clinically significant change following an abbreviated inter-disciplinary program of rehabilitation. *Journal of Pain*, 15: 101–13.

Waddell, G., Newton, M., Henderson, I., Somerville, D. and Main, C.J. (1993). A Fear-Avoidance Beliefs Questionnaire (FABQ) and the role of fear-avoidance beliefs in chronic low back pain and disability. *Pain*, 52: 157–68.

Wagner, E.H., Austin, B.T., Davis, C., Hindmarsh, M., Schaefer, J. and Bonomi, A. (2001). Improving chronic illness care: translating evidence into action. *Health Affairs*, 20 (6): 64–78.

Wald, N., Kiryluk, S., Darby, S., Doll, R., Pike, M. and Peto, R. (1988). *UK Smoking Statistics*. Oxford: Oxford University Press.

Wallace, R.K., Benson, H. and Wilson, A.F. (1971). A wakeful hypometabolic physiologic state. *American Journal of Physiology*, 221 (3): 795–9.

Waller, J., Jackowska, M., Marlow, L. and Wardle, J. (2012). Exploring age differences in reasons for nonattendance for cervical screening: a qualitative study. *BJOG*, 119 (1): 26–32.

Wallston, K.A., Burger, C., Smith, R.A. and Baugher, R.J. (1988). Comparing the quality of death for hospice and non-hospice cancer patients. *Medical Care*, 26: 177–82.

Walters, G.D. (2002). The heritability of alcohol abuse and dependence: a meta-analysis of behaviour genetic research. *American Journal of Drug & Alcohol Abuse*, 28: 557–84.

Wang, C., Burris, M. and Xiang, Y.P. (1996). Chinese village women as visual anthropologists: a participatory approach to reaching policymakers. *Social Science & Medicine*, 42: 1391–400.

Wang, Y. and Willis, E. (2016). Supporting self-efficacy through interactive discussion in online communities of weight loss. *Journal of Health Psychology*. doi:10.1177/1359105316653264.

Ward, B.W., Schiller, J.S. and Goodman, R.A. (2014). Multiple chronic conditions among US adults: a 2012 update. *Preventing Chronic Disease*, 11. doi:10.5888/pcd11.130389.

Wardle J. (2007). Eating behaviour and obesity. *Obesity Review*, 8: 73–5.

Wardle, J., McCaffery, K., Nadel, M. and Atkin, W. (2004). Socioeconomic differences in cancer screening participation: comparing cognitive and psychosocial explanations. *Social Science & Medicine*, 59: 249–61.

Wardle, J., Waller, J. and Rapoport, L. (2001). Body dissatisfaction and binge eating in obese women: the role of restraint and depression. *Obesity Research*, 9: 778–87.

Ware Jr, J.E. and Sherbourne, C.D. (1992). The MOS 36-item Short-Form Health Survey (SF-36): I. Conceptual framework and item selection. *Medical Care*, 30 (6): 473–83.

Ware, K., Davies, J., Rowse, G. and Whittaker, S. (2015). The experience of hepatitis C treatment for people with a history of mental health problems: an interpretative phenomenological analysis. *Journal of Health Psychology*, 20 (7): 990–1001.

Warr, P., Jackson, P. and Banks, M. (1988). Unemployment and mental health: some British studies. *Journal of Social Issues*, 44: 47–68.

Wassell, J., Rogers, S.L., Felmingam, K.L., Bryant, R.A. and Pearson, J. (2015). Sex hormones predict the sensory strength and vividness of mental imagery. *Biological Psychology*, 107: 61–8.

Wassertheil-Smoller, S., Shumaker, S., Ockene, J., Talavera, G.A., Greeland, P., Cochrane, B. et al. (2004). Depression and cardiovascular sequelae in postmenopausal women. *Archives of Internal Medicine*, 164: 289–98.

Waterman, A.S. (1993). Two conceptions of happiness: contrasts of personal expressiveness (eudaimonia) and hedonic enjoyment. *Journal of Personality and Social Psychology*, 64: 678–91.

Watson, J.D. and Crick, F.H.C. (1953). A structure for deoxyribose nucleic acid. *Nature*, 171: 737–8.

Webb, T., Joseph, J., Yardley, L. and Michie, S. (2010). Using the internet to promote health behavior change: a systematic review and meta-analysis of the impact of theoretical basis, use of behavior change techniques, and mode of delivery on efficacy. *Journal of Medical Internet Research*, 12 (1): e4.

Wei, Y., Schatten, H. and Sun, Q.-Y. (2015). Environmental epigenetic inheritance through gametes and implications for human reproduction. *Human Reproduction Update*, 21 (2): 194–208.

Weinman, J., Petrie, K.J., Moss-Morris, R. and Horne, R. (1996). The Illness Perception Questionnaire: a new method for assessing the cognitive representation of illness. *Psychology & Health*, 11: 431–46.

Weinstein, N.D. (1980). Unrealistic optimism about future life events. *Journal of Personality and Social Psychology*, 39 (5): 806.

Weinstein, N.D. (1993). Testing four competing theories of health-protective behavior. *Health Psychology*, 12: 324–33.

Weir, H.K., Anderson, R.N., Coleman King, S.M., Soman, A., Thompson, T.D., Hong, Y. et al. (2016). Heart disease and cancer deaths: trends and projections in the United States, 1969–2020. *Preventing Chronic Disease*, 13: E157.

Weiss, M.R. and Williams, L. (2004). The why of youth sport involvement: a developmental perspective on motivational processes. In M.R. Weiss (ed.), *Developmental Sport and Exercise Psychology: A Lifespan Perspective*. Morgantown, WV: Fitness Information Technology. pp. 223–68.

Weitkunat, R., Markuzzi, A., Vogel, S., Schlipköter, A., Koch, H.-J., Meyer, G. and Ferring, D. (1998). Psychological factors associated with the uptake of measles immunization. *Journal of Health Psychology*, 3: 273–84.

Wells, R., Steel, Z., Abo-Hilal, M., Hassan, A.H. and Lawsin, C. (2016). Psychosocial concerns reported by Syrian refugees living in Jordan: systematic review of unpublished needs assessments. *The British Journal of Psychiatry*, 209 (2): 99–106.

Wertli, M.M., Rasmussen-Barr, E., Held, U., Weiser, S., Bachmann, L.M. and Brunner, F. (2014). Fear avoidance beliefs: a moderator of treatment efficacy in patients with low back pain: a systematic review. *The Spine Journal*, 14 (11): 2658–78.

Wessely, S., Butler, S., Chalder, T. and David, A. (1991). The cognitive behavioural management of the post-viral fatigue syndrome. In R. Jenkins and J. Mowbray (Eds.), *Post-Viral Fatigue Syndrome*. Chichester: John Wiley & Sons. pp. 305–34.

Wessely, S., David, A. and Butler, S. (1989). Management of chronic (post-viral) fatigue syndrome. *Journal of the Royal College of General Practitioners*, 39 (318): 26–9.

West, R. (2005). Time for a change: putting the Transtheoretical (Stages of Change) Model to rest. *Addiction*, 100: 1036–9.

West-Eberhard, M.J. (1989). Phenotype plasticity and the origins of diversity. *Annual Review of Ecology Systematics*, 20: 249.

Wheeler, S. (2012). The significance of family culture for sports participation. *International Review for the Sociology of Sport*, 47: 235–52.

Whelehan, P., Evans, A., Wells, M. and Macgillivray, S. (2013). The effect of mammography pain on repeat participation in breast cancer screening: a systematic review. *Breast*, 22 (4): 389–94.

White, P.D., Goldsmith, K.A., Johnson, A.L., Potts, L., Walwyn, R., DeCesare, J.C. et al. (2011). Comparison of adaptive pacing therapy, cognitive behaviour therapy, graded exercise therapy, and specialist medical care for chronic fatigue syndrome (PACE): a randomised trial. *The Lancet*, 377: 823–36.

Whitehead, D.L., Strike, P., Perkins-Porras, L. and Steptoe, A. (2005). Frequency of distress and fear of dying during acute coronary syndromes and consequences for adaptation. *The American Journal of Cardiology*, 96 (11): 1512–16.

Whitlock, E.P., Polen, M.R., Green, C.A., Orleans, T. and Klein, J. (2004). Behavioural counseling interventions in primary care to reduce risky/harmful alcohol use by adults: a summary of the evidence for the US Preventive Services Task Force. *Annals of Internal Medicine*, 140: 557–68.

Whooley, M.A. and Browner, W.S. (1998). Association between depressive symptoms and mortality in older women. *Archives of Internal Medicine*, 158: 2129–35.

WHOQoL Group. (1995). The World Health Organization quality of life assessment (WHOQOL): position paper from the World Health Organization. *Social Science & Medicine*, 41 (10): 1403–9.

Widman, L., Noar, S.M., Choukas-Bradley, S. and Francis, D.B. (2014). Adolescent sexual health communication and condom use: a meta-analysis. *Health Psychology*, 33 (10): 1113.

Widom, C.S. and Kuhns, J.B. (1996). Childhood victimization and subsequent risk for promiscuity, prostitution, and teenage pregnancy: a prospective study. *American Journal of Public Health*, 86 (11): 1607–12.

Wiggins, S., Potter, J. and Wildsmith, A. (2001). Eating your words: discursive psychology and the reconstruction of eating practices. *Journal of Health Psychology*, 6: 5–15.

Wilkinson, A., Whitehead, L. and Ritchie, L. (2014). Factors influencing the ability to self-manage diabetes for adults living with Type 1 or 2 diabetes. *International Journal of Nursing Studies*, 51 (1): 111–22.

Wilkinson, J.M. and Stevens, M.J. (2014). Use of complementary and alternative medical therapies (CAM) by patients attending a regional comprehensive cancer care centre. *Journal of Complementary and Integrative Medicine*, 11 (2): 139–45.

Wilkinson, R. (1996). *Unhealthy Societies*. London: Routledge.

Wilkinson, R. and Pickett, K. (2010). *The Spirit Level: Why Equality is Better for Everyone*. London: Penguin.

Wilkinson, S. (1998). Focus groups in health research: exploring the meaning of health and illness. *Journal of Health Psychology*, 3: 329–48.

Williams, A. (2006). Perspectives on spirituality at the end of life: a meta-summary. *Palliative & Supportive Care*, 4: 407–17.

Williams, D.C., Golding, J., Phillips, K. and Towell, A. (2004). Perceived control, locus of control and preparatory information: effects on the perception of an acute pain stimulus. *Personality & Individual Differences*, 36: 1681–91.

Williams, D.M., Anderson, E.S. and Winett, R.A. (2005). A review of the outcome expectancy construct in physical activity research. *Annals of Behavioral Medicine*, 29: 70–9.

Williams, D.R. and Collins, C. (1995). US socioeconomic and racial differences in health: patterns and explanations. *Annual Review of Sociology*, 21: 349–86.

Williams, D.R., Yu, Y., Jackson, J.S. and Anderson, N.B. (1997). Racial differences in physical and mental health: socio-economic status, stress and discrimination. *Journal of Health Psychology*, 2: 335–51.

Williams, M. (2016). *Proof Positive (Revisited)*. Available: www.margaretwilliams.me/2016/proof-positive-revisited.pdf [accessed 25 March 2017].

Williams, M. (2017). *A Travesty of Science and a Tragedy for Patients: Quotable Quotes Continued 2006–2016*. Available: www.margaretwilliams.me/2017/quotable-quotes-continued.pdf [accessed on 28 August 2017].

Willig, C. (2008). A phenomenological investigation of the experience of taking part in extreme sports. *Journal of Health Psychology*, 13: 690–702.

Willig, C. (2009). 'Unlike a rock, a tree, a horse or an angel …': reflections on the struggle for meaning through writing during the process of cancer diagnosis. *Journal of Health Psychology*, 14: 181–9.

Wilshire, C.E., Kindlon, T., Matthees, A. and McGrath, S. (2017). Can patients with chronic fatigue syndrome really recover after graded exercise or cognitive behavioural therapy? A critical commentary and preliminary re-analysis of the PACE trial. *Fatigue*, 5 (1): 1–4.

Wilson, D.K., Ainsworth, B.E. and Bowles, H. (2007). Body mass index and environmental supports for physical inactivity among active and inactive. *Health Psychology*, 26: 710–17.

Wilson, J. and Jungner, G. (1968). *Principles and Practice of Screening for Disease*. World Health Organization Public Health Paper No. 34. Geneva: WHO.

Wilson, N.J., Cordier, R., Parsons, R., Vaz, S. and Buchanan, A. (2016). Men with disabilities: a cross sectional survey of health promotion, social inclusion and participation at community men's sheds. *Disability and Health Journal*, 9 (1): 118–26. doi:10.1016/j.dhjo.2015.08.013.

Wing, R.W. (2004). Behavioural approaches to the treatment of obesity. In G.A. Bray and C. Bouchard (eds.), *Handbook of Obesity* (2nd edn). New York: Marcel Dekker.

Wire, T. (2009). *Fewer Emitters, Lower Emissions, Less Cost*. London: London School of Economics.

Witkiewitz, K., Marlatt, G.A. and Walker, D. (2005). Mindfulness-based relapse prevention for alcohol and substance use disorders. *Journal of Cognitive Psychotherapy*, 19: 211–28.

Wong, D., Sullivan, K. and Heap, G. (2012). The pharmaceutical market for obesity therapies. *Nature Reviews Drug Discovery*, 11: 669–70.

Wong, J.M., Na, B., Regan, M.C. and Whooley, M.A. (2013). Hostility, health behaviors, and risk of recurrent events in patients with stable coronary heart disease: findings from the Heart and Soul Study. *Journal of the American Heart Association*, 2 (5): e000052.

Woodgate, J. and Brawley, L.R. (2008). Self-efficacy for exercise in cardiac rehabilitation: review and recommendations. *Journal of Health Psychology*, 13: 366–87.

World Bank (2002). Globalization, growth, and poverty. Available: http://documents.world bank.org/curated/en/954071468778196576/pdf/multi0page.pdf [accessed 28 August 2017].

World Health Organization. (1946). Constitution of the World Health Organization as adopted by the International Health Conference, New York, 19–22 June 1946; signed on 22 July 1946 by the representatives of 61 States (Official Records of the World Health).

World Health Organization. (1986). *The Ottawa Charter for Health Promotion*. First International Conference on Health Promotion, Ottawa, 21 November 1986. Geneva: WHO.

World Health Organization. (1989). *World Health Statistics Annual*. Geneva: WHO.

World Health Organization. (2002). *Investing in Health: A Summary of Findings of the Commission on Macroeconomics and Health*. Geneva: WHO. Available: http://apps.who.int/iris/bitstream/10665/42709/1/9241562412_eng.pdf [accessed 5 December 2014].

World Health Organization. (2004a). Immunisation posters. Available: http://apps.who.int/immunization-week-posters/

World Health Organization. (2004b). *Global Strategy on Diet, Physical Activity and Health*. Available: www.who.int/dietphysicalactivity/strategy/eb11344/strategy_english_web.pdf [accessed 5 December 2014].

World Health Organization. (2007). *World Health Organization Expert Committee Second Report on Problems Related to Alcohol Consumption*. Geneva: WHO. Available: www.who.int/substance_abuse/expert_committee_alcohol/en/ [accessed 5 December 2014].

World Health Organization. (2008). *Global Incidence and Prevalence of Selected Curable Sexually Transmitted Infections – 2008*. Geneva: WHO.

World Health Organization. (2011). *Unsafe Abortion: Global and Regional Estimates of Incidence of Unsafe Abortion and Associated Mortality in 2008*. Geneva: WHO.

World Health Organization. (2013). *Tobacco Control Economics*. Geneva: WHO. Available: www.who.int/tobacco/economics/en/ [accessed 5 December 2014].

World Health Organization. (2014a). Draft Guideline: Sugars intake for adults and children. Available: http://www.who.int/nutrition/sugars_public_consultation/en/

World Health Organization. (2014b). *10 Facts on Noncommunicable Diseases*. Geneva: WHO. Available: www.who.int/features/factfiles/noncommunicable_diseases/en/ [accessed 5 December 2014].

World Health Organization. (2014c). *Global Update of the Health Sector Response to HIV, 2014*. Geneva: World Health Organization.

World Health Organization. (2014d). *Global Status Report on Alcohol and Health 2014*. Available: www.who.int/mediacentre/news/releases/2014/alcohol-related-deaths-prevention/en/.

World Health Organization. (2015a). *Consolidated Guidelines on HIV Testing Services*. Geneva: WHO.

World Health Organization. (2015b). *Health Literacy Toolkit for Low- and Middle-Income Countries*. Available: www.searo.who.int/entity/healthpromotion/documents/hl_tookit/en/

World Health Organization. (2015c). *The WHO Framework Convention on Tobacco Control: 10 years of implementation in the African Region*. Geneva: WHO.

Wright, J., MacDonald, D. and Groom, L. (2003). Physical activity and young people: beyond participation. *Sport, Education & Society*, 8: 17–33.

Wu, G., Feder, A., Cohen, H., Kim, J.J., Calderon, S., Charney, D.S. and Mathé, A.A. (2013). Understanding resilience. *Frontiers in Behavioral Neuroscience*, 7: 10.

Wulsin, L.R. and Singal, B.M. (2003). Do depressive symptoms increase the risk for the onset of coronary disease? A systematic quantitative review. *Psychosomatic Medicine*, 65: 201–10.

Xia, Q. and Grant, S.F. (2013). The genetics of human obesity. *Annals of the New York Academy of Sciences*, 1281 (1): 178–190.

Xu, J., Tang, W., Wang, Y., Lu, L. and Lu, Y. (2020). Posttraumatic growth among 5195 adolescents at 8.5 years after exposure to the Wenchuan earthquake: roles of PTSD and self-esteem. *Journal of Health Psychology* (in press).

Yamazaki, Y. and Omori, M. (2016). The relationship between mothers' thin-ideal and children's drive for thinness: a survey of Japanese early adolescents and their mothers. *Journal of Health Psychology*, 21 (1): 100–11.

Yang, Q., Zhang, Z., Gregg, E.W., Flanders, W.D., Merritt, R. and Hu, F.B. (2014). Added sugar intake and cardiovascular diseases mortality among US adults. *JAMA Internal Medicine*, 174: 516–24.

Yehuda, R., Bell, A., Bierer, L.M. and Schmeidler, J. (2008). Maternal, not paternal, PTSD is related to increased risk for PTSD in offspring of Holocaust survivors. *Journal of Psychiatric Research*, 42: 1104–11.

Yehuda, R., Engel, S.M., Brand, S.R., Seckl, J., Marcus, S.M. and Berkowitz, G.S. (2005). Transgenerational effects of posttraumatic stress disorder in babies of mothers exposed to the World Trade Center attacks during pregnancy. *The Journal of Clinical Endocrinology and Metabolism*, 90: 4115–18.

Yeich, S. (1996). Grassroots organizing with homeless people: a participatory research approach. *Journal of Social Issues*, 52: 111–21.

Yiengprugsawan, V., Khamman, S., Seubsman, S., Lim, L.L. and Sleigh, A.C. (2011). Social capital and health in a national cohort of 82,482 Open University adults in Thailand. *Journal of Health Psychology*, 16 (4): 632–42.

Yokoyama, Y., Nishimura, K., Barnard, N.D., Takegami, M., Watanabe, M., Sekikawa, A. et al. (2014). Vegetarian diets and blood pressure: a meta-analysis. *JAMA Internal Medicine*, 174 (4): 577–87.

Yong, E. (2012). In the wake of high profile controversies, pyschologists are facing up to problems with replication. *Nature*, 483: 298–300.

Zarcadoolas, C. (2011). The simplicity complex: exploring simplified health messages in a complex world. *Health PromotInt*, 26 (3): 338–50.

Zaridze, D., Lewington, S., Boroda, A., Scélo, G., Karpov, R., Lazarev, A. et al. (2014). Alcohol and mortality in Russia: prospective observational study of 151,000 adults. *The Lancet*, 363: 1465–73.

Zerach, G., Greene, T. and Solomon, Z. (2013). Secondary traumatization and self-rated health among ex-POWs' wives: the moderating role of marital adjustment. *Journal of Health Psychology*, doi:10.1177/1359105313502563.

Zetta, S., Smith, K., Jones, M., Allcoat, P. and Sullivan, F. (2011). Evaluating the Angina Plan in patients admitted to hospital with angina: a randomized controlled trial. *Cardiovascular Therapeutics*, 29 (2): 112–24.

Ziarnowski, K.L., Brewer, N.T. and Weber, B. (2000). Present choices, future outcomes: anticipated regret and HPV vaccination. *Preventitive Medicine*, 48: 411–14.

Zigmond, A.S. and Snaith, R.P. (1983). The hospital anxiety and depression scale. *ActaPsychiatricaScandinavica*, 67: 361–70.

Zika, S. and Chamberlain, K. (1992). On the relation between meaning in life and psychological well-being. *British Journal of Psychology*, 83: 133–45.

Zlatevska, N.S., Dubelaar, C. and Holden, S.S. (2014). Sizing up the effect of portion size on consumption: a meta-analytic review. *Journal of Marketing*, 78 (3): 140–54.

Zuckerman, M. (1979). *Sensation Seeking: Beyond the Optimal Level of Arousal*. Hillsdale, NJ: Lawrence Erlbaum.

Zuckerman, M. and Antoni, M.H. (1995). Social support and its relationship to psychological, physical and immune variables in HIV infection. *Clinical Psychology & Psychotherapy*, 2: 210–19.

AUTHOR INDEX

Page numbers in *italics* refer to figures; page numbers in **bold** refer to tables.

SUBJECT INDEX

anti-vaccination movements and conspiracy theories, 328, 330, 332, 334–335
anxiety, 35, 386, 407–408, 423, 513–515
aromatherapy, 122, 124
arrhythmias, 445
arthritis, 484
asexuality, 200
assigned sex, 200
assisted suicide, 103, 104–105
asylum seekers, 128–129
atherosclerosis, 444
attachment styles, 428
attachment theory, 10, 213–214
autism, 332
autoimmune diseases, 46
automatized action schemata, 256
autonomic nervous system (ANS), 30, *30*, 32, 35–36, 357–358
autonomy, 5, 507
Ayurvedic medicine, 118–119, 122

bariatric surgery, 225
basal cell carcinomas, 420
B cells, 43–44
Beck Depression Inventory (BDI), **398**, 452
Behavioral Risk Factor Surveillance System (BRFSS), 127
behavioural. *See* health behaviour change
behavioural immunology, 26. *See also* psychoneuroimmunology (PNI)
behavioural inhibition system (BIS), 37
behavioural setting, 272–273
behavioural strategies, 412
behaviour change agents, 172–173
behaviour change techniques (BCTs), 170–172, *171*, 286–287
Behaviour Change Wheel, 168–169
behaviour genetics, 61–64
beliefs, 114
Bereavement Questionnaire, 512–513
between groups designs, 134
Big Five personality traits, 382, 390, 392
Bio-behavioural Pain Profile, **399**
biological determinism, 236
biological sex, 41–42, 200
biological therapy (BT), 426
biomedical model, 15
biomedicine (allopathic medicine), 116–117, 121, 378
biopsychosocial model (BPSM)
    overview of, 16–18, *17*, 377–379
    long-term conditions and, 484–485
    ME/CFS and, 499–502
    pain and, 400
    smoking and, 253–257, **254**
bisexuality, 200. *See also* LBGTQ people
Black Report (1982), 94–95, 96–98
blogs, 136–138, **137**
body image, 280–281
body mass index (BMI), 205, 206–208, *207*
Bogalusa Heart Study, 449–450

Bonferroni correction, 134–135
bottom-up research approaches, 154–155
bowel cancer screening, 321
brain, 31–32, *31*, 48
brain and spinal cord tumours, 421–422
brain death, 518–519
Brazil, 83–84
breast cancer screening, 314–317, 320–324
brief interventions, **243**, 244
British Psychological Society (BPS), 100, 378
Buddhism, 117

California Medical Association, 516
calorie, 209–210
cancer
    overview of, 419–422, **422**, *423*, 445, *446*
    alcohol and, 233
    caregivers and, 433–434, 512
    diagnosis of, 424
    future research on, 441
    personality–illness correlations and, 378, 388–389, 391, 392
    post-traumatic growth and, 431–432
    psychosocial interventions and, 434–441
    risk factors for, 422–424
    stress and, 371–372, 425
    survivorship and, 430–431, *431*
    treatments for, 423, 425–430
cancer screening, 314–324, *319*, 325
cannabis, 414
capabilities, 95
carcinogens, 250
carcinoid tumours, 422
carcinomas, 420
cardiac rehabilitation (CR), 453–455
cardiovascular disease (CVD), 234, 235, 367
caregivers
    cancer and, 433–434, 512
    coronary heart disease (CHD) and, 452–453
    diabetes mellitus and, 494
    ME/CFS and, 502
    stress and, 433–434, 452–453
    women as, 485
carrier testing, 324–325
case studies, 135
catastrophizing, 406
Center for Epidemiological Studies–Depression scale, 467
central circadian pacemaker, 38–40, *40*
central nervous system (CNS), 27, 30, *30*, 32, 37, 48, 65
cerebellum, 27
cerebrospinal fluid (CSF), 32
cervical cancer screening, 315–317, 321–322
chemotherapy (CT), 423, 426
childhood adversities (CAs), 364–366
children and young people
    diabetes mellitus and, 487
    immunization and, 328, 331–333, **331–332**
    pain and, 410